Contemporary Cardiology

Series Editors
Peter P. Toth
Ciccarone Ctr Prevent. Cardio. Disease,
Johns Hopkins University,
Sterling, IL, USA

For more than a decade, cardiologists have relied on the Contemporary Cardiology series to provide them with forefront medical references on all aspects of cardiology. Each title is carefully crafted by world-renown cardiologists who comprehensively cover the most important topics in this rapidly advancing field. With more than 75 titles in print covering everything from diabetes and cardiovascular disease to the management of acute coronary syndromes, the Contemporary Cardiology series has become the leading reference source for the practice of cardiac care.

Kevin C. Maki • Don P. Wilson

Editors

Cardiovascular Outcomes Research

A Clinician's Guide to Cardiovascular Epidemiology and Clinical Outcomes Trials

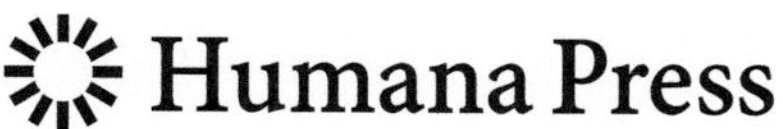 Humana Press

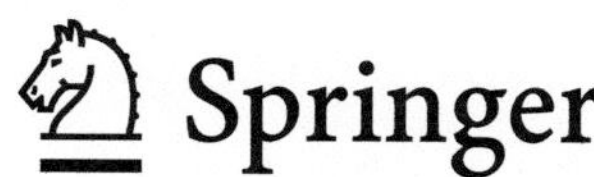 Springer

Editors
Kevin C. Maki
Midwest Biomedical Research
Addison, IL, USA

Don P. Wilson
Pediatric Endocrinology and Diabetes
Cook Children's Medical Center
Fort Worth, TX, USA

ISSN 2196-8969   ISSN 2196-8977   (electronic)
Contemporary Cardiology
ISBN 978-3-031-54962-5   ISBN 978-3-031-54960-1   (eBook)
https://doi.org/10.1007/978-3-031-54960-1

This Springer imprint is published by the registered company Springer Nature Switzerland AG
The registered company address is: Gewerbestrasse 11, 6330 Cham, Switzerland

Paper in this product is recyclable.

Foreword

Translation and implementation of evidence-based medical research into every day clinical practice is a global priority because of its potential impact on health services delivery and patient-centered outcomes. Nearly 20 years ago, the U.S. Institute of Medicine in partnership with the National Institutes of Health proposed initiating a new model for re-engineering clinical research and healthcare delivery so that evidence is available when it is needed, and applied in healthcare settings that is both more effective and more efficient than exists presently. This movement became known as a "Learning Health System" (LHS) wherein the pace, uptake, and integration of medical evidence derived from randomized clinical trials and observational studies can be accelerated more expeditiously at the point of clinical care. Because it is generally estimated that it takes an average of 17 years for published research evidence to reach clinical practice, translating scientific discoveries into patient benefit more quickly is a policy priority of many "Learning Health Systems."

Against this backdrop, most physicians, research scientists, nurse practitioners, physician assistants, and other healthcare providers are besieged with ever-expanding evidence base derived from randomized clinical trials and observational studies that challenge how such important information can be applied to bedside clinical decision-making. Yet, little time is devoted during provider training about how to read and critically interpret clinical research data and reports published from cardiovascular outcomes studies. As an academic preventive cardiologist in a teaching institution who has also been a lead investigator and Study Chair for the Veterans Affairs Non-Q-Wave Infarction Strategies in Hospital (VANQWISH) and the Clinical Outcomes Utilizing Revascularization and Aggressive Drug Evaluation (COURAGE) trials, Study Co-Chair of the Atherothrombosis Intervention in Metabolic Syndrome with Low High Density Lipoprotein/High Triglycerides: Impact on Global Health Outcomes (AIM-HIGH) trial, and a national Co-Principal Investigator for the International Study of Comparative Health Effectiveness with Medical and Invasive Approaches (ISCHEMIA) trial, these experiences have underscored both the critical importance of testing hypotheses in clinical medicine and the slow pace at which new results from such studies are incorporated into clinical practice (the so-called "T2 lag" in translational biomedical research, cited above).

Accordingly, it is abundantly clear that there is a critical, unmet need among clinicians for guidance on interpreting the medical literature surrounding cardiovascular outcomes studies and how this knowledge can be best applied to clinical decision-making. While clinical practice guidelines and recommendations can be helpful for summarizing and rating the quality of available evidence, new trial results and meta-analyses of existing pooled data with important treatment implications for clinical practice arrive with regularity, such that clinicians need to be familiar with the implications of new findings and how best to interpret them in order to provide the best care for their patients.

Cardiovascular Outcomes Research: A Clinician's Guide to Cardiovascular Epidemiology and Clinical Outcomes Trials, the latest book in Springer's Contemporary Cardiology series, edited by Maki and Wilson, is a welcome resource that busy clinicians should find as an extremely helpful guide to becoming better and more knowledgeable consumers of the medical literature relevant to prevention and management of cardiovascular diseases. In their new book, Drs. Maki and Wilson provide insightful coverage of foundational concepts in biostatistics, study design, and guideline development. In addition, an overview is provided of our current understanding of the key roles of cardiovascular risk factors, as well as both lifestyle and pharmacologic interventions for achieving optimal residual cardiovascular risk reduction related to dyslipidemias, inflammation, hypertension, obesity, diabetes, thrombosis, arrhythmias, and chronic kidney disease. This is a book that will occupy a prominent position on the bookshelf in my office and will be a valuable educational resource to advance learning for me and other readers for years to come.

Boston University Chobanian   William Edward Boden
and Avedisian School of Medicine
Harvard Medical School
Boston, MA, USA

Preface

It has been just over 75 years since the initiation of the Framingham Heart Study, which was the first study to demonstrate that risk factors, particularly elevated serum cholesterol, diabetes mellitus, hypertension, and cigarette smoking, were associated with increased incidence of myocardial infarction in a group of adults in the United States. When the Framingham Heart Study was initiated, the general view in the medical community was that "hardening of the arteries" was an unavoidable consequence of the aging process. In the space of one lifetime, a great deal of progress has been made in the identification of additional risk factors, as well as reliable methods of determining whether strategies to modify risk factors lower incidence of cardiovascular morbidity and mortality. Clinicians now have an array of tools available for reducing cardiovascular event risk and improving outcomes in both primary and secondary prevention, including lifestyle therapies and pharmacologic and surgical approaches.

The randomized controlled trial (RCT) has become the gold standard for evaluating the benefits and risks of interventions intended to affect human health. While observational studies are important for hypothesis generation, they are more subject to certain types of bias and confounding than RCTs. Due to random application of treatment, a large-scale RCT has the advantage that the treatment groups can be assumed to have similar prognoses because both known and unknown determinants of the outcome will be approximately equally distributed across treatment conditions.

At times it may not be ethical or feasible to test an intervention using an RCT to evaluate the impact on cardiovascular outcomes (e.g., bariatric surgery or cigarette smoking cessation). In such instances, clinical recommendations must rely on the best available evidence, which might include results from observational studies, short-term investigations to evaluate effects of the intervention on biomarkers of cardiovascular risk, and animal models, as well as other types of evidence such as that from Mendelian randomization. Mendelian randomization uses genetic variants to determine whether an observational association between a risk factor and an outcome is consistent with a causal effect. It relies on the natural random distribution of genetic variants in a population. Because these genetic variants are typically unassociated with confounders, differences in the outcome between those who carry the variant and those who do not can be attributed to the difference in the risk factor. Recommendations for the use of interventions that have not been rigorously tested using adequately powered RCTs should be qualified to alert clinicians to the lower quality of evidence compared with interventions that have been demonstrated to reduce cardiovascular morbidity and/or mortality in RCTs.

Clinical training typically involves a greater focus on the application of interventions than on the process by which the evidence is produced to support the use of those interventions. The focus of this book is on the process by which such evidence is generated and the basics of interpreting reports in the medical/scientific literature from observational and intervention studies to assess relationships of risk factors and interventions to cardiovascular outcomes, particularly major adverse cardiovascular events, such as myocardial infarction, stroke, revascularization, and cardiovascular death.

The book is divided into two parts. Part I describes the history and evolution of cardiovascular outcomes studies and the major roles such studies play, including pharmaceutical development, regulatory approval, and the formation of guidelines for cardiovascular disease risk reduction and clinical management of cholesterol and dyslipidemia. The challenges associated with developing evidence-based recommendations for non-pharmacological interventions for cardiovascular risk reduction, and the emerging field of implementation science, which aims to accelerate the adoption and integration of evidence-based clinical practice guidelines, are also discussed. Chapters regarding the statistical methods used in cardiovascular outcomes trials and their interpretation, and biomarkers and imaging modalities for detecting subclinical atherosclerotic disease are also included. Part II provides an overview of the evidence for categories of interventions affecting cardiovascular outcomes including chapters on lifestyle therapies and interventions affecting lipids and lipoproteins, inflammation, thrombosis and hemostasis, blood pressure, obesity, diabetes mellitus, cardiac rhythms, and chronic kidney disease.

<table>
<tr><td>Addison, IL, USA</td><td align="right">Kevin C. Maki</td></tr>
<tr><td>Fort Worth, TX, USA</td><td align="right">Don P. Wilson</td></tr>
</table>

Acknowledgments

There are many people who contributed in various ways to bringing this book to fruition, and it would be impossible to properly acknowledge all who did so. However, the Editors would like to thank Peter Toth, MD, PhD (series Editor), who encouraged us to take on this project, and Swathiga Karthikeyan from Springer, who provided logistical and technical support. We are grateful for our colleagues who generously shared their knowledge and expertise as authors. Also, the Editors are particularly indebted to Mary R. Dicklin, PhD, Midwest Biomedical Research, for her assistance with editing the chapters and communicating with the contributors throughout the publication process. Mary has been a long-time friend and colleague and has contributed in innumerable ways to this and many other projects.

Contents

Part II Overview of Current Evidence in Categories of Interventions

Contributors

Anandita Agarwala, MD Division of Cardiology, Center for Cardiovascular Disease Prevention, Baylor Scott & White Heart Hospital Baylor Plano, Plano, TX, USA

David B. Allison, PhD Department of Epidemiology and Biostatistics, Indiana University School of Public Health-Bloomington, Bloomington, IN, USA

Andrew D. Althouse, PhD Department of Medicine, Center for Research on Health Care, University of Pittsburgh, Pittsburgh, PA, USA

Medtronic, Minneapolis, MN, USA

Agastya D. Belur, MD Division of Cardiology, University of Louisville, Louisville, KY, USA

Aurelian Bidulescu, MD, PhD Department of Epidemiology and Biostatistics, Indiana University School of Public Health-Bloomington, Bloomington, IN, USA

Laurie Cavendish, PharmD, BCPS Department of Pharmacy and Medical Nutrition, Grady Health System, Atlanta, GA, USA

Mary Katherine Cheeley, PharmD, BCPS Department of Pharmacy and Medical Nutrition, Grady Health System, Atlanta, GA, USA

Harry Chiang, MD Department of Radiology, Baylor Scott and White Health, Temple, TX, USA

Gates B. Colbert, MD Division of Nephrology, Texas A&M College of Medicine, Dallas, TX, USA

Joseph A. Diamond, MD Cardiovascular Institute, Northwell, New Hyde Park, NY, USA

Mary R. Dicklin, PhD Midwest Biomedical Research, Addison, IL, USA

Mohamed Elrggal, MD Nephrology Department, AlQabbary Hospital, Alexandria, Egypt

Nephrology Department, Kidney and Urology Center, Alexandria, Egypt

Elaine Foster, PhD Department of Human Performance and Sport Studies, Idaho State University, Pocatello, ID, USA

Kishore M. Gadde, MD Department of Surgery, University of California Irvine, Irvine, CA, USA

Lovy Gaur, MD, DNB (Nephrology), SCE Department of Nephrology and Kidney Transplant, Max Superspeciality Hospital, Vaishali, Delhi-NCR, Ghaziabad, Uttar Pradesh, India

Samuel S. Gidding, MD Department of Genomic Health, Geisinger, Danville, PA, USA

Michael R. Gionfriddo, PharmD, PhD Division of Pharmaceutical, Administrative and Social Sciences, School of Pharmacy, Duquesne University, Pittsburgh, PA, USA

Kathryn A. Greaves, PhD Nutrition Outside the Box, LLC, Battle Creek, MI, USA

Western Michigan University, Kalamazoo, MI, USA

Steven A. Greenstein, MD Cardiovascular Institute, Northwell, New Hyde Park, NY, USA

Liana L. Guarneiri, PhD, RDN Midwest Biomedical Research, Addison, IL, USA

Luke Hamilton Research Data Science and Analytics, Cook Children's Hospital Health Care System, Fort Worth, TX, USA

Steven R. Horbal, PhD, MPH Department of Surgery, University of Michigan, Ann Arbor, MI, USA

Philip D. Houck, MD Division of Cardiology, Department of Internal Medicine, Baylor Scott and White Health, Temple, TX, USA

Laney K. Jones, PharmD, MPH Department of Genomic Health, Geisinger, Danville, PA, USA

Heart and Vascular Institute, Geisinger, Geisinger, Danville, PA, USA

Dinesh K. Kalra, MD Division of Cardiology, Department of Medicine, University of Louisville School of Medicine, Rudd Heart and Lung Center, Louisville, KY, USA

Ali Keramati, MD The Lankenau Institute for Medical Research, Wynnewood, PA, USA

Carol F. Kirkpatrick, PhD, RDN Midwest Biomedical Research, Addison, IL, USA

Kasiska Division of Health Science, Idaho State University, Pocatello, ID, USA

Peter R. Kowey, MD The Lankenau Institute for Medical Research, Wynnewood, PA, USA

Department of Medicine, Thomas Jefferson University, Philadelphia, PA, USA

Bahij Kreidieh, MD The Lankenau Institute for Medical Research, Wynnewood, PA, USA

Edgar V. Lerma, MD Section of Nephrology, Department of Medicine, University of Illinois at Chicago College of Medicine, Associated in Nephrology, SC, Chicago, IL, USA

Hector Madariaga, MD Lahey Hospital and Medical Center, Burlington, MA, USA

Kevin C. Maki, PhD Midwest Biomedical Research, Addison, IL, USA
Midwest Biomedical Research, Bonita Springs, FL, USA
Indiana University School of Public Health-Bloomington, Bloomington, IN, USA

Catherine J. McNeal, MD, PhD Division of Cardiology, Department of Internal Medicine, Baylor Scott and White Health, Temple, TX, USA

Reed Mszar, MPH, MS Department of Physiology, Georgetown University, Washington, DC, USA

James Murchison, MD Department of Radiology, Baylor Scott and White Health, Temple, TX, USA

Nguyen N. Nguyen, PhD Department of Pathology, Baylor Scott and White Health, Temple, TX, USA

Carl E. Orringer, MD Rooney Heart Institute at NCH, NCH Healthcare System, Naples, FL, USA

Kristina S. Petersen, PhD, APD Department of Nutritional Sciences, Pennsylvania State University, University Park, PA, USA

Munis Raza, MD Division of Cardiology, University of Louisville, Louisville, KY, USA

Alexander Sakers, MD, PhD Perelman School of Medicine, University of Pennsylvania, Philadelphia, PA, USA
Department of Medicine, Massachusetts General Hospital, Boston, MA, USA

Mitchell N. Sarkies, PhD School of Health Sciences and Sydney Health Partners, University of Sydney, Sydney, NSW, Australia
Centre for Healthcare Resilience and Implementation Science, Australian Institute of Health Innovation, Macquarie University, Sydney, NSW, Australia

Priyanka Satish, MD Department of Cardiology, Houston Methodist DeBakey Heart and Vascular Center, Houston, TX, USA

Daniel Soffer, MD Perelman School of Medicine, University of Pennsylvania, Philadelphia, PA, USA
Perelman Center for Advanced Medicine, University of Pennsylvania Health System, Philadelphia, PA, USA

Gerald F. Watts, MD, DSc School of Medicine, University of Western Australia, Perth, WA, Australia

Department of Cardiology, Royal Perth Hospital, Perth, WA, Australia

Don P. Wilson, MD Pediatric Endocrinology and Diabetes, Cook Children's Medical Center, Fort Worth, TX, USA

Shengnan Zheng, MD Division of Cardiology, University of Louisville, Louisville, KY, USA

Part I
Background and Process

Evolution of Cardiovascular Outcomes Studies

Liana L. Guarneiri, Mary R. Dicklin, and Kevin C. Maki

Key Points

- The Framingham Heart Study was the first large-scale cardiovascular epidemiology study in the USA, and observations from it pioneered the notion of cardiovascular risk factors.
- Observational studies like Framingham led to the testing of strategies to reduce cardiovascular event risk by modifying risk factors.
- Observational studies are effective at evaluating research questions that are not appropriate for an experimental design, but they are vulnerable to bias and confounding.
- Mendelian randomization is an observational method that uses genetic variation to investigate the relationship between a risk factor and a disease outcome.
- Cardiovascular outcome intervention trials have increased in size, complexity, and cost in recent decades.
- Explanatory trials are designed to test the efficacy of an intervention in optimized conditions, while pragmatic trials favor study design choices that maximize the applicability of study findings to usual care settings.
- Registry-based randomized controlled trials use patient registries to collect data and follow up with patients, which reduces the cost and enhances the generalizability of findings.

L. L. Guarneiri · M. R. Dicklin
Midwest Biomedical Research, Addison, IL, USA

K. C. Maki (✉)
Midwest Biomedical Research, Addison, IL, USA

Department of Applied Health Science, Indiana University School of Public Health, Bloomington, IN, USA
e-mail: kmaki@mbclinicalresearch.com

K. C. Maki, D. P. Wilson (eds.), *Cardiovascular Outcomes Research*, Contemporary Cardiology, https://doi.org/10.1007/978-3-031-54960-1_1

3

- In cardiovascular research, major adverse cardiovascular events (MACE) are common composite endpoints, traditionally including cardiovascular death, non-fatal myocardial infarction, and nonfatal stroke, although other endpoints are often included such as revascularization procedures, unstable angina, and hospitalization for heart failure.
- Adaptive study designs use interim statistical analyses to inform decisions on the modification of study design elements (e.g., sample size, randomization ratio, number of treatment arms, dose, and population).
- The blinding of participants/researchers, comparator groups, population, outcome variables, and follow-up duration are important considerations when designing cardiovascular outcome studies.

1   Evolution of the Study of Cardiovascular Outcomes

Prior to the mid-1900s, cardiovascular (CV) practices were based on tradition [1]. Recognizing the need to invest in research on CV disease (CVD) prevention, the U.S. Public Health Service initiated the Framingham Heart Study (FHS) in 1948 [2]. The FHS was the first large-scale CV epidemiology study in the USA; it involved 5209 mostly white men and women who were evaluated biennially through physical examinations, laboratory tests, and questionnaires. Results from the FHS were instrumental in pioneering the notion that CV risk factors could be identified that predicted risk for CVD events and that some risk factors are modifiable, which has revolutionized the prevention of CVD [3, 4]. The four key modifiable risk factors for CVD identified in the FHS were elevated levels of blood pressure, cholesterol, glucose (diabetes mellitus), and cigarette smoking.

Today, large studies that evaluate the impact of an intervention on CV outcomes (e.g., CV death, myocardial infarction (MI), stroke, and heart failure hospitalization) are termed cardiovascular outcomes trials (CVOTs) [1]. The first outcomes trial in CVD conducted in the late 1960s, the Department of Veterans Affairs (VA) Cooperative trial, evaluated the effects on the morbidity of antihypertensive treatments and laid the foundation for the management of hypertension today [1, 5]. Another instrumental study was the Lipid Research Clinics Coronary Primary Prevention Trial (LRC-CPPT) which was conducted in men with hypercholesterolemia in the 1970s and 1980s [6]. This randomized, double-blind, placebo-controlled trial demonstrated that lipid-lowering therapy with cholestyramine (a bile acid sequestrant) reduced total cholesterol and low-density lipoprotein cholesterol (LDL-C) concentrations more than placebo, which translated into reduced risk of coronary heart disease (CHD). In 2008, in response to concerns about the CV safety of certain antidiabetes compounds, the Food and Drug Administration mandated that all new hypoglycemic drugs must demonstrate CV safety, which led to the initiation of numerous CVOTs [7]. This guidance was modified in 2020 by a new approach that continued to stress the importance of CV safety data (not limited to atherosclerotic events) in the evaluation of diabetes medications but recommended basing the safety evaluation on signals of risk identified in the development program, rather than using a one-size-fits-all approach [8]. Nevertheless, CVOTs remain a key step in the evaluation of the safety and efficacy of numerous drug classes, such as those that target lipoproteins and related variables, blood pressure, glycemia, inflammation, and platelet function.

There are several challenges associated with conducting CV outcomes investigations. As medicines with the potential to improve CV risk factors and reduce CVD risk have become more effective and widely used, the level of evidence required to support the introduction of a new drug into the marketplace has increased immensely [1]. Additionally, the cost of conducting a CVOT has increased markedly due to the large sample sizes and long durations that are required. Furthermore, the importance of inclusivity in CVOTs is now recognized. To be able to generalize the results of CVOTs, the population studied needs to reasonably represent the population that will receive the drug therapy. Women and racial/ethnic minorities are disproportionately impacted by CVD, yet these participants are continually underrepresented in CVOTs, including those for lipid-lowering and hypoglycemic therapies [9–13]. For example, Avgerinos et al. systematically reviewed CVOTs that investigated the effect of hypoglycemic medications on major adverse cardiovascular events (MACE) in adults with type 2 diabetes [11]. Although women and African Americans represent 47.5% and 15.7% of patients with type 2 diabetes in the USA, only 35.1% and 4.6% of the trial participants, respectively, were drawn from these populations. Similarly, Grant et al. demonstrated that among 40 randomized controlled trials (RCTs) of lipid-lowering therapies with proven atherosclerotic cardiovascular disease (ASCVD) benefits, non-Hispanic Black participants comprised just 7.3% (median) of the total number of subjects per trial [13]. Furthermore, the calculation of the ratio of the percentage of non-Hispanic Black enrollees among trial participants to the percentage of non-Hispanic Black persons among the disease population (i.e., the participation-to-prevalence ratio [PPR]) indicated a marked underrepresentation compared with their disease burden in studies of persons with diabetes (PPR, 0.18), hypercholesterolemia (PPR, 0.33), stable coronary artery disease (PPR, 0.20), and acute coronary syndrome (PPR, 0.08). Selecting broad inclusion criteria, hiring multilingual staff, and providing flexibility in participation hours to accommodate work schedules are a few strategies to increase the enrollment of underrepresented populations in CVOTs.

2 Types of Observational Studies and Clinical Trials

Observational studies evaluate the relationship between exposures and disease outcomes in free-living populations [14]. Although useful for answering research questions that are not appropriate for experimental designs and generating hypotheses about potential interventions, observational studies are vulnerable to bias and confounding. The two main types of observational studies are case–control and cohort study designs.

In case–control designs, individuals with the outcome of interest are identified as the cases, and individuals without the outcome of interest in the population are identified as the controls. The level of historical exposure is compared between the cases and controls. Case–control designs are generally cost-effective and are most useful for studying rare outcomes and diseases for which little is known about potential causative factors [15].

In cohort designs, patients with varying levels of exposure and without the disease/outcome of interest are followed over time to evaluate the incidence of the outcome in each exposure group [14]. Cohort designs clearly establish a temporal relationship between exposure and disease, which is less clear in case–control designs since the exposure and disease have already occurred at the time of enrollment. In addition, multiple disease outcomes can be studied for a given exposure. One key limitation of cohort study designs for behavioral exposures is the self-selection of the exposure. For example, individuals who choose to exercise regularly, use dietary supplements, consume whole grains, use oral contraceptives, smoke cigarettes, and numerous other lifestyle choices may differ in material respects with relevance to disease risk from those who make different choices.

Confounding occurs when a factor is related to both the exposure and the disease under study. Although statistical methods are available to investigate potential confounding, these are far from perfect, and it is difficult to rule out residual confounding. Bias is a particular type of confounding that occurs when there are systematic differences that result in a difference in the likelihood of the outcome of interest between those with and without an exposure (or with different degrees of exposure), resulting in an inaccurate estimate of the relationship between the exposure and the outcome.

3   Mendelian Randomization Studies

Mendelian randomization is an observational method that uses genetic variation to investigate the relationship between a risk factor and a disease outcome; it is an important way to identify and validate potential targets of therapy [16]. During meiosis, offspring receive a random assortment of genetic variants from the parents. Individuals with and without genetic variants that affect risk factors (e.g., a gene variant that increases LDL-C) are observed over time for the occurrence of the outcome of interest (e.g., CHD). Because genetic variants are not affected by confounders, differences in the outcome between individuals with and without the genetic variant are more likely to be attributable to the difference in the risk factor (e.g., higher LDL-C), providing strong evidence for a causal relationship despite the study's observational nature. For example, results from a Mendelian randomization study reported that individuals with mutations in the gene for proprotein convertase subtilisin/kexin type 9 (PCSK9) that are associated with lower LDL-C throughout life had lower ASCVD risk [17].

4 Types of Cardiovascular Outcomes Trials

4.1 Randomized Controlled Trials

RCTs are prospective investigations used to examine cause-and-effect relationships between an intervention and an outcome [18]. They are considered the highest level of evidence to establish causal associations in clinical research. Because randomization balances participant characteristics between groups, including known and unknown predictors of the outcome, it generally allows the attribution of differences in the outcome to the intervention being studied. There are many RCT designs and features, some of which are described in more detail below.

4.1.1 Explanatory and Pragmatic Trials

In the late 1960s, two French statisticians proposed a distinction between trials aimed at confirming a physiological hypothesis (explanatory) and trials aimed at informing a clinical or policy decision (pragmatic) [19]. More specifically, explanatory trials are designed to test the efficacy of an intervention in optimized conditions. They include highly specific eligibility criteria and strict protocols for the assessment of safety and efficacy [20]. The interventions are often delivered by specialized research personnel with expertise in research implementation, and the trial is carefully monitored and followed up. Establishing efficacy via an explanatory trial is a hurdle that needs to be overcome before an intervention can be approved by regulators and introduced into the market. Conversely, pragmatic trials are focused on providing evidence for an intervention in the context of real-world clinical practice and often inform clinical or policy decisions [21]. Pragmatic trials were developed in response to concerns that explanatory trials are not relevant to clinical practice due to their frequent lack of generalizability, and that they may overestimate the benefits of interventions [20, 21]. Therefore, pragmatic trials combat these issues by utilizing simple study designs with minimal trial procedures and data collection (e.g., mailed questionnaires, web-based forms, etc.) [21]. The interventions are delivered by staff with typical clinical experience to a large, unselected patient population. The primary endpoints of explanatory trials are usually surrogates of physiological endpoints that indicate the efficacy of an intervention, whereas primary endpoints of pragmatic trials often focus on patient-centered outcomes (e.g., survival, quality of life, and functional status) [20].

There are several benefits to using a pragmatic approach. First, pragmatic trials optimize recruitment efforts by reducing the burden of the study protocol on practitioners and patients and including a wider pool of participants [20]. The reduced burden of the trial increases the accessibility of participation in research to historically marginalized groups with limited transportation, finances, or time. Oftentimes, pragmatic trials include entire practices or registries, resulting in large and diverse study populations that improve the generalizability of the results. Second, pragmatic trials are often cheaper to conduct than explanatory trials because fewer resources and specialized staff are required. Third, less frequent contact with participants in pragmatic trials minimizes the Hawthorne effect, in which participants change their behavior in response to their awareness of being observed [22]. However, there are also limitations to pragmatic trials. There may be more missing data in pragmatic vs. explanatory trials since follow-up in pragmatic trials is often conducted via mailed questionnaires or web-based forms, resulting in challenges for analysis and interpretation [21]. Additionally, pragmatic trials require a larger sample size for adequate statistical power due to increased nonadherence, dropouts, and crossover between groups compared to explanatory trials [20]. Since explanatory and pragmatic approaches exist on a continuum, it is important for researchers to consider design choices that will support applicability while preserving the ability to understand efficacy [23].

4.1.2   Registry-Based Randomized Controlled Trials

Registry-based RCTs use patient registries to collect data, randomize, and follow-up [24]. Eligible patients are identified prior to intervention selection when the registry is used for reporting, then the randomization service embedded in the registry randomizes participants to a treatment strategy [25]. Data in registries are typically obtained from patients, physicians, medical charts, electronic health records (EHRs), or other databases [24]. Benefits of registry-based RCTs include rapid consecutive enrollment of patients, improved completeness of follow-up, reduced cost of implementation, and enhanced generalizability. These trials tend to be pragmatic in nature since the eligibility criteria are less stringent, and the patient monitoring and follow-up reflect real-world circumstances rather than a controlled environment. The Thrombus Aspiration during ST-segment Elevation MI (TASTE) trial was one of the first registry-based trials [26]. This trial demonstrated that intracoronary thrombus aspiration plus primary percutaneous coronary intervention (PCI) vs. PCI alone did not reduce 30-day mortality in patients with ST-segment elevation MI; the cost was approximately US $50 per patient [24, 26]. Another example is the Bivalirudin Versus Heparin in ST-Segment and Non-ST-Segment Elevation MI in Patients on Modern Antiplatelet Therapy in the Swedish Web System for Enhancement and Development of Evidence-based Care in Heart Disease Evaluated According to Recommended Therapies Registry (VALIDATE-SWEDEHEART) trial. This was an open-label, registry-based RCT that demonstrated no difference in the primary composite endpoint of death, MI, and major bleeding events in patients receiving bivalirudin vs. heparin during a PCI [27].

Despite the benefits, registry-based RCTs also have challenges such as poor registry data quality, ethical issues, and methodological difficulties [24]. An example of an ethical concern is the level of informed consent that needs to be documented when all treatments administered are established and used in routine clinical practice. A methodological concern is that the registry may not include blinding, standardized implementation procedures, and/or fixed follow-up duration. Trialists should acknowledge the challenges associated with registry-based RCTs and attempt to mitigate the impact of these challenges on study quality.

4.1.3 Electronic Health Record-Enabled Trials

EHR-enabled trials are large pragmatic RCTs that are conducted through the routine clinical setting [28]. Enhanced technology allows the RCT to be embedded in the EHR without disrupting clinical workflows [29]. The result is the full integration of knowledge generation and health-care delivery. Eligibility for the RCT may be assessed in real time as data are entered into the EHR or retrospectively by backward querying of the database [28, 29]. Additionally, randomization can be programmed to occur within the EHR system, and follow-up occurs naturally when patients interact with their health-care provider [29]. The strengths of an EHR-enabled trial are similar to registry-based RCTs (rapid consecutive enrollment, low cost, and enhanced generalizability) [28]. However, there are several limitations, including the initial cost of implementing EHR infrastructure that is appropriate for research facilitation; privacy and ethical considerations; and poor standardization and quality of data. Clinical staff typically use free-text boxes to record electronic health data, which can be challenging to translate into quantifiable data for an RCT. Furthermore, the interval of contact between patients and providers is not standardized like it would be in a traditional clinical trial protocol. Finally, the detail and accuracy of the data recorded will likely vary between staff members. These limitations must be addressed to ensure high-quality data collection.

4.1.4 Time-to-Event Outcome Studies

In time-to-event (TTE) outcome studies, subjects are followed longitudinally with a clearly defined start time and end time (usually until the event of interest or the last follow-up occurs) [30]. TTE endpoints are a measure of treatment efficacy. The TTE analysis simultaneously evaluates whether an event happened (i.e., a binary outcome) and when the event happened (e.g., a continuous outcome) [31]. It is important that the event is clearly defined and mutually exclusive (e.g., alive vs. dead, or hospitalized vs. not hospitalized). If the event is not mutually exclusive (e.g., becoming symptomatic), then a threshold must be defined to differentiate an event vs. no event.

Composite endpoints are often used to increase the number of primary outcome events [32]. In CV research, MACE is used as a common composite endpoint. Traditional (3-point) MACE includes CV death, nonfatal MI, and nonfatal stroke; thus, a TTE outcome study would capture the time to any one of these events. Other MACE composites (e.g., 4- or 5-point) may include outcomes such as revascularization procedures, unstable angina, and hospitalization for heart failure.

The power needed to analyze TTE data is dependent on the number of events instead of the total sample size, and the trial may be stopped early when a prespecified minimum number of events is reached [33, 34]. When calculating sample size, first the number of events needed to detect a minimum clinically important effect size with a preselected power and alpha level (p-value to declare statistical significance) is calculated [33]. Next, the proportion of patients who are expected to experience the event is estimated. The length of follow-up is based on the frequency of events, which may result in longer than anticipated follow-up if the event rate observed is below that projected during planning or vice versa [30].

In the Further Cardiovascular Outcomes Research with PCSK9 Inhibition in Subjects with Elevated Risk (FOURIER) trial, the median follow-up period was planned to be 4 years, but the actual follow-up was 2.2 years due to a higher than postulated event rate [35]. The trial demonstrated that treatment with evolocumab resulted in a 15% reduction in the risk for the primary composite endpoint (CV death, MI, stroke, hospitalization for unstable angina, or coronary revascularization). Following the "parent trial," patients were eligible to be enrolled in the FOURIER open-label extension (FOURIER-OLE) in which all patients were treated with evolocumab, regardless of their original treatment assignment in FOURIER [36]. After a median follow-up of 5 years, patients who had been originally randomized to evolocumab in the parent trial had a 15–20% lower risk of MACE, and a 23% lower risk of CV death, compared to the patients who were originally randomized to placebo. These data suggest that there is a delay in observing the full clinical benefit of LDL-C lowering. This illustrates the importance of utilizing a sufficiently long follow-up period in CVOTs.

Patients who do not experience the event of interest prior to their last follow-up and patients that do not complete their scheduled follow-up for reasons independent of the event of interest are described as censored patients [30]. It is not appropriate to exclude censored patients from the analysis since the event might occur at an unknown future time, so TTE analysis methods must be used to account for censoring. One example is the Kaplan–Meier method, which includes data from patients who had the event of interest and those being censored to estimate the probability of survival at different time points [30, 31]. Another challenge of analyzing TTE data is that not all participants are followed for an equal amount of time. For this reason, the log-rank test is the most popular method for comparing the survival of groups since it considers the entire observed follow-up using person-time units of observation (e.g., person-years) for all participants rather than selecting an arbitrary point in time [37].

4.1.5 Adaptive Designs

Adaptive designs use accumulating data, such as those from interim statistical analyses, to inform decisions on the modification of study design elements (e.g., sample size, randomization ratio, number of treatment arms, dose, and population) [38]. Adaptive designs increase the efficiency of RCTs and improve the likelihood of identifying a benefit of the intervention, if one exists, while maintaining the integrity and validity of the trial [39]. There are two common adaptations that are applied to CVOTs [40]. First, the sample size may be re-estimated without changing the total number of events after a blinded interim review of the event rate. Second, the targeted number of events may be modified based on an unblinded review of the interim data. One strategy is to power the CVOT to demonstrate superiority, but to include an interim analysis to determine whether the trial should be continued or stopped early due to noninferiority or futility. Another strategy is to power the trial for noninferiority and then to update the study objective to superiority by increasing the total number of events and/or subjects if the interim analysis yields promising results for superiority.

There are several obstacles to implementing an adaptive design [39, 41]. Since adaptive designs are less conventional, funding and regulatory agencies often scrutinize proposals for adaptive designs more closely and require additional explanation for the rationale of the design. Additionally, the interim analyses should be conducted with care to avoid introducing bias into the trial [41]. It is best practice for an unblinded independent data monitoring committee to review interim data and then make recommendations to a blinded steering committee. All adaptation rules should be specified in the protocol prior to trial initiation. Finally, the interpretation of results from an adaptive trial will require extra care. A statistician with experience in adaptive designs should be consulted when creating the statistical analysis plan, and the trial processes and procedures that will be used to minimize potential operational bias should be described in detail.

4.2 Considerations for Designing Cardiovascular Outcomes Trials

4.2.1 Blinding

Blinding of study participants, care providers, research investigators, and outcome assessors is used in RCTs to minimize post-randomization bias (mainly performance bias and ascertainment bias) [42]. Performance bias occurs when care providers inadvertently administer different care to participants in the intervention arm. Ascertainment bias occurs when a researcher is influenced by group assignment during outcome measurement, verification, or recording. Blinding is optimal for RCTs but not always feasible due to methodological, technical, or ethical reasons. In open-label outcome trials, an external blinded outcome adjudication committee can be used to prevent differential classification of outcomes between interventions and controls [43]. In CVOTs, these committees are especially important for evaluating nonfatal endpoints such as unstable angina or revascularization procedures, which are more vulnerable to subjective evaluation [44]. However, some question whether the benefits of blinded outcome adjudication committees always outweigh the high cost and loss of efficiency in these trials.

4.2.2 Comparator Group

Placebo-controlled interventions blind participants and investigators to the allocated treatment by simulating the experience of receiving an experimental intervention without administering a therapeutic intervention [45]. The incorporation of a placebo arm controls for response bias (patients report outcomes that they believe will please the investigators) and the placebo effect (participants experience symptoms differently when receiving an intervention). Although administering a placebo is optimal for establishing the efficacy of a drug, the ethics of administering a placebo to patients with diseases for which an effective treatment has already been established come into question [46].

One option to mitigate the ethical concerns of placebos is to use historical control data to replace concurrent control data [47]. Data for historical controls often come from medical charts, published data of off-label use, registries, and previously completed trials. Using historical data is cost-efficient but requires robust justification and heavy involvement of regulatory bodies. Historical controls are most often used in trials studying rare diseases when a standard of care has not been established. A more common approach to mitigate ethical concerns of placebos in CV research is to administer a drug with established therapeutic benefits as an active control and then to test whether the new drug is noninferior to the established drug [46, 48]. The following section describes the difference between trials evaluating superiority, equivalence, and noninferiority among treatments.

4.2.3 Superiority Vs. Noninferiority Trials

The objective of a superiority (comparative) trial is to demonstrate that an investigative treatment is better than an active control or placebo [48]. The objective of equivalence trials is to show that treatment with either therapy does not differ by more than a predefined threshold in either direction, which is referred to as the equivalence margin and denoted by Δ [49, 50]. If the confidence interval that is computed around the difference between the two treatments lies within the equivalence margin ($-\Delta$ to $+\Delta$), then the two treatments are deemed equivalent [49]. The purpose of a noninferiority trial is to demonstrate that the new treatment is not worse than the active control [48]. Noninferiority trials employ one-sided hypothesis testing toward $-\Delta$ (also referred to as the noninferiority margin), while equivalence and superiority trials employ two-sided testing, highlighting the need to establish the trial goals *a priori*. Two treatments are determined to be noninferior if the lower bound of the confidence interval that is computed around the differences between the two treatments does not exceed $-\Delta$. Noninferiority trials are popular in CV research since, as described previously, it is often unethical to include a placebo arm in RCTs when a "gold standard" therapy for the disease being studied has already been established. When the efficacy of a new therapy is determined to be noninferior to the "gold standard" therapy, the new therapy should ideally have an alternative benefit such as lower cost, fewer side effects, or improved convenience.

Noninferiority testing should be designed and conducted with rigor because less rigor makes it easier to show noninferiority [49]. "Biocreep" or "technology creep" describes when an inferior therapy is erroneously deemed noninferior and becomes an active control group in a future trial, resulting in degradation over time in the efficacy of the investigational treatment. Defining the noninferiority margin is an important step in designing a rigorous noninferiority trial [50]. The margin should be based on one or more placebo-controlled trials of the active comparator or a meta-analysis of several placebo-controlled trials. Researchers must also apply clinical judgment to determine what level of loss of efficacy in a new treatment would become clinically meaningful. Selecting an unreasonably wide margin will yield a lower sample size requirement, resulting in an underpowered trial that is more likely to show noninferiority [48]. Additionally, rigorous noninferiority trials should be designed similarly to previous trials to fulfill the constancy assumption, which states that the effect of the active comparator is consistent with the effect that was previously observed [51]. It is not appropriate to draw conclusions about noninferiority when the constancy assumption is not met. Altogether, noninferiority trials provide an exceptional opportunity to advance CV research and impact clinical practice, but these trials must be expertly designed and conducted, rigorously analyzed, and carefully interpreted to avoid bias toward noninferiority [48].

4.2.4 Population

When designing a clinical trial, it is important that researchers consider the study objective, the safety of participants, the feasibility of the eligibility criteria, and the target population [52]. The purpose of early phase trials is to isolate the effects of the intervention; thus, a more homogenous population will reduce response variation. However, later phase trials should target more heterogeneous populations to ensure the trial is generalizable to the entire population in which the intervention will be utilized in clinical practice. Researchers should also consider the feasibility of eligibility criteria. Although strict eligibility criteria may be desirable, the criteria may need to be relaxed to ensure completion of the trial within a reasonable time frame. Furthermore, studies should be designed to enroll a group of participants with an increased risk that is attributable to a pathophysiological state that might be mitigated by the administration of the intervention under investigation.

4.2.5 Outcome Variables

When selecting outcome variables to measure in clinical trials, researchers should consider the clinical relevance, interpretability, sensitivity to the intervention, practicality, and affordability of the measurement [52]. In addition, clinical trials frequently use composite outcomes, which combine two or more variables into a single measure that is used to assess a treatment's efficacy, tolerability, and/or safety [53]. Composite outcomes may also be used in CVOTs to provide a more comprehensive evaluation of the variables being studied, but they can also make the interpretation of clinical trial results more difficult. A positive result for a composite outcome does not equate to positive results for all variables that make up that composite outcome. Another limitation of composite outcomes is that the time-to-first occurrence of any event in the composite is often evaluated, thus later events, that may be more severe, are ignored [54]. Therefore, the effect of the intervention on the individual components should also be evaluated as a sensitivity analysis and, ideally, total events (as opposed to the first events) should also be evaluated.

As mentioned previously, the composite outcome of MACE is frequently used in CVOTs [55]. Although there is no standard definition for MACE, the classic definition focuses on the manifestation of ASCVD in the coronary and cerebral vessels (nonfatal MI, nonfatal stroke, and CV death), sometimes referred to as three-point MACE. Additionally, four-point MACE, which also includes hospitalization for unstable angina or revascularization procedures, and five-point MACE, which also includes heart failure, are commonly reported in the literature [56]. When choosing a composite outcome, the expected outcome of the intervention should be carefully considered. For example, in the Empagliflozin Cardiovascular Outcome Event Trial in Type 2 Diabetes Mellitus Patients (EMPA-REG OUTCOME), the primary outcome was the classic three-point MACE, but the trial demonstrated no effect of empagliflozin on two of the three key MACE components, MI or stroke [57]. Conversely, the risk of hospitalization for heart failure decreased by 35%, suggesting that the main effect of empagliflozin is on myocardial function, not atherosclerosis [55]. Similarly, in the Vitamin D and Omega-3 Trial (VITAL), there was no significant difference in the primary composite endpoint of MACE (MI, stroke, and CV mortality) between the marine-omega-3 fatty acids and placebo groups, but analyses of the individual components of the primary composite endpoint indicated a significant 18% reduction in MI [58]. Unfortunately, when the primary outcome is not significantly impacted, even if the secondary outcome(s) do show a significant effect, then regulatory approval for a new drug is improbable [59]. However, the findings for the secondary outcomes may contribute to the generation of new hypotheses that can be tested in subsequent RCTs.

4.2.6 Follow-Up Duration

Since CVOTs are driven by CV event occurrence, the length of follow-up is an essential component of the study design. Shorter follow-ups are more cost-effective but are vulnerable to overestimating the effect of the intervention since the estimated treatment effect varies randomly throughout the trial [60]. For example, Silverman et al. reported that the mean follow-up for CVOTs involving statins has been ~4.5 years, while other CVOTs involving nonstatin therapies have had even shorter follow-ups [61]. As described previously, the FOURIER trial was stopped after a median follow-up of 2.2 years when evolocumab demonstrated a 15% reduction in the primary composite outcome relative to placebo [35], but an even lower risk of the primary endpoint was detected after the open-label extension when patients were followed for a median of 5 years (FOURIER-OLE) [36]. These data suggest that there is a delay in observing the full clinical benefit of LDL-C lowering, thus longer follow-up periods in CVOTs evaluating lipid-lowering therapies may be crucial.

In addition, stopping a trial early may limit evidence for important secondary and safety outcomes [60]. In the Fractional Flow Reserve versus Angiography for Multivessel Evaluation (FAME 2) trial, in which PCI was compared with medical therapy alone, the trial was stopped after randomization of 54% of the initially planned study sample when PCI showed superiority for the primary outcome (all-cause death, MI, or urgent revascularization) [62]. However, the improvement with PCI was driven by fewer urgent revascularizations, which are arguably less clinically important than the other components of the primary outcome (all-cause death and MI) [60]. The results for death and MI were lower with PCI but did not reach statistical significance [62]. If the trial had continued longer, a significantly lower rate of death or MI may have materialized, improving the relevance and confidence of the trial findings.

4.2.7   Internal and External Validities

Internal validity evaluates whether the clinical trial was designed, conducted, and analyzed in a manner that answers the research question without bias [63]. Systemic error and random error are the two main factors that threaten internal validity of a trial. Systemic error results from four sources: selection bias, performance bias, detection bias, and attrition bias [64]. Effective randomization procedures, including appropriate allocation sequence generation and allocation concealment, reduce selection bias and balance known and unknown confounding factors [65]. Furthermore, performance bias occurs when there are systemic differences in the care provided to participants in different groups, and detection bias occurs when there are systemic differences in outcome assessment between groups [64]. Blinding participants, care providers, research investigators, and outcome assessors, and selecting objective outcome measures reduce the risk of performance bias and detection bias [66]. Finally, attrition bias occurs when there are systemic differences between groups in the loss of participants from the study [64]. Using an intention-to-treat analysis, which includes all randomized participants, minimizes the risk of overestimating the clinical effectiveness of the treatment.

External validity evaluates whether results from a clinical trial can be generalized to the "real world" population [64]. Results from a trial must have internal validity before being considered for external validity. Researchers may improve external validity by recruiting diverse populations, enrolling patients with a variety of clinical features and comorbidities, implementing interventions in a manner that is feasible in routine practice, and assessing a broad range of clinical outcomes.

5 Conclusions

Since the start of the FHS in 1948, the management of CVD has transitioned from being informed by tradition and anecdotes to being based on the results of rigorous CVOTs. These CVOTs have increased in size, complexity, and cost in recent decades and their use has expanded to evaluate the safety and efficacy of drug classes beyond those traditionally considered CV related. There are several study design decisions that must be considered when designing a CVOT, including the degree of pragmatism, the source of recruitment (nontraditional sources include registries and EHRs), blinding, comparator groups, population, outcome variables, and follow-up durations. A well-designed CVOT provides invaluable evidence for the regulatory approval of new drugs and clinical decision-making, while poor design decisions may thwart the validity and applicability of the trial results.

References

1. Solomon SD, Pfeffer MA. The future of clinical trials in cardiovascular medicine. Circulation. 2016;133(25):2662–70.
2. Tsao CW, Vasan RS. The Framingham Heart Study: past, present and future. Oxford University Press; 2015. p. 1763–6.
3. Dawber TR, Moore FE, Mann GV. Coronary heart disease in the Framingham study. Am J Public Health Nations Health. 1957;47(4 Pt 2):4–24.
4. Kannel WB, et al. Factors of risk in the development of coronary heart disease—six year follow-up experience. The Framingham Study. Ann Intern Med. 1961;55:33–50.
5. Henrie AM, et al. Impact of Department of Veterans Affairs Cooperative Studies Program clinical trials on practice guidelines for high blood pressure management. Contemp Clin Trials Commun. 2019;13:100313.
6. Rifkind BM. Lipid research clinics coronary primary prevention trial: results and implications. Am J Cardiol. 1984;54(5):30–4.
7. Food and Drug Administration. Guidance for industry on diabetes mellitus-evaluating cardiovascular risk in new antidiabetic therapies to treat type 2 diabetes. 2008. [cited 2023 Jul 2] https://www.federalregister.gov/documents/2008/12/19/E8-30086/guidance-for-industry-on-diabetes-mellitus-evaluating-cardiovascular-risk-in-new-antidiabetic.
8. Food and Drug Administration. Type 2 diabetes mellitus: evaluating the safety of new drugs for improving glycemic control: guidance for industry. 2020. [cited 2023 Jul 10]. https://www.fda.gov/media/135936/download.
9. Khan SU, et al. Participation of women and older participants in randomized clinical trials of lipid-lowering therapies: a systematic review. JAMA Netw Open. 2020;3(5):e205202.
10. Sawant S, Wang N. Under-representation of ethnic and regional minorities in lipid-lowering randomized clinical trials: a systematic review and meta-analysis. Eur J Prev Cardiol. 2023;30(11):1120–31.
11. Avgerinos I, et al. Racial, ethnic and sex disparities among participants in cardiovascular outcomes trials in type 2 diabetes: a systematic review and descriptive analysis. Diabetes Obes Metab. 2023;25(2):618–22.
12. Herskind AEJ, Nørgaard B. Gender representation in drug development studies for diabetes mellitus. A systematic review. Diabetes Metab Syndr Clin Res Rev. 2023;17:102815.

13. Grant JK, et al. Under-reporting and under-representation of non-Hispanic Black subjects in lipid-lowering atherosclerotic cardiovascular disease outcomes trials: a systematic review. J Clin Lipidol. 2022;16(5):608–16.
14. Jepsen P, et al. Interpretation of observational studies. Heart. 2004;90(8):956–60.
15. Schulz KF, Grimes DA. Case-control studies: research in reverse. Lancet. 2002;359(9304): 431–4.
16. Emdin CA, Khera AV, Kathiresan S. Mendelian randomization. JAMA. 2017;318(19):1925–6.
17. Cohen JC, et al. Sequence variations in PCSK9, low LDL, and protection against coronary heart disease. N Engl J Med. 2006;354(12):1264–72.
18. Zabor EC, Kaizer AM, Hobbs BP. Randomized controlled trials. Chest. 2020;158(1S):S79–87.
19. Schwartz D, Lellouch J. Explanatory and pragmatic attitudes in therapeutical trials. J Chronic Dis. 1967;20(8):637–48.
20. Usman MS, et al. The need for increased pragmatism in cardiovascular clinical trials. Nat Rev Cardiol. 2022;19(11):737–50.
21. Ford I, Norrie J. Pragmatic trials. N Engl J Med. 2016;375(5):454–63.
22. Sedgwick P, Greenwood N. Understanding the Hawthorne effect. BMJ. 2015;351:h4672.
23. Treweek S, Zwarenstein M. Making trials matter: pragmatic and explanatory trials and the problem of applicability. Trials. 2009;10(1):1–9.
24. Li G, et al. Registry-based randomized controlled trials—what are the advantages, challenges, and areas for future research? J Clin Epidemiol. 2016;80:16–24.
25. Nyberg K, Hedman P. Swedish guidelines for registry-based randomized clinical trials. Ups J Med Sci. 2019;124(1):33–6.
26. Fröbert O, et al. Thrombus aspiration during ST-segment elevation myocardial infarction. N Engl J Med. 2013;369:1587–97.
27. Erlinge D, et al. Bivalirudin versus heparin monotherapy in myocardial infarction. N Engl J Med. 2017;377(12):1132–42.
28. McCord KA, Hemkens LG. Using electronic health records for clinical trials: where do we stand and where can we go? CMAJ. 2019;191(5):E128–33.
29. Pletcher MJ, et al. Randomized controlled trials of electronic health record interventions: design, conduct, and reporting considerations. Ann Intern Med. 2020;172(11_Supplement):S85–91.
30. Le-Rademacher J, Wang X. Time-to-event data: an overview and analysis considerations. J Thorac Oncol. 2021;16(7):1067–74.
31. Denfeld QE, Burger D, Lee CS. Survival analysis 101: an easy start guide to analysing time-to-event data. Eur J Cardiovasc Nurs. 2023;22(3):332–7.
32. Bebu I, Lachin JM. Properties of composite time to first event versus joint marginal analyses of multiple outcomes. Stat Med. 2018;37(27):3918–30.
33. Schober P, Vetter TR. Survival analysis and interpretation of time-to-event data: the tortoise and the hare. Anesth Analg. 2018;127(3):792–8.
34. Zannad F, et al. When to stop a clinical trial early for benefit: lessons learned and future approaches. Circ Heart Fail. 2012;5(2):294–302.
35. Sabatine MS, et al. Evolocumab and clinical outcomes in patients with cardiovascular disease. N Engl J Med. 2017;376(18):1713–22.
36. O'Donoghue ML, et al. Long-term evolocumab in patients with established atherosclerotic cardiovascular disease. Circulation. 2022;146(15):1109–19.
37. Singh R, Mukhopadhyay K. Survival analysis in clinical trials: basics and must know areas. Perspect Clin Res. 2011;2(4):145–8.
38. Jackson N, et al. Improving clinical trials for cardiovascular diseases: a position paper from the Cardiovascular Round Table of the European Society of Cardiology. Eur Heart J. 2016;37(9):747–54.
39. Bhatt DL, Mehta C. Adaptive designs for clinical trials. N Engl J Med. 2016;375(1):65–74.
40. Marchenko O, et al. Statistical considerations for cardiovascular outcome trials in patients with type 2 diabetes mellitus. Stat Biopharm Res. 2017;9(4):347–60.

41. Pallmann P, et al. Adaptive designs in clinical trials: why use them, and how to run and report them. BMC Med. 2018;16(1):1–15.
42. Renjith V. Blinding in randomized controlled trials: what researchers need to know? Manipal J Nurs Health Sci (MJNHS). 2017;3(1):45–50.
43. van der Ende NAM, et al. Added value of a blinded outcome adjudication committee in an open-label randomized stroke trial. Stroke. 2022;53(1):61–9.
44. Greene SJ, Butler J. Investigator-reported versus adjudicated clinical events. J Am Coll Cardiol. 2021;78(15):1538–40.
45. Laursen DRT, et al. Active placebo versus standard placebo control interventions in pharmacological randomised trials. LID—MR000055. 2020(1469-493X (Electronic)).
46. Spławiński J, Kuźniar J. Clinical trials: active control vs placebo—what is ethical? Sci Eng Ethics. 2004;10(1):73–9.
47. Ghadessi M, et al. A roadmap to using historical controls in clinical trials—by Drug Information Association Adaptive Design Scientific Working Group (DIA-ADSWG). Orphanet J Rare Dis. 2020;15(1):69.
48. Head SJ, et al. Non-inferiority study design: lessons to be learned from cardiovascular trials. Eur Heart J. 2012;33(11):1318–24.
49. Schumi J, Wittes JT. Through the looking glass: understanding non-inferiority. Trials. 2011;12:1–12.
50. Angeli F, et al. Optimal use of the non-inferiority trial design. Pharm Med. 2020;34:159–65.
51. Koopmeiners JS, Hobbs BP. Detecting and accounting for violations of the constancy assumption in non-inferiority clinical trials. Stat Methods Med Res. 2018;27(5):1547–58.
52. Evans SR. Fundamentals of clinical trial design. J Exp Stroke Transl Med. 2010;3(1):19–27.
53. Gewandter JS, et al. Composite outcomes for pain clinical trials: considerations for design and interpretation. Pain. 2021;162(7):1899.
54. Redfors B, et al. The win ratio approach for composite endpoints: practical guidance based on previous experience. Eur Heart J. 2020;41(46):4391–9.
55. Hupfeld C, Mudaliar S. Navigating the "MACE" in cardiovascular outcomes trials and decoding the relevance of atherosclerotic cardiovascular disease benefits versus heart failure benefits. Diabetes Obes Metab. 2019;21(8):1780–9.
56. Bosco E, et al. Major adverse cardiovascular event definitions used in observational analysis of administrative databases: a systematic review. BMC Med Res Methodol. 2021;21(1):241.
57. Zinman B, et al. Empagliflozin, cardiovascular outcomes, and mortality in type 2 diabetes. N Engl J Med. 2015;373(22):2117–28.
58. Manson JE, et al. Marine n-3 fatty acids and prevention of cardiovascular disease and cancer. N Engl J Med. 2019;380(1):23–32.
59. Pocock SJ, Stone GW. The primary outcome fails—what next? N Engl J Med. 2016;375(9):861–70.
60. Pocock SJ, Stone GW. The primary outcome is positive—is that good enough? N Engl J Med. 2016;375(10):971–9.
61. Silverman MG, et al. Association between lowering LDL-C and cardiovascular risk reduction among different therapeutic interventions: a systematic review and meta-analysis. JAMA. 2016;316(12):1289–97.
62. De Bruyne B, et al. Fractional flow reserve–guided PCI for stable coronary artery disease. N Engl J Med. 2014;371(13):1208–17.
63. Andrade C. Internal, external, and ecological validity in research design, conduct, and evaluation. Indian J Psychol Med. 2018;40(5):498–9.
64. Akobeng AK. Assessing the validity of clinical trials. J Pediatr Gastroenterol Nutr. 2008;47(3):277–82.
65. Sil A, et al. Selection of control, randomization, blinding, and allocation concealment. Indian Dermatol Online J. 2019;10(5):601–5.
66. Probst P, et al. Blinding in randomized controlled trials in general and abdominal surgery: protocol for a systematic review and empirical study. Syst Rev. 2016;5(1):48.

Statistical Methods for Cardiovascular Outcomes Studies

Aurelian Bidulescu, Steven R. Horbal, and Andrew D. Althouse

Key Points

- "Evidence-based medicine" is driven by well-designed research studies and statistical evidence.
- A typical epidemiologic analysis involves the summarization of variables, deriving the associations of the pertinent variables (through various regression procedures, for instance), and stratifying these estimates by groups.
- Understanding study design is important to discern the level of evidence being presented as well as the pros and cons of different modeling procedures.
- A statistical approach should be informed by the research objective, not by what the data look like.
- Multivariable analysis should be driven by proper conceptualization of the relationship between different factors, not by using all available data.
- Studies should include a sample size justification to show that the planned/available sample was/is large enough to fulfill the desired research objective.

A. Bidulescu (✉)
Department of Epidemiology and Biostatistics, Indiana University School of Public Health-Bloomington, Bloomington, IN, USA
e-mail: abidules@indiana.edu

S. R. Horbal
Department of Surgery, University of Michigan, Ann Arbor, MI, USA
e-mail: shorbal@med.umich.edu

A. D. Althouse
Department of Medicine Center for Research on Health Care, University of Pittsburgh, Pittsburgh, PA, USA

Medtronic, Minneapolis, MN, USA
e-mail: ADA62@pitt.edu

© The Author(s), under exclusive license to Springer Nature Switzerland AG 2024
K. C. Maki, D. P. Wilson (eds.), *Cardiovascular Outcomes Research*, Contemporary Cardiology, https://doi.org/10.1007/978-3-031-54960-1_2

- More complex modeling procedures offer distinct performance advantages and are paramount for clinicians to understand takeaway points and contextualize the results in the literature.
- Several statistical procedures and concepts are presented and clinically interpreted.

1 Introduction

Medical practice has advanced greatly in the last century, thanks to "evidence-based medicine" principles; it is now generally accepted that for patients to receive the best medical care, clinical practice should be informed by well-controlled research studies. Consider some of the following scenarios:

1. We have a new imaging technique for evaluating or diagnosing a particular condition. We believe that it is more accurate in determining a patient's risk of a poor clinical outcome than existing options. We should perform a research study to demonstrate that the new procedure works as advertised before it is widely used to inform therapeutic decisions. How can we empirically demonstrate the diagnostic accuracy of the new technique?
2. Patients undergoing a certain procedure (e.g., transcatheter aortic valve replacement [TAVR]) have a risk of a particular complication (e.g., periprocedural stroke). We wish to accurately estimate each patient's risk of periprocedural stroke; with this information, the patient can be properly informed of the potential risks, while the clinical team might consider whether this patient is a suitable candidate for additional preventive measures (e.g., we might consider an embolic protection device in patients with a very high risk of periprocedural stroke). How can we develop and validate tools that estimate the risk of periprocedural stroke for patients undergoing TAVR?
3. Perhaps the best-known research design is the randomized clinical trial: we have a new therapy that we wish to test against the existing standard of care in a particular patient population to determine whether the new therapy is effective in improving one or more clinical outcome(s) of interest. How can we empirically test whether the new treatment has the desired effect?

Each of these tasks may be accomplished, in part, by collecting data and applying statistical analyses to these data to answer the question at hand.

This chapter provides an overview of commonly used statistical analyses in cardiovascular medicine. Please note that there are no detailed technical descriptions of the methods described herein as this would lie beyond the scope of a single chapter in this textbook. Several of the topics addressed in single paragraphs of this book are the subject of entire chapters, or even books, of their own. Mathematical notation has been omitted entirely; this is an explanatory chapter with the aim of providing clinicians a basic understanding of how statistical analyses are performed and what they may encounter in clinical research papers. Some technical references have been provided for further consultation.

Please also note that this chapter omits the commonly seen "flowchart," which tells the reader to simply follow some arrows and symbols to choose a statistical test or model based on the data they have available. Many readers like these flowcharts and believe them to be useful in "making statistics easy"; however, they encourage memorization, but not an understanding, of the process and encourage a scientifically backward form of thinking wherein statistical tests are chosen according to data rather than according to the objective of the research. It is important for the reader to understand that choosing a statistical approach for a scientific problem should be informed by the research objective and not by what the data look like. Hopefully, this will become clearer to the reader over the course of this chapter.

Most Figures were generated in the R package "ggplot2" except the log-rank plots, which were generated using the "survminer" package [1–3].

2 Types of Variables

In cardiovascular research, most variables that we encounter may be classified into one of the following three broad categories:

1. *Continuous* variables are best described as variables that may take on any numeric value (subject to some restrictions on the reasonable range of values and precision for that measure, of course). For example, a patient's age will never be less than zero and will seldom be greater than 100 years; however, it may take on any numeric value within that range, which is sufficient for it to be treated as a "continuous" variable in most analyses. One may point out that some of these variables are analyzed as though, they are "continuous", but are often "pseudo-continuous" in practice—e.g., age is often simply recorded to the nearest year rather than more granular units (months, days, minutes, and seconds) which are theoretically possible. This is largely unavoidable for most measures that can only be recorded to a finite degree of accuracy and often will matter little in practice unless a large amount of the information contained in the variable is lost by doing so. For example, recording age to the nearest year rather than the nearest day is unlikely to make a large difference in modeling the relationship between age and risk of cardiovascular mortality.

2. *Categorical* variables are those which may only take on discrete values. Within this group, there are three categorical variables worth mentioning. The first is a *binary* variable, which is a categorical variable that only takes on two values (often "yes/no" for a particular characteristic: the patient is a current smoker, or they are not). The second is an *ordinal* variable, which is a categorical variable that has a clear ordering. An example of this is the New York Heart Association (NYHA) class for heart failure patients, which is an ordinal scale ranging from class I (no symptoms of fatigue, angina, and/or dyspnea with ordinary physical activity) to class IV (symptoms of fatigue, angina, and/or dyspnea even at rest). The NYHA class may take on four values (I, II, III, and IV) that have a clear ordering, wherein class I represents the least severe heart failure and class IV

represents the most severe heart failure; it may be appropriate to take advantage of this natural ordering in some analyses. Finally, it must also be noted that some categorical variables are created as a derivation of more granular numeric data, in some cases by choice of the investigators after the data have been collected and in some cases because it is not practical to collect the more granular data. An example of this is a question about a participant's household income; perhaps they are asked to select one of the following choices: <$20,000, $20,000–49,999, $50,000–$99,999, or >$100,000. The actual household income is more like a continuous variable, but the data collected in this fashion are best analyzed as an ordinal variable since there are only four discrete choices permitted by the structure of the question. The final case is a categorical variable that has many possible values but no clear order, something like "clinical site" or "region of the country." There are many potential values, with no clear "ordering" thus these will be recorded as discrete values without any ordering imposed for analysis.

3. *Time-to-event* variables are just what they sound like—a numeric recording of the amount of time from some "start" time to the occurrence of a clinical event. For the naïve user, it is often tempting to simply treat these as continuous variables; after all, one can simply record the time as a number. However, there are two important considerations that necessitate the treatment of these variables differently than a typical continuous variable. The first is that not all patients will be followed for an equal amount of time; a research study may enroll patients over several years (e.g., enrolling patients from 2015 to 2017) but plan to analyze the data in the year 2020. The question is how to account for the fact that some patients had five possible years of follow-up time while others only had three possible years of follow-up time? The second is that not all patients will be observed to have the event in question, so there is a different meaning for a patient who was followed for 5 years and experienced the clinical event versus a patient who was followed for 5 years without experiencing the clinical event. Consider a clinical trial testing whether a medication reduces the risk of cardio-vascular mortality; after 5 years of follow-up, about 10% of patients have died of cardiovascular causes. Simply comparing the "average" survival times between the groups is complicated because many patients are still alive at the end of the follow-up period; this is not necessarily a good representation of the true "average" survival time for the patient population. Time-to-event variables typically require the use of specialized techniques for survival analysis, discussed later in the chapter.

There are some special cases which are not fully described here. For example, a variable such as "number of hospitalizations" is likely recorded as a number and might seem to make sense as either a "continuous" variable (after all, it's a number!) or a categorical/ordinal variable (it can only take on discrete values—integers—and may practically be limited to something like 0, 1, 2, or 3 depending on the length of time and risk in that patient population). Some analyses may decide to model this as a "count" variable. There are many options for analyzing and modeling these types of variables, some of which will be briefly mentioned later in the chapter. We should also mention that sometimes readers are tempted to analyze and report ordinal variables that take on numeric values as though they are continuous values (e.g., recording the NYHA class as I, II, III, and IV and treating it as a continuous variable in further analyses); later in the chapter we will briefly discuss reasons why this should be discouraged.

2.1 Summarizing One Variable

One of the first tasks in statistical analysis is simply "describing" the data present within a single variable. This is necessary to understand for its own sake as well as building toward more complex analyses.

For a continuous variable, one typically reports a measure of *central tendency* and a measure of *spread*. The most common measures of central tendency include the *mean* (or average), the *median* (the "middle" observation when the data are sorted from lowest to highest), and the *mode* (the most common value in the set). The most common measures of spread are the *standard deviation, interquartile range* (IQR, the distance between the first quartile and third quartile), and *range* (distance between the minimum and maximum of all values). It should be noted that the IQR is actually one number and the IQR limits would be the bounds of the 25th and 75th percentiles; similarly, the range is a single number, and the range limits are the minimum and maximum values. However, the terms IQR and range are commonly used, even in peer-reviewed journals, when the results presented are actually the IQR limits or range limits. Of course, it is often useful to plot the data, when possible, as any reduction to a few summary measures will invariably tell the reader less than seeing all of the data.

Table 1 reports age and high-density lipoprotein (HDL) cholesterol for a 500-participant cohort. The distribution of age is reported as mean (standard deviation), and the distribution of HDL cholesterol is reported as median and the lower (L) and upper (U) bounds of the interquartile range (IQR:L,U). Figure 1 displays the ages of cohort participants (left) and the HDL cholesterol (right). Note that while the bounds of the IQR for measured HDL cholesterol give us an idea of the overall distribution's shape, the bin frequencies in the tail are not easily inferred.

It is commonly believed that one should test whether the data are normally distributed and then choose an appropriate summary measure based on the results of that test (e.g., mean if normally distributed, median if not normally distributed). This is well-meaning but misguided advice. First, tests of normality are extremely sensitive and tend to regard nearly any slight departure from normality as significant, even when the data are slightly asymmetric or heavy-tailed and the mean still

Table 1 Select continuous variables in 500 participant cohort

	Participants ($N = 500$)
Age, mean (SD)	55.38 (13.19)
HDL cholesterol, IQR (L,U)	50.00 (42.25, 59.00)

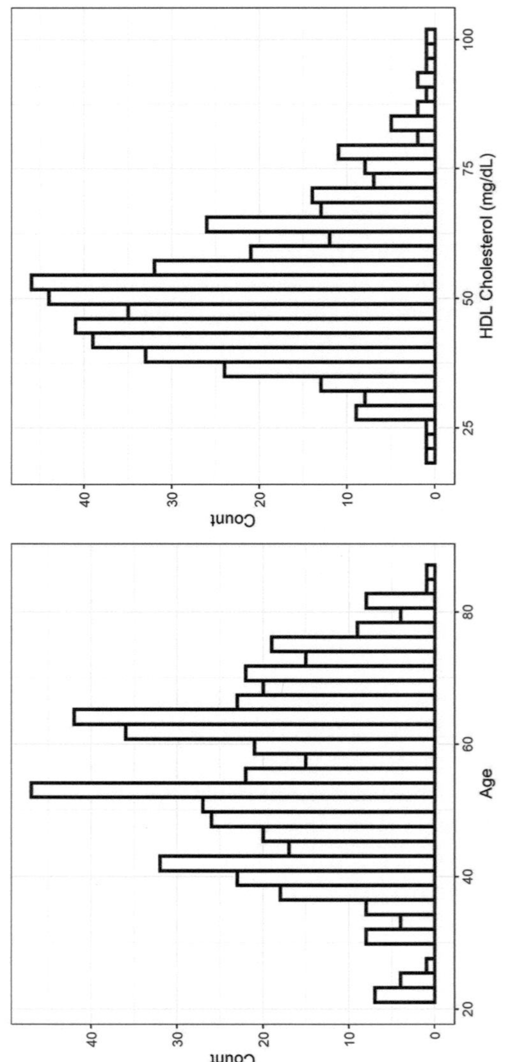

Fig. 1 Scatter plots of age (left) and high-density lipoprotein (HDL) cholesterol (right)

serves as a suitable measure of central tendency. Second, it is not always as simple as testing whether the data are normally distributed to decide which is a better measure of central tendency. Consider a dataset of 100 points with 51 zeroes and 49 values ranging from 1 up to 100. The median value of this data would be zero, but that would not be a very good representation of the central tendency. The median would also be zero in a dataset of 99 zeroes and one positive value, but the implications of those two scenarios are very different for analysis. This example illustrates why it is often necessary to plot the data and/or look at several quantiles in addition to simply looking at one measure of central tendency and one measure of spread to fully appreciate how a variable is distributed.

For a categorical variable, the description is quite simple—just report the frequency and percentage of the total patients within each category of the variable. Table 2 reports the breakdown of reported gender from a cohort of 500 participants. Among the participants, 201 (~40%) are men and 299 (~60%) are women. When looking at the proportion of participants by coronary heart disease (CHD) status, one can categorize the participants by their gender. Among men, 179 (92.23%) did not have CHD while 15 (7.73%) did. The percentages of the columns should typically add up to 100%.

For a time-to-event variable, there are two general approaches. The first is to present a survival curve (often generated using the Kaplan–Meier method) and report the proportion of patients that have experienced the event at specific time points (or, conversely, one may prefer to report the proportion that has *not* yet experienced the event—e.g., the % alive if the outcome is mortality); for example, report the number and proportion of patients that experienced the event by 30 days, 1 year, 2 years, etc. The second would be to report the estimated time at which some proportion of patients has experienced the event, e.g., the "median" survival is commonly reported in oncology studies. The latter is occasionally problematic in cardiology, where it is relatively uncommon for more than half of the study participants to experience the clinical event, in which case the "median survival" is not reached during the study time frame. In all cases, it is important to realize that differently shaped survival curves can have the same summary measure, and, as with continuous variables, there is value in using a visual representation rather than reliance on a single-number summary of the survival in a particular group.

Figure 2 displays two Kaplan–Meier Curves from a retrospective cohort investigating time to myocardial infarction. On the left, the overall survival probability over time is graphed as the outcome of interest is the occurrence of an event. On the right, event-free survival is the outcome of interest; in other words, the probability of the event not occurring. This can be modeled by taking the inverse of the Kaplan–Meier function.

Table 2 Categorical variable[a] in 500 participant cohort

	Men	Women
No CHD	179 (92.23%)	280 (92.4%)
CHD	15 (7.7%)	13 (7.6%)

[a] Reported as frequency (%)

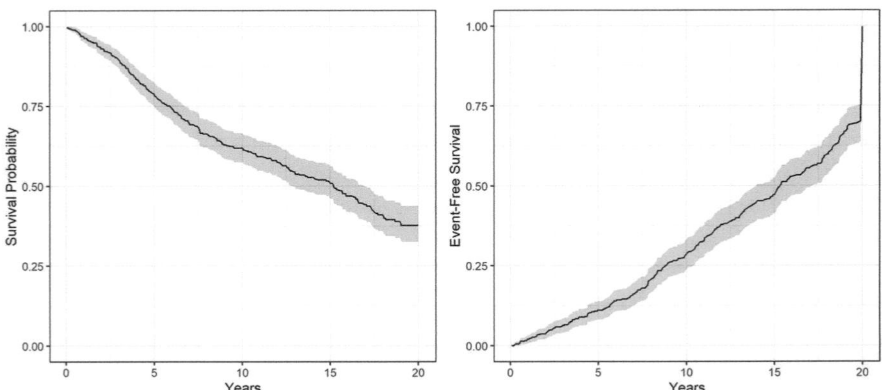

Fig. 2 Kaplan–Meier curves for myocardial infarction, survival probability (left) and event-free survival (right)

2.2 Relationships Between Two Variables

The next task after understanding how we might summarize the distribution of a single variable is to appreciate how we study relationships *between* variables. For example, suppose that we have an existing standard of measurement for fractional flow reserve (FFR) that requires an invasive assessment, and a new approach that can be performed non-invasively. If the invasive FFR measurement is considered the gold standard, we might study whether the new noninvasive measurement correlates with the gold-standard invasive measurement well enough to be considered suitable for use (either as a replacement or perhaps simply in selected cases where it is difficult to perform an invasive assessment). Such an investigation should begin with plotting the data. This may be accomplished using a *scatterplot*, which allows the reader to see all data points. The Pearson correlation coefficient is often used to provide a measure of the strength of association between two continuous variables. Note, however, that this measures only the strength of the correlation between two variables, not their agreement; two variables may be very strongly "correlated" with one another but not necessarily in "agreement" with one another. The Spearman rank correlation is sometimes used as an alternative to the Pearson correlation. This is a correlation coefficient computed based on the ranks of the data rather than the data points themselves. It has the advantage of robustness to outliers (e.g., it does not matter if the highest data point is 100 or 1000, just that it is the highest) and provides a good measure of "Do higher values of (X) tend to correspond with higher values on (Y)?" However, it still does not address the important question, which is whether the noninvasive measure tends to *agree* with the invasive FFR measure. For this, we need a *Bland–Altman plot*, which plots the difference between the two measures on the Y axis against one of the measures (or their average) on the X axis. In Fig. 3, we have plotted the difference between the two measures against the gold standard invasive FFR measurement. The blue line reflects the mean of means

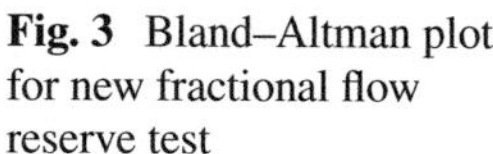

Fig. 3 Bland–Altman plot for new fractional flow reserve test

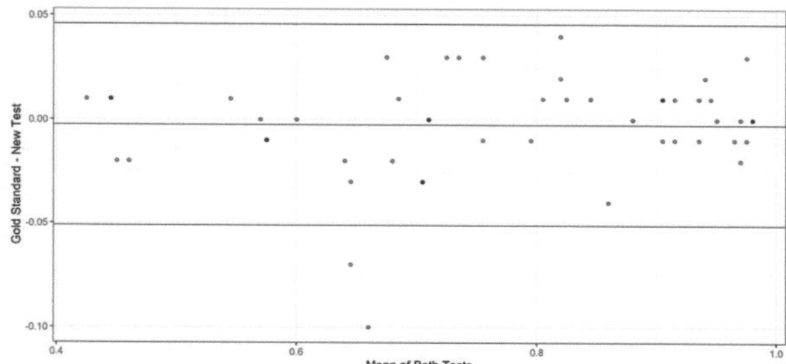

between the two tests, while the red lines indicate confidence intervals (CIs) around this mean. It should be observed that many points on the plot are outside the CIs. Using this plot, we can see that while the variables appear to be reasonably *correlated* with one another, the noninvasive measurement may not be considered exchangeable with the invasive measurement; many patients have an FFR value that is quite different when measured with the noninvasive approach versus the invasive approach. While there are differences between the gold standard and the new test, we can see that the scatter around the mean is relatively random, indicating that a measurement bias is not apparent. Although the CIs can provide statistical significance and a bias can be ruled out, it will ultimately be up to the clinician to decide the level of *clinical significance*. In this case, the clinician will need to decide whether a range of ~0.1 is a reasonable error to implement the new test.

As a second example, consider the relationship between age and systolic blood pressure (SBP). Now we are no longer concerned with "agreement" between the two variables; we just want to know if there is a relationship between the two variables, specifically whether SBP tends to be higher for older patients. Now, we are free of the concern about the "agreement" above that requires a Bland–Altman plot; a simple scatterplot will do (Fig. 4). We also might augment the scatterplot with a Pearson correlation and perhaps a simple linear regression model. Note that, in this case, the "fit" between the data points need not be perfect for the model to tell us something useful—even if there is not a perfect linear association between age and SBP, it is still possible that there is value in knowing that *in general* the mean SBP of older patients will be higher than the mean SBP of younger patients, as opposed to the prior example where the correlation and agreement would have to be very high to be meaningful for clinical practice.

Please note that rather than starting with "when we have two continuous variables…" to introduce these examples, we began with the *question* that each analysis was trying to address. Always keep in mind that the statistical analysis should be determined by the research objective, not the type of data. Note: if you are unfamiliar with hypothesis testing, it will be discussed in the context of clinical trials later in the chapter.

Please also note the omission of *p*-values and "statistical significance" above; it is necessary first to think of research objectives before asking about hypothesis tests and, in some cases, a hypothesis test may not be needed at all. The examples above provide a nice illustration of why this topic requires much nuance. It is easily

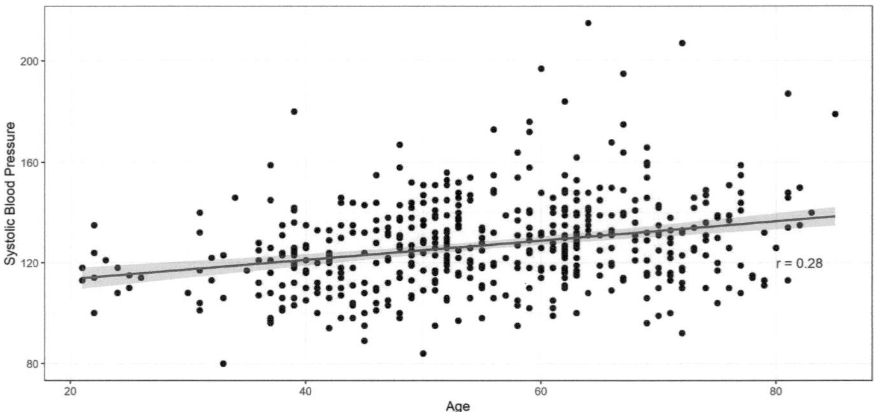

Fig. 4 Scatterplot between age and systolic blood pressure

possible in the first case to have a "significant" *p*-value for a null hypothesis test of the correlation coefficient between the FFR values measured with the noninvasive approach versus the invasive approach; however, that is not necessarily strong evidence that the correlation between the two variables is a *strong* correlation. One can have a correlation coefficient of $r = 0.3$ with $p < 0.001$ quite easily; while a sample dataset with a correlation coefficient of $r = 0.3$ certainly supports the idea that there is a non-zero correlation between the two variables, that is not the same as proving that the two variables are so strongly correlated with one another that one can predict the value of the other based solely on knowledge of the first variable. In the second case, the reverse is somewhat true; a statistically significant association indicating support for a non-zero correlation between age and SBP could be useful information even if the correlation between the two variables is relatively weak; we would not necessarily expect to perfectly *predict* a person's SBP with knowledge of their age alone, but it may be valuable simply to know that older patients tend to have higher SBPs (Fig. 4). We may also be interested in assessing the relationship between one variable and another while taking into account the effect of other observed (confounding) variables; this is discussed later in the chapter.

2.3 Comparing Two (or More) Groups

Suppose that we have an experimental medication that is intended to reduce blood pressure in patients with hypertension. We perform a randomized controlled trial where a sample of patients with hypertension is recruited and randomly assigned to receive the experimental medication or a placebo. In our hypothetical randomized, controlled trial, each patient is treated for 6 weeks, and at the conclusion of the trial, we compare the final blood pressure measurements in patients who received the experimental medication against those who received the placebo. How can we use the blood pressure data from this trial to draw a conclusion about whether the medication effectively reduces blood pressure?

If the reader has any familiarity with the field of statistics (and it is no shame if they do not), they may be aware of two broad statistical philosophies that are the subject of much debate: *frequentist* and *Bayesian* statistics. Much ink has been and will continue to be spilled on this topic; this chapter is not the place for a complete explanation of these two philosophies and the debates between the two. While Bayesian statistics are increasingly popular, frequentist statistical approaches still dominate in the biomedical sciences; therefore, the chapter will typically describe the frequentist statistical approaches first. A brief explanation of Bayesian philosophy and approaches is included later in the chapter, and some passing comments about Bayesian approaches will be interspersed throughout where practical.

Returning to our example, how can we use the data from our randomized trial to draw a conclusion about whether the experimental medication is more effective at reducing blood pressure than standard treatment? The outcome, blood pressure measured after 6 weeks of treatment, is a continuous variable. We have two groups, those treated with the experimental medication and those that received a placebo. When one wishes to compare the distribution of a continuous outcome variable between two groups, the simplest statistical approach is to use a *two-sample t-test* to compare the distribution of blood pressure measurements in patients who received the experimental medication against the distribution of blood pressure measurements in patients that received the placebo.

Here, we must briefly explain how frequentist statistical testing works. One first defines a *null hypothesis*. In our case, the null hypothesis is that the experimental medication is no more effective than standard care; statistically, this is presented as the mean blood pressure for patients treated with experimental medication being equal to the mean blood pressure for patients treated with standard care. We collect some data and use these data to compute a *test statistic*, which is essentially a measure of the compatibility between the data and null hypothesis. The test statistic may then be compared against a known distribution to obtain the infamous *p-value*. The *p*-value is very hard to define both concisely and with complete technical accuracy; for practical purposes, it may be best to think of it as "the probability we would see the observed data if the null hypothesis were true." Even this definition includes some known technical inaccuracies (the most obvious being that a *p*-value is actually the probability of obtaining data *at least as incompatible with the null hypothesis* as the observed data, not the precise probability of seeing exactly the observed data), but it is the best combination available of brevity and accuracy. A *p*-value of 0.03 in a randomized controlled trial with a null hypothesis of "patients treated with experimental medication have the same blood pressure as patients treated with placebo" means that there was a 3% probability of obtaining the study data if the experimental medication had no true effect on blood pressure (e.g., the true distribution of blood pressures for patients receiving the experimental medication is identical to the true distribution of blood pressures for patients receiving the placebo).

When this probability is very small, one might decide to *reject* the null hypothesis, concluding that the study provides evidence that the experimental treatment is effective; the small *p*-value tells us that the data would be very surprising if the null hypothesis were true. It should be briefly mentioned that the *type I error* (a notion that we will explain in detail later) occurs when a null hypothesis is rejected that should not have been rejected. This is a concept opposed to a *type II error* or a "false negative" result, where the trial concludes that the treatment does not work even though it is effective.

CIs are another approach to investigating statistical significance and provide additional information about precision. After we observe a point estimate or effect size (such as a test statistic, beta coefficient, or odds ratio), the 95% CI provides a range of observations that may include where the point estimate exists at the $\alpha = 0.05$ level. To reflect this range, an upper and lower bound of the interval is reported. Returning to our experimental blood pressure medication hypothetical, let us say that the difference in means between treatment and placebo groups was 10 mm Hg (remember that the *p*-value was 0.03). The mean difference is important, but we really do not have any information about the range of values that the difference could have been. A hypothetical mean and CI could be 10 mm Hg (95% CI 4–14). The lower bound of the confidence range is 4 mm Hg while the upper bound is 14 mm Hg. In this situation, 10 mm Hg is an appropriate guess, but there is a 5% chance that the true difference lies outside the 4–14 mm Hg range. While the 95% CI is typically chosen, we can choose parameters and report a smaller or larger band of confidence (such as a 90% or 99% CI). Keep in mind though that the greater the confidence, the wider the range.

Returning to hypothesis testing, as the hypothetical CI (95% CI 4–14) does not include 0, the null value, we can reject the null hypothesis and report that there is a significant difference between mean values in the treatment and placebo groups at the 5% level of statistical significance (i.e., alpha of 0.05). If the CI includes the null value, such as 95% CI −2, 14, then we fail to reject the null hypothesis. In this situation, a corresponding *p*-value would be greater than 0.05.

If you find all that a bit confusing, you are hardly alone. Why calculate the probability of seeing data like these given a "straw man" null hypothesis (that the drug is ineffective)? That seems a rather backward way of answering our question. Why not compute the probability that the drug is effective at reducing blood pressure based on the observed data? These philosophical questions are the central tension in the debate over whether the historically traditional frequentist statistical approach (the former) should continue, or if we should move toward the Bayesian approach (the latter). The precise reasons why the former approach has been preferred to the latter are complex and beyond the scope of this book, though a few comments will be provided later in the chapter. For now, the important thing to know is that most of what one sees in the medical literature uses the frequentist approach, and we have made an effort to explain what that does above.

Therefore, when we have two groups to compare on a measure that is represented as a continuous variable, we might use a two-sample *t*-test. Perhaps we are interested in the difference in mean age across genders in a cohort of 500 participants.

We see that the mean age in men is 54.58 years and the mean age in women is 55.90 years. The null hypothesis of the t-test is that there is not a significant difference in mean age across genders. Results of the t-test provide a t-value of -1.1 and a p-value of 0.26. Thus, we fail to reject the null hypothesis and assume that there is no difference in age across genders.

What about scenarios where there are more than two groups? This could be another randomized clinical trial, as described above, but now with multiple treatment groups; or it could be something else entirely. Perhaps we wish to assess whether the NYHA heart failure class (an ordinal variable) is a good way of classifying heart failure patients' physiologic reserve according to an objective measure of physical function. We have a set of patients that includes some with NYHA class I, some with class II, some with class III, and some with class IV heart failure; each of the patients performs a 6-min walk test to record their maximal 6-min walking distance. How can we use these data to test whether the patients from different NYHA classes do, in fact, have differences in their objectively measured physical function? The *analysis of variance* (ANOVA) is the extension of a t-test that accommodates more than two groups. This tests an overall null hypothesis that patients from the different NYHA classes have the same distribution of 6-min walking distance. A small p-value from this test tells us that the data would have been unlikely to occur if there were no difference in walking distance between the NYHA classes, but it does not tell us which groups are significantly different from one another. It only shows that we have evidence against the overall null hypothesis that all group means are equal.

Now we must point out that the t-test and ANOVA are simply specific cases of an ordinary least-squares regression model. This is often a shocking realization to people who were not taught this, but it is true. Constructing a simple linear regression model with a continuous dependent variable and one binary independent variable will give the same test statistic and p-value for that independent variable as a two-sample t-test comparing the means between the two groups. Similarly, a multivariable regression model with indicator variables for each group will give the same global test statistic and p-value as ANOVA. Linear regression models may be used to represent many of the common workhorse statistical tests as they are mathematically equivalent.

Why is this useful? Well, suppose that we want to test whether there is a difference in a continuous variable between two or more groups, but we want to be able to "adjust" the analysis for some potentially confounding variables. Multivariable regression models allow us to estimate the effect of one particular variable (perhaps a "treatment" indicator in the context of a comparison between two treatment groups, or several indicators for the NYHA class) when controlling for the effects of other variables. This will be discussed a bit more later in the chapter.

The aforementioned t-test, ANOVA, and linear regression models are all *parametric* statistical procedures, meaning that they rely on assumptions about the shape of the distribution of a variable, which may be described with *parameters* (for example, the shape of a normal distribution may be described fully with knowledge of two parameters: the mean and standard deviation). What exactly it means to "rely" on these assumptions is a bit tricky, but essentially it means that these procedures will maintain their best operating characteristics such as type I error (false positive) and type II error (false negative) rates when the data are drawn from something close to the assumed underlying distribution.

Sometimes we are concerned that the variables of interest will deviate far from the distributional assumptions of the classic statistical procedures. For example, we may know that one of our proposed outcome variables tends to follow a skewed distribution that is not assumed by our commonly used tests; perhaps, a particular biomarker tends to cluster near zero for patients with no disease but may take on very large values for patients that have severe disease (e.g., troponin in the setting of acute myocardial infarction). In such cases, one might prefer the use of *non-parametric* tests. The term non-parametric is rather difficult to define; briefly, one might say that non-parametric statistical procedures do not rely on assumptions about the shape or form of the probability distribution from which the data were drawn—but that seems a bit of a mouthful. As for how non-parametric statistical tests work, it is quite simple. Rather than comparing the distribution of the actual values between groups, typically they are based on "ranks" of the data. The Wilcoxon (for two groups) and Kruskal–Wallis (for more than two groups) procedures are the ones most analogous to the *t*-test and ANOVA, respectively. The null hypotheses tested by these procedures are slightly different than the null hypotheses tested by the *t*-test and ANOVA, but the overall objective(s) are essentially the same. They test whether the data suggest that the groups being compared have distributions that seem to be drawn from the same overarching distribution, or if they provide evidence that the groups are drawn from different distributions of the variable of interest. As an example, we will compare the HDL cholesterol levels across our theoretical 500-person cohort. The median HDL cholesterol value in men is 45 mg/dL, and the median HDL cholesterol value in women is 53 mg/dL. The computed test statistic will be much larger than the critical value, and the *p*-value is much less than 0.001. Therefore, we would reject the null hypothesis of equivalent medians.

Although nonparametric tests have the attractive feature of making fewer assumptions about the distribution of measurements in the population than parametric tests, they have two main drawbacks. The first is that they are generally less statistically powerful than the corresponding parametric test when the underlying data are approximately normal, meaning that they have a slightly lower probability of correctly rejecting the null hypothesis (i.e., concluding that there is a difference between treatment groups when one truly exists) than their parametric counterparts. If you are planning a study and trying to determine how many patients are needed, a nonparametric test will require a slightly larger sample size to have the same statistical power as the analogous parametric test. The second drawback is interpretability; the results of non-parametric tests tend to be more difficult to interpret than parametric tests. As mentioned earlier, most nonparametric tests use rankings of the values in the data rather than using the actual data. Knowing that there tends to be a difference in ranks between two groups does not really help our intuitive understanding of the data; we only learn that one group tended to be higher than the other group but are not necessarily provided an estimate of how large the difference between groups is. On the other hand, knowing that the median SBP of patients taking the experimental drug was 10 mm Hg lower than the median SBP of patients on the standard treatment is useful in quantifying the effect of the new treatment.

Two final notes on nonparametric tests and procedures. First, it is a common misuse of terminology in the biomedical literature to see statements like "parametric variables were compared using t-tests, and nonparametric variables were compared using Wilcoxon tests." Please note that variables are not "parametric" or "nonparametric" by some definitions. One may choose to use a statistical procedure that relies on parametric assumptions or a statistical procedure that does not rely on parametric assumptions, but it is not a feature of the data or the variable itself.

Second, it is a common misunderstanding that one should first test the distribution of some variables and then choose between a parametric test or a non-parametric test, using a parametric test if the data are normally distributed and a nonparametric test otherwise (note the parallel to the misunderstanding described in the prior section about testing for normality and then choosing which summary statistic to report). While it is technically true that parametric tests "rely" on parametric assumptions—meaning that their operating characteristics are best when the data are drawn from the assumed distribution—it is a myth that they cannot be used if the data show any deviation from the assumed distribution. Furthermore, one introduces a slight distortion of the operating characteristics of a statistical procedure if they are contingent on testing the distribution of the data before choosing which test to use (particularly given that the tests for normality are so sensitive that virtually any slight asymmetry or heavy-tailed distribution will test as being non-normally distributed). Please do not mistake these disclaimers for a lack of enthusiasm regarding nonparametric tests on the part of the authors. It is just worth understanding that the advertised benefit of "fewer distributional assumptions" for nonparametric tests comes at a cost, and it is advisable to consider the pros and cons of a nonparametric test versus a parametric test before looking at the data instead of choosing based on the data that you have already collected and examined. In the latter case, it opens the door for the author to make decisions that are convenient for them based on knowledge of the observed data (e.g., they perhaps are more likely to choose the test that gives a more impressive result and retroactively justify this by saying they needed to see the data to decide which test was more appropriate). Such practices compromise the intended frequentist statistical properties of controlling type I error.

2.4 Comparing Two (or More) Groups with Categorical Variables

The previous section discussed a few options for comparing the distribution of a continuous outcome variable between two or more groups. As discussed in the opening, though, not all variables that we might analyze are continuous variables; some are more properly characterized as categorical variables (which includes special cases such as binary and ordinal variables). How can we test whether the distribution of a categorical variable differs between two or more groups?

Suppose that we have a two-group randomized clinical trial where participants have now been assigned to either an experimental medication or placebo but rather than a continuous measure (e.g., blood pressure) as the primary outcome of interest we have a binary variable, perhaps "post-operative stroke within 48 h of the procedure." Patients who had a stroke within 48 h are coded as a "yes" while patients who did not have a stroke within 48 h are coded as a "no" for this variable. How can we test whether the observed data provide evidence of whether the experimental treatment reduces the risk of postoperative stroke? The most common test in this situation is a *chi-squared test for independence.* Note that I said *a* chi-squared test and not *the* chi-squared test. Many statistical tests rely on the chi-squared distribution, and it is a bit of a misnomer to refer to any test, even the most commonly used, as *the* chi-squared test. The chi-squared test for independence essentially compares the "observed" counts in each cell of a contingency table against the "expected" counts if the two variables are truly independent.

It is also commonly taught that if the expected count in one or more of the cells is very small, it would be preferable to use *Fisher's exact test* rather than the chi-squared test for independence. This is a matter of some debate in the statistical community. It is true that the chi-squared approximation is less accurate in the setting of very small, expected cell counts, potentially inflating type I (false positive) error rates; however, it should be noted that Fisher's exact test, though it gives "exact" *p*-values, will actually be slightly conservative in practice (resulting in slightly decreased power), for technical reasons a bit beyond the scope of this chapter. Therefore, perhaps the decision on which test to use in the setting of small cell counts ought to be based on a careful consideration of whether it would be worse to make a type I error (false positive) or a type II error (false negative) in a particular context.

Tables 3 and 4 report examples of a chi-squared test and a Fisher's exact test, respectively. A cohort of participants at a radiology clinic was used to investigate the proportion of patients who have CHD. An arbitrary cutoff between "older" and "younger" is established, and it was discovered that 15/50 = 30% of "younger"

Table 3 Age by coronary heart disease (CHD) status in 100-participant cohort (Chi-squared test)

	CHD	No CHD	Sum	*p*-value
Younger	15	35	50	<0.01
Older	22	28	50	
Sum	37	63		

Table 4 Age by coronary heart disease (CHD) status in 100-participant cohort (Fisher's exact test)

	CHD	No CHD	Sum	*p*-value
Younger	4	46	50	<0.01
Older	15	35	50	
Sum	19	81		

participants have CHD, while 22/50 = 44% of "older" participants have CHD. As all cell counts are above 5, a chi-squared test will tell us if there is a significant difference in proportions between the two groups. The resulting p-value from the chi-squared test indicates that there is a significant difference in proportions of CHD between the groups. Table 5 reports a similar census at a different clinic and demonstrates that 4/50 = 8% of "younger" participants have CHD while 15/35 = 30% of "older" participants have CHD. As the cell count for "younger" participants with CHD is below 5, Fisher's exact test is appropriate. The small (<0.01) p-value indicates that there is a statistically significant difference in the proportion of CHD between the age groups.

As was the case in the prior section, we should acknowledge that these tests are only suitable for comparing groups when there is no need to account for other variables in the analyses. If we want to test for a difference between groups in a binary outcome variable, several different multivariable regression options are available thanks to the family of *generalized linear models* (GLMs). This term is often misunderstood by lay readers who seem to believe that "linear regression" only refers to a regression model like that described in the previous section, where one models the relationship between two continuous variables by estimating the value of one variable as a linear function of another variable. However, GLMs provide the ability to estimate a response variable as a function of a linear combination of covariate values via a link function. *Logistic regression* is common in the medical literature. From a logistic regression model, one may estimate the *odds ratio* for experiencing the outcome of interest in one group relative to the other group. Note that the odds ratio can be computed directly for a simple 2 × 2 table with no need to use logistic regression; a simple logistic regression model with one variable only will give the same odds ratio as computed from a 2 × 2 table. An odds ratio of 1 means that the two groups have exactly the same odds of experiencing the outcome. Odds ratios are calculated by dividing the odds of the cases by the odds of the noncases. The odds of the cases are found by calculating the odds of being a case among those exposed (A/B) to the odds of being a case among those not exposed (C/D) (See Table 5). Table 6 consists of 491 participants, 263 of which have experienced a myocardial

Table 5 Setup of basic 2 × 2 table

	Outcome status	
	Positive (+)	Negative (−)
Exposure status: Positive (+)	A	B
Negative (−)	C	D

Table 6 2 × 2 for Myocardial infarction status (outcome) by smoking status (exposure)

	Myocardial infarction status		
	Positive (+)	Negative (−)	Sum
Smoking status: Positive (+)	206	120	326
Negative (−)	57	108	165
Sum	263	228	

Table 7 Ordered logistic regression results

Variable	OR	95% CI
Age	1.01	(0.99, 1.03)
Men	1.75	(1.21, 2.54)

infarction, and 228 that have not experienced a myocardial infarction. Additionally, 326 participants are smokers, while 165 are not smokers. To calculate the odds ratio, we find the odds of case status (A/B) (206/120 = 1.71) among the smokers (exposed) and the odds of case status among those who are not smokers (not exposed) (C/D) (120/108 = 0.52). Therefore, the odds ratio of cases to noncases is 1.71/0.52 = 3.25. An odds ratio greater than 1 means that the exposed group has higher odds of experiencing the outcome than the reference group; an odds ratio less than 1 means that the exposed group has lower odds of experiencing the outcome than the reference group. In the case of our example, the odds of experiencing myocardial infarction for positive smoking status are 3.25 times higher than the odds of myocardial infarction for negative smoking status.

For ordinal variables, it is commonly taught that one may use the nonparametric tests named in the first section (Wilcoxon tests and Kruskal–Wallis tests) to compare the distribution of an ordinal variable between two or more groups. Because these tests are based on ranks, they may be used for comparisons of ordinal variables as well as continuous variables. However, these do not offer the ability to account for other variables in the analysis. If a multivariable option is required to test for a difference between groups while adjusting for one or more covariates of interest, an ordered logistic regression (sometimes referred to as a *cumulative logit model* or a *proportional odds model*) may be used. This model uses cumulative probabilities up to a threshold, thereby making the whole range of ordinal categories binary at that threshold. As an example, you are investigating trends of smoking status among your patient demographics. All participants have reported to be never, previous, or current smokers. An ordered logistic regression model can be fit to investigate the relationship of age, gender, and smoking status. Table 7 illustrates the reported results of such a model. In this scenario, a significant relationship is not apparent for age, but there is a relationship for gender. From this model, the men have 1.75 times the odds of the women to be classified at the higher smoking status, after controlling for the effects of age.

2.5 Comparing Two (or More) Groups with Time-to-Event Variables

Time-to-event data require the use of specialized statistical methods often referred to as *survival analysis*. As shown briefly in a prior section, the proportion of patients surviving (or free from whatever the "event" is—survival analysis need not only refer to mortality as the endpoint, but it could also be freedom-from-hospitalization, freedom-from-disease-progression, etc.) may be presented using a Kaplan–Meier curve. How does one perform a statistical test comparing the distribution of survival times in two (or more) groups when accounting for unequal follow-up time and censoring? Of course, one could compute survival curves for each group and compare the proportions surviving at any specific point in time. However, this approach does not provide a comparison of the total survival experience of the groups but only a comparison at some arbitrary time point. The *log-rank test* is the most popular method of comparing the survival of groups that takes the entire observed follow-up into account.

The log-rank test uses the null hypothesis that there is no difference between groups in the probability of an "event" at any time point. The test statistic for the log-rank test is proportional to the difference between the observed number of events versus the expected number of events under the null hypothesis. This test statistic may be compared against a chi-squared distribution, and from this, one may compute a p-value that translates approximately to the probability we would have observed these data under the null hypothesis that the group(s) have the same underlying survival distribution. If the p-value is small, we may choose to reject the null hypothesis because it would be very surprising to see the study data if the groups had the same true underlying survival distribution; we may then conclude that the study provides evidence of a true difference in the underlying survival distribution between the groups.

The log-rank test uses the same assumptions as the Kaplan–Meier curve: that censoring is unrelated to the future outcomes (e.g., patients that drop out of the curve do so "randomly" or for administrative reasons, like the trial ending, not because they are more or less likely to experience the study outcome in the future), and that survival probabilities do not change appreciably for patients that join the study later compared to those that join the study sooner. Deviations from these assumptions matter more if they are different in the groups being compared, for example, if one group has many more patients censored than the other group.

The log-rank test is most likely to detect a difference between groups when the risk of an event is greater across the entire range of the survival curve for one group than another; it is less likely to detect a difference when survival curves cross, which is one reason why visual examination of survival data always adds something over any single-number summary or statistical test. Figure 5 demonstrates the log-rank test for a study investigating myocardial infarction hazard by gender. Results indicate a significant difference between the two groups ($p = 0.035$), and that the curves begin to diverge around year 14 of the study.

Because the log-rank test is a test of significance only, it does not provide an estimate of the effect size (difference between groups) or a CI, nor does it provide the ability to adjust the analysis for covariates. To do this, we need to use a regression model that requires some additional assumptions. The *Cox proportional-hazards model* is the most commonly used method to analyze time-to-event data in the medical literature. Survival models have two parts: an underlying baseline hazard function and the effect parameters, which summarize how the baseline hazard changes as a function of the covariates. If one is willing to assume proportional hazards, the effect parameters may be estimated even without specifying the

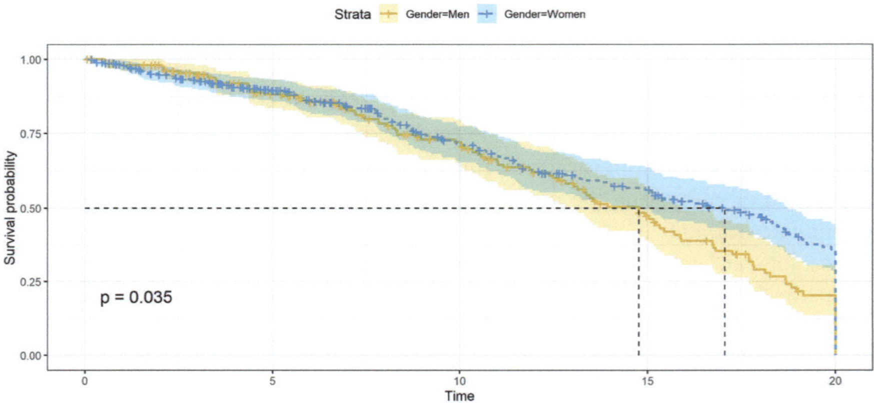

Fig. 5 Log-rank for myocardial infarction by gender

baseline hazard function; these effect parameters may be converted into the commonly seen *hazard ratio*. Although giving a precise technical definition of the hazard ratio is difficult and beyond the scope of this chapter, for the reader, the important takeaway is this: a hazard ratio of 1 means that there is no difference in the survival times between the two groups; a hazard ratio less than 1 means that the experimental group has a lower hazard (lower incidence of events) than the comparison group; a hazard ratio greater than 1 means that the experimental group has an increased hazard (higher incidence of events) versus the comparison group.

Kaplan–Meier curves can also be used to visualize the survival functions between two groups, such as in the context of clinical trial results. Visually, the researcher can decipher the relative success of one group to another. As an example, let us say we are performing a randomized controlled trial investigating whether a new treatment option will prevent reclotting events in a higher-risk, hospital-based cohort. Figure 6 demonstrates the comparative Kaplan–Meier curves among participants. Given these results, there is a clear separation in cumulative incidence between both standard treatment (blue) and new treatment (red). Thus, these results provide evidence supporting the efficacy of the new treatment option in reducing the cumulative incidence of clotting events when compared to the standard treatment option.

The Cox proportional-hazards model is ubiquitous and easily implemented in many common statistical software packages, which, no doubt, contributes to its widespread use in practice. However, critics point out that the Cox model relies on several tenuous assumptions that are difficult to verify, and in some cases obviously violated (e.g., if two survival curves cross during the course of follow-up, then the proportional-hazards assumption is violated), making the hazard ratio particularly difficult to interpret as a single-number summary measure of treatment effect. One alternative approach is the *restricted mean survival time* (RMST), which is equivalent to the area under the Kaplan–Meier curve from the beginning of the study through a specific time point. One may compute the RMST for two groups and then estimate the difference by subtracting the two to estimate the gain in survival time

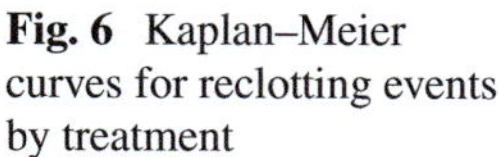

Fig. 6 Kaplan–Meier curves for reclotting events by treatment

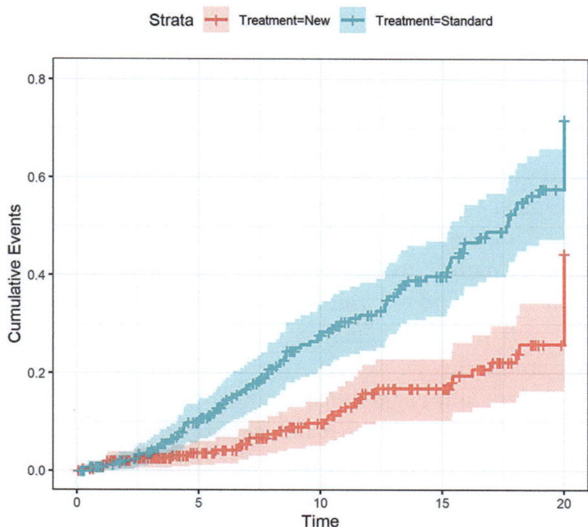

due to treatment versus the comparison group during that period (e.g., an RMST difference of 90 days over a 5-year study period means that the expected gain in survival for patients receiving treatment versus control is 90 days over the next 5 years).

It is also worth a brief mention that sometimes we may have a time-to-event variable that could occur more than once, such as heart failure hospitalization. There are statistical approaches that allow the modeling of multiple occurrences of time-to-event outcomes, including the Andersen-Gill model and joint frailty models (which allow modeling two separate but correlated processes, such as hospitalization for heart failure but with a terminal competing event of death). We will not cover these in great detail here, but the reader should at least be aware of their existence should they encounter this situation; the authors of this chapter have occasionally encountered comments from poorly informed reviewers who believed it was impossible to model recurrent events and suggested redoing the entire analysis with just the first event for each patient included for analysis. It is true that the standard application of Kaplan–Meier curves and Cox proportional-hazards models assume independence (e.g., only one period-at-risk/event per patient) but the reader should be aware that methods that allow multiple events do exist. It is worth noting that using only the index event markedly understates the burden of the disease and may understate the value of a therapy.

3 Multivariable Analysis: Know Your Objective

We have already alluded to a few different types of multivariable regression procedures in this chapter. These include "ordinary least squares" regression for continuous outcome variables, logistic regression for binary outcome variables, Cox proportional-hazards regression for time-to-event variables, and other types of regression models that we have not covered in detail.

Multivariable regression offers the ability to ask all sorts of interesting statistical questions, but it is also often misused and/or misunderstood. There seems to be a common belief that there is one and only one correct way to build a multivariable regression model: take all the variables you have, identify those with significant p-values, and feed them into a variable selection algorithm to end up with one final "true" model. This approach is likely taught and adopted because it feels like a simple "recipe" to follow and carries with it an attractive feeling that you "let the data speak" and tell you what the correct model is. Unfortunately, this approach is not well-suited to nearly any of the objectives we are trying to fulfill in medical research.

Before you begin constructing a multivariable regression model (or before you begin evaluating whether the authors of a paper that you are reading have done so correctly), you must first ask: what is the research objective that the model is trying to fulfill? Most projects that use multivariable regression seem to fit into one of the following four categories.

The first category is a study wherein the researcher wishes to estimate the causal effect of a treatment on an outcome of interest. When the goal is estimating a specific causal effect, decisions about which variables belong in the model should be made based on how the selection of additional variables affects the estimate of that treatment effect, not based on the statistical significance of individual covariates in the observed data. A deep dive into causal inference is beyond the scope of this chapter, but a few more comments will follow in the section on observational studies vs. randomized trials and the section on target trials.

The second category is a study wherein the researcher wishes to estimate the independent (possibly, but not always, causal) effect of a specific variable on an outcome of interest. For example, one may wish to study whether patients who smoke have significantly different outcomes than patients who do not smoke. Again, if this is the objective, the selection of additional variables should be based on how their inclusion affects the estimate of that primary effect of interest, not their own statistical significance in the observed data.

The third category is prediction modeling. The researcher wishes to construct a model that converts into a "risk score," which may be used to accurately estimate individual patient risk for a particular outcome and/or classify patients into groups (e.g., "low risk" versus "high risk"). When the objective is risk prediction, decisions about which variables belong in the model should be made not based on the statistical significance of individual variables but based on how the inclusion of a variable affects the accuracy of the predictions (at least, purely from the statistical perspective). There is also a slightly separate discussion about ensuring that the end product is usable in the desired setting and consideration of trade-offs in speed versus accuracy. For example, if a model that contains just a few variables offers similar accuracy to a competing model that requires far more variables, the consequences for implementation may be discussed to inform why a particular statistical decision was made. The construction of a prediction model for whether a cardiac arrest patient will be discharged from the hospital alive has a very different context than a prediction model for an "elective" operation that may be planned over the course of several weeks or months. A model that is meant for use in a time-sensitive setting obviously benefits from requiring fewer inputs and perhaps even from simplified scoring systems that allow quick at-the-bedside or on-the-fly assessment to inform clinical decisions. However, in settings that are not time-sensitive, it is arguably detrimental to patient care to use an overly simplified score if the predictive accuracy of the model could be improved by adding more inputs or a more complex calculation.

There are three important concepts to understand in evaluating the performance of a clinical prediction model: discrimination, calibration, and validation. *Discrimination* assesses how well the model differentiates between patients who experience the outcome and those who do not, commonly assessed using the c-statistic. *Calibration* is an assessment of how closely the predictions of the model match the observed outcomes in the data—do patients that have a predicted risk of 5% actually have the outcome 5% of the time? *Validation* means that the model has been established to work satisfactorily (showing good discrimination and/or calibration) on a different dataset than the one used to construct the model.

The fourth and final category is a rather ill-defined one, which is vaguely described as "identifying significant predictors." These models stop short of claiming that they are actually "predicting" the outcome, as they do not actually evaluate the model's predictions using any of the concepts above (discrimination, calibration, or validation). Rather, in many cases, this seems to consist of simply taking a set of variables, applying a stepwise variable selection algorithm, and claiming that the resulting model identifies which variables are "significant predictors" of the outcome. This is common to see in the medical literature to evaluate the feasibility of novel putative risk factors. It is not really a prediction model; it does not identify causal relationships of importance, nor does it even really give a good picture of the individual contributions of specific risk factors of interest. Some believe that authors should set out clearer objectives for their research than "identify risk factors" for a particular outcome. The identification of risk factors should be based on expert opinion, rooted in causality, and have substantial, favorable peer-reviewed evidence. This analytic approach is becoming more popular with the proliferation of machine learning in medical spaces. While the evidence of such an approach is relatively weaker, it can provide a starting point for future analyses and be strengthened through assessments of external validity.

One final concept that warrants mention in this section is the *Table 2 fallacy*, which refers to the practice of interpreting all of the estimates from a single multivariable regression model as representative of the causal effect for each individual variable. Again, an in-depth discussion of causal inference lies a bit beyond the scope of this chapter, but it is important for the reader to understand that identification of a causal effect for one specific variable requires careful consideration of the causal structures in play between all potential confounders and the outcome, and that often different multivariable models would be necessary to estimate the causal effect of individual variables on a particular outcome.

4   Observational Studies Vs. Randomized Trials

Broadly speaking, most clinical research involving interventions is either *observational* (where patients are treated as part of routine clinical care at the discretion of the treating clinician) or *experimental* (where the choice of intervention or procedure is controlled or determined by the study; these are commonly described as *clinical trials*). Many experimental studies involve some element of *randomization*, meaning that patients are randomly assigned to a treatment condition (e.g., experimental treatment versus standard care); such trials are known as *randomized trials*. While randomized trials are generally considered superior for comparing treatments/policies against one another, observational research fulfills many critical roles: characterizing incidence and prevalence of diseases and/or complications, assessing trends over time in utilization and/or outcomes for certain patients and/or procedures, monitoring newly approved drugs and/or devices for potential complications, developing and testing prediction models, and more. Furthermore, for some research questions, observational studies are the only feasible way to obtain any data because a prospectively designed randomized trial has not been done and may even be outright impossible. In such cases, a high-quality observational study may be preferable to making decisions based on no data at all. However, when it comes to comparing two or more candidate treatments against one another in a defined target population, observational research is susceptible to biases that make it difficult to accurately estimate causal treatment effects. This will be discussed at more length in a few paragraphs.

4.1   Types of Observational Studies

Cohort studies are longitudinal studies that follow a group of patients who share a defining characteristic, such as experiencing an event in a defined timeframe (birth, hospitalization, intensive care unit [ICU] admission, diagnosis with a specific condition). Cohort studies are excellent for understanding the natural history of a disease, estimating incidence and prevalence, and developing prognostic risk scores.

In a *prospective cohort study*, many of the variables that will be collected are decided before the study begins, and data are subsequently collected from all patients that enroll in the cohort after inception. Ideally, the key research question(s) to be examined should be decided before cohort inception. This ensures that investigators structure the data collection process to collect all key elements that might be needed to answer the key research questions on all study participants. Of course, it may be possible to add new data elements later in the course of long-running cohort studies, but this will likely be available only for subsets of the cohort (these essentially become sub-studies branching off from the main cohort study).

Retrospective cohort studies typically make use of data that were already collected for some other purpose (such as data collected as part of usual care and stored in electronic health records). For example, a cardiac surgeon may wonder if there is a difference in clinical outcomes between two widely available bioprosthetic aortic valves for patients that require aortic valve replacement. If there is no prospective study comparing the performance of the two valves directly against one another, the clinical investigator who wants to know if there is a meaningful difference between them may seek out an existing database that includes patients who received both valves and compare outcomes between patients that received each of the two against one another.

While it is attractive to make use of data that already exist, retrospective cohorts are often limited by incomplete data, selective reporting, and behaviors present in good clinical decision making—some of which are a sign of good clinical care but may work against efforts to use these data for research questions. Note carefully that I am not saying this is a bad thing—we want patients to receive the best possible care—but it is important to understand the effects this has when repurposing such data for research. Electronic health record data are particularly susceptible to selection and information biases (e.g., tests that may be used to make a diagnosis or identify patients for a cohort are obtained only in cases with high clinical suspicion). Automated extraction from electronic health records will often have difficulty differentiating between incident and prevalent disease, which can be problematic if one is trying to assess a temporal relationship. For example, "does pulmonary hypertension cause atrial fibrillation?" is difficult to answer if one cannot tell whether a condition was already prevalent on entry, or if it occurred during the course of a hospitalization. Without manual chart review, often all that is known is that a diagnosis code for a particular condition was recorded sometime during that hospitalization. There is an ever-present concern about patterns of missing data: patients may receive subsequent care in other systems or may fail to present for scheduled follow-up, and patients that have repeat assessments may tend to differ from those that do not have repeat assessments outside of a structured research protocol (this is true even within a structured research protocol, but much exacerbated outside a structured research protocol). Consider a possible study where one wishes to use electronic health record data to report trends in serial B-type natriuretic peptide (BNP) measurements taken on heart failure patients. Note that only patients who are doing poorly are likely to visit the hospital frequently; patients who are doing relatively well are less likely to visit the hospital, and therefore less likely to have serial BNP measurements. In this setting, it is unlikely that any estimated trend in BNP over time will be reflective of the "true" trend in BNP in heart failure patients because the patient's clinical course affects whether they are likely to have follow-up data.

Finally, there is the concern of unmeasured confounding—when factors that could influence what was observed, such as why a patient was given a therapy, are not available for inclusion in the analysis. Retrospective cohorts are limited to whatever information was collected for the intended purpose of the cohort, and investigators may not have access to data on important, recognized confounders. Consider the case study mentioned above, using electronic health record data to compare outcomes for patients who received two different bioprosthetic aortic valves.

Perhaps the choice of valve was influenced by the patient's anatomic factors (e.g., the surgeon choosing which valve seemed more suitable for the patient's anatomy), or patients requiring a concomitant coronary artery bypass graft (CABG) operation were more likely to receive one valve versus another. Maybe the surgeons at a particular hospital were of variable quality, and some of the better surgeons preferred one valve while the less proficient preferred another valve. If these factors are not recorded or captured reliably and accounted for in the data analysis, it may be difficult to get an unbiased estimate of the treatment effect one would obtain had these things been accounted for in the design or analysis.

Observational studies using electronic health records data are sometimes called "real-world evidence" and some have proposed they give a better representation of treatment effects in "real-world practice" than randomized clinical trials. It is a nice idea, but "real-world evidence" is susceptible to the potential biases described above. While there are methods that attempt to identify and adjust for these biases (e.g., multivariable models, propensity scores, and other complex approaches—some of which are discussed in this chapter), these issues can never be entirely removed with certainty. Even if all known confounders were available, unmeasured and/or unrecognized confounders are likely to affect the results. Finally, we should caution that one advertised advantage of observational studies—the ability to include large numbers of patients in an observational study—does not ensure accuracy; in fact, this is just as likely to amplify any biases as it is to mitigate them. It is rare that observational studies comparing two or more treatments are sufficiently strong to warrant changing practice on their own or convincing enough to override the evidence from high-quality clinical trials that compared the same/similar treatments as an observational study.

4.2 Randomized Trials

Clinical trials are experimental research where the receipt of the intervention is controlled by the study. As with observational research, there is a broad range of clinical trial designs, each suited to a different research question, ranging from traditional "patient-level" randomized trials (meaning each individual patient that is enrolled in the trial is randomly assigned to a treatment) to "cluster-randomized" designs that apply interventions to a collective unit (such as ICUs or hospitals). When appropriately designed, randomized trials provide the best evidence of the *average treatment effect* that will be experienced by patients who are given the studied intervention, directly informing bedside care.

When attempting to estimate treatment effects, randomized trials have several advantages over observational studies. When patients are randomly allocated to receive or not receive a given intervention, researchers do not know which group the patient will be assigned to until after randomization (*allocation concealment*), preventing selection bias and ensuring that group assignment is not related to any other factors. Randomization also has a large-sample tendency to balance all known and unknown confounders between groups. In randomized studies, small imbalances in baseline characteristics may occur by chance, but under the conditions of randomization, we can harness these known distributions to estimate the probability that any observed difference is due to a true effect of the treatment, or perhaps just the play of chance in randomization.

Randomized trials also (in some settings) make it possible to implement blinding, where patients, healthcare providers, and outcome assessors do not know the arm to which patients were randomized. This minimizes several potential biases, including the possibility that clinicians will make subsequent treatment decisions based on knowledge of group assignment (performance bias), the possibility that outcome assessments will be biased by knowledge of group assignment (information bias), and the possibility that knowledge of group assignment will affect a patient's interpretation of symptoms that are reported as adverse events. Blinding is particularly important for studies with subjective endpoints (quality of life, duration of symptoms). However, not all interventions can be blinded, particularly in interventional cardiology and/or cardiac surgery settings; one may even argue from a pragmatic standpoint that open-label trials (which may introduce some of the biases described above) are a better representation of real-world practice since treating clinicians will know what a patient has received and base any subsequent decisions about their treatment accordingly. However, even if it is impossible to blind the patients and treating clinicians, the use of blinded outcomes assessors remains desirable (when practical) to ensure that any judgments about a patient's outcome are not influenced by knowledge of what they received.

Estimating how many patients are needed for a randomized trial is a complex operation that, unfortunately, tends to involve some guesswork and judgment. Most trials are designed so that the trial will have a high probability (power) of concluding that the treatment is effective if there is a true treatment effect; however, some judgment must necessarily go into the size of this presumed treatment effect. Ideally, rather than using the effect one *hopes* to see, one should base the sample size calculation on the "minimum clinically important difference" or the smallest effect size that one would not want to miss. However, this is a rather abstract and not easily defined concept. Even relatively small absolute changes, like a 1–2% reduction in mortality, may be considered "clinically important" in some settings.

Trials should be appropriately powered, as underpowered trials are likely to waste resources by producing uninformative results. Worse, they might lead to false conclusions about the effectiveness (or lack thereof) of the tested interventions. Unfortunately, appropriately powering a trial often requires a sample size that comes as a shock to the hopeful investigator. For binary outcomes like mortality, demonstrating small but clinically important treatment effects may require enrolling more patients than can feasibly be enrolled in most traditional explanatory clinical trials. A more detailed discussion of sample size calculations is presented later in the chapter.

4.3 Target Trials

The most obvious advantage of a randomized trial (versus an observational study) for estimating treatment effect is the randomization procedure itself, which eliminates any systematic bias in the types of patients that receive the respective treatments. However, there are other advantages that are less recognized that become clear when one attempts to hold an observational study to the standards of a randomized trial.

If no randomized trial is available and one is forced to work with nonrandomized data, one strategy to mitigate these concerns is the *target trial* approach. Target trial emulation is the application of design principles from randomized trials to the analysis of observational data. The purpose is to improve the quality of observational research through the application of trial design principles when a randomized trial is not yet available or feasible, by ensuring that researchers are mindful of possible biases that may be present in an observational analysis and take steps to overcome them when possible.

In the target trial approach, the researcher explicitly writes out the entire design of the trial that they are seeking to emulate: eligibility criteria for patients, the setting in which the trial is carried out, how patients are assessed for eligibility in the cohort and when they become eligible for inclusion, the intervention(s) or group(s) that are being compared, how the assignment of treatments occurs, the period at which patients enter the trial and the follow-up period, the outcome and how it will be assessed, and the analysis which will be performed to compare the groups of interest. Doing this and then contrasting it against the available data source(s) and analysis plan will often reveal several potential biases that one must be wary of, above just the lack of randomization.

Consider the following example: suppose that we believe a particular medication may be useful in the treatment of critically ill patients admitted to the hospital. Lacking any prospective randomized data, we seek to perform a retrospective analysis that compares patients with the illness of interest who received the medication against those who did not. We see that patients who received the medication generally appeared to have better survival than patients who did not receive the medication and conclude that the medication improved survival to hospital discharge. What could be wrong here?

One potential problem is *immortal time bias*. In the example described above, the only patients that are included in the "treatment" arm are the patients who survived long enough to receive a dose of the medication. Patients in the intervention group, therefore, are "immortal" from the start of the cohort to the initiation of treatment; any patient who dies during this period cannot be assigned to the intervention group. Conversely, patients who were so critically ill that they died soon after reaching the hospital (before the medication was considered or could be administered) are all included in the comparison group by default. Most of these patients would not be included in a clinical trial (they are not alive at the time they would be assessed for enrollment), but in an observational study, they are included in the analysis as part of the control group. This effect could overestimate the true benefit of the medication in improving survival to hospital discharge.

Another potential problem is *indication bias* (or *confounding by indication*). This occurs when one of the study treatments may only be given to patients for a particular reason or in a particular setting. A darkly humorous example of this would be the use of cardiopulmonary resuscitation (CPR). In a naïve comparison of survival to hospital discharge for all patients admitted to the hospital who received CPR versus those who did not, surely an unadjusted comparison would suggest that the mortality is far higher in patients who received CPR than those who did not. One might conclude from this data that CPR kills patients and that we should cease its use in the hospital setting due to the high mortality.

Of course, with a moment's thought, that is ridiculous: CPR is only applied to patients who are dying and in need of CPR to have a chance at survival. This is where the target-trial emulation would come in handy; by explicitly writing out the randomized trial we would seem to emulate, we would realize that the control group will now include many patients in whom there was no reason to attempt CPR. One thing to keep in mind when performing observational analyses is that, ideally, all patients should have at least been able to be considered for both "treatments" that are being compared. If some of the potentially included patients could only have received one of the treatments (perhaps because the other is never performed on that type of patient), then these patients should be excluded from the analysis, as this type of patient likely would not be included in a randomized trial.

Admittedly, we cannot always emulate the core elements of an ideal trial. In some cases, even if we cannot emulate the ideal trial, we may still pursue the study while cognizant of the compromises made and possible biases they may introduce. In other cases, we may realize the trial we are able to emulate is too far removed from the ideal target trial, and we may choose to refine our questions or seek other data rather than proceed with a study that is too badly flawed to provide useful data.

Please do bear in mind that target trials are not actually randomized trials. Rather, the term indicates that the researchers have made some effort to ensure that the observational study comes as close as possible to mimicking the structure of the hypothetical trial one *would* have done if they had been able to carry out a randomized trial. In many cases working in this framework will bring the observational analysis closer to the ideal randomized trial that we would have liked to mimic; in others, the main benefit is that it makes plain what potential biases still exist that cannot be easily accounted for with design or analysis.

5 Propensity Scores

Another approach to estimating a treatment effect from observational (nonrandomized) data involves the use of propensity scores. These may be used in several different ways: matching, stratification, weighting, or covariate adjustment. The most popular in cardiovascular medicine seems to be propensity-score matching, in part because of the appearance that it recreates a randomized trial. The idea is approximately as follows: use a multivariable regression model (often logistic regression) to obtain estimates of the relationships between covariates of interest and the probability of receiving the treatment of interest (versus some comparison treatment). The resulting regression coefficients may be used to compute a propensity score, which is essentially interpreted as the "probability" that the patient received the active treatment, given their observed covariate values. With these values, it becomes possible to match patients that have similar propensity scores; there are several different matching algorithms, and often one must specify a caliper distance (a maximum distance between the propensity scores that still allows a given pair of patients to be considered a match). Depending on the size of the cohort, one may choose a 1:1 matching ratio (only matching 1 control patient to each treated patient) or an n:1 ratio; if there are many more control patients than treated patients available, one can increase the effective sample size by matching 2 or even 3 control patients to each treated patient. After matching patients from the treatment group to patients with similar propensity scores in the comparison group, one will be left with a cohort of treatment and control patients that are generally more alike (on the features used to create the propensity score, that is) than the full set of treatment and control patients were alike. From this point, it is common for authors to proceed with analyses comparing the treatment and control patients in the propensity-score matched cohort as though they came from a randomized trial, though some make additional efforts with further covariate adjustment or weighting even after restricting the analysis to the propensity-score matched cohort.

Although this approach looks appealing on the surface as it gives an appearance of recreating a randomized trial by forming (apparently) comparable groups of treated and control patients, one must be cautious. Propensity-score matching has limitations; it can only reduce confounding on measured variables, which sometimes can paradoxically increase the degree of confounding on important unmeasured variables. For example, a patient's preference for one procedure versus another is not often recorded; similarly, sometimes a patient ends up getting the procedure/medication they did because it was the only one that was available, or because the physician thought they were a poor candidate for the alternative, and these things are not always easily captured or measured in research databases. Whenever possible, propensity-score matched analyses should be restricted to include only patients that, in theory, could have received either of the two treatment options that are being compared (note that the discussion here echoes some common themes from the target trial discussion above).

Other options include weighting (most commonly inverse probability of treatment weighting [IPTW]) and covariate adjustment. Conceptually, weighting attempts to fully adjust for measured confounders by creating a pseudo-population that is balanced between the treatment groups and estimates the treatment effect based on this pseudo-population; there are many technical details that lie beyond the scope of this chapter. Another option that is sometimes used is simply adding the estimated propensity score to a multivariable regression model while performing the analysis on the full original dataset. These options have the advantage of retaining all of the original analytic set, whereas matching invariably results in discarding the information from some of the patients; however, they are less attractive to many readers because they do not give the same appearance that matching gives of recreating what looks like a randomized trial from the observational data.

6 Correlated Data

Many of the analyses learned in introductory statistics courses operate under the assumption that the data are independent. This is not true when there are multiple measurements from the same patient in a dataset, which may be the case in a longitudinal study with repeated measures, or perhaps when multiple vessels per patient may be included in a vessel-level analysis. Sometimes there is a desire to account for the correlation between patients who are treated by the same physician, or at the same hospital, in a multi-center study. It is important to know that there are statistical approaches that are specifically adapted to account for correlation between observations. These include some relatively simple approaches, such as paired t-tests, and more sophisticated ones, such as generalized estimating equations and linear mixed-effects models. We will provide just a few possible scenarios for discussion.

The simplest correlated-data problem involves paired data, such as PRE and POST measurements on the same participants. Suppose that we measured the SBP of patients 5 min before giving them a beverage, asked them to consume the beverage, and measured again 5 min after they finished drinking; we wish to test the hypothesis that drinking beverage results in a transient increase in blood pressure. If one compares the POST values against the PRE values using an independent-samples t-test to determine whether the beverage results in higher blood pressure after drinking versus before drinking, we fail to account for the dependence between repeated observations on the same person; our standard error will be too large. We might use a *paired t-test* to better account for the correlation between each participant's PRE and POST measurements rather than treating them as fully independent samples, as a standard two-sample t-test would do. By harnessing the known dependence between observations on the same person, we get a smaller standard error and, therefore, a more powerful statistical test than if we treat the data points as two fully independent samples.

Second, suppose that we are interested in studying the effect of a particular exposure on hospital length of stay in heart failure patients followed over a 5-year period in a particular health system. Since heart failure patients may be hospitalized more than once during this period, it is desirable to make use of all available data rather than using only one observation per patient; otherwise, we may discard a lot of potentially useful data. However, we must choose an analytic method that accounts for the dependency between repeated encounters with the same patient (instead of treating each encounter as a totally independent data point); if this is not done, we may not get an accurate estimate of the true impact of that exposure on length of stay. In this situation, a *linear mixed-effects model* may prove suitable; one might also consider the use of *generalized estimating equations*.

Finally, suppose that we wish to analyze the effect of a particular exposure on survival to hospital discharge in the same population as described in the previous paragraph (patients seen over a 5-year period in a particular health system). Similarly, to the previously described situation, we wish to include all of the data as we would be discarding much useful information if we only used the first hospitalization from each patient; however, again we have the problem of correlated observations between participants, this time with a binary outcome variable rather than a continuous outcome variable. In this problem, we might consider a *generalized linear-mixed effects model* (GLMM), which allows us to fit a mixed-effects model using a link function, as described earlier in the chapter for GLMs. In addition to the flexibility provided by the link function that allows us to model different response variables (e.g., binary variable for survival-to-hospital-discharge rather than a continuous variable), we also have the power of a mixed-effect model, which allows us to include subject-level random effects that account for the multiple data points from one participant.

A detailed description of these methods is beyond the scope of this chapter, but the important takeaway for the reader is that it is important to be mindful of whether the analysis contains any repeated measures on the same participants and, if so, whether this was taken into account in the analysis or whether the data have been simply treated as fully independent observations.

7 Missing Data

In typical classroom teaching examples, the datasets provided are not missing any values, so this topic is often glossed over or omitted entirely from the brief statistics education many clinicians receive; yet, in real life, this is a common problem. It is rare for a research dataset to have complete data recorded on every patient with no missing values of any kind. The implications of missing data and handling are a complex topic that lies rather beyond the scope of this book, but there are a few points worth mentioning. The first is that one must carefully evaluate what, exactly, is missing; are a few baseline values not recorded? Are there missing outcome data? If there are missing outcome data, are they likely to bias the results? For example, consider a clinical trial that compares two treatments for heart failure patients with the primary outcome of a 6-min walking distance measured 1 year after the patient begins treatment. Suppose that some patients have died in the intervening period. If the number of deaths in one arm is greater than the number of deaths in the other arm, a naïve comparison of the 6-min walking distances between the groups will be biased, because some of the sickest patients in one group have died (and will not have a recorded value) while their counterparts in the other group remain alive, though perhaps in poor health. One must consider an analytic approach that takes this into account.

A *complete case* analysis (also known as "listwise deletion") simply removes any patient with missing data and analyzes patients that have complete data for all of the values required in the analytic model of choice. The advantage is simplicity; the disadvantage is that it can be biased if the missingness is somehow related to the outcome data, such as the example above where sicker patients (i.e., those that would have had poorer 6-min walking distance if still alive) are those most likely to be missing from the analysis.

A *single-imputation* analysis is where missing values are simply replaced in the dataset by some value and, then, the analysis is carried out as though those are the observed values. Some commonly seen options are imputing the mean of all observations from similar patients to the one with the missing value, imputing the last observation from that patient (if the study is longitudinal), or in some cases preferentially assigning the "worst" value—in the example above, perhaps one would assign the worst recorded 6-min walking distance from the dataset to all patients that died before the 6-month assessment. The advantage is again simplicity; the disadvantage is that, frankly, these approaches do not provide unbiased estimates with the correct standard errors, though the degree to which this matters varies considerably based on the amount and pattern of missing data. The implications are quite different if one simply imputes the mean for a missing covariate value for a few patients in order to retain them in the overall primary analysis versus if one imputes the primary outcome data for a large number of missing values, some of which are known to be due to informative missingness.

Because the imputed data are then analyzed as though they are real observations, a single imputation does not take into account the uncertainty in the imputations. Therefore, *multiple imputation* was developed by Rubin to deal with the problem of increased error due to imputation [4]. All multiple imputation methods follow three steps: imputation, analysis, and pooling. The imputation step proceeds similarly to a single imputation; however, the imputed values are drawn multiple times from a distribution rather than just once, creating multiple datasets, each with its own set of imputed values. In the analysis step, each of the imputed datasets is then analyzed. In the pooling step, the results from all of the analyses of the imputed datasets are consolidated into one result by calculating the mean, variance, and CI for the variable(s) of interest in the model. As alluded to in the previous section, a single imputation does not account for any uncertainty in the imputations—after imputation, the data are analyzed as if they were the real values. The negligence of uncertainty will lead to inappropriately precise estimates and errors in any conclusions. By imputing multiple times, multiple imputation accounts for the uncertainty and range of values that the true value could have taken.

There are many complex efforts to develop solutions to various missing data problems, the technical details of which lie well beyond the scope of this book (indeed, there are entire books on this subject alone). The important takeaway for the purposes of this book is to be mindful of missing data, consider whether the missing data are potentially informative or likely to introduce a bias, and examine whether the authors of a given paper say anything about the presence of, and efforts to account for, missing data in their analysis.

8 Win Ratio

One emerging method in cardiovascular outcomes trials that warrants attention here is the "win ratio" approach to comparing treatment groups. The win ratio provides a way to combine several outcomes, even different types of outcome variables, into a single composite measure for the comparison of two treatments. Consider the following: suppose that we are conducting a trial in heart failure patients and that we wish to test whether a new heart failure medication results in better outcomes than standard care. Furthermore, suppose that we believe it is important not only that the medication improves mortality but also the patients' physical function in their daily lives. We propose to use a composite outcome measure of the patients' 6-min walking distance while accounting for the fact that some patients may be too sick to complete a 6-min walk test or may die before the end of the trial. We may construct a composite endpoint that first asks if the patient died before the end of the trial; if so, their outcome is the survival time. If the patient survived to the end of the trial but was too sick to attempt a 6-min walk test, this is their recorded outcome. If the patient survived to the end of the trial and completed a 6-min walk test, their outcome is the recorded 6-min walking distance. Using this composite outcome, each patient in the treated group is compared to every patient in the control group to ask which was the "winner" (see example in Table 8 below).

With this approach, one may compare every possible pairing of treated patient and control patient, then compute the number of "wins" for each group. The win ratio is then reported as the ratio of the number of wins for the treated group in comparison to the control group; a win ratio exceeding 1 indicates that the treated

Table 8 Example of a win ratio approach

Treated patient	Control patient	"Winner"
Survived to complete trial 6-min walk distance = 300 m	Survived to complete trial 6-min walk distance = 200 m	Treated patient (longer distance)
Survived to complete trial 6-min walk distance = 300 m	Survived to complete trial Did not complete 6-min walk test	Treated patient (completed 6 min-walk test while control patient was too sick to attempt test)
Survived to complete trial 6-min walk distance = 300 m	Deceased after 5 months	Treated patient (completed 6-min walk test while control patient died before the end of the trial)
Deceased after 1 month	Deceased after 5 months	Control patient (both patients died and control patient survived longer than treated patient)

group results in more wins than the control group. Similarly, as is the case for other outcome measures, one may compute a CI and p-value and conduct a statistical test for whether the data conclusively prove that the treatment is likely to result in superior outcomes when generalized to a broader population. As stated, multiple outcomes per participant are frequently observed in the context of observational and experimental studies. For example, a participant could experience a cerebrovascular event and later death. Decisions must be made on how to treat such data that can create analytic problems. Typically, a researcher using a Cox model will use the first event and ignore the death, or endpoints will be treated equally regardless of statistical weighting [5]. The win ratio is an intuitive and elegant solution to such problems.

9 Hypothesis Testing and Interim Analyses in Clinical Trials

A natural question from many readers in response to the section above is why we need to perform sample size calculations before the study at all; surely, we could just start recruiting patients and keep checking the data until we had strong evidence for or against a benefit of the treatment, right? Why do we have to decide in advance on a sample size?

We must now briefly explain some things about the philosophy of hypothesis testing in frequentist statistics. Obviously, we cannot collect an infinite amount of data. Since we will never be able to test a treatment on all patients that might 1 day be considered for this treatment, we test the treatment on a *sample* of such patients and use that data to make an informed guess as to whether the treatment seems to be beneficial. Unfortunately, if we are required to make a binary conclusion from a given trial, we will make occasional errors. The first concept is a *type I error*, where we reject a null hypothesis that should not have been rejected; in a clinical trial, this may be called a "false positive" trial result—concluding that a treatment works when it has no real effect. The opposing concept is a *type II error*—or a "false negative" result, where the trial concludes that the treatment does not work even though it actually is effective.

We now must revisit the much-maligned p-value. Recall earlier that we introduced and defined the p-value as approximately meaning "the probability of obtaining the observed data if the null hypothesis were true." In the context of a clinical trial testing for a difference between two treatments, a small p-value typically means that it would be unlikely to observe these data if the treatments were equally effective (e.g., there is no difference between the treatment groups). Requiring that clinical trials have a small p-value to declare that the treatment is effective is our way of controlling the risk of type I error. By requiring that the p-value be less than 0.05 to conclude that a treatment is effective at the final analysis, we guarantee the trial has only a 5% risk of concluding that an ineffective treatment is superior to its comparator treatment.

Suppose that we "look" at the data more than once; perhaps the trial was designed to enroll 1000 patients, but we look at the data every ten patients and compare the groups, seeking a $p < 0.05$ at each analysis. By taking many looks at the data, we now have much greater than a 5% probability of concluding that an ineffective treatment is effective. This would be somewhat akin to flipping a coin a thousand times, but stopping at the first run of five consecutive heads and declaring that the coin is weighted toward heads. To maintain the risk of false positive clinical trial findings at a desired level, one must somehow account for the fact that there were multiple looks at the data which gave it more "chances" to cross the threshold.

There are several strategies that may be considered for carrying out interim analyses while maintaining type I error control. The *group-sequential approach* to interim analyses is the most common way to plan interim analyses in trials designed using frequentist statistics. Some notable examples include the Haybittle–Peto approach, the Pocock approach, and the O'Brien–Fleming approach, explained below.

The *Haybittle–Peto approach* is pleasingly intuitive, albeit statistically imperfect; it suggests that one may perform fairly frequent interim analyses so long as they only stop the trial if a very high threshold is crossed (e.g., $p < 0.0001$). If this threshold is not crossed, the trial may continue and, furthermore, the investigators may still use the standard $p < 0.05$ threshold to declare significance at the final analysis. The main attraction of this approach is that it only stops the trial early if the evidence is truly overwhelming and it preserves the ability to use the 0.05 threshold at the final analysis, thereby maximizing the statistical power should the trial proceed to the maximum planned sample size. On the "con" side of the ledger for the Haybittle–Peto approach, some might argue that the requirement for such a high threshold to stop the trial early is a disadvantage; the practical likelihood of stopping early is quite small, and further, it technically could inflate type I error slightly beyond 0.05 if one includes many interim analyses with the $p < 0.001$ threshold and retains the 0.05 level for the final analysis rather than make any adjustment.

The *Pocock approach* uses the same significance level at each of the planned interim analyses as well as the final analysis. For example, assuming that the analyses are equally spaced, with three total analyses planned (two "interim" analyses and a final analysis) the researchers may declare a significant finding with $p < 0.0221$ at any of the three planned analysis time points while preserving the overall type I error at 0.05. This approach is more aggressive in allowing early stopping than the Haybittle–Peto approach but at the cost of reduced statistical power at the final analysis because it requires a more stringent threshold than the traditional 0.05 level.

The *O'Brien–Fleming approach* lies somewhere in between these two extremes. It uses a slightly less stringent threshold for early stopping than the Haybittle–Peto approach but preserves more for the final analysis than the Pocock approach.

An alternative to these group-sequential approaches is the *alpha-spending approach*. Unlike the group-sequential approaches, the alpha-spending approach brings with it some additional flexibility that these are lacking. In the classic group-sequential approaches, the interim analyses must be pre-specified and should be equally spaced, which can be difficult to implement; does this mean an equal number of patients recruited, an equal number of outcome events or information, or equal amounts of calendar time between analyses? The alpha-spending approach that was developed by DeMets and Lan provides a flexible approach to control the type I error while allowing a flexible schedule of interim analyses without having to specify *a priori* when and how many such interim analyses will be conducted [6].

The preceding paragraphs all deal with interim analyses that permit trials to test for and declare efficacy. We should also mention that sometimes clinical trials build in interim analyses for futility, which refers to stopping the trial because it is unlikely that the trial will proceed to meet its primary objective. This has an attraction from an ethical perspective (patients are no longer enrolled in a trial that is essentially already a foregone conclusion and may seek other treatment or perhaps enroll in a different trial) and from a sponsor's perspective (knowing that the trial is unlikely to result in a positive conclusion, they can cease exhausting further resources and redirect them to a different research program). The creation of futility-stopping rules is rather different than efficacy-stopping rules because, unlike the efficacy-stopping rules, the possibility of a futility stop does not introduce an increased possibility of a type I error. Futility-stopping rules are, therefore, typically rooted in some sort of "conditional power" calculation; essentially, this asks "based on the data observed so far, plus some assumptions about the possible treatment effect, what is the probability that the trial will meet a successful conclusion?" If the conditional power is very low, it may be recommended to stop the trial and direct the patients and resources elsewhere. Note that this is not quite the same as stopping a trial due to a safety concern that the therapy is actively harmful; rather, it is simply that the trial no longer has any realistic prospect of demonstrating that the therapy is effective. One may also stop a trial for futility based on slower-than-expected accrual of patients, not necessarily because the therapy is proven ineffective but because there simply are not enough patients being enrolled in the trial for it to conclude in a timely fashion or before the resources (money) runs out. Such trials are frustrating because they do not provide a definitive answer as to whether a treatment works, but they are common. One might even argue that if it was sufficiently difficult to enroll patients in the trial, the enthusiasm for the therapy might have been low, and/or there are not many available patients who were qualified for the therapy.

We must close this section with yet one more disclaimer, which is that all of the above text is written in the context of purely statistically driven rules, mostly focused on controlling type I error and optimizing the operating characteristics of that specific trial. However, the job of a Data and Safety Monitoring Board (DSMB) is to weigh not only the trial evidence and stopping rules in front of them but also any outside knowledge or other developments in the field. For example, if a similar trial of the same medication is completed in a similar patient population and revealed to be successful, the DSMB may recommend early termination of an ongoing trial if their trial's evidence also suggests benefit even if the formal stopping rule was not met, citing the outside evidence and ethical considerations (e.g., no longer ethical to continue randomizing patients to an inferior therapy when a seemingly superior one is now available). Or, perhaps a competing trial is stopped early due to safety concerns, such as an untoward increase in a particular adverse event with the experimental treatment; again, the DSMB may exercise discretion and could recommend a pause or early termination while their trial's data are examined to see if there is similar evidence of a safety concern.

All of this is enough to make one wonder if there could be a more efficient way of formalizing these things; some would argue that there already is.

10 Bayesian Statistical Analysis

Throughout this chapter, we have described how to approach some common research problems using a frequentist approach to statistical analysis. Frequentist statistical approaches use no outside information; they use only the observed data, and typically focus on testing a null hypothesis, subsequently providing a p-value that evaluates how incompatible the observed data are with the null hypothesis. A very small p-value indicates that the observed result is "very" incompatible with the null hypothesis. To a frequentist, it follows that because it would be very surprising to obtain such results if the null hypothesis were true, we should "reject" the null hypothesis, thereby accepting an alternative (e.g., rejecting the null hypothesis of "treatment has no effect" leads us to accept an alternative hypothesis that the treatment does have an effect).

Admittedly, the p-value provides only indirect information about what clinicians would presumably most like to know to make treatment decisions, which is some combination of the magnitude of a treatment effect and the degree of confidence in whether the observed data are likely to represent a real effect or just noise. Furthermore, frequentist studies that fail to reach significance thresholds are frequently referred to as "negative" and often incorrectly interpreted as proving that an intervention has no effect when many are better described as inconclusive. One must carefully look not only at the p-value but also at the confidence bounds for the treatment effect to determine whether a study has truly ruled out a meaningful benefit of the therapy, or if perhaps it was simply too small to provide conclusive evidence regarding the presence of a clinically meaningful effect.

The entire Bayesian philosophy and approach is quite different. Statistical inference using Bayesian methods produces a distribution of effect sizes that would be compatible with observed trial data, computed based on a combination of the study data and *prior distributions* for the parameters included in the model. To clinicians, the most appealing feature of Bayesian statistical models might be the more direct probability statement at the end. Rather than the indirect probability statement of a p-value, the probability from a Bayesian analysis may be framed as a direct answer to the clinical question: "what is the probability that the studied treatment is superior to the control treatment?"

One aspect of Bayesian analysis that is likely new to clinicians and researchers trained predominantly with frequentist methods is the concept of a "prior" distribution. The prior is a distribution of potential effect sizes estimated from prior knowledge or beliefs. In Bayesian analysis, the observed data (the "likelihood") is combined with prior knowledge or assumptions (the "prior") to produce an updated distribution of estimated effect sizes (called the "posterior" distribution). Some Bayesian analyses present the results using multiple different priors, providing posterior probability distributions for each to demonstrate the robustness of the study results to different choices of the prior distribution. For clinical trials, a skeptical prior (one that assumes the most likely treatment effect is zero and places less prior probability on a large benefit or harm) is recommended as the primary analysis as it is most analogous to the null hypothesis in a frequentist trial and aligns with the concept of clinical equipoise. One may perform a Bayesian analysis using a "flat" or "uninformative" prior for all parameters; in such cases, the Bayesian results (i.e., point estimate, credible intervals) will likely be a near-exact match for the frequentist point estimate and CI.

Bayesian statistical modeling and analysis are, of course, much richer and sophisticated than can be conveyed in the few paragraphs here, and there is increasing recognition of other applications for Bayesian statistical procedures than just 2-group comparisons in clinical trials. The most important point for readers of this book to appreciate is their potential utility and application in clinical trials. When the reader encounters a clinical trial analyzed using Bayesian methods, instead of the familiar "p-value," they will likely be presented with a "posterior probability" which may be interpreted as the probability (computed based on the prior and observed data) that the experimental treatment is superior to the comparison treatment. Rather than a small p-value telling us that, "it would be surprising to see these data if the treatment makes no difference, so instead we'll assume that the treatment does something," the Bayesian probability statement will actually tell us an estimated probability that the treatment is better, e.g., the observed trial data tell us there is a 97.8% probability that outcomes are better with the experimental treatment than the control treatment.

11   Statistical Power and Sample Size Considerations

For statisticians in medicine, a commonly encountered scenario is a researcher asking if they can "just" do a "quick" power calculation, so the researcher knows the sample size needed for a given study. This request also often comes shortly before a grant proposal is due, usually without compensation, and it is unclear whether the statistician is actively being asked to collaborate on the proposal as a colleague or just to provide a number as a one-off favor. In some cases, the statistician is effectively told, "We can afford 100 patients in the budget, so it would be great if you can make that work," or given precious little information on which to base this magical "power calculation." There are several issues with this interaction, which we will ignore for now other than to say that statistical colleagues generally prefer to be given more than a few hours' notice to complete tasks such as planning an entire grant submission, and with clear expectations regarding their capacity as a consultant or funded collaborator on the proposal. In this space, however, we will focus on the statistical topic only, which is: how do we estimate how many patients you need?

The term "statistical power" is tossed about frequently in these discussions, but it is often being applied poorly, since the concept of "power" is narrower than many people realize. We prefer to introduce a more general term, *sample size justification*, first, and then discuss how a *power calculation* fits into that concept. All studies should include a *sample size justification* to show that the planned/available sample was/is large enough to fulfill the desired research objective; this justification may benefit from including one or more power calculation(s) but, in some cases, that would be misguided or outright wrong. The easiest way to explain this is to define a power calculation, show an example in practice, and then discuss other types of studies where something other than a power calculation is needed to estimate the necessary sample size.

The power of a statistical test is simply the probability that the test will reach a particular conclusion given the planned sample size and some assumptions about the underlying data-generating process. If that seems like a mouthful, consider this specific example: we are planning to perform a randomized trial comparing the use of a new blood-pressure-lowering medication against remaining on standard treatment. Our primary outcome will be the SBP measured after 4 weeks of treatment. We know that the "typical" SBP in our targeted patient population on standard treatment is approximately 150 mm Hg, with a standard deviation of approximately 10 mm Hg. To estimate the probability that the trial concludes that the medication is effective (reject the null hypothesis that the treatments are equivalent), we must have some estimate of the distribution of blood pressure values that we will see in the group receiving the new medication. This is sometimes mistakenly thought of as our best guess of what the treatment *will* do, but that is not quite right. Here, we must introduce the concept of the "minimum clinically important difference" (MCID). A frustrating and vexing concept to fully grasp, the MCID is the smallest difference between two treatments that we would consider "clinically important" in practice. If a new medication only lowers blood pressure by 1 mm Hg, we might argue that the effect on clinical outcomes would be so small it is unlikely worth implementing this treatment anyway; therefore, we do not particularly care if our study is too small to detect this effect. Defining precisely what is "the" MCID in a particular scenario is admittedly very challenging, especially given that patient preferences and values likely vary widely (some may value small gains more than others) and may not match clinicians' beliefs as to what effect size is "clinically important." There is never just one answer to "what is an MCID" that will apply to all possible scenarios. That said, contemplating the "MCID" is still an important concept because it is better to design a research study thinking "what is the smallest effect that I would care about?" rather than "what effect do I think the treatment will have?" We will now illustrate why.

Suppose that we have a pilot study where five patients took the medication and experienced a mean reduction in their SBP of 20 mm Hg from a baseline measurement to a follow-up measurement taken 4 weeks later. Brimming with confidence from these impressive pilot results, we design our trial based on the assumption that the new medication actually reduces SBP by 20 mm Hg. Our power calculation tells us that even with just six patients per treatment group (12 total), we will have over 80% power to detect a reduction in blood pressure if the true effect of the treatment is a 20 mm Hg reduction over standard treatment. We run our clinical trial and obtain the following results: a mean SBP = 150 mm Hg in the control group (SD = 10 mm Hg) and a mean SBP = 140 mm Hg in the treated group (SD = 10 mm Hg). Our two-sample t-test returns a p-value of 0.11, and we fail to reject the null hypothesis; we have insufficient evidence that the new medication is effective in reducing blood pressure.

What happened? Is the medication ineffective? It is hard to know—the study data certainly have not ruled out the possibility that the medication reduces blood pressure; they even suggest that it might reduce blood pressure quite substantially (note that the treated patients had a mean SBP that was 10 mm Hg lower than the patients receiving standard treatment), but the study was too small to produce a definitive result. The mistake was using too optimistic an estimate of the medication's true effect to inform the power calculation. By assuming such a large effect size in the power calculation, we made the trial too small ("underpowered") to be able to detect a smaller benefit of the treatment, even if that smaller benefit would still have been worth finding.

Now suppose that instead we had decided that the MCID for a new blood pressure medication was lowering the SBP by 10 mm Hg—meaning, we want to be very confident that our trial results will lead us to conclude the medication is effective if it actually reduces blood pressure by 10 mm Hg or more. Perhaps we know that medications that reduce SBP by this amount have good track records in demonstrating clinical benefit on harder clinical endpoints. Instead of designing our trial with just six patients per arm, we consider a design with 20 patients per arm (40 patients total). If the mean SBP in patients receiving standard care is 150 mm Hg, and the mean SBP in patients receiving the new medication is 140 mm Hg, this study will have approximately 87% power to provide statistical evidence (i.e., a p-value < 0.05) that the new medication is effective in reducing SBP. We now can proceed, confident that if the medication has some clinically relevant effect of interest, our study is large enough to have a reasonably high probability of detecting that effect.

This is, of course, but one illustrative example. There are different ways of approaching these problems: one may choose to estimate the necessary sample size for a given power and effect size or one may start with a planned sample size and effect size and compute the estimated power. These quantities are all somehow related, and the basics of "what is needed for a power calculation" are essentially some estimate of the outcome in the control group and some estimate of the "treatment effect" you expect (or the outcome in the intervention group). The exact calculations also depend on the choice of study outcome: is it a continuous variable, like blood pressure; an ordinal scale, like the modified Rankin Scale used in some neurologic research; dichotomous, perhaps survival to hospital discharge in a critically ill population; or time-to-event, such as freedom from a major adverse cardiovascular event over 5 years of treatment, as commonly seen in secondary prevention trials of coronary disease? There are additional considerations for different trial designs (e.g., cluster-randomized trials must account for variation in cluster size and the potential degree to which the clusters influence outcomes; non-inferiority trials require setting a non-inferiority margin and structuring the hypotheses differently than a trial testing for superiority) and other more sophisticated analyses that we will not discuss in detail here.

One important thing that should be mentioned, though, is the more granular the primary endpoint, the greater a trial's statistical power will be to detect a treatment effect. In some cases, there is a desire to dichotomize an ordinal or continuous endpoint in a misguided effort to identify "responders" to the treatment. This is well-intentioned but problematic for several reasons, both statistical and translational to clinical practice. Consider this example: once again, we are investigating a new blood-pressure-lowering medication. Rather than comparing the mean SBP between the two groups as a continuous variable, someone proposes that we create a binary endpoint that is "yes" if the patient's final SBP is less than 140 and "no" if the final SBP is above 140. This might seem attractive at first since one might think the achievement of this threshold is "clinically relevant" as it would mean these patients no longer have an SBP above the threshold that defines a patient as having "hypertension" (depending on the current guidelines as to what defines hypertension, of course). However, this creates an awkward discontinuity in the outcome data as well as a loss of relevant information. Note that a change in SBP from 170 to 145 mm Hg will be classified as a "nonresponse" while a change in SBP from 145 to 135 mm Hg would be classified as a "response." Or, note that a patient whose SBP goes from 170 to 165 mm Hg would have the same outcome as a patient whose SBP goes from 170 to 145 mm Hg—both would be considered a "nonresponse" since neither had a final value below the threshold of 140. This treatment of an outcome variable could create silly scenarios. If all patients had an SBP of 170 mm Hg at entry, all patients that received a placebo had a final value of 165 mm Hg, and all patients that received treatment had a final value of 145 mm Hg, by the dichotomous definition we would conclude that this medication had no effect on blood pressure, even though the patients that received the medication had a mean SBP 20 mm Hg lower than patients that did not receive the medication.

Of course, there will be clinical settings where the primary endpoint of interest *is* truly binary in nature. In the setting of critical illness, one might reasonably argue that the primary objective is ensuring the patient's survival and that new treatments must demonstrate improved survival to warrant use. The authors certainly do not advocate using clinically unimportant outcomes just because they offer better statistical power. Rather, we suggest that when a more granular measure is already available and being used as the study outcome, researchers should make use of the full range of that outcome measure to determine whether the treatment is responsible for a change in that outcome. Subsequent analyses may be used to determine whether the treatment seems responsible for a "clinically relevant" change in that outcome and formalize tradeoffs of a gain in one outcome versus a loss in another (e.g., in the setting of secondary prevention trials after percutaneous coronary intervention, weighing reduction in future myocardial infarction and stent thrombosis events against the risk of additional bleeding complications from more intense antiplatelet therapy).

One final word on statistical power before we move on. There is a pervasive belief that studies that failed to demonstrate "significant" differences should be accompanied by a "post-hoc power" calculation where the authors report the power the study would have with the achieved sample size and effect size. This comes from a well-intentioned belief that it would help the reader distinguish "true negative" studies (where there is no true effect, and the study concludes that there is no effect) from "false negative" studies (where there is a true effect, but the study was unable to detect it, perhaps because it was too small). The intention is good; the execution is wrong. A posthoc power calculation that is performed using the observed effect size is simply a transformation of the p-value. Studies that found significant effects will invariably appear to have high post-hoc power, while studies that failed to find significant effects will appear to have low post-hoc power (even if they were, in fact, reasonably well-powered to detect a clinically meaningful effect). In some cases, the answer is simply "the treatment doesn't work," while in other cases, the answer is "the study was too small"—but a post-hoc power calculation based on the observed effect size in the study cannot tell you which of these was true. It may be reasonable to perform a post-hoc power calculation by using some chosen clinically meaningful effect size, not by using the observed effect size in the study data; otherwise, it becomes a wholly circular exercise with a self-fulfilling conclusion.

At the very beginning of this section, we mentioned that it was important to understand the distinction between a "power calculation" and the broader issue of "sample size justification." Hopefully, it has become clear in the preceding pages that a power calculation has a specific, narrower definition: the probability that a statistical procedure will reach a particular conclusion under a set of assumptions, usually the probability of rejecting a null hypothesis. Note that there are studies for which the objective is not chiefly to test something against a null hypothesis or at least not by what one might consider the default null hypothesis. For example, consider a study that proposes to evaluate the agreement between an existing diagnostic test and a new diagnostic test. One manner of doing this would be assessing the correlation between measures obtained from the new test and the existing test. However, if all one requires to declare that the measures "agree" with one another is that the study rejects the null hypothesis of zero correlation, the estimated sample size will be far too small to carry out a much more meaningful statistical objective, which is assessing whether the tests show a good degree of agreement with one another. Proving that a correlation is greater than zero is a different statistical objective than proving that two tests have good agreement, yet we often see papers that report p-values for tests of whether a correlation coefficient is significantly different from zero and hold them up as evidence of "agreement" between the two measures. A power calculation based on testing a null hypothesis that the correlation is equal to zero will return a sample size estimate that is too small for a good test of whether the two measures agree with one another; the sample size has been justified based on the wrong statistical target. A more appropriate sample size justification would illustrate that the study is large enough to precisely estimate the limits of agreement to some reasonable level of tolerance that allows judgment as to whether the measures may be considered in agreement with one another.

Required sample sizes can be calculated using a few select parameters and standard sample size equations or one of the many other available calculations [7]. These include the significance levels, statistical power, effect size, event rate, and

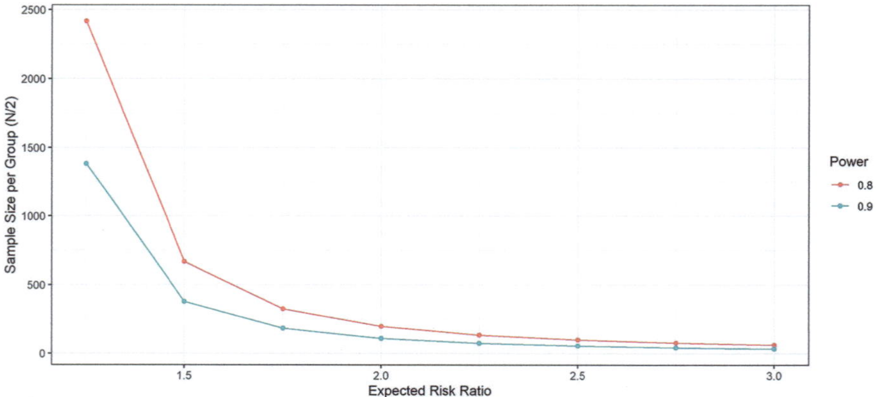

Fig. 7 Relationship of sample size estimates and expected risk ratio by power

standard deviation of the measure of interest. Let us assume that we are developing a randomized controlled trial with two independent study groups given different therapies. We anticipate that the rate of cardiovascular disease in the standard therapy group (Group 1) is 20%, and the rate of cardiovascular disease in the new therapy group (Group 2) is 14%. The expected effect size for the risk ratio (RR) = (Risk in Group 1/Risk in Group 2) = (14/20) = 0.70. We are assuming that there will be a 1:1 enrollment ratio among both groups of participants, and we will use the standard values of $\alpha = 0.05$ (significance level) and $\beta = 0.80$ (power). The resulting sample size estimate is 614 participants for each arm of the study, resulting in 1228 total participants. Figure 7 illustrates the relationship between sample size estimates and the expected RR for this study. The main takeaway should be that as the expected point estimate increases, the required sample size per group decreases. Also, take notice that relaxing the power estimate results in a lower sample size requirement.

Briefly, hypothesis testing can be performed with one-tail or two-tails. The default in biomedical research tends to be the two-tailed (two-sided) test. In two-sided tests, you are investigating an effect that could be in either direction (higher or lower) relative to the null hypothesis. The direction of effect ultimately does not matter. An example question could be: in our study population, is the mean SBP for patients taking beta blockers the same as the mean SBP for those not taking beta blockers? (the null hypothesis being that both group means are equivalent; the alternative hypothesis being that both group means are different). One-tailed tests will investigate your hypothesis in one direction. An example question would be: in our study population, do patients taking beta-blockers have an SBP lower than 120 mm Hg? The null hypothesis would be that study participants have an SBP higher than 120 mm Hg, and the alternative hypothesis is that the study participants have an SBP lower than 120 mm Hg. Note that the direction for the hypothesis test matters.

As another example, building and validating a risk prediction model is a different statistical task than testing whether one treatment seems to be superior to an alternative. There is no single "power" estimate for one significance test in building a prediction model as there are many different variables included and tests that may be performed as part of this process. Determining whether the sample size is sufficient to develop and validate a prediction model is a complex task that may be based on the ability to achieve a certain level of precision in the overall outcome along with a desired small level of prediction error. Some practical guidance is provided in papers by Riley et al. and van Smeden et al., but the details are beyond the scope of this chapter [8, 9]. The important thing the reader should understand is, in a nutshell, that a study that professes to present a prediction model should have justified that the sample size was sufficient to achieve the task. The reader should also look with skepticism at papers that present so-called prediction models, which include many predictor variables based on a relatively small number of observed outcomes. We hesitate to provide any rules of thumb, but the reader should be wary of a multivariable model developed with a cohort of 100 patients, 10 of whom experienced the clinical event, that makes strong claims about its predictive accuracy.

12 Adaptive/Platform Trials

With the challenge of enrolling large numbers of patients into randomized clinical trials (as well as financial considerations for sponsors and ethical considerations for patients), there is increasing interest in methods to increase trial efficiency. One of the simplest methods is to conduct a *factorial* clinical trial where two (or more) interventions are simultaneously assessed in a group of patients. If the trial interventions do not interact (one treatment does not affect the effect size of the other), a factorial design allows investigators to answer two different questions with approximately the same effort required to conduct one clinical trial. Assumptions of independence of the interventions, however, are often unclear before conducting the trial, leading to concerns that it may be difficult to accurately assess the independent effect of each treatment when the effect of one intervention may be influenced by the presence or absence of the other. It is also difficult to perform factorial trials of interventions that may not be well-suited to be given together or that may be contraindicated for one another.

Another promising development is the concept of a *platform trial*. Rather than testing just one treatment, such trials are designed to answer multiple clinical questions using a shared trial infrastructure to screen, consent, and monitor patients without the need to set up a new trial infrastructure for each new treatment [10]. Platform trials are typically organized around a disease/population of interest, such as "hospitalized patients with coronavirus disease of 2019 (COVID-19)," but may test many different treatments within that single data collection framework. For example, the Randomized Evaluation of COVID-19 Therapy (RECOVERY) trial has tested no fewer than nine unique treatments for hospitalized COVID-19 patients, all within the shared infrastructure of a single trial, though each treatment has its own statistical analysis to estimate its unique treatment effect. Platform trials may be designed as factorial trials (patients randomized to multiple treatment domains) or designed such that patients are only randomized to one "intervention" of interest, but all are compared against a common control group, still greatly improving efficiency over requiring each treatment to run a 1:1 allocation trial with their own control group.

Another proposed method to increase trial efficiency is *enrichment*. Prognostic enrichment refers to the recruitment of patients expected to have a high incidence of the outcome. By focusing on patients with the highest risk of the outcome, the intervention is tested on those who presumably have the most to gain from treatment, making it easier to detect a treatment benefit with a fixed number of patients enrolled in the trial. A second type of enrichment is predictive enrichment, where inclusion criteria are adjusted during the study to focus recruitment on patients that seem more likely to benefit from the treatment being tested in the trial. Because prognostic enrichment increases the baseline event rate and predictive enrichment increases the expected treatment effect, both types of enrichment reduce the number of patients needed to detect a treatment benefit. One challenge of enrichment is that the results are only generalizable to patients who meet the strict eligibility criteria; however, the benefit is that the trial has essentially focused on the population most likely to benefit and, in so doing, has effectively told the clinical community which patients are most suitable for that particular treatment. It limits generalizability by its design because the trial data tell us that these patients are most likely to benefit from the intervention under study.

Another method to improve trial efficiency is the *adaptive trial*, which involves one or more pre-specified adaptation rules. Traditional clinical trials use "fixed" designs meaning that the patient population, interventions, outcomes, and sample size are agreed upon and the trial is run to completion, at which time the data are reviewed and a decision is made based on the results. Recently, it has been acknowledged that it is possible (and even desirable) that information gathered during early portions of the trial be used to improve the conduct of the remainder of the trial. Adaptive trials may use information accrued during the trial to revise the needed sample size, modify the patient population, change the treatment allocation ratio, drop or add interventions, or change the primary analysis. It is necessary to pre-specify all potential adaptations to ensure that the operating characteristics of the trial can be established and that it does not become easier to get a "positive" result simply by fishing around for data that look better. When designed and carried out properly, adaptive trials can increase efficiency without affecting the rigor of the trial results.

Several of the methods discussed above can be combined in a single platform trial with adaptive features (e.g., dropping arms, adding new treatments, and enriching the population may all be part of a single design). Adaptive platform trials have the potential to provide robust answers to clinical questions while minimizing the number of patients exposed to less effective treatments, but they are complicated to design, analyze, and interpret. Despite these challenges, the COVID-19 pandemic has offered several examples of highly successful adaptive platform trials (e.g., RECOVERY; Randomized, Embedded, Multifactorial Adaptive Platform Trial for

Community-Acquired Pneumonia [REMAP-CAP]; World Health Organization COVID-19 Solidarity Trial for COVID-19 Treatments [SOLIDARITY]) so it is likely we will see more of these in the future.

13 Concluding Thoughts

Some readers may wonder about the necessity of more complex statistical methods, believing that any intervention that is worthwhile would have such an obvious effect that it should be evident from even the simplest of statistics. The authors have some sympathy for this view. However, it must be acknowledged that much of the "low-hanging fruit" has already been picked—interventions and/or effects that are exceedingly obvious have largely been identified already—and yet we have not and should not give up on improving clinical outcomes for patients. Interventions that are so obviously effective that they do not need a statistical test to prove their effectiveness are relatively rare in modern medicine but that does not mean we abandon the search for them altogether. As we are investigating ever smaller and/or more complex effects, it becomes necessary to use more sophisticated analyses. Furthermore, many of the analyses described herein offer significant performance advantages, such as the ability to determine whether a treatment is effective with fewer total patients exposed in a research study. They also offer the potential to use more "patient-centered" outcome measures that can include survival, hard clinical endpoints such as hospitalization or myocardial infarction, and patient-reported outcomes such as quality of life or physical function all in a single analysis to test whether a treatment has an overall clinical benefit.

References

1. Kassambara A, Kosinski M, Bieck P. survminer: Drawing survival curves using "ggplot2". Published online 2021. https://CRAN.R-project.org/package=survminer.
2. R Core Team. R: a language and environment for statistical computing. Published online 2013. http://www.R-project.org/.
3. Wickham H. Ggplot2: elegant graphics for data analysis. New York: Springer; 2016. https://ggplot2.tidyverse.org.
4. Rubin DB. An overview of multiple imputation. In: Proceedings of the survey research methods section; 1988. p. 79–84.
5. Ferreira JP, Jhund PS, Duarte K, et al. Use of the win ratio in cardiovascular trials. JACC Heart Fail. 2020;8(6):441–50. https://doi.org/10.1016/j.jchf.2020.02.010.
6. DeMets DL, Lan KK. Interim analysis: the alpha spending function approach. Stat Med. 1994;13(13–14):1341–52; discussion 1353–6. https://doi.org/10.1002/sim.4780131308.
7. Rosner B. Fundamentals of biostatistics. Cengage Learning; 2015.
8. Riley RD, Ensor J, Snell KIE, et al. Calculating the sample size required for developing a clinical prediction model. BMJ. 2020;368:m441. https://doi.org/10.1136/bmj.m441.

9. van Smeden M, de Groot JA, Moons KG, et al. No rationale for 1 variable per 10 events criterion for binary logistic regression analysis. BMC Med Res Methodol. 2016;16:163.
10. Adaptive Platform Trials Coalition. Adaptive platform trials: definition, design, conduct and reporting considerations. Nat Rev Drug Discov. 2019;18(10):797–807.

Additional Resources

Boden W, O'Rourke R. Optimal medical therapy with or without PCI for stable coronary disease. N Engl J Med. 2007;356(15):1503–16.
Friedman L, Furberg C, DeMets D. Fundamentals of clinical trials. 3rd ed. New York: Springer; 1992.
Guyatt GH, Sackett DL, Sinclair JC, Hayward R, Cook DJ, Cook RJ. Users' guides to the medical literature. IX. A method for grading health care recommendations. Evidence-Based Medicine Working Group. JAMA. 1995;274(22):1800–4. https://doi.org/10.1001/jama.274.22.1800.
Hulley SB. Designing clinical research. Philadelphia: Lippincott Williams & Wilkins; 2007.
Yusuf S, Hawken S, Ounpuu S, et al. Effect of potentially modifiable risk factors associated with myocardial infarction in 52 countries (the INTERHEART study): case-control study. Lancet. 2004;364(9438):937–52. https://doi.org/10.1016/S0140-6736(04)17018-9.

Pharmaceutical Development and Approval in the United States of Agents to Influence Cardiovascular Health

Mary Katherine Cheeley and Laurie Cavendish

Key Points

- Drug development consists of multiple steps to ensure both efficacy and safety.
- Drug discovery to identify a compound with the potential to affect a therapeutic target is followed by preclinical studies in *in vitro* and animal models to characterize its administration, absorption, distribution, metabolism, and excretion.
- Drug developers submit an Investigational New Drug Application to the Food and Drug Administration (FDA) before beginning clinical research.
- Clinical studies progress through Phases 1, 2, and 3 with FDA guidance before drug developers submit a New Drug Application to the FDA for a new chemical entity pharmaceutical (or a Biologics License Application for biological compounds).
- Phase 1 studies enroll healthy volunteers without the disease/condition under study and are primarily to demonstrate the safety of an investigational drug.
- Phase 2 studies typically enroll a relatively small cohort of participants with the disease/condition and aim to demonstrate efficacy and dose–response and collect information needed for designing Phase 3 trials.
- Phase 3 studies enroll a relatively large cohort of participants and aim to demonstrate efficacy and safety in groups with the target disease/condition.
- Phase 4 trials are conducted after the drug has already been approved and is being marketed to provide information about the long-term risks and benefits of the drug.
- A cardiovascular outcome trial is a Phase 3 trial designed to demonstrate the reduced risk of major adverse cardiovascular events.

M. K. Cheeley (✉) · L. Cavendish
Department of Pharmacy and Medical Nutrition, Grady Health System, Atlanta, GA, USA
e-mail: mcheeley@gmh.edu; lmcavendish@gmh.edu

- The FDA has provided specific guidance for the development of agents that affect cardiovascular health including lipoprotein- and lipid-altering therapies, antihypertensive agents, and agents for heart failure, type 2 diabetes mellitus, weight management, and nonalcoholic steatohepatitis.
- Drugs may be removed from the market after approval for safety reasons, either at the request of the FDA or voluntarily, or for the drug developer's own reasons.

1 Overview

As science and research grow, more potential therapeutic agents are discovered, but only a few will ever make it to market. The following chapter describes the drug development and approval process from discovery through postmarketing surveillance.

2 Drug Discovery

The first step in the drug development process is to determine which medications and therapies need to be developed. As science continues to provide a better understanding of disease processes and pathophysiology, new targets for drug development are also discovered.

Once a compound has been discovered that alters a therapeutic target, the process can begin to develop the compound into a therapeutic agent. The main categories of therapeutic agents include small molecule drugs, which are chemically synthesized, and biologics, which are made from living sources and may include vaccines, blood and blood components, therapeutic proteins, gene therapies, etc. Examples of biological compounds include monoclonal antibodies, recombinant human proteins, and small interfering RNA compounds. The process for approval of a new chemical entity pharmaceutical involves the preparation of a New Drug Application (NDA), whereas that for a biological compound uses a process known as a Biologics License Application (BLA).

Once a promising compound has been identified, the next step is to characterize the agent's administration, absorption, distribution, metabolism, and excretion. This is undertaken initially in preclinical studies that are completed *in vitro* and in animal models, followed by clinical studies in humans. The study sponsor will generally meet with the Food and Drug Administration (FDA) at each stage of the process, submit an Investigational New Drug (IND) application, and seek approval to move forward with the next stage from preclinical studies into Phase 1 clinical studies, then Phase 2, and finally Phase 3. Once the Phase 3 studies have been completed, an NDA is prepared, although this may at times occur while final Phase 3 studies are ongoing, such as seeking NDA review while a large-scale cardiovascular outcomes trial (CVOT) is underway. Phase 4 clinical trials are performed after the FDA has approved the medication, can last for many years, and are used to obtain more information about the drug's long-term safety and effectiveness.

3   Preclinical Studies

Before any medication can be tested on human subjects, it must first be shown that there is no evidence of potential for serious toxicity or harm. Preclinical studies provide detailed information regarding dosing, mechanism of action, and toxicity. These investigations include the evaluation of multiple potential toxicities (major body systems and genotoxicity), effects on reproduction, and carcinogenicity.

4   Phase 1 Clinical Trials

Phase 1 is the first phase of development that involves testing in humans. Initial testing is typically in healthy volunteers who are given the drug over a relatively short duration to determine dosing schemes. Dosage is usually studied in a stepwise, escalating manner to identify potential adverse effects and their severity at a lower dosage before moving to the next higher dosage. It should be noted that dose refers to the amount of medication taken at one time, while dosage refers to the specific amount, number, and frequency of doses employed over a specific period of time.

Information is also gathered on efficacy in Phase 1, which dictates the final dose(s) and delivery method chosen for investigation in Phase 2. Additional Phase 1 studies are employed to define the pharmacokinetics of the medication, as well as potential interactions with other medications that may be commonly used in the disease or condition for which the agent will be utilized. Slightly more than half of all drugs will advance from Phase 1 to Phase 2.

5   Phase 2 Clinical Trials

Phase 2 clinical trials begin to test the drug in a small cohort of human participants. Some Phase 2 trials may include healthy volunteers, but most are completed in participants with the disease or condition for which an indication is being sought. This group of participants is larger than that employed in Phase 1 trials. The intent is to demonstrate efficacy and dose–response and to provide information to inform the size of the group that will be needed to show meaningful efficacy in Phase 3 trials. Approximately one-third of drugs that enter Phase 2 clinical trials will advance to Phase 3.

6 Phase 3 Clinical Trials

Phase 3 trials include the largest cohort of participants, and are aimed at demonstrating efficacy, as well as continued evaluation of safety in larger and more broadly representative groups. Phase 3 development trials will often include a comparison to an existing therapy to allow evaluation of relative safety and efficacy. Participants must have the target disease or condition to be included in this phase of trials. The inclusion criteria for these trials are informed by the FDA standards, as well as by the results from Phases 1 and 2 such as dosing, duration of therapy needed to show efficacy, adverse conditions to exclude, and when to collect data for outcomes and safety. Phase 3 trial populations are intended to be broadly representative of the group for whom the drug would be prescribed in clinical practice.

In some instances, an agent may only need to show efficacy based on the effects on a surrogate marker, such as lowering the triglyceride (TG) concentration in patients with severe hypertriglyceridemia, which is a surrogate for reduction in the risk for acute pancreatitis. In other cases, the FDA may require completion of a trial to demonstrate efficacy for reducing the risk of clinical events, such as a trial to demonstrate reduced risk for major adverse cardiovascular events (MACE), which is typically referred to as a CVOT.

7 Submission of an Application for the FDA Review

Submission of an NDA or BLA to the FDA is generally done once Phase 3 trials have been completed, although, as previously mentioned, in some cases the application may be submitted for the review, while larger clinical outcomes trials are underway. Initial approval for marketing for a medication or biologic agent intended to impact cardiovascular (CV) health may be with a narrow indication that might subsequently be expanded based on CVOT results.

The key elements of an NDA or BLA include:

- Proposed labeling, including indication, route of administration and dosing, patient instructions, potential for abuse, and clinical effects;
- Integrated summaries of safety and efficacy data (preclinical studies through Phase 3 trials and results from trials that may have been conducted outside of the United States);
- Information on chemistry, manufacturing, and controls.

Once the application is accepted, the FDA has 6–10 months to make an approval or denial decision. During the review, each member of the FDA team reviews their respective section of the application. FDA inspectors also travel to clinical trial sites and determine if there is any evidence of fabrication, manipulation, or withholding of any information. Manufacturing facilities are also inspected for compliance with Good Manufacturing Practices. All the individual reviews are compiled into an "action packet." This packet is then presented for an official decision regarding the drug.

If a drug is deemed safe and effective, and all outstanding issues and questions from the FDA have been addressed and resolved, the FDA will work with the manufacturer to develop patient education, prescribing information, and marketing materials and approve the agent for marketing in the United States. On occasion, the FDA can also request additional studies, and the drug manufacturer can determine whether they would like to continue the approval process, appeal, or withdraw the application.

Another special circumstance may arise where the agency would like to obtain advice from outside experts regarding the potential benefits and risks of an agent for which approval is being sought. This occurs most often for new pharmaceutical classes or in situations where significant questions are present regarding the potential risk to benefit ratio. The FDA may convene an Advisory Committee to elicit such independent, expert advice. This forum also allows the public to provide comments, often including those from patients with the disease and advocacy organizations. In most instances the agency will follow the recommendation of the Advisory Committee regarding approval of a new medication, although the ultimate decision has historically been contrary to the majority Advisory Committee vote in some instances (~10 to 20% of reviews).

8 Key Elements of FDA Guidance for Development of Agents That Affect Cardiovascular Health

Approval of some categories of drugs requires undertaking a Phase 3 CVOT to demonstrate reduced risk of MACE and/or CV safety. The FDA has provided guidance for the development of several types of agents that affect CV health including lipoprotein- and lipid-altering therapies, antihypertensive agents, as well as agents for management of heart failure, type 2 diabetes mellitus, body weight, and nonalcoholic steatohepatitis (NASH) (Table 1).

8.1 *Lipoprotein- and Lipid-Altering Therapies*

New drugs targeting the lowering of lipoproteins continue to increase, with a number of new therapeutic targets under development. There are two main targets of therapy, low-density lipoprotein cholesterol (LDL-C) and TG, however new targets are being investigated, including lipoprotein (a) [Lp(a)] and apolipoprotein (Apo) CIII. The FDA recognizes LDL-C reduction as a surrogate for atherosclerotic cardiovascular disease (ASCVD) risk reduction, therefore therapies that target LDL-C may not be required to have completed a CVOT before initial approval. However,

Table 1 Description of Food and Drug Administration guidance documents for the development of agents that affect cardiovascular health

Disease state	FDA guidance document	Key elements	Is CVOT required for initial approval?
Hyperlipidemia	Clinical Evaluation of Lipid-Altering Agents (1998; withdrawn 2010)	• FDA works with sponsors of drugs for existing and new therapeutic targets on an individual basis	Should be in progress prior to applying for FDA approval
Hypertension	Hypertension Indication: Drug Labeling for CV Outcome Claims (March 2011)	• Recommendations on labeling verbiage and justification for adding outcome claims to labeling	No General, qualitative claim of CV outcome benefits pertains to all classes of antihypertensive drugs
	Hypertension: Conducting Studies of Drugs to Treat Patients on a Background of Multiple Antihypertensive Drugs (July 2018)	• Two paths for approval of antihypertensive drugs on a background of multiple antihypertensive drugs – Superiority to PBO in reducing BP in patients on appropriate doses of ≥ 2 drugs with different MOAs – Superiority to another (or >1) antihypertensive drug (active comparator) in reducing BP in patients already receiving maximum doses of ≥ 3 drugs with different MOAs	
	Hypertension: Developing Fixed-Combination Drug Products for Treatment (November 2018)	• Each component must contribute to claimed effects and dosage of each is such that the combination is safe and effective for the intended population • One Phase 3, double-blind randomized trial in population where initiating therapy with two drugs is appropriate is sufficient to demonstrate effectiveness of combination drug products of previously approved antihypertensive drugs	
Heart failure	Treatment for Heart Failure: Endpoints for Drug Development (2019)	• Effect on symptoms or physical function, without favorable effect on survival or risk of hospitalization can be basis for approval • Recommendations for mortality data (as efficacy or safety endpoint), symptomatic efficacy endpoints, hospitalization, outpatient metrics of acute decompensation, biomarkers and surrogate endpoints, acute heart failure, and heart failure with preserved ejection fraction • Pediatric guidance available in separate documents	Yes However, if drug being evaluated is in a class with established mortality data, additional mortality endpoints may not be required

Table 1 (continued)

Disease state	FDA guidance document	Key elements	Is CVOT required for initial approval?
Type 2 diabetes mellitus	Type 2 Diabetes Mellitus: Evaluating the Safety of New Drugs for Improving Glycemic Control (2020; previous 2008 guidance was withdrawn)	• Safety database should include data from clinical trials of sufficient duration (patient-years exposed) • Development program should include patients with stage 3/4 CKD, established CVD, and age >65 years	Not technically "Adverse CV outcomes remain an important source of morbidity and mortality for patients with diabetes mellitus. Therefore, sponsors should use rigorous methods for the collection of adverse CV events and assess them by adjudication"

	Diabetes Mellitus: Efficacy Endpoints for Clinical Trials Investigating Antidiabetic Drugs and Biological Products (2023)	• Different efficacy endpoints may be appropriate depending on clinical goal
		  – Change from baseline A1C is accepted primary endpoint to support glycemic control
		  – Reduction in risk of hypoglycemia (along with reduction or maintenance of acceptable A1C) is clinically relevant endpoint for subjects with diabetes, especially those using insulin (guidance provides definitions, trial considerations and tools to facilitate hypoglycemia-related drug claims)
		  – Other clinical endpoints can be proposed by sponsor (e.g., macrovascular or microvascular outcomes, changes in BP, serum lipids, body wt)	

Weight management	Developing Products for Weight Management (2007, Revision 1 that will replace 1996 guidance)	• Studies should include patients:
		  – At all wt classifications
		  – From various demographic backgrounds
		• Sample size adequate to assess safety endpoints (larger than size needed to assess efficacy)
		• At least 1 year duration
		• Product effective if after 1 year:
		  – Difference in mean wt loss between active and PBO groups is ≥5% and difference is statistically significant
		  – Proportion of subjects who lose ≥5% of baseline body wt in active is ≥35%, ~double the proportion in PBO, and difference between groups is statistically significant
		• Changes in common wt-related comorbidities should be factored into efficacy assessment
		• Specific inclusion criteria for patients with T2DM
		• Specific safety measures based on drug's MOA
		• Provides specific guidance for subgroups, products used in combination, medication-induced wt gain, trials in pediatric patients, labeling considerations, stand-alone indications for wt-related comorbidities, and metabolic syndrome
			No

(continued)

Table 1 (continued)

Disease state	FDA guidance document	Key elements	Is CVOT required for initial approval?

Nonalcoholic steatohepatitis	Noncirrhotic Nonalcoholic Steatohepatitis with Liver Fibrosis: Developing Drugs for Treatment (2018)	• Encourages use of animal models for NASH to screen and identify potential investigational drugs; select based on drug's MOA
		• If potential for liver toxicity, institute plan to monitor liver safety early in development
		• Exclude patients with evidence of abnormal liver synthetic function from early phase trials until the drug's tolerability and safety characterized
		• Provides detailed Phase 2 and 3 development considerations and pediatric considerations
		• Endpoints reasonably likely to predict clinical benefit and support accelerated approval include:
		  – Resolution of steatohepatitis on overall histopathological reading and no worsening of liver fibrosis on NASH CRN fibrosis score; or
		  – Improvement in liver fibrosis ≥ 1 stage and no worsening of steatohepatitis; or
		  – Both resolution of steatohepatitis and improvement of fibrosis
			Not technically "Given the growing evidence of a link between NAFLD and cardiovascular disease, cardiovascular safety should be adequately monitored in clinical trials. FDA encourages sponsors to establish an expert committee to adjudicate cases that meet protocol defined criteria for major adverse cardiac events"

	Nonalcoholic Steatohepatitis with Compensated Cirrhosis: Developing Drugs for Treatment (2019)	• Provides Phase 3 program considerations
		  – Include only patients whose cirrhosis is secondary to NASH who have histological diagnosis of NASH and other causes of chronic liver disease are ruled out; exclude patients with decompensated cirrhosis
		  – Evaluate effect relative to PBO on composite endpoint of time to complication of ascites, variceal hemorrhage, hepatic encephalopathy, worsening MELD score, liver transplantation, or death from any cause
		  – Clinical outcome trials strongly recommended because insufficient evidence to support histological improvements as surrogate endpoint
		  – Develop algorithm and specify guidelines for monitoring liver function and have expert committee to adjudicate cases of drug-induced liver injury	

A1C glycated hemoglobin, *BP* blood pressure, *CKD* chronic kidney disease, *CRN* clinical research network, *CV* cardiovascular, *CVD* cardiovascular disease, *CVOT* cardiovascular outcomes trial, *FDA* Food and Drug Administration, *MELD* model for end-stage liver disease, *MOA* mechanism of action, *NAFLD* nonalcoholic fatty liver disease, *NASH* nonalcoholic steatohepatitis, *PBO* placebo, *T2DM* type 2 diabetes mellitus, *wt* weight

https://www.fda.gov/regulatory-information/search-fda-guidance-documents

such a trial must generally be underway and "substantially" enrolled (generally at least 50%). For example, drugs targeting proprotein convertase subtilisin kexin type 9 showed reductions in LDL-C and were approved for use before the conclusion and reporting of the results from their CVOTs [1, 2].

Agents with other lipoprotein-related targets, for example Lp(a) and Apo CIII, will require outcome trials to be completed before initial approval, as lowering these targets has not been previously demonstrated to reduce MACE risk. And, as with any new agent for which FDA clearance is being sought, sponsors must show a lack of material off-target effects when a new mechanism of action or drug target is being investigated. A reduction in atherogenic lipoproteins is important, however, as in the case with torcetrapib, concurrent increases in systolic blood pressure and aldosterone were likely contributors to an increase in MACE, and clinical development was stopped [3].

Severe hypertriglyceridemia (TG $\geq$500 mg/dL) is an area with multiple drugs in development. Due to the rare nature of this disease and the even more rare consequence of acute pancreatitis, an outcomes trial showing a reduction in acute pancreatitis would be time consuming and costly, and likely limit the development of agents for this indication. Therefore, a clinically important reduction in the TG concentration and the lack of evidence for material off-target effects are sufficient to apply for FDA clearance.

8.2   Antihypertensive Agents

In 2011 most drugs that were indicated to reduce blood pressure did not include information in the label about the clinical benefits that resulted from a reduction in blood pressure. At that time, the FDA recommended a standard label for antihypertensive drugs. Their hope was that an updated label, with clinical trial data, would encourage appropriate use of these drugs and improve CV outcomes, and thus the guidelines for label information for this class were updated [4].

Data from large epidemiological data sets show an absolute increase in the risk of CV events as blood pressure increases, particularly for patients with comorbid conditions that also increase CV risk. Both placebo-controlled and active-controlled trials demonstrated primarily a reduction in risk of stroke, but also showed reductions in myocardial infarction and CV mortality. All outcome trials that have been conducted included multidrug regimens; therefore, determinations about individual drug classes have been difficult.

In light of the multimodal blood pressure-lowering approach used in clinical trials with increased doses and/or addition of one or more additional agent(s) if blood pressure was not adequately controlled, the FDA recommended manufacturers submit updated label applications which included the following information:

Indications and Usage–"DRUGNAME is a [name of pharmacologic class] indicated for the treatment of hypertension, to lower blood pressure. Lowering blood pressure reduces the risk of fatal and nonfatal cardiovascular events, primarily strokes and myocardial infarctions." They also proposed changes to the Full Prescribing Information and Clinical Studies sections, to include landmark trial results for the class of medications, along with others.

In 2018, the FDA released two additional sets of guidance regarding the conduct of studies to treat patients on a background of multiple antihypertensive drugs, and the development of fixed-combination drugs for the treatment of hypertension [5, 6].

8.3 Agents for Heart Failure

In 2019, the FDA provided guidance regarding endpoints for the development of drugs for the treatment of heart failure [7]. By doing so, the FDA aimed to make clear that even without a favorable effect on survival or risk of hospitalization, an effect on symptoms or physical function can be a pathway for drug approval to treat heart failure. The document also provides guidance on how to assess mortality effects. It is mainly intended to describe chronic heart failure, both with reduced ejection fraction and preserved ejection fraction, although sections on acute heart failure and pediatric considerations are also included.

8.4 Agents for Type 2 Diabetes Mellitus

In 2008, the FDA recommended that manufacturers demonstrate that new drugs to improve glycemic control (glycated hemoglobin, A1C) in patients with type 2 diabetes mellitus, "do not result in an unacceptable increase in CV risk" [8]. Since then, many CVOTs have been conducted, which were generally designed to show noninferiority to placebo regarding MACE. Some have demonstrated a reduction in CV events, such as selected agents in the glucagon-like peptide-1 receptor agonist and sodium-glucose cotransporter-2 inhibitor classes. Therefore, in 2020 a new FDA guidance was released which recommends that trials completed for inclusion in the NDA include the following patient characteristics and duration of therapies [9]:

- At least 4000 patient-years of exposure to the new drug in Phase 3 clinical trials (all dosing strengths);
- At least 1500 patients exposed to the new drug for at least 1 year and 500 patients for at least 2 years;
- At least 500 patients with stages 3–4 chronic kidney disease;
- At least 600 patients with established CVD (prior myocardial infarction, documented coronary artery disease, previous stroke, or peripheral vascular disease);
- At least 600 patients older than 65 years of age.

There are also recommendations pertaining to the level of rigor with which data on CV outcomes are collected. However, CVOTs are no longer required for all new agents intended to treat type 2 diabetes mellitus. In 2023, the FDA released guidance describing the efficacy endpoints for clinical trials of antidiabetic drugs and biological products, which included definitions and other considerations for A1C, hypoglycemia, and additional endpoints [10].

8.5 Agents for Body Weight Management

In 2004, the FDA sought public comment and convened an Advisory Board to update 1996 guidance regarding drugs for weight management. Their recommendations resulted in the release of an FDA guidance document in 2007 which includes all phases of the clinical trial process [11]. Some key features of the guidance for adult patients include:

- Phases 1 and 2

  - Due to excess adiposity and the impact that can have on drug absorption, distribution, metabolism, and excretion, the pharmacokinetic profile should be examined in trial participants with a body mass index (BMI) of 27–35 kg/m^2, and early phase trials should include a range of doses to identify no-effect and maximally tolerated doses.
  - Phase 2 trials should be long enough to capture the maximal or near-maximal weight loss, and consideration should be given as to whether the product will be used in a fixed-dose or dose-titration scheme which affects study design choices.

- Phase 3

  - Trials should be randomized, double-blind, and placebo-controlled; participants should have or be at significant risk for weight-related morbidity and mortality with BMI $\geq$30 kg/m^2 or $\geq$27 kg/m^2 in the presence of comorbidities.
  - All clinical trial participants should receive standard of care lifestyle/behavioral interventions aimed at producing weight loss through caloric restriction and appropriate physical activity.

- The primary efficacy endpoints should be, "a comparison of the mean absolute or percent change in body weight between the active-product and placebo-treated groups and the proportion of patients in each treatment group who lose greater than or equal to 5% of baseline weight."

8.6 Agents for Nonalcoholic Steatohepatitis

In 2018, the FDA provided guidance for a new area of therapeutic interest, noncirrhotic NASH with liver fibrosis [12]. This included guidance on the use of animal models in the development of drug therapies for NASH. The guidance recommends using an appropriate model based on the proposed mechanism of action of the investigational drug. If liver toxicity is observed in animal studies, then the sponsor is encouraged to develop a plan to monitor liver toxicity throughout the entire drug development process, although it may be challenging to determine such liver signals given the nature of the disease state that is being targeted. Lastly, since these drugs are being developed for a condition in which liver function, a major pathway for drug metabolism and excretion, is likely impaired, the FDA recommends first establishing tolerability, preliminary safety, and pharmacokinetics in patients with normal liver function. Once safety and tolerability are determined in a healthy population, a dosing trial that includes participants with all classifications of NASH is recommended.

During Phase 2 studies, sponsors may utilize noninvasive biomarkers for proof-of-concept endpoints and enroll patients without baseline histological documentation of NASH. This will allow the evaluation of endpoints in a similar population as those planned for in Phase 3 trials. As the Phase 2 program progresses, sponsors should determine the drug effect on histological endpoints (reduction in inflammation, improvement in fibrosis, or both) and, because these changes take time, Phase 2 trials should be at least 12–18 months in length. The last recommendation for Phase 2 trials includes guidance on the use of biomarkers, such as how they can be used in screening, as prognostic indicators, and as markers of progression to cirrhosis.

In Phase 3 studies, sponsors should include patients with various other metabolic conditions, given their overlap with NASH. The FDA also outlines the histologic and diagnostic criteria that would qualify a patient for enrollment in a NASH trial. This includes, but is not limited to, a model for end-stage liver disease (MELD) score ≤ 12, a NASH activity score ≥ 3, and fibrosis greater than 1 but less than 4. The guidance also provides exclusion criteria including evidence of portal hypertension, other diagnoses of chronic liver disease, and aspartate transaminase and alanine transaminase levels greater than 5 times the upper limit of normal.

Per the FDA "the ultimate goal of NASH treatment is to slow, halt, or reverse disease progression and improve clinical outcomes" [12]. Slowing the progression of a disease takes time, therefore the FDA recommends the use of surrogate endpoints, such as histological improvements or worsening MELD score, to show either benefit or detriment. With regard to safety, given the baseline hepatic dysfunction of patients with NASH, a specific algorithm to monitor liver function is important, and sponsors should establish an expert committee to adjudicate cases of hepatic decompensation. Lastly, as the link between nonalcoholic fatty liver disease and ASCVD is becoming more apparent, the FDA encourages monitoring ASCVD outcomes and establishing an expert committee to adjudicate cases of MACE. Pediatric NASH seems to be different in course and histology than adult NASH, so the FDA also comments on the need for robust adult data before pediatric trials can begin.

In 2019, the FDA released guidance for the development of drugs for the treatment of NASH with compensated cirrhosis, which has goals of halting or slowing the progression of fibrosis, preventing clinical decompensation, reducing the need for liver transplantation, and improving survival [13]. This guidance focuses on the enrollment criteria, trial design, efficacy endpoints, and safety considerations for Phase 3 trials and identifies knowledge gaps and challenges in developing drugs for this indication, but does not address clinical development of drugs for the treatment of decompensated cirrhosis resulting from NASH; it refers to the previously described guidance for topics such as using animal models and approaches for monitoring potential liver toxicity.

9 Drug Removals from the Market

When necessary, there are well-defined mechanisms for the FDA to request or require drugs to be removed from the market. This is traditionally done for safety reasons, and the manufacturer of a drug may either voluntarily remove the drug from the market pursuant to a request from the FDA or for their own reasons.

An example of an FDA requested removal was lorcaserin due to possible increased risks for pancreatic and colorectal cancers [14]. No safety signals were observed in clinical trials, however after FDA approval, trends began to emerge. The FDA reviewed safety information, warned the public of the potential risk they were investigating, and later requested that the manufacturer voluntarily remove the drug from the market, which was done. In another instance, the manufacturer voluntarily removed rofecoxib from the US market immediately upon becoming aware of results from a long-term safety study that showed an increased risk of myocardial infarction or stroke [15]. This official removal occurred after a period of increased warnings in the product labeling, which prompted further studies and surveillance. Immediate-release exenatide and albiglutide were removed from the market by the manufacturers due to a lack of sales and the availability of newer agents in the same class.

10 Conclusion

The drug approval process managed by the US FDA is a structured framework that allows rigorous evaluation of whether a drug provides benefits that outweigh its known or potential risks for the targeted population. CVOTs play a key role in the development of therapies with the potential to affect the risk of ASCVD. Understanding the purpose of a CVOT for certain drug classes is critical to conducting and appraising clinical research.

References

1. Schwartz GG, Steg PG, Szarek M, et al. Alirocumab and cardiovascular outcomes after acute coronary syndrome. N Engl J Med. 2018;379:2097–107.
2. Sabatine MS, Giugliano RP, Keech AC, et al. Evolocumab and clinical outcomes in patients with cardiovascular disease. N Engl J Med. 2017;376:1713–22.
3. Barter PJ, Caulfield M, Eriksson M, et al. Effects of torcetrapib in patients at high risk for coronary events. N Engl J Med. 2007;357:2109–22.
4. US Department of Health and Human Services. Food and Drug Administration. Center for Drug Evaluation and Research (CDER). Guidance for industry: hypertension indication: Drug labeling for cardiovascular outcome claims. 2011. https://www.fda.gov/media/134777/download#:~:text=This%20guidance%20is%20intended%20to%20assist%20applicants%20in,cardiovascular%20outcomes%20expected%20from%20such%20blood%20pressure%20reduction. Accessed 28 Jul 2023.
5. US Department of Health and Human Services. Food and Drug Administration. Center for Drug Evaluation and Research (CDER). Hypertension: conducting studies of drugs to treat patients on a background of multiple antihypertensive drugs: guidance for industry. 2018a. https://www.fda.gov/media/114731/download. Accessed 28 Jul 2023.
6. US Department of Health and Human Services. Food and Drug Administration. Center for Drug Evaluation and Research (CDER). Clinical/Medical. Hypertension: developing fixed-combination drug products for treatment. Guidance for industry. 2018b. https://www.fda.gov/media/117975/download. Accessed 1 Aug 2023.
7. US Department of Health and Human Services. Food and Drug Administration. Center for Drug Evaluation and Research (CDER). Center for Biologics Evaluation and Research (CBER). Treatment for heart failure: endpoints for drug development. Guidance for industry. 2019a. Clinical. https://www.fda.gov/media/128372/download. Accessed 1 Aug 2023.
8. US Department of Health and Human Services. Food and Drug Administration. Center for Drug Evaluation and Research (CDER). Guidance for industry: diabetes mellitus-evaluating cardiovascular risk in new antidiabetic therapies to treat type 2 diabetes. 2008. https://www.federalregister.gov/documents/2008/12/19/E8-30086/guidance-for-industry-on-diabetes-mellitus-evaluating-cardiovascular-risk-in-new-antidiabetic. Accessed 28 Jul 2023.
9. US Department of Health and Human Services. Food and Drug Administration. Center for Drug Evaluation and Research (CDER). Type 2 diabetes mellitus: evaluating the safety of new drugs for improving glycemic control: guidance for industry. 2020. https://www.fda.gov/media/135936/download. Accessed 28 Jul 2023.
10. US Department of Health and Human Services. Food and Drug Administration. Center for Drug Evaluation and Research (CDER). Diabetes mellitus: efficacy endpoints for clinical trials investigating antidiabetic drugs and biological products. Guidance for industry. 2023. Clinical/Medical. https://www.fda.gov/media/168475/download. Accessed 1 Aug 2023.
11. US Department of Health and Human Services. Food and Drug Administration. Center for Drug Evaluation and Research (CDER). Guidance for industry. Developing products for weight management. 2007. Clinical/Medical. Revision1. https://www.fda.gov/media/71252/download. Accessed 3 Aug 2023.

12. US Department of Health and Human Services. Food and Drug Administration. Center for Drug Evaluation and Research (CDER). Noncirrhotic nonalcoholic steatohepatitis with liver fibrosis: developing drugs for treatment. Guidance for industry. 2018c. https://www.fda.gov/media/119044/download. Accessed 31 Jul 2023.

13. US Department of Health and Human Services. Food and Drug Administration. Center for Drug Evaluation and Research (CDER). Nonalcoholic steatohepatitis with compensated cirrhosis: developing drugs for treatment. Guidance for industry. 2019b. https://www.fda.gov/media/127738/download. Accessed 31 Jul 2023.

14. Tak YJ, Lee SY. Long-term efficacy and safety of anti-obesity treatment: where do we stand? Curr Obes Rep. 2021;10:14–30.

15. Baron JA, Sandler RS, Bresalier RS, et al. Cardiovascular events associated with rofecoxib: final analysis of the APPROVe trial. Lancet. 2008;372:1756–64.

Biomarkers and Imaging Modalities to Detect Subclinical Atherosclerotic Cardiovascular Disease

Catherine J. McNeal, Philip D. Houck, Nguyen N. Nguyen, James Murchison, and Harry Chiang

Key Points

- Biomarkers are essential tools for early diagnosis and risk stratification, especially in subpopulations in which traditional risk scores are known to over- or underestimate risk.
- The development of biomarkers to detect subclinical atherosclerotic cardiovascular disease (ASCVD) continues to evolve as more knowledge is amassed regarding the underlying pathology of this disease.
- The pathology suggests biomarkers of endothelial function, immune-mediated inflammation, lipids and their metabolites, platelet function, hematopoietic factors, and the clotting cascade are key targets. Repair mechanisms suggest progenitor cells, natriuretic peptides, cardiac enzymes, apoptosis, and repair functions of the immune system are additional targets for biomarker discovery.
- High-sensitivity C-reactive protein (hsCRP) is a useful biomarker for predicting future cardiovascular events but it is also an important regulator of inflammatory processes; as such, it may also be elevated by any type of inflammation and/or infection; thus the relationship solely with the ASCVD risk must be interpreted with caution.
- Cardiac troponin is a frequently used biomarker in the evaluation of chest pain but has also been shown to have high prognostic utility in asymptomatic individuals for future ASCVD events.

C. J. McNeal (✉) · P. D. Houck
Division of Cardiology, Department of Internal Medicine, Baylor Scott and White Health, Temple, TX, USA
e-mail: Catherine.McNeal@bswhealth.org

N. N. Nguyen
Department of Pathology, Baylor Scott and White Health, Temple, TX, USA

J. Murchison · H. Chiang
Department of Radiology, Baylor Scott and White Health, Temple, TX, USA

K. C. Maki, D. P. Wilson (eds.), *Cardiovascular Outcomes Research*, Contemporary Cardiology, https://doi.org/10.1007/978-3-031-54960-1_4

- Measurements of brain natriuretic peptide (BNP) and N-terminal proBNP (NT-proBNP) are the gold standard for the diagnosis of heart failure. In addition, these biomarkers also provide prognostic information for mortality and first major cardiovascular events beyond traditional risk factors in individuals without ASCVD.
- A combination of biomarkers, including NT-proBNP, high sensitivity cardiac troponinT, hsCRP, and imaging studies of subclinical ASCVD, improves the prediction of both long- and short-term risk compared to standard risk factors and Pooled Cohort Equations.
- We discuss herein additional biomarkers including interleukin-6, the albumin-to-creatinine ratio, lipoprotein-associated phospholipase-A2, myeloperoxidase, and ceramides, although a number of other biomarkers have also been developed.
- Coronary artery calcium (CAC) scoring has demonstrated superiority to the Framingham Risk Score (FRS) and multiple studies have shown that approximately 20–25% of patients are more accurately classified into specific risk categories utilizing CAC scoring compared to FRS.
- The United States Preventive Services Task Force has no recommendation for the use of CAC scoring in asymptomatic patients due to insufficient evidence regarding benefit versus harm. The American College of Cardiology and American Heart Association 2019 guidelines for primary prevention state it may be reasonable to obtain CAC for asymptomatic adults aged 40–75 years with borderline risk (5% to <7.5% 10-year ASCVD risk) or intermediate risk ($\geq$7.5% to <20% 10-year ASCVD risk) if treatment remains uncertain.
- Measurements of carotid plaque and carotid artery intima-media thickness have been extensively utilized as potential screening tools in asymptomatic patients.
- Meta-analysis of ten different studies showed that carotid-femoral pulse wave velocity is a predictor of future ASCVD events independent of the FRS.
- Incidental calcium noted on chest computed tomography studies and mammograms should not be ignored since it may be an important finding to aid in the detection of subclinical ASCVD in asymptomatic patients.

1　Overview

This review summarizes the current evidence for biomarkers and imaging modalities to detect subclinical atherosclerotic cardiovascular disease (ASCVD), thereby improving the diagnosis, prognosis, and treatment outcomes for individuals without overt ASCVD. Our knowledge of this disease continues to evolve, but early detection remains a critical factor in clinical care and patient outcomes, with opportunities arising a decade or more before symptoms are present in order to prevent major adverse cardiovascular events (MACE) arising a decade or more before symptoms are present. For this reason, imaging modalities to detect the earliest pathological changes in the arterial wall, including minimal intimal thickening and arterial stiffness, are being used increasingly in clinical practice, even in children with genetic risk factors that predispose them to develop premature atherosclerosis.

This chapter focuses primarily on biomarkers and imaging modalities of subclinical ASCVD currently available for use by practicing clinicians but also describes some of the emerging biomarkers and imaging modalities that will likely soon come into use. Lipids are omitted as these are discussed in other chapters in this publication. It is worth noting that due to the multifactorial nature of atherosclerosis, there is no single marker or imaging test with high specificity, which can unambiguously assess the severity of atherosclerosis and help in the prognosis and guideline-based treatment of cardiovascular risk. Rather, a combination of biomarkers and noninvasive imaging tests better predict MACE, especially in populations where the Pooled Cohort Equations (PCE) may not be applicable (i.e., familial hypercholesterolemia), or where they may underestimate risk in other special populations described in recent guidelines, or overestimate risk in populations with protective risk conditions.

2 ASCVD and Risk Estimation

Despite significant progress over the past decades, ASCVD remains the leading cause of mortality globally and in the USA [1, 2]. Atherosclerotic plaque builds up in artery walls over many years, sometimes even starting in childhood, depending on the severity and number of risk factors. The formation of plaque is a progressive and chronic inflammatory process with no apparent symptoms for a long period of time, beginning with fatty streaks that progress into larger fibrous plaques and eventual plaque disruption [3]. Acute coronary syndrome, myocardial infarction (MI), stable or unstable angina, coronary heart disease (CHD) (with or without revascularization), other arterial revascularization, stroke, transient ischemic attack, and peripheral artery disease (PAD) (including aortic aneurysm) are all atherosclerotic in origin. MACE, which is relevant for the purpose of discussing risk assessment, is often much more narrowly defined typically as a nonfatal or fatal MI, stroke, or cardiac death; coronary revascularization and hospitalization for heart failure (HF) are also often included. The application of quantitative risk assessment tools is a critical step in identifying patients who require primary prevention of ASCVD. The first cardiovascular disease (CVD) risk score was established by the Framingham Heart Study, which assigned points corresponding to age, total and high-density lipoprotein cholesterol (HDL-C), blood pressure, smoking, diabetes status, and gender. The total score corresponds to a 10-year risk estimate for hard CHD events only (i.e., coronary death or MI). HF, PAD, and cerebrovascular disease were subsequently added to the 2008 Framingham Risk Score (FRS) [4]. Risk scores have continued to evolve with increasing accuracy and broader inclusion of race/ethnicity, as well as to provide 30-year and lifetime risk estimates [5]. In this chapter, we focus primarily on the use of the American Heart Association (AHA) and American College of Cardiology (ACC) PCE. Scores are categorized into low (<5%), borderline (5% to <7.5%), intermediate (7.5–20%), and high (>20%) risk for fatal and nonfatal CHD and stroke only. Other forms of ASCVD (PAD, aneurysmal disease, HF, etc.) are not included. The 10-year risk score is restricted to those aged 40–79 years and lifetime risk is for those aged 20–59 years [1, 5–7]. Risk-enhancing conditions are included (Table 1) to further refine the risk estimation in special populations [6]. This list is incomplete and almost certain to grow as new epidemiological and genetic studies provide evidence regarding the impact of diseases such as depression and other mental health conditions [8, 9], as well as social determinants of health that can modulate ASCVD risk [10]. The inclusion of biomarkers and imaging studies, most notably, high-sensitivity C-reactive protein (hsCRP) and coronary artery calcium (CAC) scoring, has improved the ability to predict not only the 10-year risk of hard CHD events but also the risk of subclinical atherosclerosis and the risk in younger individuals [11–13].

Table 1 Risk-enhancing factors defined in the 2019 American College of Cardiology/American Heart Association guidelines

Family history of premature ASCVD: male <55 years; female <65 years

Primary hypercholesterolemia
    LDL-C 160–189 mg/dL
    Non-HDL-C 190–219 mg/dL

Metabolic syndrome (3 criteria met from below)
    Increased waist size
    Elevated triglycerides >175 mg/dL
    High blood pressure
    High glucose
    Low HDL-C: men <40 mg/dL; women <50 mg/dL

CKD: (eGFR 15–59 mL/min/1.73 m^2 with or without albuminuria, not treated with dialysis or kidney transplant)
Chronic inflammatory conditions: psoriasis, RA, or HIV/AIDS
History of premature menopause and pre-eclampsia
South Asian ancestry

Lipid/biomarkers:
    Hypertriglyceridemia >175 mg/dL
    hsCRP >2.0 mg/L
    Lp(a) >50 mg/dL
    apoB >130 mg/dL
    ABI >0.9

ASCVD atherosclerotic cardiovascular disease, *LDL-C* low-density lipoprotein-cholesterol, *non-HDL-C* non-high-density lipoprotein-cholesterol, *HDL-C* high-density lipoprotein cholesterol, *CKD* chronic kidney disease, *eGFR* estimated glomerular filtration rate, *RA* rheumatoid arthritis, *HIV/AIDS* human immunodeficiency virus/acquired immunodeficiency syndrome, *hsCRP* high-sensitivity C-reactive protein, *Lp(a)* lipoprotein(a), *apo* apolipoprotein, *ABI* ankle brachial artery index

3   Definition and Purpose of Biomarkers

Biomarkers are essential tools for early diagnosis and risk stratification especially where the PCE may over- or underestimate risk. Despite their substantial value, in many cases, there is significant disagreement about the fundamental definitions and concepts involved in their use in research and clinical practice. Several definitions of biomarkers have been proposed by different organizations. The National Institutes of Health Biomarkers Working Group defines a biomarker as, "a characteristic that is objectively measured and evaluated as an indicator of normal biological processes, pathogenic processes, or pharmacologic responses to a therapeutic intervention," while the International Program on Chemical Safety defines a biomarker as, "any substance, structure, or process that can be measured in the body or its products and influence or predict the incidence of outcome or disease" [14]. While these definitions overlap considerably, the broad nature and diverse function of biomarkers make it difficult to create a harmonized definition that is suitable for all fields. To clarify this confusion, a number of subtypes of biomarkers were defined in 2016 and later updated in 2021 by the US Food and Drug Administration (FDA) and the National Institutes of Health Biomarker Working Group according to their putative applications [15]. It is worth noting that a single biomarker may meet multiple criteria for different uses and the same biomarker can represent multiple subtypes. Combinations of multiple biomarkers in the PCE have also been shown to improve short-term global CVD risk prediction especially for older adults [16].

The use of biomarkers is evolving. Forty-five years ago, a panel of six or seven different serum tests (glucose, kidney function, and electrolytes), a complete blood cell count, and a urine analysis constituted most of the laboratory tests that characterized the health or disease status of patients. These tests are, in essence, biomarkers. Since that time, many additional tests, images, and measurements have been developed to aid in risk assessment. The value of these biomarkers is in predicting adverse cardiovascular events, measuring therapeutic outcomes, and the acquisition of knowledge to prevent adverse outcomes or optimize their treatment. The list of potential biomarkers and imaging modalities is vast. Furthermore, two individuals, both of whom are healthy, could have very different biomarker profiles. Biomarkers are interdependent, compensating for differences in metabolism, structural activities, growth, and repair. Abnormal values represent a compensatory mechanism for a structural or environmental stressor. Every cell can contribute to the production or manifestation of a biomarker. Some cells are dedicated to the production of a biomarker and obey rules of production and cessation of production to maintain homeostasis. Biomarkers produced in response to an acute event or present chronically are eliminated after being metabolized. The nature and function of biomarkers involved in atherosclerosis were described from studies of molecular biology, identifying proteins and hormones and other measurements by blood analysis, electrical recordings discriminating disease states, and imaging demonstrating structural abnormalities.

The search for an informative biomarker begins with the pathologic nature of the disease [17]. Autopsies of individuals dying of MI suggest three potential mechanisms responsible for the fatal event: (1) plaque rupture (60–75%) is the most common cause of an MI suggesting an inflammatory process; (2) plaque erosion (25–40%) is more commonly seen in young female smokers suggesting a failure of repair of the endothelium; and (3) a ruptured nodule (2–7%) disrupting the endothelium and triggering thrombosis, which is the least common mechanism [18]. Coronary dissection and spasms are rare, and their role is controversial [19]. The pathophysiologic process that leads to these acute events should be linked to the discovery of biomarkers. All the processes implicate some form of endothelial dysfunction. Plaque rupture involves inflammatory cells, cytokines and thrombosis leading to an MI with platelet and clotting cascade activation. That being the case, measures of endothelial function, immune-mediated inflammation, lipids and their metabolism, platelet function, hematopoietic factors, and the clotting cascade appear to be good candidates for biomarkers (Table 2). Repair mechanisms suggest progenitor cells, natriuretic peptides, cardiac enzymes, apoptosis, and functions of the immune system are additional targets for biomarker discovery (Table 3). The structure relies on anatomical and physiological measurements such as echocardiography.

Table 2 Biomarkers derived from myocardial pathology

Endothelial function	Aortic pulse wave velocity	Flow-mediated dilation	Flow-mediated slowing	Pulse amplitude ratio	
Lipids	LDL-C	HDL-C	Triglycerides	Lipoprotein(a)	apoB
Immune-mediated inflammation	hsCRP	Cytokines	Lymphocytes T-helper cells 1 and 2	RDW	
Platelet function	Platelet reactivity				
Hematopoietic factors	WBC Hgb/Hct	RDW	Extracellular vesicles	Muscle enriched microRNA-133a	
Clotting cascade	Fibrinogen	D-Dimer	Tissue plasminogen activator Plasminogen activator inhibitor type 1	Von Willebrand Factor	Homocysteine
Hormones	Insulin	Estrogen Progesterone Testosterone	Growth hormone		

LDL-C low-density lipoprotein cholesterol, *HDL-C* high-density lipoprotein cholesterol, *apo* apolipoprotein, *hsCRP* high-sensitivity C-reactive protein, *RDW* red cell distribution width, *WBC* white blood cell, *Hgb* hemoglobin, *Hct* hematocrit

Table 3 Biomarkers of myocardial injury and repair

Hematopoietic	White blood cells	Progenitor cells	Th1/Th2 cells
Natriuretic peptides	Brain natriuretic peptide		
Cardiac enzymes	Creatinine phosphokinase isoenzymes	Troponin hsCRP	

Th T helper, *hsCRP* high-sensitivity C-reactive protein

4 High-Sensitivity C-Reactive Protein

CRP is one of the most accessible biomarkers in clinical practice. It is an ancient, highly conserved protein that was initially discovered in patients with pneumococcal pneumonia by Tillett and Francis in 1930 [20]. The name CRP arose because it was first identified as a substance in the serum of patients with acute inflammation that reacted with the "c" carbohydrate antigen of the capsule of pneumococcus. CRP is an acute phase protein existing in two forms: a pentameric or native CRP (nCRP) which can dissociate into a monomeric CRP (mCRP) [21]. There is mounting evidence that CRP isoforms have distinct biological properties, with nCRP often exhibiting more anti-inflammatory activities than mCRP. The nCRP isoform activates the classical complement pathway, induces phagocytosis, and promotes apoptosis, while mCRP promotes chemotaxis and recruitment of circulating leukocytes to areas of inflammation and can delay apoptosis [22]. CRP is involved in both chronic and acute atherosclerotic processes as part of the inflammatory and pro-thrombotic response. CRP is synthesized primarily by the liver and, to a lesser extent, in endothelial cells and smooth muscle cells in response to inflammatory cytokines, such as interleukin (IL)-6, IL-1, and tumor necrosis factor alpha (TNF-α). Current evidence suggests that vascular inflammation plays a critical role in the pathophysiology of atherosclerosis. Interventions that reduce inflammation decrease cardiovascular risk and events [23, 24]. A substantial number of studies have demonstrated that circulating levels of CRP are associated with atherosclerotic plaque development as well as with destabilization of plaques and the promotion of occlusive thrombi. CRP, therefore, has been shown to have utility in predicting future cardiovascular events [25, 26]. However, clinically, CRP is a sensitive and dynamic marker of trauma, inflammation, and infection. The production of CRP has been used to monitor the presence of infection and its successful treatment. Evidence suggests that CRP is not only a marker of inflammation or infection but also an important regulator of inflammatory processes; for these reasons, hsCRP values *are not related to cardiovascular risk and interpretation of hsCRP values must be done with caution.*

The standard assay measures CRP in the range from 10 to 1000 mg/L. Because the concentration of CRP increases in severe inflammatory states and infections and decreases with the resolution of the condition, the standard CRP assay (not hsCRP) is widely used to detect and monitor various inflammatory states and monitor the course of infections. To detect the low-end variations required for the prediction of vascular risk, the high-sensitivity assay was developed [27]. The hsCRP assay measures a much lower level or trace amount of CRP in the blood in the range between 0.5 and 10 mg/L. Although the use of hsCRP was pioneered in the 1990s, its utility was limited by a lack of clinical laboratories capable of reliably performing the test. The more recent standardization of hsCRP tests on several commercial platforms and its superior assay precision, accuracy, and availability have allowed it to be widely used in the clinical setting to predict future cardiovascular events [28].

The hsCRP assay has been incorporated into multiple guidelines as a biomarker to improve ASCVD risk assessment including the 2018 AHA/ACC Multi-Society Cholesterol Guidelines which listed several biomarkers shown to improve risk stratification [29]. These included hsCRP, lipoprotein(a), and apolipoprotein (apo) B. Elevation of hsCRP is also one of the risk-enhancing factors in the ACC/AHA PCE [11]. The Reynold's Risk Score highlighted the use of hsCRP to improve FRS predictions in women [30] and men [31]. According to the Centers for Disease Control and Prevention (CDC) and the AHA statement in 2003, concentrations of hsCRP of <1.0, 1.0–3.0, and >3.0 in mg/L are considered to represent a relatively low, average, or high risk of CVD (defined as MI, stroke, peripheral vascular disease, and sudden cardiac death), respectively. As an acute phase reactant, as previously outlined, levels of hsCRP are influenced by a variety of conditions, and values greater than 10 mg/L are generally attributed to an acute or resolving illness or inflammation and do not represent CVD risk [32]. For primary prevention, the CDC and AHA recommend obtaining an average of hsCRP measurements from two or more tests, optimally 2 weeks apart, fasting or nonfasting, in patients free of infection or acute illness.

Ample research has demonstrated that hsCRP is a strong independent predictor of future cardiovascular events: The Justification for the Use of Statins in Prevention: An Intervention Trial Evaluating Rosuvastatin (JUPITER) showed that participants who achieved hsCRP less than 1 mg/L and low-density lipoprotein cholesterol (LDL-C) less than 70 mg/dL had a 79% reduction in vascular events (defined as nonfatal MI, nonfatal stroke, admission for unstable angina, arterial revascularization, or cardiovascular death) over the 5-year course of the study compared to a 33% event reduction in those who achieved one or neither target [33]. An individual with an average hsCRP level higher than 3 mg/L has an increased risk of CHD [34], and this risk increases in those with type 2 diabetes [35]. The Atherosclerosis Risk in Communities (ARIC) study involving 9784 participants found hsCRP predicted ASCVD risk independently of the lipid profile [36]. An inhibitor of IL-1β (canakinumab) has been shown to reduce levels of hsCRP and IL-6, and notably reduce ASCVD events without lowering LDL-C, which provided proof of concept of the role of inflammation in atherogenesis independent of lipids [37]. In the Improved Reduction of Outcomes: Vytorin Efficacy International Trial (IMPROVE IT) [38] and the Pravastatin or Atorvastatin Evaluation and Infection Therapy Thrombolysis in Myocardial Infarction 22 (PROVE IT-TIMI 22) [39] trial, residual hsCRP elevation was associated with increased risk of events despite achievement of LDL-C control (LDL-C <70 mg/dL); this has led some experts to advocate for achievement of "dual targets" of both LDL-C <70 mg/dL and hsCRP <2 mg/dL. In the Women's Health Study (WHS), LDL-C, an established causative biological marker of atherosclerosis, was compared with hsCRP in 27,939 healthy women who were followed for an average of 8 years for MI, ischemic stroke, coronary revascularization, or cardiovascular death. After adjustment for age and conventional risk factors, hsCRP was a stronger predictor of cardiovascular events than LDL-C. The primary endpoint was twice as likely in those with hsCRP in the fourth quintile between 2.10 and 4.19 mg/L as compared with levels of 0.49 mg/L (relative risk [RR]: 2.0; 95% confidence interval [CI]: 1.3–3.0). LDL-C levels in the fourth quintile (132–154 mg/dL) had a 30% excess risk of cardiovascular events as compared with those with LDL-C <96 mg/dL (RR: 1.3; 95% CI: 1.0–1.7) [40, 41].

Ethnicity influences baseline hsCRP levels [42]. In a systematic review and meta-analysis of 221,287 individuals from 89 studies, the geometric mean of hsCRP levels varied significantly depending on ethnic background [43]: 2.6 mg/L in Black subjects, 2.5 mg/L in Hispanic subjects, 2.3 mg/L in South Asian subjects, 2.0 mg/L in non-Hispanic White subjects, and 1.0 mg/L in East Asian subjects ($n = 39,521$). There can also be considerable intraindividual variability due to the acute phase properties of CRP as discussed above. A myriad of other factors can affect an individual's baseline level besides elevations associated with inflammatory and infectious etiologies, including smoking, osteoarthritis, and obesity [32]. An example of the clinical variability in a patient is shown in Fig. 1.

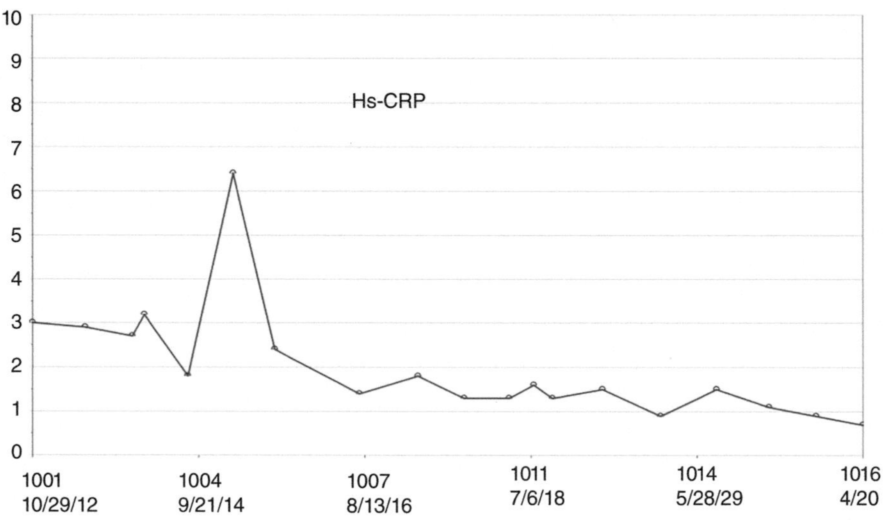

Fig. 1 Example of high-sensitivity C-reactive protein (Hs-CRP) variations in a patient

5 Cardiac Troponin and High-Sensitivity Cardiac Troponin

Cardiac troponin (cTn) is the most frequently utilized biomarker due to its role in assessing individuals experiencing chest pain, one of the top ten reasons for seeking emergency care. Troponin exists in muscle cells and is an inhibitor of the binding of actin and myosin. When calcium enters the cell, actin and myosin bind together and, with the addition of adenosine triphosphate (ATP), muscle contraction ensues. After the calcium is removed from the cell, troponin inhibits binding so the muscle cell can relax to its initial configuration. The cTn complex consists of three subunits, cTnC which is an 18 kDa protein that binds calcium; cTnI which is a 26.5 kDa actomyosin-ATP-inhibiting protein; and cTnT which is a 39 kDa protein that binds tropomyosin. Both cTnI and cTnT are released in response to acute cardiac myocyte injury from ischemia or infection and as a consequence are considered "the biochemical gold standard for diagnosing cardiac injury" [44]. The normal range for cTn is <0.04 ng/mL, but a high-sensitivity troponin assay is preferred to detect even lower levels (below 14 ng/L) in asymptomatic individuals, which has high prognostic utility for future CVD events [45]. A number of population studies in CVD-free populations have validated the importance of this biomarker in subclinical ASCVD. The ARIC trial [46] found that elevated high-sensitivity TnI (hs-TnI) was an independent risk predictor for disease, HF, hospitalization, global CVD, and total mortality in individuals without a prior history of CVD. Differences were observed between Black and White individuals; Black ARIC participants had higher hs-TnI but fewer events than the White population. Sex differences occurred with women having a stronger association with hs-TnI than men. The Age, Gene/Environment Susceptibility—Reykjavik Study (AGES-Reykjavik) [47] showed similar findings in an older population free of ASCVD (mean age 77 years) followed for 10 years examining all-cause death and incidence of CVD and CHD. The authors found that hs-cTnI concentrations within normal limits of the assay were highly correlated with mortality and incident CVD. The rates of mortality and major adverse cardiac events increased with increasing concentrations of hs-cTnI and there was a strong association of hs-cTnI with age, irrespective of any history of CVD. Most importantly, the study found that hs-cTnI offered "incremental predictive power over traditional risk factors for prediction of CHD and CVD."

A reliable and clinically relevant biomarker should also be changed by an intervention that improves clinical outcomes. This was demonstrated for hs-cTnI in the West of Scotland Coronary Prevention Study [48], a primary prevention study in men aged 45–64 years randomized to receive pravastatin or placebo for an average of 5 years. Like in AGES-Reykjavik, baseline hs-TnI concentrations were associated with an increased risk of CHD (nonfatal MI or death from CHD) at the 5- and 15-year follow-up visits. Compared to placebo, pravastatin reduced the hs-TnI by 10–15% and was associated with the lowest risk for future coronary events proving that this biomarker can be used to monitor the impact of therapeutic interventions.

6   Brain Natriuretic Peptide and N-Terminal Pro B-Type Natriuretic Peptide

Brain natriuretic peptide (BNP) is a peptide that is produced in the ventricular myocardium in response to increased wall stress [49]. It is secreted as a prehormone (proBNP) which is cleaved into the active hormone (BNP) and N-terminal pro B-type natriuretic peptide (NT-proBNP), an inactive peptide, in equimolar amounts. Because of the way they are cleared from circulation, these products have different half-lives: 1–2 h for NT-proBNP vs 20 min for BNP [50]. Therefore levels of NT-proBNP are higher in plasma than BNP, but NT-proBNP is impacted more by renal dysfunction than BNP because it is cleared by renal excretion. Both assays have shown similar sensitivity and specificity, at least with respect to diagnosing HF [51], although recent clinical studies are more inclined to utilize NT-proBNP, likely because of the higher measurable levels. Assays for both peptides are commonly available in clinical laboratories as well as point-of-care testing [52]. Both are useful and reliable biomarkers and are considered the "gold standard" for diagnosing HF, as well as for assessing prognosis and monitoring the therapeutic response to HF medications [53]. Despite not being included as a risk-enhancing factor for ASCVD, these assays, especially NT-proBNP, have been increasingly utilized in the risk assessment for ASCVD events [36]. In an asymptomatic older population, NT-proBNP improves risk prediction not only of HF but also of CVD beyond classic risk factors, resulting in a substantial reclassification of participants to a lower or higher risk category [54]. Levels of NT-proBNP are positively associated with the risk of thromboembolic, ischemic, or hemorrhagic stroke, independently of several other risk factors and conditions [55, 56]. A number of studies have shown that NT-proBNP is useful in the risk stratification of individuals with type 2 diabetes mellitus, a population where standard approaches to CVD risk stratification have fallen short [57–59]. Measurement of NT-proBNP provides prognostic information, beyond traditional risk factors, for mortality and first MACE [60, 61]. Importantly, a combination of biomarkers including NT-proBNP, hs-cTnT, and hsCRP, and imaging studies described below, has proven to better predict short-term (3-year) risk compared to standard risk factors and PCE [62].

7   Cytokines

The inflammatory response has a key role in the progression of coronary artery disease (CAD) as noted above in our discussion of hsCRP. An additional biomarker of inflammation, IL-6, is a pro-inflammatory cytokine secreted along with other stimulatory and inhibitory interleukins such as IL-1, IL-8, IL-12, IL-18, and

TNF-α. These cytokines either stimulate or inhibit leukocytes through T-cell-mediated processes and effects on monocytes. IL-6 is the most studied inflammatory marker for atherosclerotic aggregation and inflammation. IL-6 binds to the IL-6 receptor in the classic signaling pathway, which leads to the synthesis of acute phase proteins such as plasminogen activator inhibitor, CRP, fibrinogen, and serum amyloid A protein in the liver [63]. IL-6 also has an effect on the trans-signaling inflammatory pathway and has been shown to be associated with future cardiovascular events [64]. In a patient cohort undergoing coronary angiography, a serum IL-6 level elevated above 1 pg/mL was predictive of CAD; and IL-6 was shown to be a better predictor than hs-CRP by the receiver operating characteristics analysis [65]. Others have shown that the polymorphism of the IL-6 gene also contributes significantly to CAD. In a meta-analysis, the C allele of the -174G/C polymorphism of the IL-6 promoter region was noted to trigger the progression of CAD among Caucasians [34]. These observations suggest that inflammatory markers such as IL-6 and/or their genetic polymorphism should be considered in the detection of subclinical ASCVD as well as the assessment of therapeutic efficiencies of novel anticoagulants and antiplatelet and anti-inflammatory agents. Standardized testing assays and reference intervals are increasingly available in many clinical laboratories.

8 Albuminuria

A very simple and commonly measured test is the spot urine albumin-to-creatinine concentration ratio (ACR) (instead of the traditional 24-h urine collection), which has been positively associated with subclinical atherosclerosis and predicted risks of cardiovascular events and all-cause death [66]. As such, the evaluation of ACR levels is a useful biomarker that can easily be integrated into risk stratification and prevention of cardiovascular events and all-cause deaths, especially among those with pre-existing subclinical atherosclerosis and cardiometabolic abnormalities. Daily creatinine excretion is dependent upon an individual's muscle mass. Assuming an average value of 10 mmol creatinine per day, the albumin loss can be estimated by multiplying the ACR by a factor of 10. Albuminuria, defined as an ACR value higher than 5 mg/g, is associated with an increased risk of cardiovascular mortality. To be valid, the ACR should be confirmed by testing in at least two out of three urine samples collected in the absence of infection, acute metabolic crisis, or other factors that might artificially increase albumin loss, including upright posture collection, menstrual contamination, vaginal discharge, hypertension, urinary tract infection, HF, or strenuous exercise. Monitoring urinary albumin may improve the personalized cardiovascular risk assessment from a microvascular perspective in nondiabetic, low-to-moderate cardiovascular risk individuals with or without hypertension [67].

9   Lipoprotein-Associated Phospholipase A2

Lipoprotein-associated phospholipase A2 (Lp-PLA2 or often just PLA2) is an enzyme associated with both traditional (cholesterol-linked) and novel (inflammatory) pathways of atherosclerosis [68]. Lp-PLA2 is synthesized by monocytes and lymphocytes and is thought to cleave oxidized lipids to produce lipid fragments that increase endothelial adhesion. It should be noted that hsCRP, a marker of systemic inflammation, can improve risk stratification but that it is not specific to CVD. On the other hand, Lp-PLA2 is a specific marker of vascular inflammation associated with atherosclerosis [69]. A 2008 consensus panel recommended testing Lp-PLA2 as an adjunct to traditional risk factor assessment in individuals with moderate or high risk of CVD as defined by FRS [70]. The panel found that an Lp-PLA2 level >200 ng/mL indicates an individual's risk is actually higher than that determined using FRS, and more intensive therapy is appropriate. Because Lp-PLA2 is a highly specific biomarker for vascular inflammation, its measurement has been recommended for those with a family history of premature ASCVD [71]. However, in a large-scale human genetic study, none of a series of Lp-PLA2-lowering alleles was related to CHD risk, suggesting that Lp-PLA2 is unlikely to be a causal risk factor [72]. This assay is approved by the FDA with a range from 120 to 342 ng/mL for females and 131–376 ng/mL for males; the normal range determined for Lp-PLA2 is <200 ng/mL. Lp-PLA2 testing is often available through reference laboratories (e.g., Cleveland Clinic, Quest, and LabCorp).

10   Myeloperoxidase

Myeloperoxidase (MPO) is another key element in the innate immune system. MPO is a heme peroxidase highly expressed in neutrophils and monocytes when cells undergo oxidative stress and aggregation. It is found in the granules of myeloid cells. When MPO oxidizes apoA-1, the HDL function is disabled. Oxidized apoA-1 inactivates the cholesterol efflux ability of the membrane-associated ATP-binding cassette transporter A1 and, at the same time, disables the ability of lecithin:cholesterol acyltransferase to convert free cholesterol to cholesteryl ester [73]. There are a number of studies that show the association of MPO to CAD and CAD severity, from stable CAD to non-ST-segment elevation of acute coronary syndrome and acute MI

[75]. MPO concentration increases when patients present with acute coronary syndrome. In fact, a single initial plasma MPO measurement can predict early MI as well as the risk of MACE in the next 30-day and 6-month periods in the absence of myocardial necrosis [74, 75]. Quantitation and imaging of MPO are useful in the assessment of atherosclerotic plaque instability and rupture [76, 77]. These findings suggest that MPO can be a biomarker of short- and long-term risk of cardiovascular events. Like Lp-PLA2, this assay is available through many reference laboratories, but assay standardization and reference ranges have not been established for routine clinical use.

11 Ceramides

Ceramides are sphingolipids involved with cellular signaling. Synthesis of ceramides occurs in all tissues. Ceramides accumulate within tissues and the blood plasma during metabolic dysfunction, dyslipidemia, and inflammation. Elevations of ceramides are predictive of cardiovascular mortality and are independently associated with MACE in patients with and without CAD [78]. Elevated plasma concentrations of ceramides are associated with multiple risk factors of ASCVD, and comorbidities including obesity, insulin resistance, and diabetes mellitus, and may perhaps explain the risk associated with the metabolic syndrome [79]. Furthermore, atherosclerotic plaques are highly enriched with ceramides. Increases in ceramide content may accelerate atherosclerosis development by promoting LDL infiltration into the endothelium and aggregation within the intima of artery walls. Thus, ceramides appear to play a key role in the development of cardiometabolic disease due to their central location in major metabolic pathways that intersect lipid and glucose metabolism [80]. Recently published data have shown that ceramides are not only of scientific interest but may also have diagnostic values. Furthermore, their independent prognostic values for future cardiovascular outcomes over and above LDL-C and other traditional risk factors have consistently been shown in numerous clinical studies [81–84]. Based on abundant published data, a risk score using the concentrations of circulating ceramides has been developed and adapted for routine clinical practice [80].

Although not discussed in this review, it is important to note that the list of biomarkers for ASCVD continues to expand and includes a number of additional candidates such as exosomal microRNAs [85], biomarkers of oxidative stress [86], glycan N-acetylglucosamine [36], serum amyloid protein A, pregnancy-associated plasma protein A, oxidized LDL, matrix metalloproteinases, monocyte chemotactic protein, tissue plasminogen activator, isoprostanes, urinary thromboxane, and adhesion molecules among others. A summary of the biomarkers described above can be found in Table 4.

Table 4 Summary of biomarkers

Biomarker	Pathophysiology	Guideline	References
hsCRP	Protein made by the liver which increases when there is inflammation or infection or in high-risk ASCVD patients	Multi-Society AHA/ACC cholesterol treatment guideline	[6, 21–25, 27–29, 32, 33, 37, 38, 40–43]
Troponins	Troponin protein in the heart muscles released after a heart attack or in high-risk ASCVD patients	Multi-Society AHA/ACC cholesterol treatment guideline	[6, 44–48]
BNP/NT-pro-BNP	Hormones from myocardial cells that are released due to volume expansion and wall stress	ACC/AHA guideline for the management of heart failure	[6, 49–52, 54–61]
Cytokines	Pro- and anti-inflammatory markers that regulate atherosclerosis formation	NA	[34, 63–65]
Albuminuria	A spot urine albumin-to-creatinine concentration ratio	NA	[65–67]
Lp-PLA2	Lp-PLA2 enzyme associated with cholesterol and inflammatory pathways of atherosclerosis	NA	[68–72]
Myeloperoxidase	Heme peroxidase expressed in neutrophils and monocytes that is released when cells undergo oxidative stress and aggregation	NA	[73–77]
Ceramides	Sphingolipids that increase during metabolic dysfunction, dyslipidemia, and inflammation	NA	[78–84]

hsCRP high-sensitivity C-reactive protein, *AHA* American Heart Association, *ACC* American College of Cardiology, *ASCVD* atherosclerotic cardiovascular disease, *BNP* B-type natriuretic peptide, *NT-pro-BNP* N-terminal-pro hormone BNP, *NA* not available, *Lp-PLA2* lipoprotein-associated phospholipase A2

12   Imaging Modalities

Noninvasive imaging can be a powerful tool in the detection of subclinical ASCVD. CAC scoring is the most widely recognized and studied of these tools and utilizes computed tomography (CT) imaging to estimate an individual's risk. Additional modalities utilizing nonionizing radiation have also demonstrated benefits in selecting patients who may be at higher risk for subclinical ASCVD through the use of ultrasound to measure carotid intima-media thickness (CIMT) and arterial tonometry for the measurement of pulse wave velocity (PWV). Finally, more recent studies have shown a correlation between vascular calcification seen incidentally on routine chest CTs and mammograms and a patient's risk for subclinical ASCVD. Each of these tools, summarized in Table 5, and their utility for the clinician will be further discussed in detail at the end of this chapter.

Table 5 Summary of imaging modalities to detect subclinical ASCVD

Imaging modality	Description	Guideline	References
Coronary artery calcium (CAC) scoring	Specialized noncontrast CT exam of the heart that identifies calcium in major epicardial vessels	AHA/ACC states it may be reasonable to obtain CAC for asymptomatic adults aged 40–75 with borderline or intermediate risk if treatment remains uncertain	[1, 87, 88]
Carotid intima-media thickness (CIMT)	Ultrasound measurement of carotid plaque and carotid intima-media thickness	AHA/ACC states CIMT has no benefit and is not recommended for routine use in clinical practice	[100, 103]
Pulse wave velocity (PWV)	Ultrasound measurement of arterial stiffness through aortic pulse wave velocity	NA	[105]
Incidental calcium on chest CT and mammography	Identification of subclinical ASCVD based on prior imaging to improve risk stratification without additional cost	SCCT and STR recommend reporting quantitative CAC scores for all noncontrast CT chest examinations ACR recommends reporting all moderate and severe CAC on routine chest CT examinations	[113, 114, 119]

ASCVD atherosclerotic cardiovascular disease, *CAC* coronary artery calcium, *CT* computed tomography, *AHA* American Heart Association, *ACC* American College of Cardiology, *CIMT* carotid intima-media thickness, *PWV* pulse wave velocity, *NA* not available, *SCCT* Society of Cardiovascular Computed Tomography, *STR* Society of Thoracic Radiology, *ACR* American College of Radiology

13 Coronary Artery Calcium Scoring

CAC scoring utilizes noncontrast CT of the heart to identify calcium within the major epicardial vessels through postprocessing [87]. The study is performed during a quick single breath-hold exam and has very low radiation exposure comparable to screening mammography. The Agatston method is the most widely accepted quantification tool used to interpret CAC scoring due to its high reproducibility. CAC scores are classified as follows: 0 = none, 1–10 = minimal, 11–100 = mild, 101–400 = moderate, 401–1000 = severe, and >1000 = very severe. These CAC scores are then compared to age, gender, and ethnicity-matched asymptomatic individuals using the Multi-Ethnic Study of Atherosclerosis (MESA) database and result in an individual CAC percentile score that aids in determining a patient's cardiovascular risk [88]. Compared to a CAC score of 0, patients with scores of 1–100 have a hazard ratio of 3.61 for any cardiac event that increases to 7.73 and 9.67 for CAC scores of 101–300 and >300, respectively [89].

CAC scoring has demonstrated superiority to FRS for the classification of patients in multiple large-scale studies [87]. Multiple studies have shown that approximately 20–25% of patients are more accurately classified into specific risk

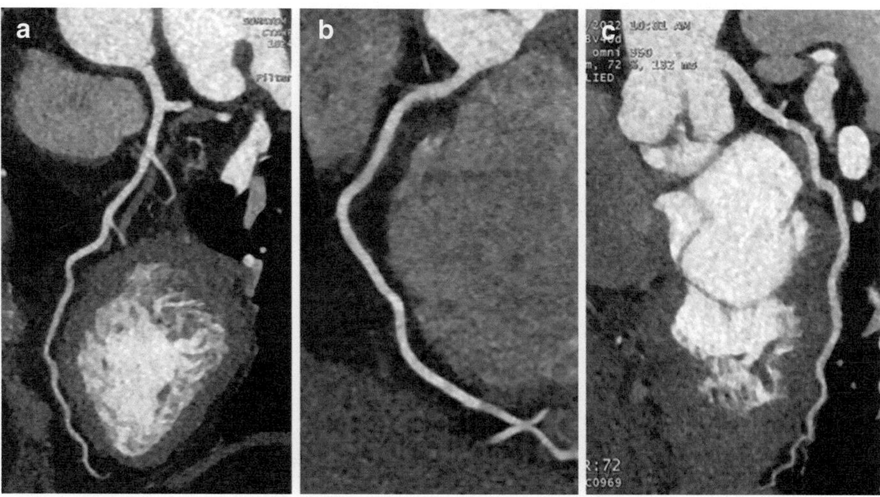

Fig. 2 Sixty-year-old female presenting with atypical chest pain and past medical history of hyperlipidemia and hypertension. Coronary artery calcium score was calculated to be zero. Multiplanar reconstructed images of the left anterior descending artery (**a**), right coronary artery (**b**), and the left circumflex artery (**c**)

categories utilizing CAC scoring compared to FRS [90–92]. However, the most consistent and important finding of CAC scoring is the low 10-year cardiovascular risk of approximately 1% in patients with a CAC score of 0 irrespective of the underlying risk factors [93, 94]. As a result, CAC scoring provides an opportunity to avoid unnecessary treatment in patients with very low ASCVD risk (i.e., CAC = 0) (Fig. 2).

CAC CT examinations are relatively inexpensive. However, the cost of the exam is not routinely covered by insurance companies and results in an additional out-of-pocket expense for patients. In addition to the exam cost, it is also important to consider subsequent expenses related to the findings. In the Early Identification of Subclinical Atherosclerosis by Noninvasive Imaging Research (EISNER) study, patients with minimal or no CAC did not frequently obtain additional cardiovascular testing [95]. This resulted in a significant reduction in overall healthcare costs that outweighed additional testing and costs in patients with higher CAC scores including invasive coronary angiography and revascularization in patients with severely elevated CAC scores ≥1000 (Fig. 3). Results of CAC scoring have also been shown to increase adherence to recommendations for primary prevention to optimize blood pressure, LDL-C, and waist circumference in patients with higher CAC scores [96]. In addition, CAC scores can aid in the determination of low-dose aspirin use as patients with a CAC of 0 had net harm as opposed to benefit in patients with a CAC ≥100 [97].

The 2018 update of the US Preventive Services Task Force (USPSTF) made no recommendation for the use of CAC scoring in asymptomatic patients due to insufficient evidence regarding benefit versus harm [98]. The ACC/AHA 2019 guidelines

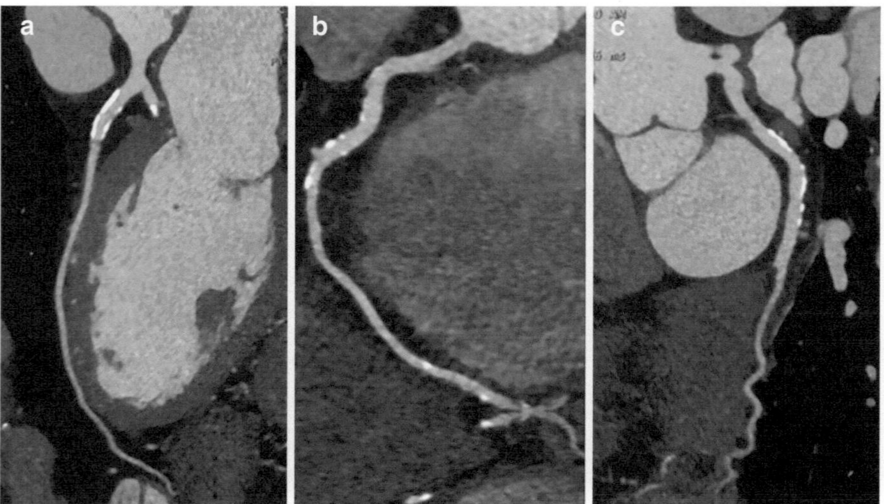

Fig. 3 Seventy-five-year-old male with a past medical history of hypertension and hyperlipidemia presenting for coronary artery disease screening. The patient's calculated calcium score was 1251. Multiplanar reconstructed images demonstrate eccentric calcification seen primarily within the proximal left anterior descending artery (**a**), diffusely throughout the right coronary artery (**b**), and within the proximal to mid-left circumflex artery (**c**)

for primary prevention state it may be reasonable (Class IIb) to obtain CAC for asymptomatic adults aged 40–75 years with borderline risk (5% to <7.5% 10-year ASCVD risk) or intermediate risk (≥7.5% to <20% 10-year ASCVD risk) if treatment remains uncertain [1]. The American College of Radiology Appropriateness Criteria have similar recommendations as the ACC/AHA stating CAC is usually appropriate for asymptomatic patients with intermediate but not low risk [99].

14 Carotid Intima-Media Thickness

Ultrasound measurement of carotid plaque and CIMT has been extensively studied as a potential tool for screening individuals who are asymptomatic [89]. This type of imaging is particularly attractive as it does not require ionizing radiation and is widely available. The American Society of Echocardiography recommends CIMT be measured at the far wall of the distal common carotid artery and supplemented with carotid plaque screening of the common carotid artery, carotid bulb, internal carotid artery, and external carotid artery [100].

A consensus on the use of ultrasound has been hampered by heterogeneity among data sets for CIMT and plaque screening limits. In the ARIC study, for patients aged 45–64 years, the best predictive model for cardiovascular events during approximately a 15-year period included traditional risk factors, CIMT, and plaque [101]. The inclusion of plaque is of particular importance in both this study and in meta-analyses as it significantly improves risk prediction in both men and women [102]. A comparison of risk assessment with CAC and CIMT for cardiovascular events shows that CAC is significantly better at classifying a patient's risk. Net reclassification for CAC is consistently >20% for cardiovascular events and reaches approximately >50% in intermediate-risk individuals compared to <10% for carotid plaque measurements [89]. As a result, the 2013 ACC/AHA prevention guidelines stated CIMT has no benefit (Class III) and is not recommended for routine use in clinical practice [103].

15   Pulse Wave Velocity

One of the earliest markers of arteriosclerotic structural changes in the arterial wall is loss of elasticity, as arteries become thicker and stiffer with age-related remodeling [104]. Atherosclerosis, a subtype of arteriosclerosis, is characterized by plaque deposition. Arterial stiffness is associated with cardiovascular morbidity independent of additional risk factors [105]. A large number of commercial ultrasound devices are available to measure PWV and perform an analysis of pulse pressure waveform. Details of this technique have been well described [106]. PWV calculates the speed of arterial pressure waves along the aorta and large vessels by measuring the transit time between two points and dividing it by the distance [104]. The most commonly targeted arteries used for the measurement of transit times are the carotid-femoral PWV (cfPWV) and brachial-ankle PWV (baPWV). cfPWV is considered the gold standard and has the most clinical data as a measure of arterial stiffness although the procedure can be uncomfortable for patients [107]. baPWV is more convenient for patients as it only requires the use of two blood pressure cuffs but measurements tend to be less accurate due to assumptions made for calculation [108]. However, the ease of access of baPWV makes it a more likely candidate for mass screening than cfPWV [105]. The fPWV has been demonstrated in the general population to be an independent predictor of CAD and stroke [109]. Meta-analysis of ten studies showed that cfPWV is a predictor of future CVD independent of FRS [110]. Meta-analyses of elevated baPWV have also demonstrated increased risks of CVD [111, 112].

16   Incidental Calcium on Chest Computed Tomography and Mammography

Identifying patients with subclinical ASCVD based on prior imaging is ideal as it allows for improved risk stratification without the additional cost to the patient or healthcare system. Atherosclerotic calcifications are commonly noted on routine CT studies of the chest and abdomen but are often ignored by providers because they are considered "incidental findings," i.e., unrelated to the reason the test was

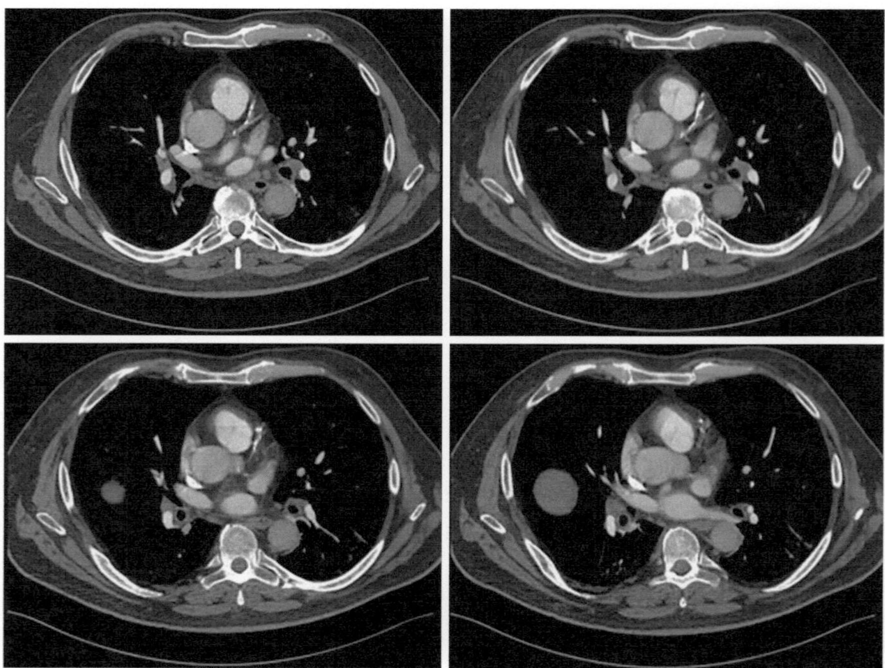

Fig. 4 Sixty-eight-year-old male with a past medical history of hypertension, hyperlipidemia, and diabetes mellitus type 2. Sequential contrast-enhanced axial CT slices of the chest demonstrate heavy to severe atherosclerotic calcification involving the proximal to distal left anterior descending artery (arrow). Coronary artery calcifications classified as heavy or severe should be further evaluated

ordered. Current guidelines from the American College of Radiology recommend reporting all moderate and severe CAC scores on routine chest CT examinations that are performed (Fig. 4) [113]. The 2016 guidelines from the Society of Cardiovascular Computed Tomography and the Society of Thoracic Radiology recommend reporting quantitative CAC scores for all noncontrast CT chest examinations, not only exams tailored for CAC scoring, but also as a method for assessing incidentally noted CAC [114]. Typically CAC scoring on CT is performed with noncontrast CT that is EKG-gated to improve resolution of the coronary vasculature. However, multiple studies have shown good correlation and accuracy with nongated noncontrast chest CT examinations, including low-dose CT chest examinations performed for lung cancer screening [115–117]. Implementation of CAC scoring on all nongated chest CTs could represent a significant improvement in the detection of subclinical ASCVD in asymptomatic patients [114].

Mammography is another opportunity to assess ASCVD burden. Breast arterial calcifications (BAC), which can be seen on routine screening mammograms, represent medial calcinosis and are indicative of arteriosclerosis (Fig. 5). Multiple studies have demonstrated a correlation between BAC and CAC scoring; however, these results should be interpreted cautiously due to small sample sizes and possible

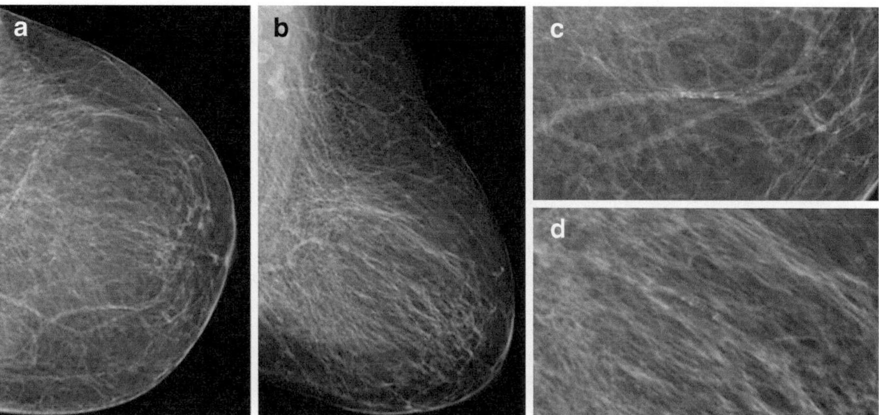

Fig. 5 Fifty-four-year-old asymptomatic female with a past medical history of hypertension and diabetes mellitus type 2. Craniocaudal (**a**) and mediolateral oblique (**b**) views of the right breast demonstrate vascular calcifications within the breast. Enlarged craniocaudal view (**c**) and enlarged mediolateral oblique view (**d**) demonstrate a linear, tram-track pattern of calcification consistent with vascular calcifications

selection bias since the studies include women who had already been referred for CT scoring [118]. Longitudinal studies evaluating cardiovascular risks and BAC have been scarce, but recent results from the Multiethnic Study of Breast Arterial Calcium Gradation and Cardiovascular Risk (MINERVA) cohort study demonstrated a threshold effect for very high BAC burden (>95th percentile) with global CVD [119]. The MINERVA cohort is large (>5000 patients) and diverse and may offer further insights into ethnic differences among patients with BAC in the coming years.

17 Summary

Atherosclerosis, the underlying cause of CVD, exists at a subclinical level a decade or more before the onset of sudden and unpredictable cardiovascular events. The plaque burden is the substrate of these debilitating and sometimes deadly occurrences. There is a substantial window of opportunity to diagnose and intervene to prevent MACE. Biomarkers and imaging modalities are useful tools to augment risk predictions in an asymptomatic population although they are somewhat less useful in actually predicting an event. Many promising markers are in development. The biology of inflammation, repair, failure to repair, and blood vessel remodeling will likely be the major targets of new biomarker identification and evaluation.

Acknowledgments The authors are grateful to Drs. Hosea Matel and Xinhua Dong for their assistance with early versions of this chapter and Dr. Stephen Heard for his editorial assistance.

References

1. Arnett DK, Blumenthal RS, Albert MA, Buroker AB, Goldberger ZD, Hahn EJ, Himmelfarb CD, Khera A, Lloyd-Jones D, McEvoy JW, Michos ED. 2019 ACC/AHA guideline on the primary prevention of cardiovascular disease: executive summary: a report of the American College of Cardiology/American Heart Association Task Force on clinical practice guidelines. J Am Coll Cardiol. 2019;74(10):1376–414.
2. Ahmad FB, Cisewski JA, Anderson RN. Provisional mortality data—United States, 2021. Morb Mortal Wkly Rep. 2022;71(17):597.
3. Fan J, Watanabe T. Atherosclerosis: known and unknown. Pathol Int. 2022;72(3):151–60.
4. Tsao CW, Vasan RS. The Framingham Heart Study: past, present and future. Int J Epidemiol. 2015;44(6):1763–6.
5. Wong ND, Budoff MJ, Ferdinand K, Graham IM, Michos ED, Reddy T, Shapiro MD, Toth PP. Atherosclerotic cardiovascular disease risk assessment: an American Society for Preventive Cardiology clinical practice statement. Am J Prev Cardiol. 2022;10:100335.
6. Grundy SM, Stone NJ, Bailey AL, et al. 2018 AHA/ACC/AACVPR/AAPA/ABC/ACPM/ADA/AGS/APhA/ASPC/NLA/PCNA guideline on the management of blood cholesterol: a report of the American College of Cardiology/American Heart Association Task Force on clinical practice guidelines. Circulation. 2019;139(25):e1082–143.
7. Lloyd-Jones DM, Braun LT, Ndumele CE, et al. Use of risk assessment tools to guide decision-making in the primary prevention of atherosclerotic cardiovascular disease: a special report from the American Heart Association and American College of Cardiology. J Am Coll Cardiol. 2019;73(24):3153–67.
8. Harshfield EL, Pennells L, Schwartz JE, Willeit P, Kaptoge S, Bell S, Shaffer JA, Bolton T, Spackman S, Wassertheil-Smoller S, Kee F. Association between depressive symptoms and incident cardiovascular diseases. JAMA. 2020;324(23):2396–405.
9. Xu L, Zimmermann M, Forkey H, Griffin J, Wilds C, Morgan WS, Byatt N, McNeal CJ. How to mitigate risk of premature cardiovascular disease among children and adolescents with mental health conditions. Curr Atheroscler Rep. 2022;24(4):253–64.
10. Al Rifai M, Jia X, Pickett J, Hussain A, Navaneethan SD, Birtcher KK, Ballantyne C, Petersen LA, Virani SS. Social determinants of health and comorbidities among individuals with atherosclerotic cardiovascular disease: the behavioral risk factor surveillance system survey. Popul Health Manag. 2022;25(1):39–45.
11. Stone NJ, Smith SC Jr, Orringer CE, Rigotti NA, Navar AM, Khan SS, Jones DW, Goldberg R, Mora S, Blaha M, Pencina MJ. Managing atherosclerotic cardiovascular risk in young adults: JACC state-of-the-art review. J Am Coll Cardiol. 2022;79(8):819–36.
12. McClelland RL, Jorgensen NW, Budoff M, Blaha MJ, Post WS, Kronmal RA, Bild DE, Shea S, Liu K, Watson KE, Folsom AR. 10-year coronary heart disease risk prediction using coronary artery calcium and traditional risk factors: derivation in the MESA (Multi-Ethnic Study of Atherosclerosis) with validation in the HNR (Heinz Nixdorf Recall) study and the DHS (Dallas Heart Study). J Am Coll Cardiol. 2015;66(15):1643–53.
13. Gidding SS, Colangelo LA, Nwabuo CC, Lewis CE, Jacobs DR Jr, Schreiner PJ, Lima JA, Allen NB. PDAY risk score predicts cardiovascular events in young adults: the CARDIA study. Eur Heart J. 2022;43(30):2892–900.
14. Strimbu K, Tavel JA. What are biomarkers? Curr Opin HIV AIDS. 2010;5(6):463–6.
15. Califf RM. Biomarker definitions and their applications. Exp Biol Med. 2018;243(3):213–21.
16. Osei AD, Blaha MJ. Combining biomarkers and imaging for short-term assessment of cardiovascular disease risk in apparently healthy adults: a paradigm-shifting approach? J Am Heart Assoc. 2020;9(15):e017790.
17. Pepe MS, Etzioni R, Feng Z, et al. Phases of biomarker development for early detection of cancer. J Natl Cancer Inst. 2001;93(14):1054–61.
18. Bentzon JF, Otsuka F, Virmani R, Falk E. Mechanisms of plaque formation and rupture. Circ Res. 2014;114(12):1852–66.

19. Adlam D, Tweet M, Gulati R, et al. Spontaneous coronary artery dissection. J Am Coll Cardiol Intv. 2021;14(16):1743–56.
20. Tillett WS, Francis T Jr. Serological reactions in pneumonia with a non-protein somatic fraction of pneumococcus. J Exp Med. 1930;52(4):561.
21. Melnikov IS, Kozlov SG, Saburova OS, Avtaeva YN, Prokofieva LV, Gabbasov ZA. Current position on the role of monomeric C-reactive protein in vascular pathology and atherothrombosis. Curr Pharm Des. 2020;26(1):37–43.
22. Boncler M, Wu Y, Watala C. The multiple faces of C-reactive protein—physiological and pathophysiological implications in cardiovascular disease. Molecules. 2019;24(11):2062.
23. Libby P. Inflammation and cardiovascular disease mechanisms. Am J Clin Nutr. 2006;83(2):456S–60S.
24. Tuñón J, Bäck M, Badimón L, et al. Interplay between hypercholesterolaemia and inflammation in atherosclerosis: translating experimental targets into clinical practice. Eur J Prev Cardiol. 2018;25(9):948–55.
25. Alfaddagh A, Martin SS, Leucker TM, et al. Inflammation and cardiovascular disease: from mechanisms to therapeutics. Am J Prev Cardiol. 2020;4:100130. https://doi.org/10.1016/j.ajpc.2020.100130.
26. Libby P, Ridker PM, Hansson GK. Progress and challenges in translating the biology of atherosclerosis. Nature. 2011;473(7347):317–25.
27. Bassuk SS, Rifai N, Ridker PM. High-sensitivity C-reactive protein: clinical importance. Curr Probl Cardiol. 2004;29(8):439–93.
28. Aday AW, Ridker PM. Targeting residual inflammatory risk: a shifting paradigm for atherosclerotic disease. Front Cardiovasc Med. 2019;6:16.
29. Agarwala A, Liu J, Ballantyne CM, Virani SS. The use of risk-enhancing factors to personalize ASCVD risk assessment: evidence and recommendations from the 2018 AHA/ACC Multi-society Cholesterol guidelines. Curr Cardiovasc Risk Rep. 2019;13(7):18.
30. Ridker PM, Buring JE, Rifai N, Cook NR. Development and validation of improved algorithms for the assessment of global cardiovascular risk in women: the Reynolds Risk Score. JAMA. 2007;297(6):611–9.
31. Ridker PM, Paynter NP, Rifai N, Gaziano JM, Cook NR. C-reactive protein and parental history improve global cardiovascular risk prediction: the Reynolds Risk Score for men. Circulation. 2008;118(22):2243–51.
32. Ockene IS, Matthews CE, Rifai N, Ridker PM, Reed G, Stanek E. Variability and classification accuracy of serial high-sensitivity C-reactive protein measurements in healthy adults. Clin Chem. 2001;47(3):444–50.
33. Ridker PM, Danielson E, Fonseca FA, Genest J, Gotto AM, Kastelein JJ, Koenig W, Libby P, Lorenzatti AJ, MacFadyen JG, Nordestgaard BG. Reduction in C-reactive protein and LDL cholesterol and cardiovascular event rates after initiation of rosuvastatin: a prospective study of the JUPITER trial. Lancet. 2009;373(9670):1175–82.
34. Hou H, Wang C, Sun F, Zhao L, Dun A, Sun Z. Association of interleukin-6 gene polymorphism with coronary artery disease: an updated systematic review and cumulative meta-analysis. Inflamm Res. 2015;64(9):707–20.
35. Shao B, Oda MN, Oram JF, Heinecke JW. Myeloperoxidase: an oxidative pathway for generating dysfunctional high-density lipoprotein. Chem Res Toxicol. 2010;23(3):447–54.
36. Sweeney T, Quispe R, Das T, Juraschek SP, Martin SS, Michos ED. The use of blood biomarkers in precision medicine for the primary prevention of atherosclerotic cardiovascular disease: a review. Expert Rev Precis Med Drug Dev. 2021;6(4):247–58.
37. Ajala ON, Everett BM. Targeting inflammation to reduce residual cardiovascular risk. Curr Atheroscler Rep. 2020;22(11):66.
38. Bohula EA, Giugliano RP, Cannon CP, Zhou J, Murphy SA, White JA, Tershakovec AM, Blazing MA, Braunwald E. Achievement of dual low-density lipoprotein cholesterol and high-sensitivity C-reactive protein targets more frequent with the addition of ezeti-

mibe to simvastatin and associated with better outcomes in IMPROVE-IT. Circulation. 2015;132(13):1224–33.

39. Rouleau J. Improved outcome after acute coronary syndromes with an intensive versus standard lipid-lowering regimen: results from the Pravastatin or Atorvastatin Evaluation and Infection Therapy–Thrombolysis in Myocardial Infarction 22 (PROVE IT–TIMI 22) trial. Am J Med. 2005;118(12):28–35.

40. Ridker PM, Rifai N, Rose L, Buring JE, Cook NR. Comparison of C-reactive protein and low-density lipoprotein cholesterol levels in the prediction of first cardiovascular events. N Engl J Med. 2002;347(20):1557–65.

41. Yousuf O, Mohanty BD, Martin SS, Joshi PH, Blaha MJ, Nasir K, Blumenthal RS, Budoff MJ. High-sensitivity C-reactive protein and cardiovascular disease: a resolute belief or an elusive link? J Am Coll Cardiol. 2013;62(5):397–408.

42. Albert MA, Ridker PM. C-Reactive protein as a risk predictor: do race/ethnicity and gender make a difference? Circulation. 2006;114(5):e67–74.

43. Shah T, Newcombe P, Smeeth L, Addo J, Casas JP, Whittaker J, Miller MA, Tinworth L, Jeffery S, Strazzullo P, Cappuccio FP. Ancestry as a determinant of mean population C-reactive protein values: implications for cardiovascular risk prediction. Circ Cardiovasc Genet. 2010;3(5):436–44.

44. Lippi G, Cervellin G, Sanchis-Gomar F. Prognostic value of troponins in patients with or without coronary heart disease: is it dependent on structure and biology? Heart Lung Circ. 2020;29(3):324–30.

45. Park KC, Gaze DC, Collinson PO, Marber MS. Cardiac troponins: from myocardial infarction to chronic disease. Cardiovasc Res. 2017;113(14):1708–18.

46. Jia X, Sun W, Hoogeveen RC, Nambi V, Matsushita K, Folsom AR, Heiss G, Couper DJ, Solomon SD, Boerwinkle E, Shah A. High-sensitivity troponin I and incident coronary events, stroke, heart failure hospitalization, and mortality in the ARIC study. Circulation. 2019;139(23):2642–53.

47. Thorsteinsdottir I, Aspelund T, Gudmundsson E, Eiriksdottir G, Harris TB, Launer LJ, Gudnason V, Venge P. High-sensitivity cardiac troponin I is a strong predictor of cardiovascular events and mortality in the AGES-Reykjavik community-based cohort of older individuals. Clin Chem. 2016;62(4):623–30.

48. Ford I, Shah A, Zhang R, et al. High-sensitivity cardiac troponin, statin therapy, and risk of coronary heart disease. J Am Coll Cardiol. 2016;68(25):2719–28.

49. Cao Z, Jia Y, Zhu B. BNP and NT-proBNP as diagnostic biomarkers for cardiac dysfunction in both clinical and forensic medicine. Int J Mol Sci. 2019;20(8):1820.

50. Kasahara S, Sakata Y, Nochioka K, Miura M, Abe R, Sato M, Aoyanagi H, Fujihashi T, Yamanaka S, Shiroto T, Sugimura K. Conversion formula from B-type natriuretic peptide to N-terminal proBNP values in patients with cardiovascular diseases. Int J Cardiol. 2019;280:184–9.

51. McCullough PA, Neyou A. Comprehensive review of the relative clinical utility of B-type natriuretic peptide and N-terminal pro-B-type natriuretic peptide assays in cardiovascular disease. Open Heart Fail J. 2009;2(1)

52. Shimizu N, Kotani K. Point-of-care testing of (N-terminal pro) B-type natriuretic peptide for heart disease patients in home care and ambulatory care settings. Pract Lab Med. 2020;22:e00183.

53. Heidenreich PA, Bozkurt B, Aguilar D, Allen LA, Byun JJ, Colvin MM, Deswal A, Drazner MH, Dunlay SM, Evers LR, Fang JC. 2022 AHA/ACC/HFSA guideline for the management of heart failure: executive summary: a report of the American College of Cardiology/American Heart Association Joint Committee on clinical practice guidelines. J Am Coll Cardiol. 2022;79(17):1757–80.

54. Rutten JHW, Mattace-Raso FUS, Steyerberg EW, et al. Amino-terminal pro-B-type natriuretic peptide improves cardiovascular and cerebrovascular risk prediction in the population: the Rotterdam study. Hypertension. 2010;55(3):785–91.

55. Folsom AR, Nambi V, Bell EJ, Oluleye OW, Gottesman RF, Lutsey PL, Huxley RR, Ballantyne CM. Troponin T, N-terminal pro–B-type natriuretic peptide, and incidence of stroke: the Atherosclerosis Risk in Communities Study. Stroke. 2013;44(4):961–7.
56. Di Castelnuovo A, Veronesi G, Costanzo S, Zeller T, Schnabel RB, de Curtis A, Salomaa V, Borchini R, Ferrario M, Giampaoli S, Kee F. NT-proBNP (N-terminal pro-B-type natriuretic peptide) and the risk of stroke: results from the BiomarCaRE consortium. Stroke. 2019;50(3):610–7.
57. Prausmüller S, Resl M, Arfsten H, Spinka G, Wurm R, Neuhold S, Bartko PE, Goliasch G, Strunk G, Pavo N, Clodi M. Performance of the recommended ESC/EASD cardiovascular risk stratification model in comparison to SCORE and NT-proBNP as a single biomarker for risk prediction in type 2 diabetes mellitus. Cardiovasc Diabetol. 2021;20(1):34.
58. Wijkman MO, Claggett BL, Malachias MV, Vaduganathan M, Ballantyne CM, Kitzman DW, Mosley T, Matsushita K, Solomon SD, Pfeffer MA. Importance of NT-proBNP and conventional risk factors for prediction of death in older adults with and without diabetes mellitus—a report from the Atherosclerosis Risk in Communities (ARIC) study. Diabetes Res Clin Pract. 2022;194:110164.
59. Bayes-Genis A. Diabetes and NT-proBNP: partners in crime. Diabetes Res Clin Pract. 2022;194:110165.
60. Alpert MA. Natriuretic peptides as predictors of cardiovascular events and all-cause mortality. J Am Coll Cardiol. 2021;77(5):572–4.
61. Kistorp C, Raymond I, Pedersen F, Gustafsson F, Faber J, Hildebrandt P. N-terminal pro-brain natriuretic peptide, C-reactive protein, and urinary albumin levels as predictors of mortality and cardiovascular events in older adults. JAMA. 2005;293(13):1609–16.
62. Gore MO, Ayers CR, Khera A, Defilippi CR, Wang TJ, Seliger SL, Nambi V, Selvin E, Berry JD, Hundley WG, Budoff M. Combining biomarkers and imaging for short-term assessment of cardiovascular disease risk in apparently healthy adults. J Am Heart Assoc. 2020;9(15):e015410.
63. Libby P, Rocha VZ. All roads lead to IL-6: a central hub of cardiometabolic signaling. Int J Cardiol. 2018;259:213–5.
64. Ziegler L, Gajulapuri A, Frumento P, et al. Interleukin 6 trans-signalling and risk of future cardiovascular events. Cardiovasc Res. 2019;115(1):213–21.
65. Wainstein MV, Mossmann M, Araujo GN, et al. Elevated serum interleukin-6 is predictive of coronary artery disease in intermediate risk overweight patients referred for coronary angiography. Diabetol Metab Syndr. 2017;9:67.
66. Liu S, Niu J, Wu S, et al. Urinary albumin-to-creatinine ratio levels are associated with subclinical atherosclerosis and predict CVD events and all-cause deaths: a prospective analysis. BMJ Open. 2021;11(3):e040890.
67. Szabóová E, Lisovszki A, Fatľová E, Kolarčik P, Szabó P, Molnár T. Prevalence of microalbuminuria and its association with subclinical carotid atherosclerosis in middle aged, nondiabetic, low to moderate cardiovascular risk individuals with or without hypertension. Diagnostics (Basel). 2021;11(9):1716.
68. Pantazi D, Tellis C, Tselepis AD. "SI: PAF" Oxidized phospholipids and lipoprotein-associated phospholipase A2 (Lp-PLA2) in atherosclerotic cardiovascular disease: an update. Biofactors. 2022;48(6):1257–70.
69. Jenny NS, Solomon C, Cushman M, et al. Lipoprotein-associated phospholipase A(2) (Lp-LA(2)) and risk of cardiovascular disease in older adults: results from the Cardiovascular Health Study. Atherosclerosis. 2010;209:528–32.
70. Tsimikas S, Willeit J, Knoflach M, et al. Lipoprotein-associated phospholipase A2 activity, ferritin levels, metabolic syndrome, and 10-year cardiovascular and non-cardiovascular mortality: results from the Bruneck study. Eur Heart J. 2009;30:107–15.
71. Davidson MH, Corson MA, Alberts MJ, et al. Consensus panel recommendation for incorporating lipoprotein-associated phospholipase A2 testing into cardiovascular disease risk assessment guidelines. Am J Cardiol. 2008;101(12A):51F–7F.

72. Gregson JM, Freitag DF, Surendran P, et al. Genetic invalidation of Lp-PLA2 as a therapeutic target: large-scale study of five functional Lp-PLA2-lowering alleles. Eur J Prev Cardiol. 2017;24(5):492–504.

73. Ndrepepa G, Braun S, Mehilli J, Von Beckerath N, Schömig A, Kastrati A. Myeloperoxidase level in patients with stable coronary artery disease and acute coronary syndromes. Eur J Clin Investig. 2008;38(2):90–6.

74. Li J, Cao T, Wei Y, et al. A review of novel cardiac biomarkers in acute or chronic cardiovascular diseases: the role of soluble ST2 (sST2), lipoprotein-associated phospholipase A2 (Lp-PLA2), myeloperoxidase (MPO), and procalcitonin (PCT). Dis Markers. 2021;2021:6258865.

75. Brennan ML, Penn MS, Van Lente F, et al. Prognostic value of myeloperoxidase in patients with chest pain. N Engl J Med. 2003;349(17):1595–604.

76. Teng N, Maghzal GJ, Talib J, Rashid I, Lau AK, Stocker R. The roles of myeloperoxidase in coronary artery disease and its potential implication in plaque rupture. Redox Rep Commun Free Radic Res. 2017;22(2):51–73.

77. Rashid I, Maghzal GJ, Chen YC, et al. Myeloperoxidase is a potential molecular imaging and therapeutic target for the identification and stabilization of high-risk atherosclerotic plaque. Eur Heart J. 2018;39(35):3301–10.

78. Hilvo M, Vasile VC, Donato LJ, Hurme R, Laaksonen R. Ceramides and ceramide scores: clinical applications for cardiometabolic risk stratification. Front Endocrinol. 2020;11:570628.

79. Berkowitz L, Cabrera-Reyes F, Salazar C, Ryff CD, Coe C, Rigotti A. Sphingolipid profiling: a promising tool for stratifying the metabolic syndrome-associated risk. Front Cardiovasc Med. 2022;8:2177.

80. Zietzer A, Düsing P, Reese L, Nickenig G, Jansen F. Ceramide metabolism in cardiovascular disease: a network with high therapeutic potential. Arterioscler Thromb Vasc Biol. 2022;42(10):1220–8.

81. Havulinna AS, et al. Circulating ceramides predict cardiovascular outcomes in the population-based FINRISK 2002 cohort. Arterioscler Thromb Vasc Biol. 2016;36(12):2424–30.

82. Mantovani A, Dugo C. Ceramides and risk of major adverse cardiovascular events: a meta-analysis of longitudinal studies. J Clin Lipidol. 2020;14(2):176–85.

83. Choi RH, et al. Ceramides and other sphingolipids as drivers of cardiovascular disease. Nat Rev Cardiol. 2021;18(10):701–11.

84. Meeusen JW, et al. Plasma ceramides: a novel predictor of major adverse cardiovascular events after coronary angiography. Arterioscler Thromb Vasc Biol. 2018;38(8):1933–9.

85. Wu J, Wang J. Research advances on circulating exosomal microRNAs as novel biomarkers of atherosclerotic cardiovascular diseases. Chin J Lab Med. 2021:558–62.

86. Petrucci G, Rizzi A, Hatem D, Tosti G, Rocca B, Pitocco D. Role of oxidative stress in the pathogenesis of atherothrombotic diseases. Antioxidants. 2022;11(7):1408.

87. Weber LA, Cheezum MK, Reese JM, Lane AB, Haley RD, Lutz MW, Villines TC. Cardiovascular imaging for the primary prevention of atherosclerotic cardiovascular disease events. Curr Cardiovasc Imaging Rep. 2015;8(9):36.

88. Budoff MJ, Nasir K, McClelland RL, Detrano R, Wong N, Blumenthal RS, Kondos G, Kronmal RA. Coronary calcium predicts events better with absolute calcium scores than age-sex-race/ethnicity percentiles: MESA (Multi-Ethnic Study of Atherosclerosis). J Am Coll Cardiol. 2009;53(4):345–52.

89. Detrano R, Guerci AD, Carr JJ, Bild DE, Burke G, Folsom AR, Liu K, Shea S, Szklo M, Bluemke DA, O'Leary DH. Coronary calcium as a predictor of coronary events in four racial or ethnic groups. N Engl J Med. 2008;358(13):1336–45.

90. Polonsky TS, McClelland RL, Jorgensen NW, Bild DE, Burke GL, Guerci AD, Greenland P. Coronary artery calcium score and risk classification for coronary heart disease prediction. JAMA. 2010;303(16):1610–6.

91. Elias-Smale SE, Proença RV, Koller MT, Kavousi M, van Rooij FJ, Hunink MG, Steyerberg EW, Hofman A, Oudkerk M, Witteman JC. Coronary calcium score improves classifica-

tion of coronary heart disease risk in the elderly: the Rotterdam study. J Am Coll Cardiol. 2010;56(17):1407–14.

92. Erbel R, Möhlenkamp S, Moebus S, Schmermund A, Lehmann N, Stang A, Dragano N, Grönemeyer D, Seibel R, Kälsch H, Bröcker-Preuss M. Coronary risk stratification, discrimination, and reclassification improvement based on quantification of subclinical coronary atherosclerosis: the Heinz Nixdorf Recall study. J Am Coll Cardiol. 2010;56(17):1397–406.

93. Blaha M, Budoff MJ, Shaw LJ, Khosa F, Rumberger JA, Berman D, Callister T, Raggi P, Blumenthal RS, Nasir K. Absence of coronary artery calcification and all-cause mortality. JACC Cardiovasc Imaging. 2009;2(6):692–700.

94. Nasir K, Rubin J, Blaha MJ, Shaw LJ, Blankstein R, Rivera JJ, Khan AN, Berman D, Raggi P, Callister T, Rumberger JA. Interplay of coronary artery calcification and traditional risk factors for the prediction of all-cause mortality in asymptomatic individuals. Circul Cardiovasc Imaging. 2012;5(4):467–73.

95. Tummala R, Han D, Friedman J, Hayes S, Thomson L, Gransar H, Slomka P, Rozanski A, Dey D, Berman D. Association between plaque localization in proximal coronary segments and MACE outcomes in patients with mild CAC: results from the EISNER study. Am J Prev Cardiol. 2022;12:100423.

96. Meah MN, Dweck MR, Newby DE. Cardiovascular imaging to guide primary prevention. Heart. 2020;106(16):1267–75.

97. Miedema MD, Duprez DA, Misialek JR, Blaha MJ, Nasir K, Silverman MG, Blankstein R, Budoff MJ, Greenland P, Folsom AR. Use of coronary artery calcium testing to guide aspirin utilization for primary prevention: estimates from the multi-ethnic study of atherosclerosis. Circ Cardiovasc Qual Outcomes. 2014;7(3):453–60.

98. Curry SJ, Krist AH, Owens DK, Barry MJ, Caughey AB, Davidson KW, Doubeni CA, Epling JW, Kemper AR, Kubik M, Landefeld CS. Risk assessment for cardiovascular disease with nontraditional risk factors: US preventive services task force recommendation statement. JAMA. 2018;320(3):272–80.

99. Earls JP, Woodard PK, Abbara S, Akers SR, Araoz PA, Cummings K, Cury RC, Dorbala S, Hoffmann U, Hsu JY, Jacobs JE. ACR appropriateness criteria asymptomatic patient at risk for coronary artery disease. J Am Coll Radiol. 2014;11(1):12–9.

100. Stein JH, Korcarz CE, Hurst RT, Lonn E, Kendall CB, Mohler ER, Najjar SS, Rembold CM, Post WS. Use of carotid ultrasound to identify subclinical vascular disease and evaluate cardiovascular disease risk: a consensus statement from the American Society of Echocardiography Carotid Intima-Media Thickness Task Force endorsed by the Society for Vascular Medicine. J Am Soc Echocardiogr. 2008;21(2):93–111.

101. Nambi V, Chambless L, Folsom AR, He M, Hu Y, Mosley T, Volcik K, Boerwinkle E, Ballantyne CM. Carotid intima-media thickness and presence or absence of plaque improves prediction of coronary heart disease risk: the ARIC (Atherosclerosis Risk In Communities) study. J Am Coll Cardiol. 2010;55(15):1600–7.

102. Inaba Y, Chen JA, Bergmann SR. Carotid plaque, compared with carotid intima-media thickness, more accurately predicts coronary artery disease events: a meta-analysis. Atherosclerosis. 2012;220(1):128–33.

103. Goff DC Jr, et al. 2013 ACC/AHA guideline on the assessment of cardiovascular risk: a report of the American College of Cardiology/American Heart Association Task Force on practice guidelines. Circulation. 2014;129(25 Suppl 2):S49–73.

104. Cavalcante JL, Lima JA, Redheuil A, Al-Mallah MH. Aortic stiffness: current understanding and future directions. J Am Coll Cardiol. 2011;57(14):1511–22.

105. Kim HL, Kim SH. Pulse wave velocity in atherosclerosis. Front Cardiovasc Med. 2019;6:41.

106. Pereira T, Correia C, Cardoso J. Novel methods for pulse wave velocity measurement. J Med Biol Eng. 2015;35(5):555–65.

107. Podolec P, Kopeć G, Podolec J, Wilkołek P, Krochin M, Rubiś P, Cwynar M, Grodzicki T, Żmudka K, Tracz W. Aortic pulse wave velocity and carotid-femoral pulse wave velocity: similarities and discrepancies. Hypertens Res. 2007;30(12):1151–8.

108. Munakata M. Brachial-ankle pulse wave velocity in the measurement of arterial stiffness: recent evidence and clinical applications. Curr Hypertens Rev. 2014;10(1):49–57.
109. Mattace-Raso FU, van der Cammen TJ, Hofman A, van Popele NM, Bos ML, Schalekamp MA, Asmar R, Reneman RS, Hoeks AP, Breteler MM, Witteman JC. Arterial stiffness and risk of coronary heart disease and stroke: the Rotterdam study. Circulation. 2006;113(5):657–63.
110. Van Sloten TT, Sedaghat S, Laurent S, London GM, Pannier B, Ikram MA, Kavousi M, Mattace-Raso F, Franco OH, Boutouyrie P, Stehouwer CD. Carotid stiffness is associated with incident stroke: a systematic review and individual participant data meta-analysis. J Am Coll Cardiol. 2015;66(19):2116–25.
111. Vlachopoulos C, Aznaouridis K, Stefanadis C. Prediction of cardiovascular events and all-cause mortality with arterial stiffness: a systematic review and meta-analysis. J Am Coll Cardiol. 2010;55(13):1318–27.
112. Ohkuma T, Ninomiya T, Tomiyama H, et al. Brachial-ankle pulse wave velocity and the risk prediction of cardiovascular disease: an individual participant data meta-analysis. Hypertension. 2017;69(6):1045–52.
113. Munden RF, Carter BW, Chiles C, MacMahon H, Black WC, Ko JP, McAdams HP, Rossi SE, Leung AN, Boiselle PM, Kent MS. Managing incidental findings on thoracic CT: mediastinal and cardiovascular findings. A white paper of the ACR incidental findings committee. J Am Coll Radiol. 2018;15(8):1087–96.
114. Hecht HS, Cronin P, Blaha MJ, Budoff MJ, Kazerooni EA, Narula J, Yankelevitz D, Abbara S. 2016 SCCT/STR guidelines for coronary artery calcium scoring of noncontrast noncardiac chest CT scans: a report of the Society of Cardiovascular Computed Tomography and Society of Thoracic Radiology. J Cardiovasc Comput Tomogr. 2017;11(1):74–84.
115. Kim SM, Chung MJ, Lee KS, Choe YH, Yi CA, Choe BK. Coronary calcium screening using low-dose lung cancer screening: effectiveness of MDCT with retrospective reconstruction. Am J Roentgenol. 2008;190(4):917–22.
116. Wu MT, Yang P, Huang YL, Chen JS, Chuo CC, Yeh C, Chang RS. Coronary arterial calcification on low-dose ungated MDCT for lung cancer screening: concordance study with dedicated cardiac CT. Am J Roentgenol. 2008;190(4):923–8.
117. Xie X, et al. Validation and prognosis of coronary artery calcium scoring in nontriggered thoracic computed tomography: systematic review and meta-analysis. Circ Cardiovasc Imaging. 2013;6(4):514–21.
118. Suh JW, La Yun B. Breast arterial calcification: a potential surrogate marker for cardiovascular disease. J Cardiovasc Imaging. 2018;26(3):125–34.
119. Iribarren C, Chandra M, Lee C, Sanchez G, Sam DL, Azamian FF, Cho HM, Ding H, Wong ND, Molloi S. Breast arterial calcification: a novel cardiovascular risk enhancer among postmenopausal women. Circ Cardiovasc Imaging. 2022;15(3):e013526.

An Overview of the Guideline Development Process for Atherosclerotic Cardiovascular Disease Risk Reduction with an Emphasis on Guidelines for Cholesterol and Dyslipidemia Management

Carl E. Orringer

Key Points

- Clinical practice guidelines for lipid management of atherosclerotic cardiovascular disease (ASCVD) are to be used in combination with clinical judgement to improve patient care and cardiovascular outcomes.
- The process for creating ASCVD prevention guidelines varies widely depending on the overall philosophy and instructional approach of the sponsoring organization(s).
- The methodology and standards for the guideline creation process described by the American Heart Association (AHA) and the American College of Cardiology (ACC) include a system to classify recommendations using the designation of class of recommendation (COR), which reflects the magnitude of benefit over risk associated with a given recommendation, and a level of evidence (LOE) rating, which reflects the quality of the types of studies and supporting data on which the recommendation is based.
- Current ACC/AHA guidelines utilize a "knowledge chunk format" to present recommendations; these include a table of the recommendations, synopsis, supporting text, and flow diagrams or additional tables for each "chunk" of information.
- The development of ASCVD risk reduction guidelines is affected by decisions regarding the types of evidence that will be considered, e.g., limiting to evidence from randomized controlled trials (RCTs) vs. placing the focus on lowering atherogenic lipoproteins including both RCT evidence and high-quality observational and mechanistic data.

C. E. Orringer (✉)
Rooney Heart Institute at NCH, NCH Healthcare System, Naples, FL, USA
e-mail: carl.orringer@nchmd.org

© The Author(s), under exclusive license to Springer Nature Switzerland AG 2024
K. C. Maki, D. P. Wilson (eds.), *Cardiovascular Outcomes Research*, Contemporary Cardiology, https://doi.org/10.1007/978-3-031-54960-1_5

- Guideline development is also affected by the ASCVD risk assessment tools available in the country for which the guideline is intended, e.g., Pooled Cohort Equations in the United States vs. Systematic Coronary Risk Estimation in Europe.
- A guideline development process limited to RCT data minimizes the key role of lifestyle intervention, the support of which is largely dependent on observational data.
- To date, most ASCVD risk reduction guidelines have focused on low-density lipoprotein cholesterol as the primary target of therapy, despite evidence that non-high-density lipoprotein cholesterol and apolipoprotein B are better predictors of risk.
- While consideration of risk-enhancing factors is recommended to further evaluate ASCVD risk and guide treatment decisions in intermediate-risk populations, their utility in individual patient management remains largely a matter of clinical judgment.
- The rapid pace of new drug development supports the need for a process that favors more frequent update of lipid management guidelines.
- Guideline development should be complemented by advances in implementation science to close the gap between recommendations and real-world application.

Clinical practice guidelines for lipid management for atherosclerotic cardiovascular disease (ASCVD) risk reduction are patient care recommendations that inform the clinician–patient discussion in the context of shared decision-making. They are not intended to be mandates for patient care, nor to replace clinical judgment, since concomitant co-morbidities or differences in responsiveness of individual patients may result in different outcomes as compared to those reported in clinical trials. Their application to patient care is intended to result in improved outcomes, reduced risk, or both.

The process of guideline creation varies from organization to organization and depends on the expertise and integrity of the chairs and members of the writing committee, adherence to process, the absence of relationships, at the very least in the chair or co-chair, that could alter the credibility of the recommendations, and a high level of transparency throughout the writing process. These standards are most clearly stated in the guideline writing process of the American Heart Association (AHA) and the American College of Cardiology (ACC).

The ACC/AHA Task Force on Practice Guidelines, in response to publication of two reports by the Institute of Medicine in 2011 [1, 2], convened their own methodology recommendations [3] in which stakeholder organizations were invited to participate as partners or collaborators, a Guidelines Writing Committee (GWC) Chair was selected and an appropriate and diverse panel of experts, including lay representatives, was selected. To promote transparency, the ACC/AHA requested that panel authors submit disclosures of relevant relationships with industry that would be documented in the Guideline document. The GWC was charged with defining the document content, performing detailed and specific evidence acquisition and review, and drafting recommendations that were based on the strength and quality of the evidence.

While the cholesterol treatment guidelines provided in the National Heart, Lung, and Blood Institute (NHLBI)-sponsored Adult Treatment Panels I–III [4–6] used a diverse body of evidence to create an extensive compendium of clinical information supporting their guidelines, the 2013 ACC/AHA Cholesterol Treatment Guideline, in an attempt to adhere to the recommendations of the NHLBI Advisory Council, addressed selected critical questions on each topic, and, unlike the previous guidelines, used an evidence review exclusively employing high-quality randomized controlled trials (RCTs) and meta-analyses of those trials. The highest quality RCTs were characterized as those having adequate randomization, blinding, and allocation concealment, being adequately powered, using intention-to-treat analyses, and having high follow-up rates. The Guideline, with few exceptions, provided recommendations only in those areas in which RCT data were available. Consequently, the scope of recommendations was considerably more limited than that of previous Guidelines. This 2013 Guideline, which was initiated by the NHLBI and subsequently transferred to the ACC and AHA, was reviewed by 23 expert reviewers and representatives of federal agencies and by four expert reviewers nominated by the ACC and the AHA [7].

The ACC/AHA proposed in 2014 [3] and affirmed in 2016 [8] a Guideline Recommendation Classification System that has been adopted for all subsequent Guidelines produced by those organizations. Recommendations are ranked by class of recommendation (COR) that reflects the magnitude of benefit over risk. Class I recommendations are considered strong and indicate that treatment should be given in most patients under most circumstances. Class II ranking connotes that benefit generally exceeds risk, with a IIa ranking suggesting a moderate, and IIb a weak, recommendation. Class III recommendations are designated as being associated either with no benefit or harm.

Quality of evidence ratings range from level A, characterized by high-quality evidence from >1 RCT, meta-analyses of high-quality RCTs, or 1 or more RCTs corroborated by high-quality registry studies; level B-R, supported by moderate quality evidence from 1 or more RCTs or meta-analyses of moderate quality RCTs; level B-NR, in which the supporting evidence is of moderate quality and from 1 or more well-designed, well-executed, non-randomized studies, observational studies or registry studies or meta-analyses of such studies; level C-LD, in which evidence is derived from randomized or non-randomized observational or registry studies with limitations of design or execution, meta-analyses of such studies, or physiologic or mechanistic studies in humans; and level C-EO, representing consensus of expert opinion based on clinical observations without additional supporting data.

To improve clinical utility and shorten their guidelines, the ACC and AHA, beginning in 2017, made formatting modifications in which their guidelines were presented in a "knowledge chunk format," in which each chunk has a table of recommendations, a brief synopsis, recommendation-specific supporting text and, as appropriate, flow diagrams or additional tables to enhance reader understanding. Hyperlinked references facilitate rapid access and review. Word limits for the contributing authors are used to emphasize the importance of brevity and clarity.

The 2018 AHA/ACC/Multi-Society Cholesterol Guideline [9], sponsored by 12 stakeholder organizations maintained the focus of the 2013 Guideline on the primacy of well-executed RCTs in providing treatment guidelines, but employed the knowledge chunk format, and increased the scope of the Guideline by allowing recommendations that employed a broader evidence base, including observational and mechanistic studies. This approach allowed the authors to provide recommendations for the management of selected disorders, such as hypertriglyceridemia, in which most of the available evidence for treatment was derived from observational studies, or the management of special populations, such as older or younger patients or those of under-represented minorities, in whom there are limited RCT data to support treatment recommendations.

Guideline development may also be affected by the philosophical underpinnings supported by the sponsoring organization's writing group and by the risk assessment tools that are applicable to the patients to which the guidelines are applied in the countries in which they reside [10]. For example, the 2018 AHA/ACC/Multi-Society Guideline was written based on the premise that the best outcomes are achieved by providing recommendations that are supported by RCT outcomes data, whereas the 2019 European Society of Cardiology (ESC)/European Atherosclerosis Society (EAS) Lipid Guidelines [11], while recognizing the high value of RCT evidence, promoted a central philosophy that the best ASCVD outcomes are achieved by those with lower concentrations of low-density lipoprotein cholesterol (LDL-C), even when RCT data may not be available in certain patient groups. This central philosophy is informed by evidence from a variety of sources in addition to RCTs, including observational research, particularly Mendelian randomization studies that show associations between genetic variants affecting lipoprotein lipid levels and subsequent ASCVD outcomes, as well as results from studies in animal models.

The AHA/ACC Guideline's risk assessment for primary prevention is based on the outcome of fatal or nonfatal myocardial infarction or stroke as estimated by the Pooled Cohort Equations (PCEs), whereas the 2019 ESC/EAS Guideline bases its primary prevention recommendations on 10-year country-specific estimates of cardiovascular death, as advocated by the Systematic Coronary Risk Estimation (SCORE) chart for European populations.

It must be acknowledged that there are a number of limitations to the approach to guideline creation employed by the AHA/ACC. The focus on RCTs necessarily drives the discussion toward drug therapy, as pharmaceutical companies have the financial support necessary to sponsor such trials. Conversely, trials of lifestyle intervention have mostly been focused on assessing changes in biomarkers with few evaluating effects on incidence of major adverse cardiovascular events, resulting in a lower strength of supporting evidence as compared to pharmacological interventions. This is paradoxical, as guidelines for ASCVD prevention and management consistently recognize lifestyle change as the necessary underpinning to all drug therapy recommendations. Furthermore, despite the recognition that non-high-density lipoprotein cholesterol (non-HDL-C) and apolipoprotein (Apo) B levels are better predictors of risk than LDL-C [12, 13], ASCVD outcomes trials have mainly focused on LDL-C as the pre-specified target of therapy. This approach may result in undertreatment in subgroups with discordance between the LDL-C level and the circulating concentration of atherogenic lipoproteins, such as patients with elevated triglycerides or low HDL-C, who often have a predominance of small, dense LDL particles and a higher level of Apo B-containing lipoprotein for a given level of LDL-C. Furthermore, most cardiovascular outcomes trials have been designed to test the effects of a medication against a control condition such as placebo, usual care, or a less intensive treatment regimen. This has resulted in a reluctance to specify goals for levels of LDL-C (as well as non-HDL-C and Apo B), since few trials tested a treat-to-goal approach.

The 2018 AHA/ACC Blood Cholesterol Guideline, as well as its 2013 predecessor, employs the use of the PCEs, the validity and clinical utility of which has been based on observational studies, but not on RCTs. The PCEs are recognized to overestimate risk in healthier populations with greater access to preventive health care and to underestimate risk in those with lesser access and in certain racial/ethnic groups. Regarding the clinical utility of the risk-enhancing factors, the high prevalence of individual risk-enhancing factors in intermediate risk populations, the potential for risk miscalibration based on their use [14], and the recognition that multiple risk-enhancing factors must be present for refinement of ASCVD risk [15] serve to complicate preventive treatment decision-making for the clinician. The American Heart Association released in 2024 a new risk calculator based on the Predicting Risk of CVD EVENTs (PREDICT) risk equations [16]. This calculator provides race-independent estimates for total cardiovascular disease, atherosclerotic cardiovascular disease and heart failure with a 10-year risk estimate for those 30-79 years of age and 30-year estimate for those 30-59 years of age. These equations are based on a far larger and more contemporary derivation and validation cohort than was used for the PCE. The utility of this new risk calculator remains to be determined.

The traditional pace of creation of lipid treatment guidelines, which in the past had been approximately every 5–7 years, will have to be modified in future iterations to account for the increasingly rapid pace of new drug development. The use of newer approaches that favor more concise, knowledge chunk formatting and employ on-line annual or biannual updates will promote more rapid incorporation of newer data into traditional treatment paradigms and will serve to provide clinicians with the latest advances in preventive care. These innovations must be complemented by advances in implementation science to help to close the gap between guideline creation and real-world application.

In summary, the guideline creation process depends on the philosophy and instructional approach that is most representative of the sponsoring organization. The process represents an integration of the scientific underpinnings of the data supporting the recommendations and of the perceived optimal methods for maximizing clinician utilization.

References

1. Committee on Standards for Developing Trustworthy Clinical Practice Guidelines, Institute of Medicine. Clinical practice guidelines we can trust. Washington, DC: The National Academies Press; 2011.
2. Committee on Standards for Systematic Reviews of Comparative Effectiveness Research, Institute of Medicine. Finding what works in health care: standards for systematic reviews. Washington, DC: The National Academies Press; 2011.
3. Jacobs AK, Anderson JL, Halperin JL. The evolution and future of ACC/AHA clinical practice guidelines: a 30-year journey: a report of the American College of Cardiology/American Heart Association Task Force on practice guidelines. J Am Coll Cardiol. 2014;64(13):1373–84.
4. Report of the National Cholesterol Education Program Expert Panel on detection, evaluation, and treatment of high blood cholesterol in adults. The Expert Panel. Arch Intern Med. 1988;148(1):36–69.
5. National Cholesterol Education Program. Report of the Expert Panel on Population Strategies for Blood Cholesterol Reduction: executive summary. National Heart, Lung and Blood Institute, National Institutes of Health. Arch Intern Med. 1991;151(6):1071–84.
6. Expert Panel on Detection, Evaluation, and Treatment of High Blood Cholesterol in Adults. Executive summary of the third report of the National Cholesterol Education Program (NCEP) Expert Panel on detection, evaluation, and treatment of high blood cholesterol in adults (Adult Treatment Panel III). JAMA. 2001;285(19):2486–97.
7. Stone NJ, Robinson JG, Lichtenstein AH, et al. 2013 ACC/AHA guideline on the treatment of blood cholesterol to reduce atherosclerotic cardiovascular risk in adults: a report of the American College of Cardiology/American Heart Association Task Force on practice guidelines. Circulation. 2014;129(25 Suppl 2):S1–45.
8. Halperin JL, Levine GN, Al-Khatib SM, et al. Further evolution of the ACC/AHA clinical practice guideline recommendation classification system: a report of the American College of Cardiology/American Heart Association Task Force on clinical practice guidelines. Circulation. 2016;133(14):1426–8.
9. Grundy SM, Stone NJ, Bailey AL, et al. 2018 AHA/ACC/AACVPR/AAPA/ABC/ACPM/ADA/AGS/APhA/ASPC/NLA/PCNA guideline on the management of blood cholesterol: a report of the American College of Cardiology/American Heart Association Task Force on clinical practice guidelines. Circulation. 2019;139(25):e1082–143.
10. Orringer CE, Tokgozoglu L, Maki KC, et al. Transatlantic lipid guideline divergence: same data but different interpretations. J Am Heart Assoc. 2020;9(21):e018189.
11. Mach F, Baigent C, Catapano AL, et al. 2019 ESC/EAS guidelines for the management of dyslipidaemias: lipid modification to reduce cardiovascular risk. Eur Heart J. 2019;41(1):111–88.
12. Johannesen CDL, Mortensen MB, Langsted A, Nordestgaard BG. Apolipoprotein B and non-HDL cholesterol better reflect residual risk than LDL cholesterol in statin-treated patients. J Am Coll Cardiol. 2021;77(11):1439–50.
13. Sniderman AD, Williams K, Contois JH, et al. A meta-analysis of low-density lipoprotein, cholesterol non-high-density lipoprotein cholesterol, and apolipoprotein B as markers of cardiovascular risk. Circ Cardiovasc Qual Outcomes. 2011;4:337–45.
14. Stern RH, Brook RD. Do risk-enhancing factors enhance risk estimation? Circ Cardiovasc Qual Outcome. 2019;12:e006078.
15. Vega GL, Wang J, Grundy SM. Prevalence and significance of risk enhancing biomarkers in the United States population at intermediate risk for atherosclerotic disease. J Clin Lipidol. 2022;16:66–74.
16. Khan SS, Matsushita K, Sang Y, et al. Development and validation of the american heart association's PREVENT equations. Circulation. 2024;149(6):430–49.

Implementation Science: Strategies to Improve Adoption and Adherence to Clinical Practice Guidelines

Laney K. Jones, Mitchell N. Sarkies, Michael R. Gionfriddo, Samuel S. Gidding, and Gerald F. Watts

Key Points
- Implementation science provides tools to improve translation of evidence-based practice and is highly relevant to cardiology.
- Incorporation of implementation science methods into the development and dissemination of clinical practice guidelines can improve the translation and uptake of evidence-based findings.

L. K. Jones (✉)
Department of Genomic Health, Geisinger, Danville, PA, USA

Heart and Vascular Institute, Geisinger, Danville, PA, USA
e-mail: Ljones14@geisinger.edu

M. N. Sarkies
School of Health Sciences and Sydney Health Partners, University of Sydney,
Sydney, NSW, Australia

Centre for Healthcare Resilience and Implementation Science, Australian Institute of Health
Innovation, Macquarie University, Sydney, NSW, Australia
e-mail: mitchell.sarkies@sydney.edu.au

M. R. Gionfriddo
Division of Pharmaceutical, Administrative and Social Sciences, School of Pharmacy,
Duquesne University, Pittsburgh, PA, USA
e-mail: gionfriddom@duq.edu

S. S. Gidding
Department of Genomic Health, Geisinger, Danville, PA, USA
e-mail: ssgidding@geisinger.edu

G. F. Watts
School of Medicine, University of Western Australia, Perth, WA, Australia

Department of Cardiology, Royal Perth Hospital, Perth, WA, Australia
e-mail: gerald.watts@uwa.edu.au

© The Author(s), under exclusive license to Springer Nature
Switzerland AG 2024
K. C. Maki, D. P. Wilson (eds.), *Cardiovascular Outcomes Research*,
Contemporary Cardiology, https://doi.org/10.1007/978-3-031-54960-1_6

- Conducting a needs assessment helps identify barriers to and facilitators of care and the development of implementation strategies.
- Select an implementation science theory, model, or framework that best fits the project goals.
- Implementation strategies should be developed to fit local context and are evaluated using rigorous methods.
- The success of implementation strategies in improving adoption of and adherence to clinical practice guidelines is variable.
- The measurement of adherence and maintenance to a proposed strategy can be complex, and new assessment tools are needed.

1 Introduction to Implementation Science

Evidence-based practices take, on average, 17 years to be incorporated into routine general practice in health care [1, 2]. This delay creates an "evidence-to-practice" gap where evidence exists about a particular subject, but individuals do not act on it. Implementation science offers theoretical and practical approaches to understanding barriers to and improving the translation of evidence into practice. For example, guideline developers can improve the translation of evidence into practice by engaging experts in implementation science and including guidance on how to adapt the recommendations to the local contexts (Fig. 1) [3]. Several recent guidelines in cardiology have included sections on implementation, such as the most recent American Heart Association (AHA) and American College of Cardiology (ACC) Cholesterol Guidelines released in 2018 [4]. Once guidelines are developed, strategies to facilitate their implementation should be tailored to overcome local barriers to practice change. Following successful implementation, monitoring and evaluation is important for sustainability and feedback of new evidence into future clinical practice guidelines.

The incorporation of implementation science into guidelines and practice in cardiology is urgently needed as evidence-based therapies are not being received by a

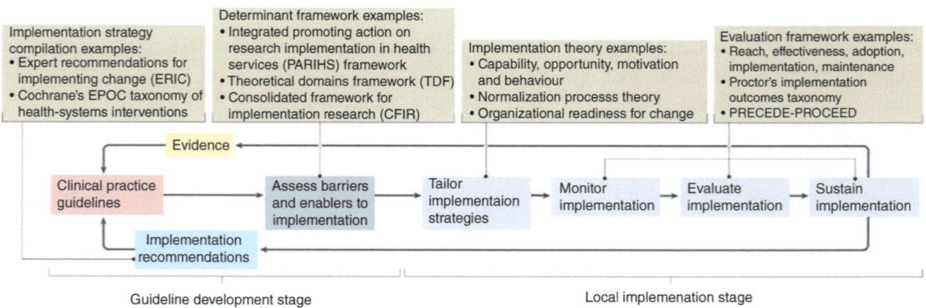

Fig. 1 Embedding implementation science into the guideline development and translation processes. Source: Reproduced from Sarkies and Jones et al. [3] with permission by Springer Nature Rights

large proportion of patients across a range of disease states, including acute coronary syndrome [5], atrial fibrillation [6], hypertension [7, 8], and hyperlipidemia [9]. The failure to utilize evidence-based therapies in practices has multiple etiologies, such as a lack of awareness of the evidence among clinicians, discordance in guideline recommendations, or a belief that recommendations are not applicable to specific clinical settings [10]. Clinicians who do follow the advice given in guidelines may be confused when multiple guidelines provide disparate advice, especially in patients with multimorbidity [11]. Further, clinicians, especially in low resource settings, may lack the resources to implement certain evidence-based practices [12]. Even in high resource settings, however, clinicians may not implement certain evidence-based practices owing to the challenges of balancing the many competing needs that arise when caring for a patient during a time-limited clinical encounter [13].

Recommended and prescribed therapies must be adhered to for benefits to be realized. Patients may not agree with the recommendation from their clinician or may struggle with finding ways to make the recommendation fit into their lives. This may be due to a lack of resources, capabilities, or support necessary to implement the intervention with fidelity. As a result of these challenges, many interventions are not implemented by patients, with rates of adherence to lipid lowering therapies, for example, often suboptimal [14].

In this chapter, we review key terminology in implementation science and provide an overview of steps to consider when utilizing implementation science in practice. The steps include: (1) defining the evidence-based practice or intervention, (2) choosing a theory, model, or framework, (3) assessing determinants, barriers, enablers, and context with respect to the evidence-based practice or intervention, (4) selecting implementation strategies, and (5) selecting options for monitoring and evaluating implementation. Finally, we provide examples of implementation strategies that have been used in the literature to improve adoption of and sustained adherence to evidence-informed recommendations in clinical practice.

1.1 Definitions

While implementation science has emerged as its own field of study, it draws from a diverse set of disciplines and intellectual traditions. These fields include philosophy, sociology, science and technology studies, improvement science, organizational science, knowledge translation, program science, and delivery science, among others [15, 16]. Reporting on the foundational concepts of implementation science, Rapport et al. identified that not all stakeholders view implementation science with the same lens [17]. For example, some stakeholders focus on conducting clinical trials to solidify evidence created by medical advances. Others are concerned with synthesizing evidence, developing technology, or providing supportive infrastructure to enable the knowledge-translation process [18–22]. This cross-disciplinary heritage and applications have added to the richness of implementation science, but have also led to challenges in developing a common language. Promoting a good understanding of terminology is essential for the success of the science and practice of implementation across academic disciplines [17]. The field of knowledge translation, well integrated with organizational and management studies, is notorious for the plethora of terms and phrases used to describe processes across disciplines and countries [23, 24]. Variation in nomenclature is important for depth of understanding within fields, but risks creating barriers between researchers, practitioners, health professionals, managers, and policy makers by driving misunderstandings between stakeholders [17]. Further, inconsistency and diversity of terminology potentially prevent synthesis and application of information [25].

Consistent use of foundational terms in implementation science must be promoted to clarify intent and meaning between stakeholders. To ensure information is accessible for non-specialists, researchers and practitioners should ensure rich descriptive explanations of a concept are provided in language that is relevant to clinicians, managers, policy makers, and recipients of care. For this chapter, and to facilitate an introduction to implementation science, we have provided a set of definitions drawn from the literature (Table 1).

Table 1 Key terms in implementation science with definitions. Source: Adapted from Livet et al. [26]

Term	Definition
Clinical practice guidelines	Clinical practice guidelines are systematically developed statements to assist practitioner and patient decisions about appropriate health care for specific clinical circumstances [27]
Dissemination science	The scientific study of the targeted distribution of information and intervention materials to a specific public health, clinical practice, or policy audience
Evidence-based practice or intervention	A specific treatment or therapeutic regimen that has been shown to be effective, to some degree and in some context, through outcome evaluations
Framework	A graphical or narrative representation of the key factors, concepts, or variables to explain the phenomenon of implementation
Implementation taxonomy/ compilation	System for categorizing implementation methods [28]
Implementation outcomes	The effects of deliberate and purposive actions to implement new treatments, practices, and services [29]
Implementation practice	Refers to the "doing" or "how to" of implementation. Focused on the application of evidence-based knowledge and strategies to enhance the quality of implementation to drive intervention effectiveness in real-world settings
Implementation research	Refers to the scientific study of implementation. Focused on understanding how and why interventions work or fail to work in real-world settings, with the goal of producing generalizable knowledge
Implementation science	The scientific study of methods to promote the systematic uptake of research findings and other evidence-based practices into routine practice

Table 1 (continued)

Term	Definition
Implementation strategies	Methods or techniques used to enhance the adoption, implementation, and sustainability of a clinical program or practice [30]
Model	Deliberate simplification of a phenomenon or a specific aspect of a phenomenon [31]
Theory	An ordered set of assertions about a generic behavior or structure assumed to hold throughout a significantly broad range of specific instances [32]

1.1.1 Step 1: Defining an Evidence-Based Practice or Intervention

An important first step is to identify the evidence-based practice or intervention that a team is proposing to implement. The evidence-based practice or intervention could be (1) a screening, assessment, or diagnostic procedure, (2) a treatment program, individual therapeutic interventions, or models of care/pathways including multiple interventions, (3) a clinical practice guideline covering many components of care, (4) an administrative intervention, (5) a policy or technology, or (6) monitoring of outcomes [33]. These practices may be drawn from rigorously designed studies, evidenced-based guidelines, or local contexts. Different levels of evidence can be considered prior to implementation. There is no exact definition for how much evidence is required to determine that your practice is evidence-based. It should, however, be one that is implementable and could improve patient care or outcomes based on published literature or known successful prior implementation strategies.

Where multiple "evidence-to-practice" gaps are present, prioritizing one or two to focus on is likely to be more successful than tackling all of them together. There are different criteria to prioritize implementation, including (1) close gaps between practice and policy/recommendation/guideline, (2) close research evidence to practice gaps, (3) improve access to services, (4) cost-effectiveness of service delivery, (5) improve effectiveness of services, (6) current imbalance between service supply and demand, (7) amount of resources involved in service delivery, (8) extent of the health problem, (9) areas of care futility, and (10) equality of workload across professionals [34]. The selected evidence-based practice needs to be defined clearly. This facilitates fidelity and outcome assessment. The action, actor, context, target, time (AACTT) framework can be used to help define the evidence-based practice (Table 2) [35]. When defining the action, it is important to specify the behavior, the dose or intensity of the action, and the evidence behind the evidence-based practice.

1.1.2 Step 2: Choosing a Theory, Model, or Framework

After stakeholders have identified and defined the evidence-based practice they propose to implement, the next step is to select the appropriate theory, model, or framework. Theories, models, and frameworks have an important role in implementation

Table 2 Action, actor, context, target, time (AACTT): a framework for specifying behavior. Source: Reproduced under the CC-BY license from Presseau J et al. [35]

Domain	Definition	Examples
Action	A discrete observable behavior	Prescribing antihypertensives, providing a referral to a specialist, washing hands, setting a policy
Actor	The individual or group of individuals who perform (or should/could) the Action	Primary care physician, pharmacist, social worker, resident, administrator, middle manager, head of unit, policy maker
Context	The physical, emotional, or social setting in which the Actor performs (or should/could) the Action	Examination room, doctor's office, outside a patient room, in a boardroom, stressful vs. calm situation, when patients' relatives are present or not
Target	The individual or group of individuals for/with/on behalf of whom the Actor performs the Action	Patient with diabetes and blood pressure above 140/80 mm Hg, patient wanting to quit smoking
Time	The time period and duration that the Actor performs the Action in the Context with/for the Target	At annual review, next time a patient visits, every week, over the next 6 months

science. They are essential for guiding the design, implementation, and evaluation of evidence-based practices [36–41]. To improve their use, the next section describes how to select the appropriate theory, model, or framework and how to apply them to improve an implementation project.

Determining how the theory, model, or framework will be used will aid in the selection of the most appropriate theory, model, or framework [31, 42, 43]. For example, Tabak et al. [42] lists frameworks based on their focus on implementation, dissemination, or both (Table 3); while, if searching for an evaluation framework, Nilsen's list is more appropriate (Table 4) [31, 42, 43]. Depending on the context where the evidence-based practice will be implemented, multiple theories, models, or frameworks at different stages of implementation may be employed.

There are also websites that help selecting the theory, model, or framework that best fits an implementation project (e.g., https://dissemination-implementation. org). Two recent publications provide excellent examples on how theories, models, and frameworks can be applied to help translate evidence into practice [36, 38]. An example specific to cardiology is the use of the Conceptual Model of Implementation Research [29, 51] to develop focus group guides to understand the acceptability, appropriateness, and feasibility of Automated Screening Approaches and Family Communication Methods aimed at improving identification of familial hypercholesterolemia [52]. Figure 2 provides an overview of the analytic framework for how the domains of the model were used for the purposes of this study [52].

Table 3 Selection of implementation science theories, models, or frameworks according to focus on dissemination/implementation, flexibility, and socio-ecological criteria and purpose. Source: from Tabak et al. with permission [42]

Model	Dissemination (D) and/or Implementation (I)	Construct flexibility: broad to operational	Socio-ecological level				
			System	Community	Organization	Individual	Policy
Promoting Action on Research Implementation in Health Services [44]	I-only	3		x	x	x	
Conceptual framework for implementation research [45]	I-only	4		x	x		
Reach, Effectiveness, Adoption, Implementation, Maintanance [46, 47]	D = I	4		x	x	x	
Conceptual model of implementation research [29]	I-only	3	x	x	x	x	

Table 4 Five categories of theories, models, and frameworks used in implementation science. Source: Adapted and reproduced under the CC-BY license from Nilsen [31]

Implementation science approach	Category	Definition	Selected examples of theories, models, and frameworks
Guide the development of implementing the evidence-based practice into clinical care	Process model	Specify steps (stages, phases) in the process of translating research into practice, including the implementation and use of research. The aim of process models is to describe and/or guide the process of translating research into practice. An action model is a type of process model that provides practical guidance in the planning and execution of implementation endeavors and/or implementation strategies to facilitate implementation	Knowledge-to-Action Model [48]
Understanding factors that affect the implementation outcomes	Determinant framework	Specify types (also known as classes or domains) of determinants and individual determinants, which act as barriers and enablers (independent variables) that influence implementation outcomes (dependent variables). Some frameworks also specify relationships between some types of determinants. The overarching aim is to understand and/or explain influences on implementation outcomes, e.g., predicting outcomes or interpreting outcomes retrospectively	Conceptual framework for implementation research [45]
	Classic theories	Originate from fields external to implementation science, e.g., psychology, sociology, and organizational theory, which can be applied to provide understanding and/or explanation of aspects of implementation	Theory of Diffusion [49]
	Implementation theories	Developed by implementation researchers (from scratch or by adapting existing theories and concepts) to provide understanding and/or explanation of aspects of implementation	Capability, Opportunity, Motivation, Behavior (COM-B) Model [50]
Evaluation of implementing the evidence-based practice	Evaluation framework	Specify aspects of implementation that could be evaluated to determine implementation success	Reach, Effectiveness, Adoption, Implementation, Maintanance [46, 47]; Conceptual model of implementation research [29]

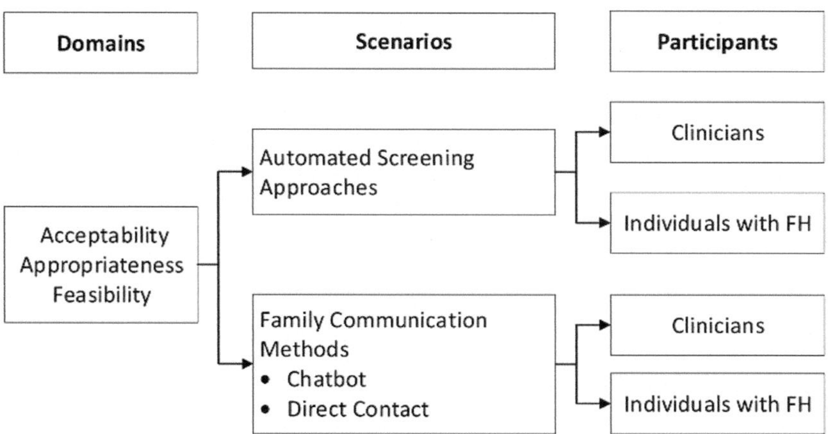

Fig. 2 Analytic framework for reviewing domains of implementation outcomes including acceptability, appropriateness, and feasibility by scenarios including automated screening approaches and family communications methods and participants including clinicians and individuals with FH. Source: Reproduced under the CC-BY license from Jones et al. [52] FH, familial hypercholesterolemia

1.1.3 Step 3: Assessing Determinants, Barriers, Enablers, and Contexts

To understand why an evidence-based practice has had poor adoption, it is important to assess barriers to and enablers of implementation. This assessment allows the selection of strategies to address those challenges that can be tailored to meet the specific needs and context of the site. It is also important to understand the barriers and enablers at different ecological levels (e.g., patient, clinician, healthcare system, community, and policy levels). These different levels allow viewpoints of all stakeholders to guide the development of context-specific implementation strategies targeting the site of intervention.

For example, recent studies of individuals with familial hypercholesterolemia used the Reach, Effectiveness, Adoption, Implementation, and Maintenance (RE-AIM) Framework and the Practical, Robust, Implementation, and Sustainability Model (PRISM) [46] to develop implementation strategies to improve uptake of guideline-recommended care [53]. RE-AIM was utilized to evaluate the implementation strategy selected (Table 5) [53]. The study then used PRISM to develop interview and focus group guides to understand barriers and facilitators to familial hypercholesterolemia care and develop solutions to address these identified barriers [54]. Finally, the study used the RE-AIM framework to evaluate the implementation of a multidisciplinary lipid clinic that was identified as a solution in the previous study [55].

Table 5 RE-AIM framework, outcome measures, and data sources from a protocol paper to evaluate an implementation strategy deployed to improve familial hypercholesterolemia care. Source: Reproduced with permission from Jones et al. [53]

RE-AIM framework dimension	Definition	Example measure	Example data source
Reach	Impacted by the implementation strategy	Of individuals targeted by the implementation strategy, how many are impacted by it?	Electronic health record (EHR)
Effectiveness	Impact of the implementation strategy on health behavior or outcome	Measure change in knowledge, attitude, and behavior to be impacted by the implementation strategy	Survey, EHR
Adoption	Reach at the setting level	Of setting targeted by the implementation strategy, how many adopt it?	–
Implementation	Fidelity to the implementation strategy	How consistently is the implementation strategy delivered over time/ setting?	–
	Cost of implementation strategy	Personnel and implementation cost for the implementation strategy	Administrative data (e.g., number of staff, cost of additional equipment)
Maintenance	Not evaluated in this study		

1.1.4   Step 4: Selecting Implementation Strategies

Implementation strategies provide the "how to" for implementing the evidence-based practice. To identify possible implementation strategies, there are currently two compilations [56, 57]. These compilations provide a list of commonly used implementation strategies with a standardized definition and explanation of each strategy. The Expert Recommendation for Implementation Change (ERIC) compilation provides nine categories of implementation strategies. These include (1) using evaluative and iterative strategies, (2) providing interactive assistance, (3) adapting and tailoring to the context, (4) developing stakeholder relationships, (5) training and educating stakeholders, (6) supporting clinicians, (7) engaging consumers, (8) utilizing financial strategies, and (9) changing infrastructure. The Effective Practice and Organization of Care (EPOC) taxonomy of health systems interventions provides strategies on delivery, financial, and governance arrangements [58].

It is important to clearly specify the implementation strategy (or strategies) and how it is used to implement the evidence-based practice, so that the work may be reproduced. Table 6 provides guidance for specifying implementation strategies [30], and includes an example of specifying an implementation strategy in cardiology [55].

Table 6 Proctor's domains and definitions for specifying implementation strategies. Source: Reproduced under the CC-BY license from Proctor et al. [30] and under Creative Commons Attribution 4.0 International License from Jones et al. [55]

Domain	Definition	Example from Jones et al. [55]
Name it	Name the strategy, preferably using language that is consistent with existing literature; such as the ERIC or EPOC compilations	Creation of new clinical teams (e.g., a multidisciplinary lipid clinic)
Define it	Define the implementation strategy and any discrete components operationally	A multidisciplinary clinical team that has complementary roles (i.e., diagnosis and treatment) with lipid expertise that is formed to improve patient care
Specify it		
The actor	Identify who enacts the strategy	*Cardiologist* *Pharmacist* *Genetic counselor*
The action	Use active verb statements to specify the specific actions, steps, or processes that need to be enacted	*Cardiologist*—evaluates the patient's symptoms, lifestyle, medications, and past lab results during an initial in-person visit; recommends a treatment plan; orders subsequent testing; requests follow-up visits as needed *Pharmacist*—evaluates the patient's current medications; offers input/suggests changes to medications; performs medication reconciliation; completes medication counseling and education; ensures prior authorizations are submitted *Genetic counselor*—evaluates the patient's past medical and family histories; assesses the patient's risk; provides pre-test genetic counseling; provides genetic testing result disclosure and post-test genetic counseling; discusses cascade testing of at-risk relatives
Action target	Specify targets according to conceptual models of implementation. Identify unit of analysis for measuring implementation outcomes	*All clinicians*—expertise caring for patients with a high-risk lipid condition and knowledge of guideline-recommended treatment for lipid conditions *Cardiologist*—diagnosis of lipid conditions, monitors clinical symptoms *Pharmacist*—optimizes treatment and follow-up on prior authorizations *Genetic counselor*—knowledge of familial cardiovascular conditions, improvement of identification methods for concerning past medical/family history, and reassurance to the patient that the testing results will benefit the patient no matter if the result is positive or negative

(continued)

Table 6 (continued)

Domain	Definition	Example from Jones et al. [55]
Temporality	Specify when the strategy is used	Patients should be referred as soon as the provider identifies a patient with a high-risk lipid condition who would benefit from the evaluation at the clinic. The initial visit to the clinic should take place as soon as scheduling allows after the patient has been referred. Subsequent visits should be scheduled on an as needed basis
Dose	Specify dosage of implementation strategy	*Cardiologist*—once at an hour-long initial visit. Subsequent visits at 6–8 weeks post-initial visit and further if needed. The cardiologist will be available to the patient via phone or through patient portal *Pharmacist*—once at an hour-long initial visit. The pharmacist will be available to the patient via phone or patient portal *Genetic counselor*—once at an hour-long initial visit. The genetic counselor will be available to the patient via phone or patient portal
Implementation outcome affected	Identify and measure the implementation outcome(s) likely to be affected by each strategy	Uptake of guideline-recommended testing and treatment for high-risk lipid clinic patients; adoption among primary care providers and other providers; penetration among eligible patients; fidelity to the protocol of the clinic; sustainability of the clinic and its expansion
Justification	Provide empirical, theoretical, or pragmatic justification for the choice of the implementation strategy	Multidisciplinary lipid clinics improve patient outcomes

ERIC Expert Recommendation for Implementing Change, *EPOC* Effective Practice and Organization of Care

1.1.5 Step 5: Selecting Options for Monitoring and Evaluation

Implementation monitoring and evaluation differs from clinical research, which generally focuses on determining the health benefits of a particular evidence-based intervention or practice. Implementation evaluation redirects attention to the adoption of practice change in routine care. For example, while therapeutic goals for low-density lipoprotein cholesterol (LDL-C) have been well established [59], they are infrequently achieved in clinical practice [60]. It is important to disentangle the impact of implementation strategies from the intervention being implemented. Implementation research has found, for example, that nurse-led telephone-based follow-up can improve translation of these guidelines into practice [61]. Distinguishing an implementation strategy (nurse telephone follow-up) from the intervention being implemented (LDL-C reduction) is an important first step to ensure clear hypotheses and selection of appropriate evaluation end points and designs [15, 62]. While LDL-C reduction remains the desired outcome, implementation research should identify the best strategy to achieve this and its mechanisms [63, 64].

Often the first step is to conduct a feasibility study to determine if it is possible to deploy the implementation strategy in the local context. It is important to use knowledge gained from subsequent steps to determine barriers and facilitators to use of an evidence-based intervention, and understand why there has been limited adoption. Engaging with stakeholders is important to determine the best way to incorporate the evidence-based practice into their workflow.

After feasibility is determined, implementation of the selected strategy must be monitored and evaluated. These processes can be formative and/or summative. Formative evaluations occur during the process of implementation, allowing information to be fed back to clinicians in a way that enables adaptations and improvements to be made in real time. This early feedback measures the fidelity of an intervention and whether the "stopping rules" of a trial are met. Summative evaluation measures the impact of implementation on care processes at the end of an implementation project seeking to understand "what works, why, and under what circumstances?" This type of evaluation is known as realist evaluation which focuses on understanding how and why interventions work under different circumstances, by considering the interaction between contextual circumstances, theoretical change mechanisms and impacts on the outcomes of processes for improving care delivery [65].

There are multiple evaluation designs that can be used in implementation science. Randomized, controlled, parallel-group trials are the mainstay of clinical research and are commonly used in implementation science. These designs can be employed to evaluate the success of an implementation in changing care processes. However, parallel trials can be challenging in implementation research [66], as implementation studies often have small sample sizes. Subjects are usually clinicians or organizations rather than patients, resulting in low statistical power (i.e., limited ability to detect differences) [67]. Furthermore, some individuals and organizations are more amenable to changing practice than others, introducing the risk

Fig. 3 Stepped wedge and counterbalanced trial designs that are commonly used in implementation research to evaluate the implementation strategies. Reproduced under Creative Commons Attribution Non Commercial (CC BY-NC 4.0) license from Sarkies et al. [71]

Stepped-wedge

Time

Cluster	1	2	3	4	5
1	A	B	B	B	B
2	A	A	B	B	B
3	A	A	A	B	B
4	A	A	A	A	B

Counterbalanced

Context

Cluster	1	2	3	4
1	A	B	C	D
2	D	A	B	C
3	C	D	A	B
4	B	C	D	A

of baseline imbalance between study groups [68, 69]. Novel, innovative designs, such as stepped wedge [70], counterbalanced [66, 71], and sequential multiple assignment randomized trials (SMART) [72] have been used to overcome these challenges. Stepped wedge trials stagger the introduction of implementation supports to participants or participating sites over time resembling traditional incomplete block designs (Fig. 3); whereas counterbalanced designs randomize participants to alternative evidence-based interventions, with different levels applied in various contexts to reduce the risk of contamination. SMART trials or adaptive intervention designs employ sequential multiple randomized assignment, which form the structure for switching or modifying interventions at certain time points if benefits are not being achieved.

Quasi-experimental studies can also be used in situations where randomized implementation trials are not feasible, such as large-scale policy changes [73–75]. Interrupted time series is a common evaluative design being applied to implementation evaluations [76]. These studies measure outcomes at multiple time points before and after an intervention is implemented, allowing the identification of an "interruption" in the time series to measure changes in outcomes. Another option is "difference in difference" studies, which measure the effect of an implementation strategy on care processes by comparing the average change over time to the average change over time in a control site [77].

2 Sustained Adoption and Adherence: Maintenance

While short-term monitoring and evaluation of implementation strategies are important to establish and ensure fidelity and effectiveness, maintaining these practices over the long term is difficult [78]. However, sustained adoption, or maintenance, of and adherence to clinical practice recommendations, are important to both clinicians and patients to improve health outcomes and reduce healthcare costs. Maintenance is one of the most underreported implementation outcomes [79]. This is because its assessment is difficult, requiring measurement of outcomes years after the intervention has been implemented. Strategies presented in the previous two sections, which evaluate the process of creating the strategies and their initial use may be inadequate to study maintenance. Generalizability of a given implementation strategy and use of multiple strategies may be the most important factors to overcome stagnation. Efforts should be made to continuously examine the implementation effort, make adaptations, and update recommendations to maintain success.

3   Adoption of Guidelines by Clinicians into Practice

While the value of implementation science in facilitating translation of evidence into practice is increasingly recognized and called for in guideline development, it is not yet universal [80, 81]. Recent guidelines that incorporate implementation science recommendations include those related to lipidology [4, 82–85], hypertension [86–88], heart failure [89], and atrial fibrillation [90]. For example, the 2018 AHA/ACC Cholesterol Guidelines included a section on implementation with recommended methods for improving patient adherence to prescribed therapy, identification of those not receiving guideline-based therapy, initiation of appropriate therapy, and promotion of shared decision making [4].

There are several barriers to the adoption or adherence to guidelines by clinicians. These barriers include time constraints, limited staffing resources, skepticism, low awareness and knowledge of guidelines, and clinician age. Facilitators that have helped improve the implementation of guidelines include clinical pathways, multidisciplinary teams and multifaceted interventions, end-user involvement, stakeholder engagement, leadership support, wider scope of implementation, organizational culture, and electronic decision support systems within the electronic health records [91, 92]. Current research suggests education, audit, and feedback have more consistently favorable effects than strategies such as reminders and incentives [91].

4   Patient Adherence to Clinical Practice Recommendations

Patient adherence to health recommendations provided by their clinicians is variable. Poor adherence can result in poor health outcomes for patients. Clinicians should work with patients to ensure treatment plans make intellectual, practical, and emotional sense [93] and are able to be implemented in the context of the patient's capacity and capability [94]. This shared-decision making conversation should help uncover potential challenges to implementing the regimen including whether or not it is acceptable to the patient [93]. After the barriers are identified, clinicians can work with patients to identify which implementation strategy(ies) would be best to address the challenge(s). Systematic reviews have found that coordinated care, specialist support, pharmacist consultation, combination pills, reminder services, community health workers, and team-based care can all improve medication adherence

[95–102]. Using multiple strategies targeting different socio-ecological levels are needed to meaningfully improve patient adherence, rather than finding one "best" approach [95, 100, 103]. It is important to remember that each strategy or set of strategies must be adapted to fit a patient's situation and must make intellectual, practical, and emotional sense to maximize the chance of success.

5 Mapping Current Strategies in Cardiovascular Disease to the ERIC Compilation

In this section, studies have been mapped to strategies designed to improve adherence to the ERIC compilation to show how using implementation science has helped improve adherence.

5.1 Financial Strategies

Cost is a common barrier to patient adherence. Many financial approaches have been tried to prevent cost-based non-adherence with variable results, some studies suggest a positive effect on adherence while others fail to demonstrate an effect [104, 105]. A more recent review found that financial assistance, including co-payments, had a positive impact on medication adherence and persistence over 1 year [106]. Incentivizing patients to adhere to treatment improved rates of adherence to cardiac rehabilitation [107], but the evidence for adherence specifically to statin therapy has been less consistent [108, 109].

5.2 Support for Clinicians

Strategies to support clinicians, such as expanding the scope of practice to include other healthcare team members, have been shown to improve adherence. Systematic reviews have documented favorable effects on medication adherence by pharmacists [101, 102], nurses [110], and community health workers [97].

5.3 Technology-Based Strategies

Technology-based strategies offer a variety of different approaches [111]. A number of systematic reviews have confirmed the positive effects of using mobile device applications for health interventions [112–115]. Telehealth interventions have been found to improve patient adherence to medication [116–118].

5.4 Educating Patients

Educating patients is a key strategy for improving treatment adherence. Having the treatment make intellectual, practical and emotional sense to the patient is a critical component of both shared decision making [93] and implementation. The General Theory of Implementation has four key constructs (Potential, Capacity, Capability, and Contribution), each with multiple sub-dimensions. Education can contribute to multiple dimensions across the constructs, but perhaps most directly to the coherence (or sense making) dimension of Contribution [94]. Through education the clinician can work with the patient to understand why adherence is important, what it means to adhere, and what is required for successful adherence to treatment. Aligned with this theoretical basis for the benefit of education, several systematic reviews have found that education can improve treatment adherence, including in conditions in the field of cardiovascular medicine, such as hypertension, hyperlipidemia, myocardial infarction, and heart failure [119–122].

6 Summary

Implementation of clinical practice guidelines does not happen spontaneously; implementation science and practice provide approaches to close this gap. This chapter introduces implementation science and provides a five-step process to guide its use and application. This approach can improve adherence to clinical guidelines and interventions by clinicians and patients, respectively. Future work should focus on increasing the incorporation of the principles of implementation science into the development of clinical guidelines, acknowledging the complexities of clinical practice and healthcare delivery. Implementation strategies should be tailored to implementing clinical recommendations. The utilization of theories, models, and frameworks can expand the scope of clinical guidelines by considering various barriers to and facilitators of their implementation. Involvement of patient advocates and multiple stakeholders at all levels of the implementation process is essential [123, 124]. Training in implementation science is strongly advised for all guideline developers [125]. Additional research is needed to better understand the determinants of sustained adoption of clinical practices and interventions to improve the rates adherence to and sustained use of clinical recommendations.

References

1. Balas EA, Boren SA. Managing clinical knowledge for health care improvement. Yearb Med Inform. 2000;9(01):65–70.
2. Morris ZS, Wooding S, Grant J. The answer is 17 years, what is the question: understanding time lags in translational research. J R Soc Med. 2011;104(12):510–20. (In Eng). https://doi.org/10.1258/jrsm.2011.110180.

3. Sarkies MN, Jones LK, Gidding SS, Watts GF. Improving clinical practice guidelines with implementation science. Nat Rev Cardiol. 2022;19(1):3–4. (In Eng). https://doi.org/10.1038/s41569-021-00645-x.

4. Grundy SM, Stone NJ, Bailey AL, et al. 2018 AHA/ACC/AACVPR/AAPA/ABC/ACPM/ADA/AGS/APhA/ASPC/NLA/PCNA guideline on the management of blood cholesterol: a report of the American College of Cardiology/American Heart Association Task Force on clinical practice guidelines. Circulation. 2019;139(25):e1082–143. (In Eng). https://doi.org/10.1161/cir.0000000000000625.

5. Huynh LT, Chew DP, Sladek RM, Phillips PA, Brieger DB, Zeitz CJ. Unperceived treatment gaps in acute coronary syndromes. Int J Clin Pract. 2009;63(10):1456–64. (In Eng). https://doi.org/10.1111/j.1742-1241.2009.02182.x.

6. Buck J, Kaboli P, Gage BF, Cram P, Vaughan Sarrazin MS. Trends in antithrombotic therapy for atrial fibrillation: data from the Veterans Health Administration Health System. Am Heart J. 2016;179:186–91. (In Eng). https://doi.org/10.1016/j.ahj.2016.03.029.

7. Eapen ZJ, Liang L, Shubrook JH, et al. Current quality of cardiovascular prevention for Million Hearts: an analysis of 147,038 outpatients from The Guideline Advantage. Am Heart J. 2014;168(3):398–404. (In Eng). https://doi.org/10.1016/j.ahj.2014.06.007.

8. Schaffer AL, Pearson SA, Buckley NA. How does prescribing for antihypertensive products stack up against guideline recommendations? An Australian population-based study (2006-2014). Br J Clin Pharmacol. 2016;82(4):1134–45. (In Eng). https://doi.org/10.1111/bcp.13043.

9. Ray KK, Molemans B, Schoonen WM, et al. EU-wide cross-sectional observational study of lipid-modifying therapy use in secondary and primary care: the DA VINCI study. Eur J Prev Cardiol. 2021;28(11):1279–89. (In Eng). https://doi.org/10.1093/eurjpc/zwaa047.

10. Glasziou P, Haynes B. The paths from research to improved health outcomes. Evid Based Nurs. 2005;8(2):36–8. (In Eng). https://doi.org/10.1136/ebn.8.2.36.

11. Guthrie B, Payne K, Alderson P, McMurdo ME, Mercer SW. Adapting clinical guidelines to take account of multimorbidity. BMJ (Clinical Research Ed). 2012;345:e6341. (In Eng). https://doi.org/10.1136/bmj.e6341.

12. Guyatt GH, Oxman AD, Kunz R, et al. Incorporating considerations of resources use into grading recommendations. BMJ (Clinical Research Ed). 2008;336(7654):1170–3. (In Eng). https://doi.org/10.1136/bmj.39504.506319.80.

13. Ghazi L, Desai NR, Simonov M, et al. Rationale and design of a cluster-randomized pragmatic trial aimed at improving use of guideline directed medical therapy in outpatients with heart failure: PRagmatic trial of messaging to providers about treatment of heart failure (PROMPT-HF). Am Heart J. 2022;244:107–15. (In Eng). https://doi.org/10.1016/j.ahj.2021.11.010.

14. Naderi SH, Bestwick JP, Wald DS. Adherence to drugs that prevent cardiovascular disease: meta-analysis on 376,162 patients. Am J Med. 2012;125(9):882–7.e1. (In Eng). https://doi.org/10.1016/j.amjmed.2011.12.013.

15. Bauer MS, Damschroder L, Hagedorn H, Smith J, Kilbourne AM. An introduction to implementation science for the non-specialist. BMC Psychol. 2015;3(1):32. (In Eng). https://doi.org/10.1186/s40359-015-0089-9.

16. Bauer MS, Kirchner J. Implementation science: what is it and why should I care? Psychiatry Res. 2020;283:112376. (In Eng). https://doi.org/10.1016/j.psychres.2019.04.025.

17. Rapport F, Braithwaite J, Mitchell R, Westbrook J, Churruca K. Transitional care in a federated landscape. In: Researching quality in care transitions. Springer; 2017. p. 179–200.

18. Grimshaw GM, Szczepura A, Hultén M, et al. Evaluation of molecular tests for prenatal diagnosis of chromosome abnormalities. Health Technol Assess. 2003;7(10):1–146. (In Eng). https://doi.org/10.3310/hta7100.

19. Grol R, Grimshaw J. From best evidence to best practice: effective implementation of change in patients' care. Lancet. 2003;362(9391):1225–30. (In Eng). https://doi.org/10.1016/s0140-6736(03)14546-1.

20. Pai M, Lloyd NS, Cheng J, et al. Strategies to enhance venous thromboprophylaxis in hospitalized medical patients (SENTRY): a pilot cluster randomized trial. Implement Sci. 2013;8:1. (In Eng). https://doi.org/10.1186/1748-5908-8-1.

21. Grol R. Successes and failures in the implementation of evidence-based guidelines for clinical practice. Med Care. 2001;39(8 Suppl 2):Ii46–54. (In Eng). https://doi.org/10.1097/00005650-200108002-00003.

22. Rapport F, Seagrove AC, Hutchings HA, et al. Barriers and facilitators to change in the organisation and delivery of endoscopy services in England and Wales: a focus group study. BMJ Open. 2012;2(3):e001009. (In Eng). https://doi.org/10.1136/bmjopen-2012-001009.

23. McKibbon KA, Lokker C, Wilczynski NL, et al. A cross-sectional study of the number and frequency of terms used to refer to knowledge translation in a body of health literature in 2006: a Tower of Babel? Implement Sci. 2010;5:16. (In Eng). https://doi.org/10.1186/1748-5908-5-16.

24. Davis D. Continuing education, guideline implementation, and the emerging transdisciplinary field of knowledge translation. J Contin Educ Heal Prof. 2006;26(1):5–12. (In Eng). https://doi.org/10.1002/chp.46.

25. Colquhoun H, Leeman J, Michie S, et al. Towards a common terminology: a simplified framework of interventions to promote and integrate evidence into health practices, systems, and policies. Implement Sci. 2014;9:51. (In Eng). https://doi.org/10.1186/1748-5908-9-51.

26. Livet M, Haines ST, Curran GM, et al. Implementation science to advance care delivery: a primer for pharmacists and other health professionals. Pharmacotherapy. 2018;38(5):490–502. (In Eng). https://doi.org/10.1002/phar.2114.

27. Institute Medicine. Clinical practice guidelines we can trust. Washington, DC: National Academies Press; 2011.

28. Leeman J, Baernholdt M, Sandelowski M. Developing a theory-based taxonomy of methods for implementing change in practice. J Adv Nurs. 2007;58(2):191–200. (In Eng). https://doi.org/10.1111/j.1365-2648.2006.04207.x.

29. Proctor E, Silmere H, Raghavan R, et al. Outcomes for implementation research: conceptual distinctions, measurement challenges, and research agenda. Admin Pol Ment Health. 2011;38(2):65–76.

30. Proctor EK, Powell BJ, McMillen JC. Implementation strategies: recommendations for specifying and reporting. Implement Sci. 2013;8(1):139. https://doi.org/10.1186/1748-5908-8-139.

31. Nilsen P. Making sense of implementation theories, models and frameworks. Implement Sci. 2015;10:53. (In Eng). https://doi.org/10.1186/s13012-015-0242-0.

32. Kislov R, Pope C, Martin GP, Wilson PM. Harnessing the power of theorising in implementation science. Implement Sci. 2019;14(1):103. https://doi.org/10.1186/s13012-019-0957-4.

33. Lengnick-Hall R, Gerke DR, Proctor EK, et al. Six practical recommendations for improved implementation outcomes reporting. Implement Sci. 2022;17(1):16. https://doi.org/10.1186/s13012-021-01183-3.

34. Wenzel L-A, White J, Sarkies MN, et al. How do health professionals prioritize clinical areas for implementation of evidence into practice? A cross-sectional qualitative study. JBI Evid Implement. 2020;18(3):288–96. https://doi.org/10.1097/xeb.0000000000000217.

35. Presseau J, McCleary N, Lorencatto F, Patey AM, Grimshaw JM, Francis JJ. Action, actor, context, target, time (AACTT): a framework for specifying behaviour. Implement Sci. 2019;14(1):102. https://doi.org/10.1186/s13012-019-0951-x.

36. Davidoff F, Dixon-Woods M, Leviton L, Michie S. Demystifying theory and its use in improvement. BMJ Qual Saf. 2015;24(3):228–38. https://doi.org/10.1136/bmjqs-2014-003627.

37. Damschroder LJ. Clarity out of chaos: use of theory in implementation research. Psychiatry Res. 2020;283:112461. https://doi.org/10.1016/j.psychres.2019.06.036.

38. Ridde V, Pérez D, Robert E. Using implementation science theories and frameworks in global health. BMJ Glob Health. 2020;5(4):e002269. https://doi.org/10.1136/bmjgh-2019-002269.

39. Birken SA, Powell BJ, Shea CM, et al. Criteria for selecting implementation science theories and frameworks: results from an international survey. Implement Sci. 2017;12(1):124. https://doi.org/10.1186/s13012-017-0656-y.

40. Oxman AD, Fretheim A, Flottorp S. The OFF theory of research utilization. J Clin Epidemiol. 2005;58(2):113–6; discussion 117–20. (In Eng). https://doi.org/10.1016/j.jclinepi.2004.10.002.

41. Bhattacharyya O, Reeves S, Garfinkel S, Zwarenstein M. Designing theoretically-informed implementation interventions: fine in theory, but evidence of effectiveness in practice is needed. Implement Sci. 2006;1:5. (In Eng). https://doi.org/10.1186/1748-5908-1-5.

42. Tabak RG, Khoong EC, Chambers DA, Brownson RC. Bridging research and practice: models for dissemination and implementation research. Am J Prev Med. 2012;43(3):337–50. (In Eng). https://doi.org/10.1016/j.amepre.2012.05.024.

43. Moullin JC, Dickson KS, Stadnick NA, et al. Ten recommendations for using implementation frameworks in research and practice. Implement Sci Commun. 2020;1:42. (In Eng). https://doi.org/10.1186/s43058-020-00023-7.

44. Rycroft-Malone J, Bucknall T. Models and frameworks for implementing evidence-based practice: linking evidence to action. Wiley; 2010.

45. Damschroder LJ, Aron DC, Keith RE, Kirsh SR, Alexander JA, Lowery JC. Fostering implementation of health services research findings into practice: a consolidated framework for advancing implementation science. Implement Sci. 2009;4:50. (In Eng). https://doi.org/10.1186/1748-5908-4-50.

46. Glasgow RE, Harden SM, Gaglio B, et al. RE-AIM planning and evaluation framework: adapting to new science and practice with a 20-year review. Front Public Health. 2019;7:64). (Mini Review) (In English). https://doi.org/10.3389/fpubh.2019.00064.

47. Glasgow RE, Vogt TM, Boles SM. Evaluating the public health impact of health promotion interventions: the RE-AIM framework. Am J Public Health. 1999;89:1322–7. https://doi.org/10.2105/AJPH.89.9.132.

48. Graham ID, Logan J, Harrison MB, et al. Lost in knowledge translation: time for a map? J Contin Educ Heal Prof. 2006;26(1):13–24. (In Eng). https://doi.org/10.1002/chp.47.

49. Rogers EM, Singhal A, Quinlan MM. Diffusion of innovations. An integrated approach to communication theory and research. Routledge; 2014. p. 432–48.

50. Michie S, van Stralen MM, West R. The behaviour change wheel: a new method for characterising and designing behaviour change interventions. Implement Sci. 2011;6:42. (In Eng). https://doi.org/10.1186/1748-5908-6-42.

51. Proctor EK, Landsverk J, Aarons G, Chambers D, Glisson C, Mittman B. Implementation research in mental health services: an emerging science with conceptual, methodological, and training challenges. Admin Pol Ment Health. 2009;36(1):24–34. (In Eng). https://doi.org/10.1007/s10488-008-0197-4.

52. Jones LK, Walters N, Brangan A, et al. Acceptability, appropriateness, and feasibility of automated screening approaches and family communication methods for identification of familial hypercholesterolemia: stakeholder engagement results from the IMPACT-FH Study. J Pers Med. 2021;11(6):587. (In Eng). https://doi.org/10.3390/jpm11060587.

53. Jones LK, Gidding SS, Seaton TL, et al. Developing implementation strategies to improve uptake of guideline-recommended treatments for individuals with familial hypercholesterolemia: a protocol. Res Social Adm Pharm. 2020;16(3):390–5. (In Eng). https://doi.org/10.1016/j.sapharm.2019.06.006.

54. Jones LK, Sturm AC, Seaton TL, et al. Barriers, facilitators, and solutions to familial hypercholesterolemia treatment. PLoS One. 2020;15(12):e0244193. (In Eng). https://doi.org/10.1371/journal.pone.0244193.

55. Jones LK, McMinn M, Kann D, et al. Evaluation of a multidisciplinary lipid clinic to improve the care of individuals with severe lipid conditions: a RE-AIM framework analysis. Implement Sci Commun. 2021;2(1):32. (In Eng). https://doi.org/10.1186/s43058-021-00135-8.

56. Powell BJ, Waltz TJ, Chinman MJ, et al. A refined compilation of implementation strategies: results from the Expert Recommendations for Implementing Change (ERIC) project. Implement Sci. 2015;10(1):1–14.
57. Mowatt G, Grimshaw JM, Davis DA, Mazmanian PE. Getting evidence into practice: the work of the Cochrane Effective Practice and Organization of Care Group (EPOC). J Contin Educ Health Prof. 2001;21(1):55–60.
58. Effective Practice and Organisation of Care (EPOC) Group. EPOC taxonomy. https://epoc.cochrane.org/.
59. Perk J, De Backer G, Gohlke H, et al. European guidelines on cardiovascular disease prevention in clinical practice (version 2012). The Fifth Joint Task Force of the European Society of Cardiology and Other Societies on Cardiovascular Disease Prevention in Clinical Practice (constituted by representatives of nine societies and by invited experts). Eur Heart J. 2012;33(13):1635–701. (In Eng). https://doi.org/10.1093/eurheartj/ehs092.
60. Kotseva K, Wood D, De Bacquer D, et al. EUROASPIRE IV: a European Society of Cardiology survey on the lifestyle, risk factor and therapeutic management of coronary patients from 24 European countries. Eur J Prev Cardiol. 2016;23(6):636–48. (In Eng). https://doi.org/10.1177/2047487315569401.
61. Jakobsson S, Huber D, Björklund F, Mooe T. Implementation of a new guideline in cardiovascular secondary preventive care: subanalysis of a randomized controlled trial. BMC Cardiovasc Disord. 2016;16:77. (In Eng). https://doi.org/10.1186/s12872-016-0252-0.
62. Sarkies MN, Skinner EH, Bowles K-A, Taljaard M, Cheng W, Haines TP. The efficacy implementation ratio: a conceptual model for understanding the impact of implementation strategies using health outcomes. Glob Implement Res Appl. 2021;1(4):258–66.
63. Lewis CC, Boyd MR, Walsh-Bailey C, et al. A systematic review of empirical studies examining mechanisms of implementation in health. Implement Sci. 2020;15(1):21. (In Eng). https://doi.org/10.1186/s13012-020-00983-3.
64. Lewis CC, Klasnja P, Powell BJ, et al. From classification to causality: advancing understanding of mechanisms of change in implementation science. Front Public Health. 2018;6:136.
65. Sarkies MN, Francis-Auton E, Long JC, Pomare C, Hardwick R, Braithwaite J. Making implementation science more real. BMC Med Res Methodol. 2022;22(1):1–8.
66. Sarkies MN, Skinner EH, Bowles KA, et al. A novel counterbalanced implementation study design: methodological description and application to implementation research. Implement Sci. 2019;14(1):45. (In Eng). https://doi.org/10.1186/s13012-019-0896-0.
67. Wilson MG, Grimshaw JM, Haynes RB, et al. A process evaluation accompanying an attempted randomized controlled trial of an evidence service for health system policymakers. Health Res Policy Syst. 2015;13:78. (In Eng). https://doi.org/10.1186/s12961-015-0066-z.
68. Ingersoll GL, Kirsch JC, Merk SE, Lightfoot J. Relationship of organizational culture and readiness for change to employee commitment to the organization. J Nurs Adm. 2000;30(1):11–20. (In Eng). https://doi.org/10.1097/00005110-200001000-00004.
69. Backer TE. Assessing and enhancing readiness for change: implications for technology transfer. NIDA Res Monogr. 1995;155:21–41. (In Eng).
70. Hemming K, Haines TP, Chilton PJ, Girling AJ, Lilford RJ. The stepped wedge cluster randomised trial: rationale, design, analysis, and reporting. BMJ (Clinical Research Ed). 2015;350:h391. (In Eng). https://doi.org/10.1136/bmj.h391.
71. Sarkies MN, Maloney S, Symmons M, Haines TP. Video strategies improved health professional knowledge across different contexts: a helix counterbalanced randomized controlled study. J Clin Epidemiol. 2019;112:1–11. (In Eng). https://doi.org/10.1016/j.jclinepi.2019.04.003.
72. Kilbourne AM, Almirall D, Eisenberg D, et al. Protocol: Adaptive Implementation of Effective Programs Trial (ADEPT): cluster randomized SMART trial comparing a standard versus enhanced implementation strategy to improve outcomes of a mood disorders program. Implement Sci. 2014;9:132. (In Eng). https://doi.org/10.1186/s13012-014-0132-x.

73. Caporaso JA, Roos LL. Quasi-experimental approaches: testing theory and evaluating policy. Evanston: Northwestern University Press; 1973.

74. Miller CJ, Smith SN, Pugatch M. Experimental and quasi-experimental designs in implementation research. Psychiatry Res. 2020;283:112452.

75. Handley MA, Lyles CR, McCulloch C, Cattamanchi A. Selecting and improving quasi-experimental designs in effectiveness and implementation research. Annu Rev Public Health. 2018;39:5–25.

76. Taljaard M, McKenzie JE, Ramsay CR, Grimshaw JM. The use of segmented regression in analysing interrupted time series studies: an example in pre-hospital ambulance care. Implement Sci. 2014;9:77. (In Eng). https://doi.org/10.1186/1748-5908-9-77.

77. Geng EH, Peiris D, Kruk ME. Implementation science: relevance in the real world without sacrificing rigor. PLoS Med. 2017;14(4):e1002288. (In Eng). https://doi.org/10.1371/journal.pmed.1002288.

78. Shelton RC, Cooper BR, Stirman SW. The sustainability of evidence-based interventions and practices in public health and health care. Annu Rev Public Health. 2018;39:55–76. (In Eng). https://doi.org/10.1146/annurev-publhealth-040617-014731.

79. Klaic M, Kapp S, Hudson P, et al. Implementability of healthcare interventions: an overview of reviews and development of a conceptual framework. Implement Sci. 2022;17(1):10. (In Eng). https://doi.org/10.1186/s13012-021-01171-7.

80. Nieuwlaat R, Schwalm JD, Khatib R, Yusuf S. Why are we failing to implement effective therapies in cardiovascular disease? Eur Heart J. 2013;34(17):1262–9. (In Eng). https://doi.org/10.1093/eurheartj/ehs481.

81. Bonner C, Fajardo MA, Doust J, McCaffery K, Trevena L. Implementing cardiovascular disease prevention guidelines to translate evidence-based medicine and shared decision making into general practice: theory-based intervention development, qualitative piloting and quantitative feasibility. Implement Sci. 2019;14(1):86. (In Eng). https://doi.org/10.1186/s13012-019-0927-x.

82. Mach F, Baigent C, Catapano AL, et al. 2019 ESC/EAS guidelines for the management of dyslipidaemias: lipid modification to reduce cardiovascular risk: the Task Force for the management of dyslipidaemias of the European Society of Cardiology (ESC) and European Atherosclerosis Society (EAS). Eur Heart J. 2020;41(1):111–88.

83. Parini P, Frikke-Schmidt R, Tselepis AD, et al. Taking action: European Atherosclerosis Society targets the United Nations Sustainable Development Goals 2030 agenda to fight atherosclerotic cardiovascular disease in Europe. Atherosclerosis. 2021;322:77–81.

84. Averna M, Banach M, Bruckert E, et al. Practical guidance for combination lipid-modifying therapy in high-and very-high-risk patients: a statement from a European Atherosclerosis Society Task Force. Atherosclerosis. 2021;325:99–109.

85. Uchmanowicz I, Hoes A, Perk J, et al. Optimising implementation of European guidelines on cardiovascular disease prevention in clinical practice: what is needed? Eur J Prev Cardiol. 2020;28(4):426–31. (In Eng). https://doi.org/10.1177/2047487320926776.

86. Wang TD, Chiang CE, Chao TH, et al. 2022 guidelines of the Taiwan Society of Cardiology and the Taiwan Hypertension Society for the Management of Hypertension. Acta Cardiol Sin. 2022;38(3):225–325. (In Eng). https://doi.org/10.6515/acs.202205_38(3).20220321a.

87. Williams B, Mancia G, Spiering W, et al. 2018 ESC/ESH guidelines for the management of arterial hypertension: the Task Force for the management of arterial hypertension of the European Society of Cardiology (ESC) and the European Society of Hypertension (ESH). Eur Heart J. 2018;39(33):3021–104. https://doi.org/10.1093/eurheartj/ehy339.

88. Whelton PK, Carey RM, Aronow WS, et al. 2017 ACC/AHA/AAPA/ABC/ACPM/AGS/APhA/ASH/ASPC/NMA/PCNA guideline for the prevention, detection, evaluation, and management of high blood pressure in adults: a report of the American College of Cardiology/American Heart Association Task Force on clinical practice guidelines. Hypertension. 2018;71(6):e13–e115. https://doi.org/10.1161/HYP.0000000000000065.

89. Heidenreich PA, Bozkurt B, Aguilar D, et al. 2022 AHA/ACC/HFSA guideline for the management of heart failure: a report of the American College of Cardiology/American Heart Association Joint Committee on clinical practice guidelines. Circulation. 2022;145(18):e895–e1032. https://doi.org/10.1161/CIR.0000000000001063.

90. January CT, Wann LS, Calkins H, et al. 2019 AHA/ACC/HRS focused update of the 2014 AHA/ACC/HRS guideline for the management of patients with atrial fibrillation: a report of the American College of Cardiology/American Heart Association Task Force on clinical practice guidelines and the Heart Rhythm Society in collaboration with the Society of Thoracic Surgeons. Circulation. 2019;140(2):e125–51. https://doi.org/10.1161/CIR.0000000000000665.

91. Chan WV, Pearson TA, Bennett GC, et al. ACC/AHA special report: clinical practice guideline implementation strategies: a summary of systematic reviews by the NHLBI Implementation Science Work Group: a report of the American College of Cardiology/American Heart Association Task Force on clinical practice guidelines. Circulation. 2017;135(9):e122–37. (In Eng). https://doi.org/10.1161/cir.0000000000000481.

92. Shanbhag D, Graham ID, Harlos K, et al. Effectiveness of implementation interventions in improving physician adherence to guideline recommendations in heart failure: a systematic review. BMJ Open. 2018;8(3):e017765. (In Eng). https://doi.org/10.1136/bmjopen-2017-017765.

93. Hargraves IG, Montori VM, Brito JP, et al. Purposeful SDM: a problem-based approach to caring for patients with shared decision making. Patient Educ Couns. 2019;102(10):1786–92. (In Eng). https://doi.org/10.1016/j.pec.2019.07.020.

94. May C. Towards a general theory of implementation. Implement Sci. 2013;8(1):18. https://doi.org/10.1186/1748-5908-8-18.

95. Gebreyohannes EA, Mill D, Salter S, Chalmers L, Bereznicki L, Lee K. Strategies for improving guideline adherence of anticoagulants for patients with atrial fibrillation in primary healthcare: a systematic review. Thromb Res. 2021;205:128–36. (In Eng). https://doi.org/10.1016/j.thromres.2021.07.014.

96. Kini V, Ho PM. Interventions to improve medication adherence: a review. JAMA. 2018;320(23):2461–73. (In Eng). https://doi.org/10.1001/jama.2018.19271.

97. Fuller RH, Perel P, Navarro-Ruan T, Nieuwlaat R, Haynes RB, Huffman MD. Improving medication adherence in patients with cardiovascular disease: a systematic review. Heart. 2018;104(15):1238–43. (In Eng). https://doi.org/10.1136/heartjnl-2017-312571.

98. Mills KT, Obst KM, Shen W, et al. Comparative effectiveness of implementation strategies for blood pressure control in hypertensive patients: a systematic review and meta-analysis. Ann Intern Med. 2018;168(2):110–20. (In Eng). https://doi.org/10.7326/m17-1805.

99. Ruppar TM, Cooper PS, Mehr DR, Delgado JM, Dunbar-Jacob JM. Medication adherence interventions improve heart failure mortality and readmission rates: systematic review and meta-analysis of controlled trials. J Am Heart Assoc. 2016;5(6):e002606. (In Eng). https://doi.org/10.1161/jaha.115.002606.

100. Jones LK, Tilberry S, Gregor C, et al. Implementation strategies to improve statin utilization in individuals with hypercholesterolemia: a systematic review and meta-analysis. Implement Sci. 2021;16(1):40. (In Eng). https://doi.org/10.1186/s13012-021-01108-0.

101. Morgado M, Rolo S, Castelo-Branco M. Pharmacist intervention program to enhance hypertension control: a randomised controlled trial. Int J Clin Pharm. 2011;33(1):132–40. (In Eng). https://doi.org/10.1007/s11096-010-9474-x.

102. Chabot I, Moisan J, Grégoire JP, Milot A. Pharmacist intervention program for control of hypertension. Ann Pharmacother. 2003;37(9):1186–93. (In Eng). https://doi.org/10.1345/aph.1C267.

103. Tajouri TH, Driver SL, Holmes DR Jr. 'Take as directed'—strategies to improve adherence to cardiac medication. Nat Rev Cardiol. 2014;11(5):304–7. (In Eng). https://doi.org/10.1038/nrcardio.2013.208.

104. Volpp KG, Troxel AB, Long JA, et al. A randomized controlled trial of co-payment elimination: the CHORD trial. Am J Manag Care. 2015;21(8):e455–64. (In Eng).

105. Choudhry NK, Avorn J, Glynn RJ, et al. Full coverage for preventive medications after myocardial infarction. N Engl J Med. 2011;365(22):2088–97. (In Eng). https://doi.org/10.1056/NEJMsa1107913.

106. Hung A, Blalock DV, Miller J, et al. Impact of financial medication assistance on medication adherence: a systematic review. J Manag Care Spec Pharm. 2021;27(7):924–35. (In Eng). https://doi.org/10.18553/jmcp.2021.27.7.924.

107. Gaalema DE, Savage PD, Rengo JL, Cutler AY, Higgins ST, Ades PA. Financial incentives to promote cardiac rehabilitation participation and adherence among Medicaid patients. Prev Med. 2016;92:47–50. (In Eng). https://doi.org/10.1016/j.ypmed.2015.11.032.

108. Barankay I, Reese PP, Putt ME, et al. Effect of patient financial incentives on statin adherence and lipid control: a randomized clinical trial. JAMA Netw Open. 2020;3(10):e2019429. (In Eng). https://doi.org/10.1001/jamanetworkopen.2020.19429.

109. Garza KB, Owensby JK, Braxton Lloyd K, Wood EA, Hansen RA. Pilot study to test the effectiveness of different financial incentives to improve medication adherence. Ann Pharmacother. 2016;50(1):32–8. (In Eng). https://doi.org/10.1177/1060028015609354.

110. Verloo H, Chiolero A, Kiszio B, Kampel T, Santschi V. Nurse interventions to improve medication adherence among discharged older adults: a systematic review. Age Ageing. 2017;46(5):747–54. (In Eng). https://doi.org/10.1093/ageing/afx076.

111. Chun-Yun Kang G. Technology-based interventions to improve adherence to antihypertensive medications—an evidence-based review. Digit Health. 2022;8:20552076221089725. (In Eng). https://doi.org/10.1177/20552076221089725.

112. Armitage LC, Kassavou A, Sutton S. Do mobile device apps designed to support medication adherence demonstrate efficacy? A systematic review of randomised controlled trials, with meta-analysis. BMJ Open. 2020;10(1):e032045. (In Eng). https://doi.org/10.1136/bmjopen-2019-032045.

113. Al-Arkee S, Mason J, Lane DA, et al. Mobile apps to improve medication adherence in cardiovascular disease: systematic review and meta-analysis. J Med Internet Res. 2021;23(5):e24190. (In Eng). https://doi.org/10.2196/24190.

114. Mikulski BS, Bellei EA, Biduski D, De Marchi ACB. Mobile health applications and medication adherence of patients with hypertension: a systematic review and meta-analysis. Am J Prev Med. 2022;62(4):626–34. (In Eng). https://doi.org/10.1016/j.amepre.2021.11.003.

115. Palmer MJ, Machiyama K, Woodd S, et al. Mobile phone-based interventions for improving adherence to medication prescribed for the primary prevention of cardiovascular disease in adults. Cochrane Database Syst Rev. 2021;3(3):Cd012675. (In Eng). https://doi.org/10.1002/14651858.CD012675.pub3.

116. Bingham JM, Black M, Anderson EJ, et al. Impact of telehealth interventions on medication adherence for patients with type 2 diabetes, hypertension, and/or dyslipidemia: a systematic review. Ann Pharmacother. 2021;55(5):637–49. (In Eng). https://doi.org/10.1177/1060028020950726.

117. Sua YS, Jiang Y, Thompson DR, Wang W. Effectiveness of mobile phone-based self-management interventions for medication adherence and change in blood pressure in patients with coronary heart disease: a systematic review and meta-analysis. Eur J Cardiovasc Nurs. 2020;19(3):192–200. (In Eng). https://doi.org/10.1177/1474515119895678.

118. Chan AHY, Foot H, Pearce CJ, Horne R, Foster JM, Harrison J. Effect of electronic adherence monitoring on adherence and outcomes in chronic conditions: a systematic review and meta-analysis. PLoS One. 2022;17(3):e0265715. (In Eng). https://doi.org/10.1371/journal.pone.0265715.

119. Viswanathan M, Golin CE, Jones CD, et al. Interventions to improve adherence to self-administered medications for chronic diseases in the United States: a systematic review. Ann Intern Med. 2012;157(11):785–95. (In Eng). https://doi.org/10.7326/0003-4819-157-11-201212040-00538.

120. Srisuk N, Cameron J, Ski CF, Thompson DR. Heart failure family-based education: a systematic review. Patient Educ Couns. 2016;99(3):326–38. (In Eng). https://doi.org/10.1016/j.pec.2015.10.009.
121. Ampofo AG, Khan E, Ibitoye MB. Understanding the role of educational interventions on medication adherence in hypertension: a systematic review and meta-analysis. Heart Lung. 2020;49(5):537–47. (In Eng). https://doi.org/10.1016/j.hrtlng.2020.02.039.
122. Rash JA, Campbell DJ, Tonelli M, Campbell TS. A systematic review of interventions to improve adherence to statin medication: what do we know about what works? Prev Med. 2016;90:155–69. (In Eng). https://doi.org/10.1016/j.ypmed.2016.07.006.
123. Blackwood J, Armstrong MJ, Schaefer C, et al. How do guideline developers identify, incorporate and report patient preferences? An international cross-sectional survey. BMC Health Serv Res. 2020;20(1):458. (In Eng). https://doi.org/10.1186/s12913-020-05343-x.
124. Petkovic J, Riddle A, Akl EA, et al. Protocol for the development of guidance for stakeholder engagement in health and healthcare guideline development and implementation. Syst Rev. 2020;9(1):21. (In Eng). https://doi.org/10.1186/s13643-020-1272-5.
125. Gifford W, Graham ID, Ehrhart MG, Davies BL, Aarons GA. Ottawa Model of Implementation Leadership and Implementation Leadership Scale: mapping concepts for developing and evaluating theory-based leadership interventions. J Healthc Leadersh. 2017;9:15–23. (In Eng). https://doi.org/10.2147/jhl.S125558.

Challenges in Developing Evidence-Based Recommendations for Non-Pharmacological Interventions for Atherosclerotic Cardiovascular Disease Risk Reduction

Kristina S. Petersen

Key Points

- Evidence-based guidelines recommend non-pharmacological lifestyle management as first-line therapy for reducing atherosclerotic cardiovascular disease (ASCVD) risk.
- Developing lifestyle-related evidence-based guidelines is challenging because of complexities associated with conducting the type of high-quality research favored in the evidence-based guideline development process.
- Evidence evaluation methodologies and frameworks used for developing pharmacological guidelines are used for developing lifestyle-related guidelines.
- Randomized controlled trials (RCTs) provide the highest level of evidence for establishing causal relationships between exposures and outcomes; however, RCTs may not be feasible or ethical for investigating the efficacy or effectiveness of lifestyle interventions for ASCVD risk reduction.
- When evidence from RCTs is available, it can be difficult to distinguish exactly what was tested and how the intervention may have differed among multiple similar studies, the common effect, and the likelihood that replication of the lifestyle intervention at a population, community, or individual level would meaningfully affect ASCVD risk.
- Evidence-based guidelines for lifestyle interventions are often general and nonspecific because of the heterogeneity in the interventions evaluated in RCTs and difficulty in quantifying exactly what was tested to inform prescriptive evidence-based recommendations.
- Limited availability of RCT evidence results in reliance upon data from observational studies in the development of lifestyle-related evidence-based guidelines.

K. S. Petersen (✉)
Department of Nutritional Sciences, Pennsylvania State University, University Park, PA, USA
e-mail: kup63@psu.edu

K. C. Maki, D. P. Wilson (eds.), *Cardiovascular Outcomes Research*, Contemporary Cardiology, https://doi.org/10.1007/978-3-031-54960-1_7

- Observational evidence is at high risk of bias from residual confounding, measurement error, and imprecise exposure assessment, which results in evidence being rated as lower quality in the guideline development process.
- Shifts in how evidence-based guidelines for lifestyle interventions are constructed may need to occur to better capture the complexity of lifestyle exposures, the efficacy of specialized clinical care interventions (e.g., medical nutrition therapy provided by registered dietitian nutritionists), and the individualized behavior change counseling needed to achieve lifestyle-related behavior change.

1 Introduction

Non-pharmacological interventions are the cornerstone of atherosclerotic cardiovascular disease (ASCVD) risk reduction. Evidence-based guidelines for ASCVD risk reduction consistently recommend following a healthy lifestyle throughout the lifespan, including a healthy dietary pattern, engaging in physical activity and limiting sedentary time, tobacco product avoidance, and moderate alcohol intake if choosing to drink [1–8]. However, developing these recommendations can be challenging because of the complexities associated with conducting the type of high-quality research favored in the evidence-based guideline development process.

For pharmacological interventions, guidance on conducting clinical trials is issued by regulatory agencies and, in some cases, regulatory or statutory requirements must be met. The U.S. Food and Drug Administration publishes a comprehensive list of clinical trial guidance documents [9] that outline general considerations for clinical studies [10], as well as guidance on specific issues, such as control group choice [11], statistical principles [12], and multiple endpoints [13]. While these documents can be used to guide the design and execution of trials testing non-pharmacological interventions, not all methods used in pharmacological trials can be feasibly implemented in trials of non-pharmacological interventions, and other factors need to be accounted for in the design and conduct of these trials. For example, a key design feature of pharmacological trials is selection of an appropriate dose and dosing regimen for the test and control drugs [11]. For trials of non-pharmacological interventions, intervention design is typically more complex than defining the "dose" and "regimen" because lifestyle-related behaviors are complex, interdependent, and interrelated. Despite these issues, less guidance is available for conducting non-pharmacological trials assessing the efficacy or effectiveness of lifestyle interventions. In the field of nutrition, the Nutrition Intervention Research (NURISH) group published a series of papers on best practices for conducting clinical trials [14–18]. These could serve as a model for other fields that primarily study non-pharmacological interventions.

The relative lack of guidance for designing and conducting clinical trials examining non-pharmacological interventions, coupled with the complexity of these trials, presents challenges to the synthesis and evaluation of the evidence base to develop recommendations for non-pharmacological interventions. This chapter will summarize key challenges in developing evidence-based recommendations for non-pharmacological interventions for ASCVD risk reduction. While the definition of non-pharmacological interventions is broad [19], this chapter will focus on lifestyle-related non-pharmacological interventions because a healthy lifestyle is recommended for first-line management of ASCVD risk, and lifestyle-related guidelines are a prominent component of recommendations issued by authoritative organizations for ASCVD risk reduction [1].

2 Guideline Development Process for Lifestyle Interventions for ASCVD

Authoritative organizations that make recommendations for lifestyle interventions for ASCVD risk reduction apply similar methodologies and frameworks to those used for pharmacological interventions. Briefly, systematic literature searches are conducted to identify all the available evidence that meets pre-defined inclusion and exclusion criteria. The results of these systematic reviews are used to formulate evidence-based recommendations. Each recommendation is then designated with a rating based on the expected clinical benefit and the quality of evidence available. These rating systems vary across organizations and evolve over time.

The American College of Cardiology (ACC)/American Heart Association (AHA) Task Force on Clinical Practice Guidelines developed a classification system involving both a Class of Recommendation (COR) and a Level of Evidence (LOE) rating that is used for all practice guidelines issued by these organizations [20–22]. The COR rates the strength of the recommendation, including the estimated magnitude and certainty of benefit in proportion to risk. The LOE describes the quality of scientific evidence supporting the intervention, and is based on the type, quantity, and consistency of data from clinical trials and other sources. The ACC/AHA Clinical Practice Guideline Recommendation Classification System has evolved over time [20–22]; Table 1 summarizes the current version [22]. Other organizations that issue evidence-based recommendations for ASCVD risk reduction, such as the National Lipid Association, have adopted the ACC/AHA Clinical Practice Guideline Recommendation Classification System in recent times [23].

The Grading of Recommendations Assessment, Development, and Evaluation (GRADE) methodology is another system used to evaluate evidence quality when conducting systematic reviews or developing evidence-based guidelines [24]. In the GRADE system, evidence quality for a specific outcome measured in several studies is rated for domains, including study design, risk of bias, imprecision, inconsistency, indirectness, and magnitude of effect. In the final evaluation for GRADE, bodies of randomized controlled trial (RCT) evidence start with the highest rating and are downgraded based on study limitations, imprecision, inconsistency of results, indirectness of evidence, and likely publication bias. Conversely, bodies of observational evidence start with the lowest rating and are upgraded if there is a large magnitude of effect, dose–response relationship, and confounders likely minimize the effect. The overall quality of the evidence is rated from very low to high

Table 1 The ACC/AHA recommendation system for applying class of recommendation and level of evidence to clinical strategies, interventions, treatments, or diagnostic testing in patient care[a]

Class (strength) of recommendation (COR)		Level (quality) of evidence (LOE)[b]	
Class I (strong)	Benefit ≫ risk	Level A	
A treatment, procedure, or intervention is useful and effective and should be performed or administered for most patients under most circumstances Recommendation language used: • Is recommended • Is indicated/useful/effective/beneficial • Should be performed/administered • Comparative-effectiveness phrases[c]: • Treatment/strategy A is recommended/indicated in preference to treatment/strategy B • Treatment A should be chosen over treatment B		• High quality evidence[b] from >1 RCT • Meta-analyses of high-quality RCTs • ≥1 RCT corroborated by high-quality registry studies	
Class IIa (moderate)	Benefit ≫ risk	Level B-R	(Randomized)
A treatment, procedure, or intervention can be useful and effective, and it is reasonable under some circumstances Recommendation language used: • Is reasonable • Can be useful/effective/beneficial • Comparative-effectiveness phrases[c]: • Treatment/strategy A is probably recommended/indicated in preference to treatment/strategy B • It is reasonable to choose treatment A over treatment B		• Moderate quality evidence[b] from ≥1 RCTs • Meta-analyses of moderate-quality RCTs	
Class IIb (weak)	Benefit ≥ risk	Level B-NR	(Non-randomized)
Implementation should be selective and based on careful consideration of individual patient factors and, for invasive procedures, available expertise Recommendation language used: • May/might be reasonable • May/might be considered • Usefulness/effectiveness is unknown/unclear/uncertain or not well established		• Moderate-quality evidence[b] from ≥1 well-designed, well-executed non-randomized studies, observational studies, or registry studies • Meta-analyses of such studies	
Class III: no benefit (moderate)	Benefit = risk	Level C-LD	(Limited data)
(Generally, LOE A or B use only)			
Actions are specifically not recommended because studies have found no evidence of benefit Recommendation language used: • Is not recommended • Is not indicated/useful/effective/beneficial • Should not be performed/administered/other		• Randomized or non-randomized observational or registry studies with limitations of design or execution • Meta-analyses of such studies • Physiological or mechanistic studies in human subjects	

Table 1 (continued)

Class (strength) of recommendation (COR)		Level (quality) of evidence (LOE)[b]	
Class III: harm (strong)	Risk > benefit	Level C-ED	(Expert opinion)
Actions are specifically not recommended because studies have found the intervention causes harm Recommendation language used: • Potentially harmful • Causes harm • Associated with excess morbidity/mortality • Should not be performed/administered/other		• Consensus of expert opinion based on clinical experience	

COR and LOE are determined independently (any COR can be paired with any LOE)

A recommendation with LOE C does not imply a recommendation is weak. Many important clinical questions addressed in guidance do not lend themselves to clinical trials. Although RCTs are unavailable, there may be very clear clinical consensus that a particular test or therapy is useful or effective

Abbreviations: *ACC* American College of Cardiology, *AHA* American Heart Association, *COR* Class of Recommendation, *LOE* Level of Evidence, *RCT* randomized controlled trial

Adapted from [22]

[a]The outcome or result of the intervention should be specified (an improved clinical outcome or increased diagnostic accuracy or incremental prognostic information)

[b]The method of assessing quality is evolving, including the application of standardized, widely used, and preferably validated evidence grading tools; and for systematic reviews, the incorporation of an Evidence Review Committee

[c]For comparative-effectiveness recommendations (COR I and IIa; LOE A and B only), studies that support the use of comparator verbs should involve direct comparisons of the treatments or strategies being evaluated

based on the rating given to each domain and the lowest quality rating among designated critical outcomes [24].

These classification systems are well-suited to evaluating the evidence base for pharmacological recommendations; however, application to evidence for lifestyle interventions can be more complex and may result in these interventions being rated at a lower level. For example, to receive a LOE "A" rating, data from more than one high-quality RCT is needed. For lifestyle interventions, a paucity of RCTs may be available because of the infeasibility of this study design for many lifestyle-related research questions. Thus, observational studies are frequently the source of evidence, which results in a LOE "B-NR" rating [22].

3 Challenges to Developing Evidence-Based Guidelines for Lifestyle Interventions for ASCVD Risk Reduction

Many challenges exist to developing evidence-based guidelines for lifestyle interventions for ASCVD risk reduction. Most of these challenges originate from the quantity, type, and quality of evidence available for lifestyle interventions. In the following sections, these issues will be summarized by exploring the feasibility of conducting the RCTs needed to inform evidence-based guidelines, the RCT evidence base available, and the reliance on observational evidence.

3.1 Infeasibility of Definitive RCTs

RCTs provide the highest quality data for establishing causal relationships between exposures and outcomes. However, conducting RCTs may not be feasible or ethical for investigating the efficacy or effectiveness of lifestyle interventions for ASCVD risk reduction. Specifically, challenges to conducting RCTs for lifestyle interventions include: (1) the lengthy exposure time and protracted clinical course of ASCVD; (2) small effect sizes for lifestyle interventions; (3) the complexity of designing a testable, reproduceable intervention; (4) the difficulty in identifying a suitable control; and (5) problems with attaining high participant adherence and poor accuracy of adherence measurement/assessment tools.

Long exposure time: To meaningfully investigate the effect of lifestyle interventions on ASCVD risk, RCTs of substantial duration are required. ASCVD results from many years of exposure to accruing risk factors; from the initiation of the atherosclerotic process, it may be up to four decades before an ASCVD event occurs [25]. In parallel, lifestyle exposures may take many years to impact the clinical course of ASCVD. Furthermore, lifestyle exposures do not typically affect disease risk through a single mechanism. Rather, cumulative exposure over long periods of time affects disease risk through multiple mechanisms, which is in stark contrast to pharmacological agents that are designed to have targeted effects on specific pathways implicated in a disease. Thus, establishing the efficacy of pharmacological agents requires detecting a very targeted effect; whereas, lifestyle interventions may affect many different mechanisms to impact disease risk and therefore it can be more difficult to establish efficacy.

RCTs investigating the effect of lifestyle interventions on ASCVD events generally require long durations, which results in high participant burden and significant expense. For example, the Salt Substitute and Stroke Study (n = 20,995), which examined the effect of a salt substitute (75% sodium chloride and 25% potassium chloride) on risk of stroke (primary outcome) and major cardiovascular events and death from any cause (secondary outcomes), had a mean duration of 4.74 years [26]. The Prevención con Dieta Mediterránea (PREDIMED) study (*n* = 7447), which investigated the effect of Mediterranean diets with extra virgin olive oil or nuts compared to a control diet (advice to follow AHA dietary guidelines), on major cardiovascular events (myocardial infarction, stroke, or death from cardiovascular causes) had a similar mean duration of 4.8 years, although this study was stopped prematurely because of an interim analysis that showed benefit; originally it was planned that the trial would run for 5+ years [27]. The Women's Health Initiative (*n* = 48,835) examined the effect of a dietary intervention designed to be low in fat and high in vegetables, fruits, and grains compared to a control group (received written materials on healthy eating and no nutrition education) on fatal and nonfatal coronary heart disease (CHD), fatal and nonfatal stroke, and total CVD (composite of CHD and stroke) and had a mean follow-up of 8.1 years [28]. These landmark RCTs demonstrate the long duration required when examining the effect of diet on ASCVD events.

Given the long duration and burdensome, costly nature of clinical ASCVD event trials, it is generally more feasible to conduct RCTs examining ASCVD risk factors, e.g., blood pressure or blood lipid/lipoprotein concentrations. However, when ASCVD risk factors are examined, questions may arise about whether observed changes in the risk factors translate into clinically relevant reductions in ASCVD event risk. This is an issue that has plagued investigations of saturated fat intake and ASCVD risk. Most studies in this area have relied on low-density lipoprotein (LDL) cholesterol as a surrogate outcome for ASCVD risk [29], and some question whether the reductions in LDL-cholesterol with lower saturated fat intake translate into ASCVD risk reduction [30]. However, because of the long duration and large sample sizes needed for RCTs examining the effect of lifestyle interventions on hard ASCVD endpoints, most of the RCT evidence available to inform evidence-based guidelines evaluates ASCVD risk factor outcomes.

Small intervention effect sizes: Generally, lifestyle interventions have modest effects on ASCVD-related endpoints. To detect these small effect sizes, large sample sizes are needed, which increases the resources and costs required for studies. Of additional consideration, the health status or baseline susceptibility of a cohort will affect the expected effect size. For example, in the Dietary Approaches to Stop Hypertension (DASH) Trial, the DASH diet lowered systolic and diastolic blood pressure by 5.5 mm Hg (95% confidence interval [CI] −7.4, −3.7 mm Hg) and 3.0 mm Hg (95% CI −4.3, −1.6 mm Hg), respectively, compared to the control diet in the whole cohort ($n = 459$) [31]. However, in participants that were hypertensive at baseline ($\geq$140/$\geq$90 mm Hg), substantially greater reductions in systolic (−11.4 mm Hg; 95% CI −15.9, −6.9 mm Hg) and diastolic (−5.5 mm Hg; 95% CI −8.2, −2.7 mm Hg) blood pressures were observed. In the absence of an adequate sample size to provide sufficient statistical power to detect the expected effect, the null hypothesis is likely to be supported. Thus, small underpowered studies do not provide a true test of the hypothesis to inform evidence-based guidelines.

Intervention design issues: The traditional hypothesis testing framework for RCTs relies on only one factor differing between the intervention group and the control group. In a randomized, placebo-controlled trial of a pharmacological intervention, one group is exposed to a specific dose of a well-characterized active ingredient(s) at a defined frequency, while the control group is given a placebo at the same frequency. Thus, the only difference between the intervention group and the control group is intake of a known quantity of the drug, if randomization assumptions are met. However, when the effect of a lifestyle intervention is tested, it can be very challenging, if not impossible, to ensure only one variable differs between the study groups. These complexities are related to the interrelationships between lifestyle behaviors, the difficulty in exposing participants to a well-defined quantity and frequency of a lifestyle intervention, delivery of the intervention as intended (i.e., intervention fidelity), background exposure to lifestyle behaviors, and adherence promotion and assessment.

Lifestyle-related behaviors are complex exposures that encompass many interdependent and interrelated constituents. For example, activity levels are defined by time spent being active, type and intensity of activity, as well as sedentary time. Prior to the commencement of an RCT, all individuals have a level of exposure to activity. Therefore, implementation of the intervention being tested might involve increasing the duration of current activities with a concomitant decrease in sedentary time, changing the type of activity done (additive to current activity or displacing current activity), changing the intensity of activity, or a combination of all these activity-related exposures, which will likely be non-uniform across the cohort unless strict inclusion and exclusion criteria are used to enroll a cohort with homogenous activity behaviors at baseline. Therefore, when intervening on a specific lifestyle-related behavior, the complex nature of the exposure and the interrelationships that exist with other lifestyle-behaviors need to be considered in the intervention design. This is unlike a pharmacological intervention that can be added to an individual's life without changing any other lifestyle-related factors.

The potential for the intervention being tested to result in addition or subtraction of an exposure, and the concomitant changes to affect the outcome of interest, is particularly relevant to RCTs investigating dietary interventions. Dietary exposure comprises nutrients and non-nutritive components that are consumed as foods, beverages, or supplements that, in totality, make up a dietary pattern. In addition, time and frequency of consumption, as well as many other behaviors that surround eating, define dietary exposure. Thus, when designing a dietary intervention, all of these levels of detail need to be considered to minimize the potential for the trial results to be confounded by an unintended exposure(s). For example, if an intervention involves higher consumption of a particular food(s), whether that food(s) is added to the usual diet or it replaces, completely or partially, a food(s) that is currently consumed needs to be considered because this will have implications for energy, macronutrient and micronutrient intakes, as well as overall diet quality. An additional complexity is that, unless the intervention involves food provision or clear instructions about how to implement the dietary change(s), heterogeneity will be observed across individuals in how the dietary change is made, which will affect the results. Therefore, it is critical that all these issues are addressed in the design phase of a clinical trial, so that results can be interpreted considering the dietary changes made and, importantly, the *"relative to what?"* question can be answered.

In trials of lifestyle interventions, the exposures of the comparator group need to be considered because, unlike in trials of pharmacological interventions, these groups are rarely given a placebo. A lack of attention to the exposures of the comparator group and a sole focus on the exposures of the intervention group can result in an incomplete understanding of the results of a trial. This issue can also result in inconsistent findings for a given intervention between studies; however, often, upon careful evaluation of the differences in the intervention group relative to the control group, results are more consistent. For example, RCTs examining the effect of lowering saturated fat intake show heterogenous effects on LDL-cholesterol and

ASCVD outcomes [32]. Subsequent analyses have revealed that the effect of lowering saturated fat on LDL-cholesterol and ASCVD risk depends on the replacement nutrient [29, 33, 34]. Replacing saturated fat with unsaturated fat (polyunsaturated fat or monounsaturated fat) is associated with reductions in ASCVD risk, whereas replacing saturated fat with refined carbohydrates is associated with increased risk of ASCVD [29].

When considering the exposures of the intervention and control groups in an RCT of a lifestyle intervention, requisite attention needs to be given to the complexity of the exposures. Often, to fit within the traditional RCT framework, reductionist approaches are applied, where one component of the exposure is the focal point. For example, historically, dietary recommendations to lower ASCVD risk focused on nutrient-based recommendations, such as limiting intake of total and saturated fat, sodium, and cholesterol [35–38]. Therefore, many trials examining nutrient-based hypotheses focused on the nutrient of interest with little or no attention on the nutrient(s) being displaced or the foods, beverages, and dietary patterns within which these nutrients were consumed. More recently, recommendations have shifted to focus on the totality of intake or dietary patterns [6, 39, 40]. This recognizes that nutrients and foods are not consumed in isolation, and synergistic and/or antagonistic interactions occur between dietary constituents [41]. From a behavioral perspective, food choices are interdependent and a change in intake of a single or few dietary constituents will have implications for the whole dietary pattern. From an interventional perspective, these changes may be expected and planned for, or they may be unintended. Thus, it is critical to measure the effect the intervention has on the whole dietary pattern, relative to the control group, and not reduce an intervention to its parts, to enable proper inference.

Considering the totality of a lifestyle intervention in the interpretation of the results from a trial may appear counter to the core tenet of RCTs that one independent variable is assessed so that causality between the exposure and the outcomes can be established. However, for lifestyle interventions, the independent variable encompasses all the components tested that differ from the control group. Therefore, reductionist approaches whereby an effect is attributed to one part of the intervention without considering other between-group differences in parallel cannot be applied. Instead, it needs to be acknowledged that we cannot determine how each component of an intervention affected the ASCVD outcome of interest, but rather the intervention as a whole had a particular effect. For example, in the DASH trial, three dietary patterns were examined, a combination diet (now called the DASH diet), a fruit and vegetable diet, and a control diet that represented average American intake at the time. In the original controlled feeding study, the combination diet reduced blood pressure to a greater extent than the fruit and vegetable diet (−2.7/1.9 mm Hg) and the control diet (−5.5/3.0 mm Hg) after 8 weeks in participants with elevated blood pressure. The authors concluded that "a diet rich in fruits, vegetables, and low-fat dairy foods with reduced saturated and total fat can substantially lower blood pressure" in recognition that the *dietary pattern* exerted the observed effect, not any one isolated part. In a trial of this nature, it is not possible to disentangle which component of the combination diet was responsible for the blood pressure-lowering effect since many components of this diet differed from both the control and fruit and vegetable diets.

Lack of a suitable comparator/control: A key characteristic of RCTs is a control group. A control group comprises individuals that have approximately the same characteristics as the intervention group and the same level of exposure to factors that are not inherent to the intervention being tested. Specifically, the control group enables estimation of the effect of certain other factors that the participants in a trial are exposed to that are not part of the intervention being tested, e.g., being in a trial, attending a clinical/health facility on a regular basis, receiving attention from the study staff, usual changes in health status over time, and seasonality. Thus, comparison of the change in an outcome between the intervention group and the control group enables isolation of the intervention effect and reduces the likelihood that the results are because of factors that were not part of the intervention (i.e., confounding). In RCTs of pharmacological agents, placebo pills are usually given to the control group. Placebos are comprised of inert ingredients that do not have any therapeutic effect and, therefore, control for factors associated with regularly taking a medication in a trial that could confound the effect of a drug being tested. However, often in the investigation of lifestyle interventions, a true control group is unethical, and, furthermore, it is challenging to identify a meaningful comparator.

There are ethical considerations to depriving individuals from evidence-based care that lowers disease risk. Currently, lifestyle management is recommended as first-line therapy for ASCVD risk reduction [1]. Therefore, having a control group that is not advised to follow any lifestyle-related behaviors that lower risk of ASCVD, i.e., a true control, presents ethical issues. In parallel, all individuals in a population are exposed to some amount of the characteristics that define a healthy lifestyle. For example, all individuals engage in a level of activity and eat foods, which is dissimilar to trials of pharmacological therapies where individuals have no exposure to a drug unless it is prescribed. Thus, in trials of lifestyle interventions, it is often more meaningful to have a comparator group rather than a true control. The comparator group may be randomized to a usual level of exposure to the lifestyle-factor(s) of interest that is different from the exposure level in the intervention group. Typically, these comparators are defined as "habitual" or "usual" behavior control groups. Comparators may also represent the care usually given to patients/clients with a particular condition or disease; these are often reported as a "usual care" control group. In some cases, a control is not the most meaningful comparator, and two active interventions will be compared to examine superiority of one intervention over another. Therefore, RCTs of lifestyle interventions can rarely be designed as double-blinded, placebo-controlled trials, which is the study design with the least bias providing the highest level of evidence to establish causation.

Blinding: Blinding of participants, outcomes assessors, study personnel administering or providing the intervention, and statisticians is implemented to minimize potential bias from differences in the management, treatment, or assessment of participants, or the interpretation of results that could arise because of participant or study personnel knowledge of the randomization scheme. Blinding study personnel who assess outcomes limits conscious or unconscious bias in how data are collected or interpreted, especially for subjective assessments. Blinding of study personnel administering or providing the active and control/comparator interventions reduces the likelihood that the interventions are delivered in different ways. Blinding the study participants to their allocation reduces the chance that behavior changes will be made based on knowledge of their study group allocation or that self-reporting will be influenced by randomization knowledge. Finally, blinding of the statistician minimizes the risk that data analyses or interpretation will be influenced by randomization knowledge. In a double-blinded trial, both study personnel and participants are blinded to the randomization. In trials of lifestyle interventions, it can be challenging to blind study participants and personnel providing the intervention. Unless dietary supplements are being investigated and a color- and taste-matched placebo is available, participants will know their study group allocation. In some cases, the study purpose is concealed from the study participants to minimize the influence of any prior knowledge they may have about the intervention being studied. However, in most studies testing lifestyle interventions, participants will be aware of their allocation group. For example, in a dietary RCT, it is generally not possible to conceal the taste, appearance, texture, or smell of foods or a diet. Thus, RCTs of lifestyle interventions are rarely double-blinded, which increases the risk of bias and may result in the evidence being downgraded in the evidence-based guideline development process.

Participant adherence: When investigating the effect of lifestyle interventions, there are many challenges related to participant adherence. First, to provide a true test of a hypothesis about the effect of a lifestyle intervention, participants must implement the intervention as intended by the investigators. If the intervention is not implemented as intended and results are consistent with the null hypothesis, it will remain unclear whether the intervention did not have the hypothesized effect or, instead, if adherence was suboptimal so the hypothesized effect simply could not be detected. The Multiple Risk Factor Intervention Trial [42] and the Women's Health Initiative [28] serve as examples of trials in which the hypothesis remained untested because poor adherence to the interventions resulted in the planned contrasts between the intervention and control groups not being achieved [43].

A second complexity is that participant adherence is generally not constant and varies with time. Adherence is generally highest at the beginning of a study and wanes over time. It is well-established that adherence to interventions designed to change behavior declines as the frequency of contact decreases [44]. Therefore, incorporating a greater number of follow-up sessions, or opportunities for contact with study personnel, is a strategy used to promote sustained adherence, although this has resource and financial implications.

Another challenge is measurement of participant adherence. In some cases, an objective method for measuring adherence may be available. For example, for measurement of physical activity, actigraphy (a wearable device that senses motion used to measure sleep, sedentary time, and activity) can be used, as well as wearable devices available in the consumer marketplace, that capture various data related to activity time, activity type, and sedentary time. In the case of dietary interventions, an objective biomarker that approximates near complete intake may be available, e.g., 24-h urinary sodium excretion generally reflects >90% of ingested sodium [45]. Alternatively, compounds may be added to a study food(s)/diet that have a known excretion, e.g., para-aminobenzoic acid is a recovery biomarker excreted in urine. A biomarker that reflects relative dietary change but does not provide exact intake estimates may also be used. For example, red blood cell omega-3 fatty acid index (eicosapentaenoic acid [EPA] plus docosahexaenoic acid [DHA] as a percentage of total fatty acids) increases in a dose–response manner with higher EPA and/or DHA intake but large inter-individual variability is observed in response to a given EPA or DHA dose [46]. However, in many cases, an objective method of assessing adherence to lifestyle interventions is not available or feasible.

Questionnaire/survey-based methods are commonly used to assess adherence to lifestyle interventions. This may include behavior checklists completed at a given frequency (e.g., daily, weekly) or other paper or electronic survey methods. Typically for dietary interventions, diet assessment methods will be used to measure dietary intake or intake of specific dietary components of interest (e.g., 24-h recalls, food records, and food frequency questionnaires). All of these methods are limited by recall bias, which is error from reporting that deviates from true intake. In addition, social desirability bias, or the tendency for respondents to provide information that they perceive will be favorably viewed, such as over-reporting intake of foods perceived as healthy and under-reporting of foods perceived as unhealthy, is a limitation of all diet assessment methods. Some diet assessment methods also have the potential to change behavior [47]. Ecological momentary assessment may also be used to measure behaviors in real time in the participant's natural environment, which reduces recall bias. Thus, sustained implementation of the intervention as intended for the duration of the study, as well as being able to accurately measure adherence, can be challenges in RCTs of lifestyle interventions. In many cases, it is difficult, if not impossible, to measure adherence accurately and precisely; therefore, regardless of whether the hypothesis is supported or rejected, the exact cause of the results can remain unclear.

Summary: A key challenge in developing evidence-based guidelines is distinguishing exactly what was tested and how the intervention may have differed among multiple similar studies, the common effect, and the likelihood that replication of a certain lifestyle intervention at a population, community, or individual level would meaningfully affect ASCVD risk. In many cases, quantifying what was tested to inform prescriptive evidence-based recommendations is not possible, which leads to general, non-specific recommendations. For example, the 2019 ACC/AHA Guideline on the Primary Prevention of Cardiovascular Disease includes the following diet and nutrition recommendation: *"A diet emphasizing intake of vegetables, fruits, legumes, nuts, whole grains, and fish is recommended to decrease ASCVD risk factors"* [1]. However, for reasons described throughout this section, research to investigate the exact quantities/proportions of each of these food groups, as well as specific food types within these groups, needed for ASCVD risk reduction to inform more prescriptive guidelines is largely infeasible.

In the 2020–2025 Dietary Guidelines for Americans, quantitative recommendations are provided for each food group and represented as healthy dietary patterns

[7]. These recommendations are based on empirical evidence about the link between foods and food combinations and health outcomes, as well as achieving nutritional adequacy by meeting the Dietary Reference Intakes (DRIs) [48]. Specifically, the 2020 Dietary Guidelines Advisory Committee conducted systematic reviews to evaluate evidence on foods and combinations of foods that are associated with lower risk of all-cause mortality and other important health outcomes across the lifespan [48]. In addition, food modeling was conducted to determine the types and amounts of food groups that meet the DRIs at various energy levels for age-sex groups 2 years and older. DRIs are a set of reference values used to plan and assess nutrient intakes of healthy people and include: (1) Recommended Dietary Allowances (RDA) that are mean daily intake levels sufficient to meet the nutrient requirements of nearly all (97–98%) healthy people; (2) Adequate Intake (AI) levels that are established when evidence is insufficient to develop an RDA and are set at a level assumed to ensure nutritional adequacy; (3) Tolerable Upper Intake Levels (UL) that are maximum daily intakes unlikely to cause adverse health effects [49]. This approach is taken for the Dietary Guidelines for Americans because of the wide generalizability of these guidelines and the focus on general health for the American population. Such an approach is more challenging for recommendations aimed at disease prevention or management because of the paucity of evidence on intakes of most nutrients associated with disease risk reduction. When the sodium and potassium DRIs were updated in 2019, a Chronic Disease Risk Reduction Intake (CDRR) was established for the first time [50]. The sodium CDRR reflects the lowest level of intake for which there was sufficient strength of evidence to characterize chronic disease risk reduction. Thus, quantitative evidence-based guidelines are developed based on multiple lines of evidence with consideration of the collective health effects, not isolated effects.

3.2 Available Clinical Trial Evidence Base

For many lifestyle-related recommendations, data from RCTs are not available. In the 2019 ACC/AHA Guideline on the Primary Prevention of Cardiovascular Disease, none of the nutrition and diet recommendations were rated as LOE "A", one recommendation had an LOE rating of "B-R", and the other four recommendations were rated as "B-NR" [1]. Similarly, none of the exercise and physical activity recommendations had an "A" LOE rating; for three of the four recommendations, only evidence from non-randomized trials was available [1]. For the treatment of tobacco use, three of the six recommendations had an "A" LOE rating. The limited number of lifestyle-related evidence-based guidelines that have a LOE "A" rating highlights the lack of RCTs examining lifestyle interventions for the primary prevention of ASCVD.

More RCT evidence is available for the effect of lifestyle interventions on risk factors for ASCVD. In the 2019 ACC/AHA Guideline on the Primary Prevention of Cardiovascular Disease, the following recommendation for adults with high blood pressure or hypertension was given an LOE "A" rating: *"In adults with elevated blood pressure or hypertension, including those requiring antihypertensive medications, nonpharmacological interventions are recommended to reduce blood pressure. These include weight loss, a heart-healthy dietary pattern, sodium restriction, dietary potassium supplementation, increased physical activity with a structured exercise program, and limited alcohol"* [1]. For this recommendation, evidence from several well-conducted RCTs was evaluated. Many of these trials were published in the 1990s and early 2000s, including Trials of Hypertension Prevention, Phase I [51] and Phase II [52], Trial of Nonpharmacologic Interventions in the Elderly [53], DASH [31], and DASH-Sodium trials [54] and remain some of the most rigorous RCTs conducted to date on non-pharmacological interventions for ASCVD risk reduction.

3.3   Reliance on Observational Studies

Because of the many challenges to conducting RCTs to test hypotheses related to the efficacy or effectiveness of lifestyle interventions for ASCVD risk reduction, data from observational studies are the primary source of evidence used in the development of evidence-based guidelines. Commonly, the findings of prospective cohort studies are used to inform lifestyle-related evidence-based guidelines because this is the strongest level of evidence available. In a prospective cohort study, assessment of lifestyle-related exposures occurs before the onset of clinical signs and symptoms of disease. Therefore, the direction of the association can be estimated with more confidence. In addition, for exposures that rely on self-reporting methods, recall bias and social desirability bias related to disease onset can be minimized. However, prospective cohort studies do have several limitations that increase the risk of bias and result in evidence being downgraded by guideline development committees. These include the potential for residual confounding, measurement error and imprecise exposure assessment, collinearity among lifestyle exposures, effect modification, differences in the health status of individuals that engage in a lifestyle-related behavior vs. those that do not, and substitution/displacement effects. Maki et al. described how each of these factors affects the results and interpretation of diet-related observational studies [55]. However, these authors also acknowledged the critically important role that observational studies, particularly prospective cohort studies, have in identifying diet–disease relationships and informing evidence-based guidelines.

Epidemiology often suffers from the criticism that observed associations fail to replicate in RCTs. This is frequently attributed to the limitations of observational evidence and, typically, the conclusion drawn is that the exposure–outcome relationship was not causal. However, given the reliance on epidemiological studies because of the relative flexibility, cost-effectiveness, large representative sample sizes, and long-term follow-up, greater investigation of discordant findings between RCTs and epidemiological studies is warranted. In the field of nutrition, inherently different questions are being asked in RCTs vs. in epidemiological studies, which may, to some degree, explain divergent study findings [56].

In an evaluation of bodies of evidence from RCTs and cohort studies in nutrition research, Schwingshackl et al. showed that study populations (inclusion and exclusion criteria and comparison groups), exposure levels (dose, duration, sources), outcomes, sample sizes, and follow-up durations differed between the two study designs [57]. In the 97 diet–disease outcome pairs examined, none were more or less similar with regard to population, intervention or exposure, comparator, and outcomes. When cohort studies and RCTs examined identical exposures, estimates were similar and low statistical heterogeneity was observed [57]. These analyses provide insight into possible reasons for discordance among findings from cohort studies and RCTs and suggest that, when an identical research question is asked, the results from an RCT or observational study both designed to answer the question should be similar. Tobias and Lajous suggested that, when appropriate, nutritional epidemiologists should begin formulating their hypotheses by asking, *"what would the trial be?"* [58]. Given the reliance on observational evidence in the formulation of lifestyle-related evidence-based guidelines, this type of approach may result in an evidence base from observational studies and RCTs that is complementary and better suited to informing evidence-based guidelines.

4   Future Directions

In fields where the feasibility of conducting RCTs to answer questions of clinical or public health relevance are low, observational studies are generally relied on to inform evidence-based guidance. However, this reliance on observational evidence is viewed by some as undermining the evidence-based guidelines in the field. For example, the Nutritional Recommendations and Accessible Evidence Summaries Composed of Systematic Reviews (NutriRECS) consortium, a group of clinical, nutrition, and public health scientists, apply the GRADE methodology to rate the certainty of evidence for nutrition- and disease-related topics [59]. Given the reliance on observational evidence in the field of nutrition and the rating algorithm used for GRADE, NutriRECs often concludes there is low or very low quality evidence for topics such as reducing processed and unprocessed meat intake for cancer and CVD risk reduction [60–65]. In the publication series the NutriRECS consortium produced on red and processed meat intake [60–65], the evidence reviewed showed that reducing unprocessed and processed meat intake by 3 servings/week was associated with reduced risk of overall cancer mortality (relative risk [RR] 0.93, 95% CI 0.91–0.94; RR 0.92, 95% CI 0.89–0.94, respectively) and CVD mortality (RR 0.90, 95% CI 0.88–0.91; RR 0.90, 95% CI 0.84–0.97, respectively) [63, 65]. However, these associations were disregarded in their conclusions because the evidence was from predominately observational studies and consequently rated as low or very low quality. In contrast to all similar current evidence-based guidelines [6, 7, 66] NutriRECs "recommended": *"adults continue current unprocessed red meat consumption (weak recommendation, low-certainty evidence). Similarly, the panel suggests adults continue current processed meat consumption (weak recommendation, low-certainty evidence)."* Rather than disregarding or denigrating observational evidence in fields where RCTs are not always feasible, approaches are needed to leverage observational research when developing evidence-based guidelines.

In general, multiple lines of evidence are considered when developing evidence-based guidelines and, when there is consistency among different evidence types, this strengthens the recommendation. For the field of nutrition, Maki et al. state that the strongest recommendations should be reserved for areas in which observational and RCT results align [55]. This type of approach is much more realistic than aiming to have a particular type of evidence for all guidelines. To overcome some of the barriers associated with conducting RCTs for lifestyle interventions, innovative approaches to emulate hypothetical target trials using observational datasets are being developed. Recently, Chui et al. used this approach to estimate the effects of sustained implementation of the AHA's 2020 food-based goals using three large datasets of U.S. health professionals (Health Professionals Follow-up Study [HPFS], Nurses' Health Study [NHS], and Nurses' Health Study II [NHS II]). In this hypothetical trial of 165,411 participants, the dietary intervention, compared with no intervention, reduced 20-year all-cause mortality risks by 15–21% across the cohorts (HPFS: RR 0.85, 95% CI 0.81–0.88; NHS: RR 0.79, 95% CI 0.75–0.85; NHS II: RR 0.86, 95% CI 0.78–0.96) [67]. This hypothetical target trial approach was also used in an analysis of middle aged women from the NHS in which it was estimated that sustained lifestyle modification (smoking cessation, weight loss, physical activity, and dietary changes) would reduce 26-year risk of total stroke by 25% and ischemic stroke by 36% [68]. A strength of these analytical approaches is that the estimated effect of multiple lifestyle interventions can be examined in one hypothetical trial, which is rarely possible in real-world RCTs. Thus, in the future, lifestyle-related evidence-based guidelines may be informed by evidence that does not fit into the traditional study design classifications, which will require evidence rating systems to be adapted.

As described throughout this chapter, one of the key difficulties in the development of evidence-based guidelines for lifestyle interventions is that the pharmacological model of developing evidence-based guidelines is applied, despite substantial differences in methodologies used for researching lifestyle interventions. RCTs of pharmacological agents examine specific doses and dose regimens of drugs, which can be used to make prescriptive evidence-based guidelines. On the other hand, RCTs of lifestyle interventions typically test more heterogenous interventions with less exact quantification of the intervention components, which results in the development of more general evidence-based guidelines. For example, the 2018 AHA/ACC/Multisociety Guideline on the Management of Blood Cholesterol includes the following primary prevention recommendation for adults aged 40–75 years with LDL-cholesterol levels of 70–189 mg/dL: *"In adults at intermediate-risk, statin therapy reduces risk of ASCVD, and in the context of a risk discussion, if a decision is made for statin therapy, a moderate-intensity statin should be recommended"* (COR 1, LOE A) [4]. Moderate-intensity statin therapy is outlined in the guideline by specific statins and doses, e.g., atorvastatin 10 mg. It is unlikely that lifestyle-related evidence-based guidelines will ever be as specific and prescriptive as guidelines for pharmacological agents, and this presents challenges for physicians that are advising patients on lifestyle-related behavior change.

Lifestyle counseling does not routinely occur during physician visits and one cited reason is that physicians report feeling unprepared or lack confidence to provide adequate lifestyle counseling [69]. While this is a complex problem requiring changes to medical education and other aspects of clinical care, greater consideration for developing more prescriptive lifestyle-related evidence-based guidelines that may aid clinical implementation is warranted. Therefore, rather than focusing on the intervention components like pharmacological therapy, the focus may be on who delivers the intervention, when, and for how long. For example, prescriptive guidelines for dietary intervention could be based on referring patients to a registered dietitian nutritionist for medical nutrition therapy when they are at a specific ASCVD risk level.

The 2015 National Lipid Association Recommendations for Patient-Centered Management of Dyslipidemia-Part 2 include the following as part of the nutrition recommendations (rated as strength A, moderate quality evidence): *"Nutritional counseling and follow-up/monitoring by a registered dietitian nutritionist is recommended whenever possible to individualize a patient's dietary pattern"* [5]. Recommendations like this that are more prescriptive about when a referral is required may assist in the clinical non-pharmacological management of ASCVD; however, implementation of this type of guidance will require that patients have access to specialized clinical care and that it is reimbursed by insurance companies. In summary, to overcome some of the challenges in developing evidence-based guidelines for lifestyle-related interventions for ASCVD risk reduction, some evolution of the traditional medical models of evidence-based guidance development may be needed for non-pharmacological guideline development.

5   Conclusions

First-line therapy for ASCVD risk reduction is non-pharmacological intervention to follow a healthy lifestyle throughout the lifespan, which is supported by multiple lines of consistent evidence [1]. However, developing evidence-based recommendations for components of a healthy lifestyle, including dietary and physical activity recommendations, can be challenging because of the complexities associated with conducting high-quality research on the efficacy or effectiveness of these types of interventions. Conducting randomized, double-blinded placebo-controlled trials, the highest quality of evidence for establishing causation, to examine the effect of lifestyle interventions on ASCVD events is largely infeasible. Therefore, lifestyle-related evidence-based guidelines are informed by some large RCTs examining clinical ASCVD events but predominately smaller RCTs assessing ASCVD risk factors as well as observational research. In many cases, observational evidence is relied on when making diet and physical recommendations. Given that observational evidence is prone to many sources of bias, guidelines based on observational evidence have lower quality of evidence ratings. Innovative methodologies are being used to emulate hypothetical target trials using observational datasets, which offer promise for leveraging epidemiological data to answer questions that cannot be feasibly investigated in RCTs. Shifts in how evidence-based guidelines for lifestyle interventions are constructed may need to occur to better capture the complexity of lifestyle exposures, the efficacy of specialized clinician care (e.g., registered dietitians nutritionists), and the individualized counseling needed to achieve lifestyle-related behavior change [70]. Thus, rather than formulating general guidelines about components of a healthy lifestyle associated with lower ASCVD risk reduction, specific guidelines focused on when (e.g., level of ASCVD risk) and how (e.g., referral to specialized clinician) patients should be given the counseling, tools, and resources needed to make lifestyle-related behavior change may improve clinical implementation and patient outcomes.

References

1. Arnett DK, Blumenthal RS, Albert MA, Buroker AB, Goldberger ZD, Hahn EJ, et al. 2019 ACC/AHA guideline on the primary prevention of cardiovascular disease: a report of the American College of Cardiology/American Heart Association Task Force on clinical practice guidelines. Circulation. 2019;140(11):e596–646.
2. Eckel RH, Jakicic JM, Ard JD, Hubbard VS, de Jesus JM, Lee I-M, et al. 2013 AHA/ACC guideline on lifestyle management to reduce cardiovascular risk: a report of the American College of Cardiology/American Heart Association Task Force on practice guidelines. Circulation. 2014;129(25 Suppl 2):S76–99.
3. Whelton PK, Carey RM, Aronow WS, Casey DE, Collins KJ, Himmelfarb CD, et al. 2017 ACC/AHA/AAPA/ABC/ACPM/AGS/APhA/ASH/ASPC/NMA/PCNA guideline for the prevention, detection, evaluation, and management of high blood pressure in adults: a report of the American College of Cardiology/American Heart Association Task Force on clinical practice guidelines. J Am Coll Cardiol. 2018;71(19):e127–248.
4. Grundy SM, Stone NJ, Bailey AL, Beam C, Birtcher KK, Blumenthal RS, et al. 2018 AHA/ACC/AACVPR/AAPA/ABC/ACPM/ADA/AGS/APhA/ASPC/NLA/PCNA guideline on the management of blood cholesterol: a report of the American College of Cardiology/American Heart Association Task Force on clinical practice guidelines. Circulation. 2019;139(25):e1082–143.
5. Jacobson TA, Maki KC, Orringer CE, Jones PH, Kris-Etherton P, Sikand G, et al. National Lipid Association recommendations for patient-centered management of dyslipidemia: part 2. J Clin Lipidol. 2015;9(6):S1–122.
6. Lichtenstein AH, Appel LJ, Vadiveloo M, Hu FB, Kris-Etherton PM, Rebholz CM, et al. 2021 Dietary guidance to improve cardiovascular health: a scientific statement from the American Heart Association. Circulation. 2021;144:e472. https://doi.org/10.1161/CIR.0000000000001031.
7. U.S. Department of Agriculture, U.S. Department of Health and Human Services. Dietary guidelines for Americans, 2020-2025. 9th ed. [Internet]. 2020. [Cited 2021 Jan 2]. http://www.dietaryguidelines.gov.
8. U.S. Department of Health and Human Services. Physical activity guidelines for Americans. 2nd ed. Washington, DC: U.S.; 2018.

9. U.S. Food and Drug Administration. Clinical trials guidance documents [Internet]. [Cited 2021 Dec 6]. https://www.fda.gov/regulatory-information/search-fda-guidance-documents/clinical-trials-guidance-documents.

10. U.S. Food and Drug Administration, Center for Drug Evaluation and Research (CDER), Center for Biologics Evaluation and Research (CBER). E8(R1) general considerations for clinical studies [Internet]. 2019. [Cited 2021 Dec 6]. https://www.fda.gov/media/129527/download.

11. U.S. Department of Health and Human Services, Food and Drug Administration, Center for Drug Evaluation and Research (CDER), Center for Biologics Evaluation and Research (CBER). Guidance for Industry E 10. Choice of control group and related issues in clinical trials [Internet]. 2001. [Cited 2021 Dec 6]. https://www.fda.gov/media/71349/download.

12. US Department of Health and Human Services, Food and Drug Administration, Center for Drug Evaluation and Research (CDER), Center for Biologics Evaluation and Research (CBER). Guidance for Industry. E9 statistical principles for clinical trials [Internet]. 1998. [Cited 2021 Dec 6]. https://www.fda.gov/media/71336/download.

13. US Department of Health and Human Services, Food and Drug Administration, Center for Drug Evaluation and Research (CDER), Center for Biologics Evaluation and Research (CBER). Guidance for Industry. Multiple endpoints in clinical trials [Internet]. 2017 [Cited 2021 Dec 6]. https://www.fda.gov/media/102657/download.

14. Weaver CM, Lichtenstein AH, Kris-Etherton PM. Perspective: guidelines needed for the conduct of human nutrition randomized controlled trials. Adv Nutr. 2021;12(1):1–3.

15. Lichtenstein AH, Petersen K, Barger K, Hansen KE, Anderson CAM, Baer DJ, et al. Perspective: design and conduct of human nutrition randomized controlled trials. Adv Nutr. 2020;12(1):4–20.

16. Weaver CM, Fukagawa NK, Liska D, Mattes RD, Matuszek G, Nieves JW, et al. Perspective: US Documentation and regulation of human nutrition randomized controlled trials. Adv Nutr. 2021;12(1):21–45.

17. Maki KC, Miller JW, McCabe GP, Raman G, Kris-Etherton PM. Perspective: laboratory considerations and clinical data management for human nutrition randomized controlled trials: guidance for ensuring quality and integrity. Adv Nutr. 2021;12(1):46–58.

18. Petersen KS, Kris-Etherton PM, McCabe GP, Raman G, Miller JW, Maki KC. Perspective: planning and conducting statistical analyses for human nutrition randomized controlled trials: ensuring data quality and integrity. Adv Nutr. 2021;12(5):1610–24.

19. Ninot G. Defining non-pharmacological interventions (NPIs). In: Non-pharmacological interventions: an essential answer to current demographic, health, and environmental transitions. Cham: Springer; 2021. p. 1–46.

20. Gibbons RJ, Smith S, Antman E. American College of Cardiology/American Heart Association clinical practice guidelines: part I: where do they come from? Circulation. 2003;107(23):2979–86.

21. Jacobs AK, Kushner FG, Ettinger SM, Guyton RA, Anderson JL, Ohman EM, et al. ACCF/AHA clinical practice guideline methodology summit report: a report of the American College of Cardiology Foundation/American Heart Association Task Force on practice guidelines. Circulation. 2013;127(2):268–310.

22. Halperin JL, Levine GN, Al-Khatib SM, Birtcher KK, Bozkurt B, Brindis RG, et al. Further evolution of the ACC/AHA clinical practice guideline recommendation classification system: a report of the American College of Cardiology/American Heart Association Task Force on clinical practice guidelines. Circulation. 2016;133(14):1426–8.

23. Kirkpatrick CF, Bolick JP, Kris-Etherton PM, Sikand G, Aspry KE, Soffer DE, et al. Review of current evidence and clinical recommendations on the effects of low-carbohydrate and very-low-carbohydrate (including ketogenic) diets for the management of body weight and other cardiometabolic risk factors: a scientific statement from the Nati. J Clin Lipidol. 2019;13(5):689–711.

24. Guyatt G, Oxman AD, Akl EA, Kunz R, Vist G, Brozek J, et al. GRADE guidelines: 1. Introduction—GRADE evidence profiles and summary of findings tables. J Clin Epidemiol. 2011;64(4):383–94.
25. Hirahatake KM, Dicklin MR, Maki KC. Epidemiology of atherosclerotic cardiovascular disease. In: Davidson M, Toth P, Maki K, editors. Therapeutic lipidology. 2nd ed. Springer Nature; 2021. p. 91–105.
26. Neal B, Wu Y, Feng X, Zhang R, Zhang Y, Shi J, et al. Effect of salt substitution on cardiovascular events and death. N Engl J Med. 2021;385:1067–77.
27. Estruch R, Ros E, Salas-Salvadó J, Covas M-I, Corella D, Arós F, et al. Primary prevention of cardiovascular disease with a Mediterranean diet supplemented with extra-virgin olive oil or nuts. N Engl J Med. 2018;378(25):e34.
28. Howard BV, Van Horn L, Hsia J, Manson JE, Stefanick ML, Wassertheil-Smoller S, et al. Low-fat dietary pattern and risk of cardiovascular disease: the Women's health initiative randomized controlled dietary modification trial. JAMA. 2006;295(6):655–66.
29. Sacks FM, Lichtenstein AH, Wu JHY, Appel LJ, Creager MA, Kris-Etherton PM, et al. Dietary fats and cardiovascular disease: a presidential advisory from the American Heart Association. Circulation. 2017;136(3):e1–23.
30. Krauss RM, Kris-Etherton PM. Public health guidelines should recommend reducing saturated fat consumption as much as possible: NO. Am J Clin Nutr. 2020;112(1):19–24.
31. Appel LJ, Moore TJ, Obarzanek E, Vollmer WM, Svetkey LP, Sacks FM, et al. A clinical trial of the effects of dietary patterns on blood pressure. N Engl J Med. 1997;336(16):1117–24.
32. Hooper L, Martin N, Abdelhamid A, Davey Smith G. Reduction in saturated fat intake for cardiovascular disease. Cochrane Database Syst Rev [Internet]. 2015;(6). https://doi.org/10.1002/14651858.CD011737.
33. Mozaffarian D, Micha R, Wallace S. Effects on coronary heart disease of increasing polyunsaturated fat in place of saturated fat: a systematic review and meta-analysis of randomized controlled trials. PLoS Med. 2010;7(3):e1000252.
34. Hooper L, Martin N, Jimoh OF, Kirk C, Foster E, Abdelhamid AS. Reduction in saturated fat intake for cardiovascular disease. Cochrane Database Syst Rev [Internet]. 2020;5:CD011737. https://doi.org/10.1002/14651858.CD011737.pub2.
35. Krauss RM, Deckelbaum RJ, Ernst N, Fisher E, Howard BV, Knopp RH, et al. Dietary guidelines for healthy American adults. Circulation. 1996;94(7):1795–800.
36. American Heart Association. Dietary guidelines for healthy Americans adults: a statement for physicians and health professionals by the Nutrition Committee. Circulation. 1986;74:1465A–8A.
37. American Heart Association. Dietary guidelines for healthy American adults: a statement for physicians and health professionals by the Nutrition Committee. Circulation. 1988;77(3):721A–4A.
38. American Heart Association. Diet and coronary heart disease: a statement for physicians and other health professionals. Circulation. 1978;54:762A–6A.
39. Lichtenstein AH, Appel LJ, Brands M, Carnethon M, Daniels S, Franch HA, et al. Diet and lifestyle recommendations revision 2006: a scientific statement from the American Heart Association Nutrition Committee. Circulation. 2006;114(1):82–96.
40. Van Horn L, Carson JAS, Appel LJ, Burke LE, Economos C, Karmally W, et al. Recommended dietary pattern to achieve adherence to the American Heart Association/American College of Cardiology (AHA/ACC) guidelines: a scientific statement from the American Heart Association. Circulation. 2016;134(22):e505–29.
41. Tapsell LC, Neale EP, Satija A, Hu FB. Foods, nutrients, and dietary patterns: interconnections and implications for dietary guidelines. Adv Nutr. 2016;7(3):445–54.
42. Multiple Risk Factor Intervention Trial. Risk factor changes and mortality results. JAMA. 1982;248(12):1465–77.
43. Willett WC. The WHI joins MRFIT: a revealing look beneath the covers. Am J Clin Nutr. 2010;91(4):829–30.

44. Artinian NT, Fletcher GF, Mozaffarian D, Kris-Etherton P, Van Horn L, Lichtenstein AH, et al. Interventions to promote physical activity and dietary lifestyle changes for cardiovascular risk factor reduction in adults: a scientific statement from the American Heart Association. Circulation. 2010;122(4):406–41.
45. Birukov A, Rakova N, Lerchl K, Olde Engberink RH, Johannes B, Wabel P, et al. Ultra-long-term human salt balance studies reveal interrelations between sodium, potassium, and chloride intake and excretion. Am J Clin Nutr. 2016;104(1):49–57.
46. Harris WS, Von Schacky C. The Omega-3 Index: a new risk factor for death from coronary heart disease? Prev Med (Baltim). 2004;39(1):212–20.
47. Thompson FE, Kirkpatrick SI, Subar AF, Reedy J, Schap TE, Wilson MM, et al. The National Cancer Institute's dietary assessment primer: a resource for diet research. J Acad Nutr Diet. 2015;115(12):1986–95.
48. Dietary Guidelines Advisory Committee. Scientific report of the 2020 Dietary Guidelines Advisory Committee: advisory report to the Secretary of Agriculture and the Secretary of Health and Human Services. Washington, DC: Agricultural Research Service; 2020.
49. U.S. Department of Health & Human Services, National Institutes of Health, Office of Dietary Supplements. Nutrient recommendations: dietary reference intakes (DRI) [Internet]. [Cited 2021 Dec 6]. https://ods.od.nih.gov/HealthInformation/Dietary_Reference_Intakes.aspx.
50. National Academies of Sciences. Engineering, and medicine. Dietary Reference Intakes for sodium and potassium. National Academies Press; 2019.
51. Whelton PK, Appel L, Charleston J, Dalcin AT, Ewart C, Fried L, et al. The effects of nonpharmacologic interventions on blood pressure of persons with high normal levels: results of the Trials of Hypertension Prevention, phase I. JAMA. 1992;267(9):1213–20.
52. The Trials of Hypertension Prevention Collaborative Research Group. Effects of weight loss and sodium reduction intervention on blood pressure and hypertension incidence in overweight people with high-normal blood pressure: the trials of hypertension prevention, phase II. JAMA Intern Med. 1997;157(6):657–67.
53. Whelton PK, Appel LJ, Espeland MA, Applegate WB, Ettinger Walter H, Kostis JB, et al. Sodium reduction and weight loss in the treatment of hypertension in older persons: a randomized controlled trial of nonpharmacologic interventions in the elderly (TONE). JAMA. 1998;279(11):839–46.
54. Sacks FM, Svetkey LP, Vollmer WM, Appel LJ, Bray GA, Harsha D, et al. Effects on blood pressure of reduced dietary sodium and the dietary approaches to stop hypertension (DASH) diet. N Engl J Med. 2001;344(1):3–10.
55. Maki KC, Slavin JL, Rains TM, Kris-Etherton PM. Limitations of observational evidence: implications for evidence-based dietary recommendations. Adv Nutr. 2014;5(1):7–15.
56. Satija A, Stampfer MJ, Rimm EB, Willett W, Hu FB. Perspective: are large, simple trials the solution for nutrition research? Adv Nutr. 2018;9(4):378–87.
57. Schwingshackl L, Balduzzi S, Beyerbach J, Bröckelmann N, Werner SS, Zähringer J, et al. Evaluating agreement between bodies of evidence from randomised controlled trials and cohort studies in nutrition research: meta-epidemiological study. BMJ. 2021;374:n1864.
58. Tobias DK, Lajous M. What would the trial be? Emulating randomized dietary intervention trials to estimate causal effects with observational data. Am J Clin Nutr. 2021;114:416.
59. Johnston BC, Alonso-Coello P, Bala MM, Zeraatkar D, Rabassa M, Valli C, et al. Methods for trustworthy nutritional recommendations NutriRECS (Nutritional Recommendations and accessible Evidence summaries Composed of Systematic reviews): a protocol. BMC Med Res Methodol. 2018;18(1):162.
60. Johnston BC, Zeraatkar D, Han MA, Vernooij RWM, Valli C, El Dib R, et al. Unprocessed red meat and processed meat consumption: dietary guideline recommendations from the Nutritional Recommendations (NutriRECS) Consortium. Ann Intern Med. 2019;171(10):756–64.
61. Zeraatkar D, Johnston BC, Bartoszko J, Cheung K, Bala MM, Valli C, et al. Effect of lower versus higher red meat intake on cardiometabolic and cancer outcomes: a systematic review of randomized trials. Ann Intern Med. 2019;171(10):721–31.

62. Vernooij RWM, Zeraatkar D, Han MA, El Dib R, Zworth M, Milio K, et al. Patterns of red and processed meat consumption and risk for cardiometabolic and cancer outcomes: a systematic review and meta-analysis of cohort studies. Ann Intern Med. 2019;171(10):732–41.

63. Han MA, Zeraatkar D, Guyatt GH, Vernooij RWM, El Dib R, Zhang Y, et al. Reduction of red and processed meat intake and cancer mortality and incidence: a systematic review and meta-analysis of cohort studies. Ann Intern Med. 2019;171(10):711–20.

64. Valli C, Rabassa M, Johnston BC, Kuijpers R, Prokop-Dorner A, Zajac J, et al. Health-related values and preferences regarding meat consumption: a mixed-methods systematic review. Ann Intern Med. 2019;171(10):742–55.

65. Zeraatkar D, Han MA, Guyatt GH, Vernooij RWM, El Dib R, Cheung K, et al. Red and processed meat consumption and risk for all-cause mortality and cardiometabolic outcomes: a systematic review and meta-analysis of cohort studies. Ann Intern Med. 2019;171(10):703–10.

66. World Cancer Research Fund, American Institute for Cancer Research. Diet, nutrition, physical activity and cancer: a global perspective: a summary of the Third Expert Report [Internet]. World Cancer Research Fund International; 2018. http://www.dietandcancerreport.org/.

67. Chiu Y-H, Chavarro JE, Dickerman BA, Manson JE, Mukamal KJ, Rexrode KM, et al. Estimating the effect of nutritional interventions using observational data: the American Heart Association's 2020 Dietary Goals and mortality. Am J Clin Nutr. 2021;114(2):690–703.

68. Jain P, Suemoto CK, Rexrode K, Manson JE, Robins JM, Hernán MA, et al. Hypothetical lifestyle strategies in middle-aged women and the long-term risk of stroke. Stroke. 2020;51(5):1381–7.

69. Hivert M-F, Arena R, Forman DE, Kris-Etherton PM, McBride PE, Pate RR, et al. Medical training to achieve competency in lifestyle counseling: an essential foundation for prevention and treatment of cardiovascular diseases and other chronic medical conditions: a scientific statement from the American Heart Association. Circulation. 2016;134(15):e308–27.

70. Laddu D, Ma J, Kaar J, Ozemek C, Durant RW, Campbell T, et al. Health behavior change programs in primary care and community practices for cardiovascular disease prevention and risk factor management among midlife and older adults: a scientific statement from the American Heart Association. Circulation. 2021;144(24):e533–49.

Part II
Overview of Current Evidence in Categories of Interventions

Lifestyle Interventions and Atherosclerotic Cardiovascular Disease Outcomes

Carol F. Kirkpatrick, Kathyrn A. Greaves, and Elaine Foster

Key Points

- A healthy lifestyle is the foundation for the prevention of atherosclerotic cardiovascular disease (ASCVD).
- Lifestyle interventions that have been associated with reduced risk of ASCVD include a healthy dietary pattern, physical activity, reducing excess adiposity, sleep hygiene, management of psychosocial stress, and tobacco cessation.
- Healthy lifestyle behaviors positively impact cardiovascular risk factors, including body weight, lipids and lipoproteins, glucose, and blood pressure.
- Evidence-based nutrition recommendations for ASCVD prevention and management include reduction of saturated fatty acids with replacement by unsaturated fatty acids, reduction of sugar-sweetened beverages, low-to-moderate alcohol consumption if a person chooses to drink, and consuming a dietary pattern that encompasses these recommendations.
- Evidence-based physical activity recommendations for ASCVD prevention and management include ≥ 150 min/week of moderate-intensity aerobic activity, ≥ 75 min/week of vigorous-intensity aerobic activity, or an equivalent combination of both, and resistance training at least two times/week.

C. F. Kirkpatrick (✉)
Midwest Biomedical Research, Addison, IL, USA

Kasiska Division of Health Sciences, Idaho State University, Pocatello, ID, USA
e-mail: carolkirkpatrick@isu.edu

K. A. Greaves
Nutrition Outside the Box, LLC, Battle Creek, MI, USA

Western Michigan University, Kalamazoo, MI, USA

E. Foster
Department of Human Performance and Sport Studies, Idaho State University, Pocatello, ID, USA
e-mail: elainefoster@isu.edu

© The Author(s), under exclusive license to Springer Nature Switzerland AG 2024
K. C. Maki, D. P. Wilson (eds.), *Cardiovascular Outcomes Research*, Contemporary Cardiology, https://doi.org/10.1007/978-3-031-54960-1_8

- The relationship between body weight and ASCVD outcomes is complex and excess adiposity, particularly visceral adipose tissue and increased waist circumference, appear to be better indicators of risk than body mass index.
- Adequate quantity and quality of sleep and psychosocial health are emerging as important risk factors for ASCVD.
- Tobacco abstinence is fundamental for promotion of cardiovascular health.
- Although there are randomized controlled trials examining the impact of lifestyle interventions on ASCVD risk factors, observational studies are the primary source of evidence for the majority of lifestyle interventions and ASCVD outcomes, with the exception of the Mediterranean dietary pattern.
- Despite the limitations inherent with observational evidence, the totality of the available data supports the view that lifestyle interventions can beneficially impact cardiovascular health and are essential in the prevention and management of ASCVD.

1 Introduction

Cardiovascular disease (CVD) is an umbrella term to describe disorders of the heart and blood vessels, which includes atherosclerotic CVD (ASCVD) [1]. Atherosclerosis results from the accumulation of inflammatory cells, lipids and lipoproteins, extracellular matrix, and other materials in the artery wall [2]. ASCVD includes coronary artery disease (CAD), which is also known as coronary heart disease (CHD), of which clinical manifestations can be acute coronary syndrome, myocardial infarction (MI), stable or unstable angina, or coronary or other arterial revascularization; cerebrovascular disease (ischemic stroke, transient ischemic attack, and carotid artery stenosis); peripheral artery disease (intermittent claudication); renal atherosclerotic disease; and aortic atherosclerotic disease (abdominal aortic aneurysm and descending thoracic aneurysm) [3, 4].

The major modifiable risk factors for ASCVD include elevated blood pressure, abnormal lipoprotein lipid levels, hyperglycemia, and cigarette smoking [4–6]. A person's 10-year and lifetime ASCVD risk can be estimated using the American College of Cardiology/American Heart Association (AHA) Pooled Cohort Equations [4, 7]. The factors used in the Pooled Cohort Equations include age, sex, race, total cholesterol, high-density lipoprotein cholesterol (HDL-C), systolic and diastolic blood pressures, use of blood pressure-lowering medication, diabetes mellitus status, and smoking status [8]. Other ASCVD risk factors include obesity/excess adiposity, chronic inflammation, unhealthy dietary patterns, excess alcohol consumption, physical inactivity, and psychosocial factors [4–7, 9–12], all of which are modifiable.

A healthy lifestyle is the foundation for ASCVD prevention [4–7, 10–13], which influences risk by positively impacting major risk factors [6, 7, 10], as well as other contributing risk factors. Non-pharmacological interventions specific to lifestyle include dietary interventions, adequate and consistent physical activity, tobacco

Table 1 Life's Essential 8 [12]

Behaviors for Achieving Optimal Scores	Metrics for Optimal Scores
Healthy eating pattern—high adherence to Mediterranean- or DASH-style eating pattern	**BMI**—BMI <25 kg/m^2
Physical activity—≥150 min/week of moderate or 75 min/week of vigorous physical activity	**Blood lipids**—non-HDL-C <130 mg/dL to reduce ASCVD risk
Nicotine exposure—self-reported "never smoker"; encourage patients to seek assistance for cessation, as needed	**Fasting blood glucose and HbA1c**—no history of diabetes and FBG <100 mg/dL or HbA1c <5.7%
Sleep health—self-reported 7 to <9 h of sleep each night	**Blood pressure**—systolic and diastolic blood pressure <120 and <80 mm Hg, respectively

Abbreviations: *ASCVD* atherosclerotic cardiovascular disease, *BMI* body mass index, *DASH* Dietary Approaches to Stop Hypertension, *FBG* fasting blood glucose, *HbA1c* glycated hemoglobin, *non-HDL-C* non-high-density lipoprotein cholesterol

abstinence or cessation, addressing psychosocial health, and adequate sleep [5–7, 12]. Excess adiposity may result from unhealthy habits related to nutrition, physical activity, and sleep. The AHA summarized key metrics for cardiovascular (CV) health in its Presidential Advisory, Life's Essential 8 [12], which is an update to the Life's Simple 7 CV health components and includes health behaviors that impact CV health metrics (Table 1). Improved health behaviors and CV health metrics have been associated with reduced risk of CVD, as well as longevity and higher quality of life [12].

Although there is randomized controlled trial (RCT) evidence to support the beneficial effects of lifestyle interventions on ASCVD risk factors, such as lipids and lipoproteins, blood pressure, glycemic control, and excess adiposity, evidence for the effect of lifestyle on ASCVD outcomes, such as decreased incidence of events and mortality, is limited and is primarily from observational studies. The purpose of this chapter is to review the currently available evidence on the effects of lifestyle interventions on ASCVD outcomes, specifically dietary interventions, physical activity, reducing excess adiposity, healthy sleep habits, psychosocial health and stress management, and tobacco cessation. The available evidence will be summarized for each of these interventions, which will focus on RCTs when available and observational studies when RCT evidence is limited.

2 Dietary Interventions and ASCVD Outcomes

Cardioprotective dietary interventions are emphasized in ASCVD prevention and risk factor reduction guidelines from the United States (U.S.) and internationally [5–7, 9–13]. There is consensus on the nutrition recommendations for ASCVD

Table 2 Evidence-based nutrition recommendations for ASCVD risk reduction and prevention [5–7, 9–11, 13]

Increase consumption of vegetables, fruits, legumes (pulses), nuts, and whole grains
Choose healthy protein foods: minimally processed fish and seafood, poultry, and lean unprocessed red meat, and plant-based proteins
Replace SFAs with dietary MUFAs and PUFAs; use plant-based non-tropical oils in place of solid fats
Reduce amounts of cholesterol and salt/sodium
Minimize intake of processed meats, refined carbohydrates, foods and beverages with added sugars, and alcohol
Avoid *trans* fatty acids
Adopt a Mediterranean, or similar, dietary pattern

Abbreviations: *ASCVD* atherosclerotic cardiovascular disease, *MUFAs* monounsaturated fatty acids, *PUFAs* polyunsaturated fatty acids, *SFAs* saturated fatty acids

prevention (Table 2). These recommendations are based primarily on the results of RCTs that examined the effect of dietary interventions on ASCVD risk factors (i.e., lipids and lipoproteins, blood pressures, glycemic control) or observational studies of the effect on risk factors and CV outcomes. An overview of the evidence for selected dietary intervention components listed in Table 2 is discussed below.

2.1 Dietary Patterns and ASCVD Outcomes

A healthy dietary pattern is an essential component of a lifestyle for ASCVD prevention. It is apparent that the totality of foods and dietary components consumed likely has a more substantial impact on ASCVD risk than individual foods and food components [14]. This is reflected by the transition from focusing on individual dietary components, such as saturated fatty acids (SFAs) and salt, to overall healthy dietary patterns in recent dietary guidance for ASCVD prevention and general health [5–7, 10, 11, 13, 15]. The recommended dietary patterns for ASCVD prevention include the Mediterranean, Dietary Approaches to Stop Hypertension (DASH), Healthy U.S.-Style, and healthy plant-based dietary patterns (e.g., vegetarian and vegan). Figure 1 illustrates the commonalities of these dietary patterns, which encompass the evidence-based nutrition recommendations for ASCVD risk reduction and prevention outlined in Table 2.

There is substantial evidence that a high adherence to healthy dietary patterns is associated with reduced ASCVD risk. Of the recommended dietary patterns for ASCVD prevention, only the Mediterranean dietary pattern has both RCT and observational evidence for its beneficial impact on ASCVD outcomes. In 2018, Dinu et al. published an umbrella review of the effect of the Mediterranean dietary pattern on various outcomes, which included meta-analyses of RCTs that examined the effect of the dietary pattern on ASCVD outcomes [16]. Although there were

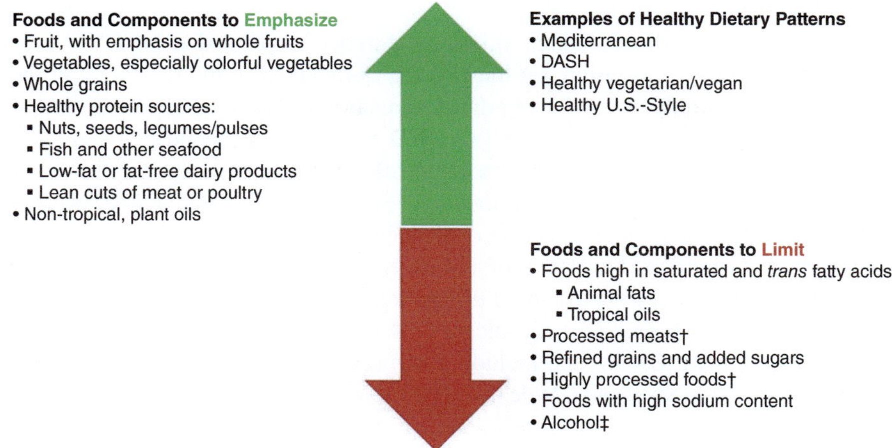

Fig. 1 Commonalities of recommended dietary patterns for ASCVD prevention* [13]. *Although healthy dietary patterns share commonalities, they emphasize different components, e.g., DASH has a greater emphasis on fruits, vegetables, and low-fat dairy, and the Mediterranean dietary pattern has a greater emphasis on a higher intake of foods rich in MUFAs, such as nuts and extra-virgin olive and canola oils. Foods and dietary components to emphasize or limit are recommended regardless of where food is prepared or consumed. †Examples of processed meats to limit include bacon, sausage, salami, ham, pepperoni, and deli meats. Examples of highly processed foods to limit include ready-to-eat and quick service meals, refined breads and baked goods, fruit juices, commercially prepared foods and beverages with added sugar or salt, sauces, and condiments. ‡If individuals choose to drink alcohol, intake should be moderate: ≤1 drink/day for women; ≤2 drinks/day for men. 1 drink = 12 fl. oz. regular beer, 8–10 fl. oz. malt beverage, 5 fl. oz. table wine, 3–4 fl. oz. fortified wine, 2–3 fl. oz. liqueur, 1.5 fl. oz. brandy/cognac, or 1.5 fl. oz. distilled spirit. **Abbreviations:** *ASCVD* atherosclerotic cardiovascular disease, *DASH* Dietary Approaches to Stop Hypertension, *MUFAs* monounsaturated fatty acids

small numbers of studies for each of the outcomes, the authors of the review reported that the results of the meta-analyses suggested a significant 38–41% reduced risk of CVD incidence and mortality, as well as a significant 36–40% reduced risk of MI and stroke incidence with a Mediterranean dietary pattern [16]. Additionally, Rees et al. conducted a Cochrane systematic review in 2019 to examine the effect of Mediterranean-style dietary patterns on primary and secondary prevention of CVD [17] of which the Prevención con Dieta Mediterránea (PREDIMED) study was the only primary prevention study that examined clinical endpoints that fit the inclusion criteria of the Cochrane review. PREDIMED included two Mediterranean diet interventions (supplemented with extra-virgin olive oil or mixed nuts) compared to a traditional Mediterranean diet in which the participants were instructed to reduce their intake of total fat. The results of the study demonstrated ~30% significant reduced risk of the primary endpoint (composite major CV event defined as MI, stroke, or CV death) with both Mediterranean dietary interventions compared with the control intervention (a lower fat traditional Mediterranean diet) [17, 18], which appeared to be driven primarily by stroke [17].

In their Cochrane review, Rees et al. also reviewed RCTs that examined a Mediterranean-style dietary intervention compared to control diet on CVD endpoints in secondary prevention. Of the two RCTs included in the review, only the Lyon Diet Heart Study showed a significant reduction in the composite endpoint of CVD deaths and nonfatal MI, as well as CVD mortality, in secondary prevention patients [17, 19]. Since the publication of the 2019 Cochrane review, the results of the CORonary Diet Intervention with Olive oil and cardiovascular PREVention (CORDIOPREV) study were published. CORDIOPREV was a secondary prevention study that examined the effects of a Mediterranean dietary pattern compared to a low-fat dietary pattern in secondary prevention patients [20]. After a median follow-up of 7 years, there was a significant 25% reduction in the primary endpoint (composite of major CV events, including MI, revascularization, ischemic stroke, peripheral artery disease, and CV death). The CORDIOPREV study provided additional evidence that the Mediterranean dietary pattern reduces ASCVD risk in secondary prevention patients.

Observational evidence also supports the benefits of the Mediterranean dietary pattern on ASCVD prevention. In their umbrella review, Dinu et al. reviewed meta-analyses of observational studies that examined the association between adherence to a Mediterranean dietary pattern and ASCVD outcomes and reported that higher adherence to the Mediterranean dietary pattern was associated with statistically significant reductions of 11–33% in the incidence of CVD, CHD, MI, and stroke, as well as CVD mortality, in prospective cohort studies [16]. These results were supported by other meta-analyses of observational studies that examined associations between a Mediterranean diet score and ASCVD and found that a higher Mediterranean diet score or adherence was consistently associated with lower risks for ASCVD-related outcomes [21, 22].

There is currently no RCT evidence for the DASH or plant-based dietary patterns and ASCVD outcomes. However, evidence from RCTs has demonstrated favorable effects for both dietary patterns on ASCVD risk factors, including significant reductions in total cholesterol, low-density lipoprotein cholesterol (LDL-C), systolic and diastolic blood pressures, hemoglobin A1c (HbA1c), fasting insulin, and body weight [23–26]. The Healthy U.S.-Style dietary pattern, which is outlined in the Dietary Guidelines for Americans, has many of the same characteristics as the DASH dietary pattern [15]. The results of RCTs that have used a dietary intervention with the food components included in the Healthy U.S.-Style pattern, compared to the typical American diet, have indicated clinically meaningful impacts on CVD risk factors, such as lipoprotein lipids and blood pressures [14]. Thus, RCT evidence available on the effect of these dietary patterns on ASCVD risk factors provides a plausible biological explanation for the favorable relationships in observational studies.

The observational evidence for the DASH dietary pattern and ASCVD outcomes indicates that a higher adherence to the dietary pattern is associated with an ~20% significant decreased incident of CHD, stroke, and CVD mortality [23]. Similarly, higher adherence to a vegetarian diet (defined as vegan or lacto-ovo-vegetarian) compared to non-vegetarian diets was associated with a significant 15–30% reduced risk for CVD, ischemic heart disease, and ischemic heart disease mortality but no significant association with stroke [27, 28]. The 2020 Dietary Guidelines Advisory Committee reported that there was strong and consistent evidence that dietary patterns with the food components that are included in the Healthy U.S.-Style dietary pattern are associated with a significantly reduced risk of all-cause mortality [14].

2.2 Dietary Pattern Quality and ASCVD Outcomes

The quality of dietary patterns can affect associations with health outcomes. The quality of a dietary pattern refers to its overall healthfulness based on its food components, nutrients, and bioactive compounds and reflects that the totality of a dietary pattern likely has a greater effect on health outcomes than individual dietary components [29]. In general, dietary pattern assessment tools favorably score higher intakes of whole grains, fruits, vegetables, seafood and plant proteins, nuts, mono-unsaturated fatty acids (MUFAs), and polyunsaturated fatty acids (PUFAs), and lower intakes of processed meats, refined grains, SFAs and animal fats, sodium, and added sugars [29]. There are no RCTs available that have examined the effects of the quality of dietary patterns per se on ASCVD outcomes. However, numerous observational studies have examined the relationships between dietary pattern quality and ASCVD outcomes, including CVD incidence, CVD mortality, and all-cause mortality. The tools used to examine the relationships between dietary pattern quality and ASCVD events in observational studies include the Healthy Eating Index (HEI), the Alternative Healthy Eating Index (AHEI), the alternate Mediterranean diet (aMedDiet) score, the DASH score, and the Healthful Plant-Based Diet Index (HPDI) [29–32]. The results of several studies using data from large cohorts found that higher scores for the HEI-2015, AHEI-2010, aMedDiet, DASH, and HPDI were associated with significant reductions in CVD incidence (14–21% reduction), CVD mortality (21–34% reduction), and all-cause mortality (12–24% reduction) [30–32].

Mente et al. developed a healthy diet score based on food components that are associated with health outcomes in the Prospective Urban Rural Epidemiology (PURE) study cohort to examine the association of the PURE Healthy Diet Score with major CV events (CVD, MI, and stroke) and all-cause mortality in the PURE cohort [33]. The investigators found that a higher score, compared to a lower score, was associated with significantly lower risks for CVD (18%), MI (14%), stroke (19%), and all-cause mortality (30%). Furthermore, the PURE Healthy Diet Score had slightly stronger associations with mortality or CVD compared to the HEI, Mediterranean, DASH, and Planetary Health diet scores. While the PURE Healthy Diet Score is simpler compared to the other dietary pattern scores, it adds to the evidence base supporting the view that an eating pattern high in fruit, vegetables, nuts, legumes, fish, and dairy is associated with a reduced risk of ASCVD. Results were similar when an alternative scoring method was used that also incorporated consumption of whole grains and unprocessed meats.

Although both RCT and observational evidence for dietary patterns supports the favorable associations and effects of the recommended dietary patterns for ASCVD prevention and risk factors, RCTs with CV event endpoints are needed to strengthen the quality of the evidence for dietary recommendations. Furthermore, the beneficial associations between dietary patterns and ASCVD outcomes are generally larger than can be explained by the effects on traditional risk factors, suggesting that the mechanisms responsible are not fully understood and/or that high diet quality is also a marker for other behaviors and characteristics associated with favorable health outcomes. Despite these limitations, the totality of the evidence discussed above supports the view that the dietary patterns recommended by scientific organizations and health authorities (Fig. 1) are associated with reduced risk for ASCVD. Healthcare professionals should feel confident in recommending the Mediterranean, DASH, Healthy U.S.-Style, and healthy plant-based dietary patterns to clients and patients to promote CV health and reduce risk of ASCVD.

2.3 *Dietary Fatty Acids and ASCVD Outcomes*

There is consensus among several professional and scientific organizations that replacing foods rich in SFAs with foods rich in MUFAs and PUFAs can reduce ASCVD risk (Table 2). Both RCT and observational evidence supports this recommendation. Hooper et al. conducted a meta-analysis of 15 RCTs on the effects of reducing SFA intake compared to usual intake of SFAs on CV events [34]. The results of the meta-analysis demonstrated that reducing SFA intake was associated with reduced combined CV events by 17%, although individual CV event components, including CVD and CHD events, and all-cause mortality showed favorable trends but did not show significant differences in pooled analyses from the control conditions. The results of the Hooper et al. meta-analysis have been criticized because an unconventional definition was used for combined CV events that included types of events that do not necessarily result from ASCVD, such as heart failure and atrial fibrillation. Thus, the significant reduction in combined CV events found in the Hooper et al. meta-analysis should be interpreted with caution [35].

As part of an AHA Presidential Advisory on dietary fats and CVD, Sacks and colleagues conducted a meta-analysis of four RCTs that examined the effects of replacing SFAs with PUFAs on CHD. The results of their meta-analysis showed a 29% lower risk of CHD when SFAs were replaced with PUFAs [36]. In the Hooper et al. meta-analysis discussed above, a subgroup analysis that examined replacement of SFAs with PUFAs found a statistically significant 21% reduction for CV events but no significant effect on CVD mortality [34].

It is important to acknowledge the limitations of the RCTs that examined the effects of SFAs on ASCVD outcomes. For many of the RCTs, the sample sizes were small, and the interventions were of relatively short durations, which limited statistical power. Furthermore, in the dietary interventions that altered SFA intake, other aspects of the participants' diets were likely altered, such as reduced total fat and salt intakes; increased consumption of fruits, vegetables, and dietary fibers; and/or increased intakes of unsaturated fatty acids. Therefore, some of the CV benefits of reducing SFAs demonstrated in RCTs may be attributable to the increased intakes of the replacement foods and nutrients [35].

The results from observational studies provide support for the likely benefits of replacing SFAs with unsaturated fatty acids, primarily PUFAs. Results from modeling analyses using data from large cohort studies indicate that substitution of 5% of energy from SFAs with PUFAs was associated with a significant 25% reduction in CHD risk [37], a 9% lower risk of CHD events, and a 13% lower risk of CHD mortality [38]. Furthermore, Li et al. found that modeling replacement of SFAs with whole grain carbohydrates was associated with a significant 9% lower risk of CHD, but replacement with carbohydrates from refined starches/added sugars was associated with a non-significant increased risk of CHD risk [37]. In the AHA Presidential Advisory, Sacks et al. concluded that, based on the overall evidence, replacement of SFAs with PUFAs (primarily omega-6 PUFA, linoleic acid) reduces the risk for CHD more than MUFAs (primarily oleic acid), whereas replacement of SFAs with unspecified carbohydrates does not reduce CHD risk [36].

The reduction of SFAs and replacement with PUFAs, MUFAs, and whole grain carbohydrates should be done in conjunction with consuming an overall healthy dietary pattern (discussed above; see Fig. 1). Table 3 illustrates the recommended amount of daily SFA intake and replacement nutrients from several international scientific organizations and health authorities.

Table 3 Recommended SFA intake and replacement nutrients [5–7, 10, 13, 15]

Organization	SFAs, %TDE	Replacement macronutrient
2019 ACC/AHA Primary Prevention of CVD	Limit	MUFAs, PUFAs
2019 ESC/EAS Management of Dyslipidemias	<10%[a]	MUFAs, PUFAs
2021 Canadian Cardiovascular Society	<9%[a]	MUFAs, PUFAs, complex CHO[b]
2020–2025 Dietary Guidelines for Americans	<10%	MUFAs, PUFAs
2021 ESC Guidelines on CVD Prevention	<10%	MUFAs, PUFAs, complex CHO[b]
2022 NLA NIAD	Limit	MUFAs, PUFAs, protein

Abbreviations: *ACC* American College of Cardiology, *AHA* American Heart Association, *CHO* carbohydrates, *CVD* cardiovascular disease, *EAS* European Atherosclerosis Society, *ESC* European Society of Cardiology, *MUFAs* monounsaturated fatty acids, *NIAD* Nutrition Interventions for Adults with Dyslipidemia, *NLA* National Lipid Association, *PUFAs* polyunsaturated fatty acids, *SFAs* saturated fatty acids, *TDE* total daily energy

[a] For patients with hypercholesterolemia, the recommendation is <7% TDE
[b] Complex carbohydrates from whole grains

2.4 Added Sugar Intake and ASCVD Outcomes

Although it has been suggested that a high intake of foods and beverages with added sugars increases the risk of ASCVD, there have been no RCTs that examined the effect of reducing added sugar intake on ASCVD outcomes [39]. Results of meta-analyses of RCTs that examined the effects of added sugars on cardiometabolic risk factors have sometimes shown an increase in TG levels with higher vs. lower intakes of added sugars [39, 40]. However, the authors of another meta-analysis found that fructose consumption (alone or as a component of sucrose or sweeteners, such as corn syrup) increased TG levels only when accompanied by excess caloric intake (+21–35% energy), with no effect after isocaloric substitution for other carbohydrates [41]. The results of a third meta-analysis showed increased hepatic insulin resistance in participants without diabetes when fructose was isocalorically substituted for other carbohydrates (glucose, sucrose, starch) [42]. The findings from these meta-analyses should be interpreted with caution because the authors assessed the RCTs included as low quality [41, 42].

The most consistent association between added sugar intake and ASCVD outcomes in observational studies has been seen with sugar-sweetened beverages (SSBs). The results of meta-analyses of large cohort studies showed that the highest vs. lowest SSB consumption was associated with a significant 19% increased risk of MI [43, 44], as well as a significantly linear association between each additional serving of SSB/day and an increased risk of CVD, CHD, stroke, and CVD mortality (7–17% increases) [43, 45–47].

It is important to note that, using the Grading of Recommendations, Assessment, Development and Evaluation (GRADE) framework, the RCTs included in the meta-analyses discussed above were assessed as low-quality evidence for the CHD and MI outcomes and very-low quality for the stroke, CVD, and CVD mortality outcomes [43]. However, these results were supported by a meta-analysis of 64 prospective cohort studies that examined the potential dose–response relationship between CVD, CHD, and stroke incidence, and CVD mortality and a variety of food sources of fructose (SSBs, fruit, fruit juice, yogurt, breakfast cereals, and cakes and cookies) to determine whether all fructose-containing foods contributed to ASCVD risk [48]. The results of the dose–response analyses showed that only SSB intake was associated with a significant increased risk of incident CVD, CHD, and stroke, and CVD mortality. Conversely, fruit consumption was associated with a reduced risk of CVD incidence, and fruit, yogurt, and breakfast cereals were associated with a significantly reduced risk for CVD mortality. The authors of the meta-analysis suggested that the food matrix may modify the association between fructose and CV outcomes [48].

The totality of the evidence supports the current dietary guidance to limit the intake of added sugars overall, especially those from SSBs, for ASCVD prevention [5–7, 10, 11, 13]. This is consistent with the conclusions and recommendations from the AHA in their scientific statements on added sugars and CVD for both children and adults [49, 50]. The AHA and 2020 Dietary Guidelines Advisory

Committee emphasized that limiting foods and beverages with added sugar to <10% of total daily energy will increase the likelihood that a dietary pattern is nutritionally adequate while avoiding excess energy intake from added sugars [14, 49, 50], thus increasing the likelihood of the consumption of foods associated with improved CV health, i.e., fruits, vegetables, whole grains, nuts, seeds, and legumes.

2.5 *Alcohol Consumption and ASCVD Outcomes*

The evidence on alcohol consumption and ASCVD outcomes is primarily from observational studies. RCTs have been conducted to examine the effect of alcohol consumption on ASCVD risk biomarkers, including lipoprotein lipids, inflammatory markers, endothelial factors, and hemostatic factors. The results of meta-analyses of RCTs that examined the effects of alcohol consumption on ASCVD risk biomarkers among adults without ASCVD demonstrated that consumption of alcohol significantly increased HDL-C, apolipoprotein A-I, and adiponectin levels, and significantly decreased fibrinogen levels [51, 52]. Alcohol consumption did not materially affect levels of total cholesterol, triglycerides (TGs), lipoprotein(a), selected inflammatory markers (C-reactive protein [CRP], tumor necrosis factor-α), endothelial factors (intracellular adhesion molecule 1, vascular cellular adhesion molecule), or hemostatic factors other than fibrinogen (tissue plasminogen activator) [51, 52]. The authors of the meta-analyses found inconsistent results for LDL-C, interleukin-6 (IL-6), and plasminogen activator inhibitor 1 levels with the results of one meta-analysis finding no effect of alcohol consumption on any of these biomarkers [51], whereas the results of another found significant decreases in LDL-C and IL-6 levels and a significant increase in plasminogen activator inhibitor 1 levels [52]. The beneficial effects of alcohol on the ASCVD biomarkers provide a plausible explanation for the association between moderate alcohol consumption and reduced adverse ASCVD outcomes.

The results of single cohort studies [53, 54] and a meta-analysis of cohort studies [55] that examined the association between alcohol consumption and all-cause mortality have generally shown a J-shaped relationship when comparing non-drinkers to current drinkers, i.e., lower mortality in moderate alcohol consumers than in non-consumers and heavy consumers. In those studies, as well as in a 2018 meta-analysis that examined a dose–response association between alcohol intake and all-cause mortality in current drinkers [56], the lowest risk of all-cause mortality was associated with consumption of 1 drink/day (~14 g alcohol).

The results of prospective cohort studies examining the association between alcohol consumption and ASCVD outcomes suggest a possible benefit with lower amounts of alcohol. The results of the 2018 dose–response analysis of current drinkers demonstrated a J-shaped association with an aggregate of CVD outcomes [56]. When CVDs were disaggregated, the dose–response analysis showed that each 100 g/week increase of alcohol above a typical intake of 100 g/week was significantly associated with an increased risk for stroke, heart failure, and fatal hypertensive disease but inversely associated with MI, after adjustment for age, sex, smoking, and history of diabetes [56]. Furthermore, dose–response analyses results published in 2022 and 2023 from two large prospective cohort studies found a J-shaped relationship between alcohol consumption and incident CAD, MI, stroke [57], and CVD mortality [54] with the lowest risk associated with 1–2 drinks/day in both cohorts, after controlling for several confounding factors (education, marital status, smoking, BMI, red meat intake, vegetable intake, physical activity, and self-reported health).

The recommended alcohol intake for adults who choose to drink according to U.S. guidelines for both general health and ASCVD prevention is ≤2 drinks/day for men and ≤1 drink/day for women, which is considered moderate intake [7, 9, 15], whereas in the European guidelines for dyslipidemia management and ASCVD prevention it is ≤10 g/day (<1 drink/day) [10] or no more than 100 g/week (≤7 drinks/week) [6] for both men and women. In the U.S., one alcoholic drink equivalent is defined as containing 14 g (0.6 fluid ounces) of pure alcohol, which equates to 12 fluid ounces of regular beer (5% alcohol), 5 fluid ounces of wine (12% alcohol), or 1.5 fluid ounces of 80 proof distilled spirits (40% alcohol) [58]. The 2020–2025 Dietary Guidelines for Americans emphasized that adults may choose to abstain from alcohol but continued to recommend limiting consumption to moderate alcohol intake (≤2/day for men, ≤1/day for women) in adults who choose to drink [15]; however, the 2020 Dietary Guidelines Advisory Committee concluded that both men and women who choose to drink should consume ≤1 drink per day [14]. Based on the totality of the available evidence, individuals who are not currently drinking should not be encouraged to start, and those who do choose to drink should limit their intake to ≤1 drink/day to balance the risk of detrimental health effects with the potential ASCVD-related benefits.

3 Physical Activity Interventions and ASCVD Outcomes

There is a large body of evidence supporting beneficial effects of physical activity on various ASCVD risk factors and its association with reduced incidence of ASCVD. The current physical activity recommendations for ASCVD prevention, as well as other chronic diseases, from several international scientific organizations and health authorities are illustrated in Table 4.

Additional guidance on the frequency, intensity, time (or duration), and types of physical activity (e.g., aerobic vs. muscle-strengthening) are provided in the physical activity recommendations as follows:

- **Frequency:** Individuals should participate in aerobic endurance activity throughout the week, preferably some amount each day, and resistance training activities, at moderate- to vigorous-intensity, at least twice per week.

Table 4 Evidence-based physical activity recommendations for ASCVD risk reduction and prevention [5–7, 9, 10, 59, 60]

Counsel patients to optimize a physically active lifestyle
Participate in at least 150 min/week of accumulated moderate-intensity or 75 min/week of vigorous-intensity aerobic physical activity (or equivalent combination of both)
Engage in some moderate- or vigorous-intensity physical activity, even if not the recommended amount
Decrease sedentary behavior
Perform resistance exercise 2+ days/week to reduce all-cause mortality

Abbreviation: *ASCVD* atherosclerotic cardiovascular disease

Table 5 Examples of physical activity and corresponding metabolic equivalents [62]

Activity level	METs	Examples
Sedentary	≤1.5 METs	Sitting
Light	1.6–2.9 METs	Standing and slow walking
Moderate	3.0–6.0 METs	Walking at 4 mph, heavy cleaning, light bicycling
Vigorous	≥6.0 METs	Jogging at 6 mph, bicycling fast, carrying heavy loads

Note: MET codes use an average RMR, which poses an issue since RMR varies based on sex, weight, and age

Abbreviations: *METs* metabolic equivalents (1 MET = energy expenditure at rest in a supine position), *mph* miles per hour, *RMR* resting metabolic rate

- **Intensity:** Recommendations encourage participation in moderate- to vigorous-intensity physical activity (MVPA) for individuals without limitations. MVPA is the commonly used descriptor for exercise intensity as a higher exercise intensity requires a higher metabolic energy demand [61]. Researchers often use MVPA as the parameter for exercise intensity regardless of the exercise modality (e.g., walking, biking, swimming). MVPA is translated into metabolic equivalents (METs) as illustrated in Table 5.
- **Time (duration):** There is consensus across the guidelines that individuals should accomplish 150–300 min/week of moderate-intensity aerobic activity, 75 min/week of vigorous-intensity aerobic activity, or a combination of both, to increase the likelihood of achieving the most health benefits. However, recommendations also emphasize the importance of replacing sedentary time with physical activity of any intensity and that any amount of physical activity is better than none.
- **Type:** Physical activity guidelines recommend a combination of aerobic and resistance training activity due to the health benefits provided by each. Additionally, there are recommendations for specific populations, such as balance training for older adults to prevent falls [59, 60].

3.1   Evidence for the Effects of Physical Activity on ASCVD Outcomes

There are no RCTs that have examined the impact of physical activity on ASCVD outcomes; however, RCTs have investigated the effects of physical activity on various ASCVD risk factors. The results of these studies consistently support beneficial effects of both aerobic and resistance training on improving lipoprotein lipids [63, 64], blood pressure [65–67], and on glycemic control in individuals with prediabetes and/or type 2 diabetes (T2D) [68, 69]. More recently, researchers have examined the effects of physical activity on coronary plaque changes, which is evolving as a surrogate marker of underlying processes that result in ASCVD events [70]. The results of RCTs that examined the effect of physical activity on coronary plaque demonstrated reduced plaque volume in patients with acute coronary syndrome participating in cardiac rehabilitation programs [71], especially those achieving ≥7000 steps/day [72], and patients with stable CAD who participated in high-intensity interval training [73]. The evidence from RCTs on the beneficial effects of physical activity on ASCVD risk factors provides biologic plausibility for the results found in observational studies.

The results of cohort studies that have examined the association between physical activity measured using accelerometry and incident CVD have shown a significantly reduced risk of CVD when the minimum 150 min/week of aerobic activity was achieved [74–76], particularly when it resulted in reduced sedentary time [76], and even if the activity was isolated to weekend days [77]. Additionally, the results of observational studies support a positive association between achieving the recommended amount of physical activity and ASCVD incidence and mortality [78–80]. This favorable association was observed regardless of age [81, 82], sex [82, 83], or family history of CVD [84].

The results of observational studies included in a systematic review conducted to inform the 2018 Physical Activity Guidelines Advisory Committee suggested that any time spent participating in MVPA is associated with improved ASCVD outcomes, but rapid and significant health gains are achieved when individuals transition from inactivity to even small amounts of physical activity [78]. Increasing physical activity from no activity to the minimum recommended amount of physical activity (150 min/week) was associated with a significant reduction in CVD incidence and mortality; however, the greatest reduction in risk occurred when activity increased from zero to ~45 min/week with continued benefit as the number of minutes of MVPA/week increased [78]. These results support the view that achieving the minimum recommended amount of aerobic physical activity (≥150 min/week of MVPA) is an appropriate goal for reducing the risk of ASCVD, although being active ≤150 min/week provides benefit, and participating in MVPA ≥300 min/week may provide additional benefit [78].

The findings from other observational studies that examined the frequency and intensity of physical activity provide further evidence to support a beneficial association with ASCVD outcomes. Participating in either moderate- or vigorous-intensity activity at least once per week was associated with a significantly reduced risk for CVD and stroke with the magnitude of the associations increasing with higher frequencies for both moderate- and vigorous-intensity physical activity. Conversely, there was no significant association between participating in either moderate- or vigorous-intensity physical activity only one to three times/month and CVD or stroke incidence [85]. However, the results of other studies suggested that participating in higher intensity physical activity (i.e., MVPA) is associated with the most benefit for reducing CVD incident and mortality [78, 83].

Banach et al. published a systematic review and meta-analysis of 17 cohort studies and demonstrated a significant inverse association between daily step count and all-cause mortality and CV mortality [86]. Every 1000-step increment was associated with a 15% decreased risk of all-cause mortality and a 500-step increment was associated with 7% decrease of CV mortality [86]. Although these studies have examined accelerometer-measured steps/day, favorable associations between physical activity and incident CVD and CVD mortality have been found with multiple types of exercise, including walking, running, cycling, and resistance exercise [78, 87].

The totality of the evidence available for the relationship between physical activity and ASCVD supports the recommendations from several scientific organizations and health authorities outlined in Table 4. The evidence from RCTs supports the biologic plausibility for the benefits of physical activity. The evidence from observational studies consistently shows that any amount or type of physical activity is associated with reductions in CVD incidence and mortality, and that higher amounts of physical activity generally confer greater benefits, which supports a dose–response effect. Therefore, healthcare professionals should encourage and support patients in their efforts to strive toward achieving the physical activity recommendations for ASCVD risk reduction and prevention.

4 Body Weight, Adiposity, and ASCVD Outcomes

Excess body weight is considered a risk factor for a variety of health concerns, including ASCVD. Body mass index (BMI) was developed as a quick and easy way to measure relative weight that correlated with many indicators of health and disease. BMI is a measure of body weight adjusted for height and, although it is often considered an indicator of obesity or adiposity, it measures excess weight rather than excess fat [88]. Although BMI is widely used as a measure of obesity status, particularly for its convenience and ease of use in epidemiologic research and clinical settings, it does not come without controversy. An example is the obesity paradox in which individuals classified as overweight based on BMI have a better prognosis for some health outcomes compared to individuals classified as underweight or normal weight. Although overweight and obesity have been associated with a significantly increased risk of developing CVD compared with a normal BMI [89], the results of meta-analyses of observational studies demonstrate that the relationship between BMI and all-cause mortality is "U-shaped," with the lowest mortality rate observed at a mildly overweight BMI [90]. The authors of another meta-analysis of 27 prospective studies found that, compared with participants with normal weight (BMI 18.5–24.9 kg/m^2), participants with overweight (BMI 25–29.9 kg/m^2) and obesity (BMI ≥30 kg/m^2) had an associated significant 14–15% lower risk of post-MI mortality, while there was no difference with participants with severe obesity (BMI ≥35 kg/m^2) and an associated 42% increased risk for participants who were underweight (BMI <18.5 kg/m^2) [91]. Additionally, compared to a normal BMI, a higher BMI has been associated with lower mortality in patients with CAD, including following percutaneous coronary intervention and acute coronary syndrome [92]. However, very high BMIs have been associated with an increased risk of CVD mortality. In the Aerobics Center Longitudinal Study cohort, compared to a medium BMI (15th–85th percentile), a high (85th–95th percentile), and very high BMI (>95th percentile) were associated with a 1.8- and 2.7-fold increased risk of CVD mortality, respectively [93]. The results of other prospective cohort studies that examined the association between BMI and CVD found that, compared to individuals with overweight, increasing severity of obesity was associated with an increased incidence of CVD, as well as CVD and all-cause mortality [94, 95].

Weight loss in the presence of excess adiposity is recommended to reduce ASCVD risk; however, there is a paucity of evidence that shows that weight loss achieved through lifestyle interventions results in a decrease in the incidence of ASCVD. Researchers have conducted RCTs that examined the effects of intensive lifestyle interventions (ILI) to reduce body weight on CVD or T2D risk, which demonstrated improvements in all cardiometabolic risk factors (i.e., LDL-C, TGs, HDL-C, systolic blood pressure, and HbA1c) [96–98]. These improvements did not result in a reduced risk of ASCVD. In two large lifestyle intervention trials, the Diabetes Prevention Program (DPP), which examined the effects of weight loss on T2D incidence in people at high risk of developing T2D [96], and the Look AHEAD trial, which examined the effects of weight loss on CV outcomes in people with T2D [97], the participants in the ILI group in both studies successfully lost an average of 6% body weight by study end. Although there was a significant reduction in T2D incidence in the ILI group in the DPP study, and improvement in cardiometabolic risk factors in the ILI participants in both the DPP and Look AHEAD studies, compared to the placebo groups, no significant reductions were observed for major adverse CV events (MACE), heart failure, CV mortality, or all-cause mortality in ILI participants in either study [97, 99, 100]. Furthermore, Ma et al. conducted a systematic review and meta-analysis of RCTs to examine the effects of ILI on weight loss, CV events, and mortality and found no significant reductions in MACE and CV mortality, although all-cause mortality was reduced by 18% [101]. The results of these studies suggest that, although lifestyle interventions produce modest weight loss (3–8%) that contributes to improved ASCVD risk factors, the weight loss achieved does not appear to have been sufficient to reduce the risk of ASCVD events. In contrast, bariatric surgery, which reduces body weight by 20–30%, is associated with marked reductions in ASCVD risk in observational studies [100]. Additionally, the results of studies using glucagon-like peptide 1 (GLP-1) receptor agonists (e.g., semaglutide) with a background ILI demonstrated a 15–20% weight loss and significantly reduced ASCVD risk in patients with T2D [100]. The results of the Semaglutide Effects on Cardiovascular Outcomes in People With Overweight or Obesity (SELECT) trial showed 20% lower MACE risk in patients with overweight or obesity and established CVD given 2.4 mg/week semaglutide, the dosage used for weight loss [102]. This dosage in combination with ILI has been associated with a reduction of ~15% in body weight. The degree to which the reduced risk of CV events with GLP-1 receptor agonists and bariatric surgery has been due to weight loss per se vs. other effects has been unclear [100]. A more detailed discussion of the ASCVD risk reduction with obesity management through lifestyle, pharmacotherapy, and surgical interventions is available in the chapter entitled, "Pharmacotherapy for Obesity: Recent Evolution and Implications for Cardiovascular Risk Reduction."

The association between body weight, BMI, and ASCVD may be more complex than a simple overall assessment of adiposity (i.e., weight or BMI), and the location of adipose tissue in the body may be an important determinant of ASCVD risk. Subcutaneous adipose tissue (SAT) is typically beneath the skin and located in the abdominal and gluteo-femoral areas, as well as the back [103]. Abdominal adipose tissue is comprised of both SAT and intra-abdominal adipose tissue, which is also called visceral adipose tissue (VAT). VAT surrounds such tissues as the liver, heart, skeletal muscle, and the mesentery and omentum [103, 104]. The adipocytes in SAT, abdominal SAT, and VAT have physiologic and metabolic differences that contribute to differences in ASCVD risk. The adipocytes in both abdominal SAT and VAT synthesize and secrete adipokines that perpetuate a chronic inflammatory state, have receptors for various endocrine hormones, and contribute to abnormal lipoprotein lipid metabolism [103, 104]. Adipocytes in VAT are larger than those in SAT, which contributes to metabolic dysfunction and increased ASCVD risk compared to SAT. VAT has a high uptake of free-fatty acids (FFAs) from TGs, as well as a high rate of lipolysis, which results in a high flux of FFAs being drained into the portal circulation directly from the VAT. The increase in hepatic exposure to FFAs contributes to an increased production of apolipoprotein B-containing lipoproteins. The result is increased very-low-density lipoprotein-TG levels [103, 104]. In addition, chronically elevated exposure of hepatic and skeletal muscle tissue to FFAs produces insulin resistance in those tissues [103, 104]. Abdominal SAT also has a high uptake of TGs and increased release of FFAs compared to SAT located in the gluteo-femoral area, albeit less than that of VAT per kg of adipose [104]. Thus, excess abdominal SAT can also promote elevated very-low-density lipoprotein-TG levels and insulin resistance.

Researchers have examined the associations between the distribution of excess adiposity and ASCVD risk factors and found that both VAT and abdominal SAT were associated with increased total cholesterol, TG, and glycemia levels, increased systolic and diastolic blood pressures, low HDL-C levels, and insulin resistance [105–109].

Neither body weight nor BMI differentiate adipose tissue location; therefore, neither detect whether individuals have a high amount VAT or abdominal SAT, which would contribute to potentially harmful metabolic consequences. Additionally, neither body weight changes nor BMI distinguish whether weight changes are due to gains in lean body mass or fat mass; therefore, neither differentiate between the effect of lean body mass gains and the harmful effect of fat mass gains, especially increased VAT mass. Therefore, some researchers and medical organizations, including the American Medical Association, recommend against using BMI alone as an assessment for a healthy weight and acknowledge that alternative measures of adiposity, such as waist circumference (WC) or waist-to-hip ratio (WHR), may be better indicators for ASCVD risk [92, 110]. Quantification of abdominal fat using dual energy x-ray absorptiometry can also be helpful for assessing the degree of abdominal adiposity [107–109].

In an ancillary study of the Look AHEAD trial, weight change and WC were strongly correlated with changes in total adipose tissue, VAT, and SAT volumes or areas [111]. Additionally, the results of a meta-analysis of 18 cohort studies from the Obesity in Asia Collaboration showed that higher values for WC and WHR, as well as BMI and waist-height ratio, were similarly and significantly associated with a higher likelihood of abnormal lipid and lipoprotein levels, particularly elevated TGs and reduced HDL-C, in both men and women of Asian and non-Asian decent [112].

Both an elevated WC and WHR have been consistently associated with CVD and all-cause mortality, especially in the presence of T2D [113], and even in the presence of a normal BMI [114] and after adjusting for total body fat [115]. An increased WC remained significantly associated with all-cause mortality after adjustment for selected lifestyle factors (e.g., smoking, alcohol intake, participation in sports). Additionally, adjustment for WC attenuated the association between a BMI >25 kg/m^2, but a BMI <25 kg/m^2 remained significantly associated with all-cause mortality [116]. Furthermore, the results of a systematic review and meta-analysis of 12 case-control studies found that an elevated WHR was significantly associated with an increased risk of MI and was a stronger predictor in women compared to men [117].

The results of the studies discussed above suggest that WC and WHR, which are surrogate markers of abdominal adiposity, are stronger predictors of ASCVD risk and outcomes compared to body weight and BMI. Barriers need to be overcome for healthcare professionals to universally accept that WC or WHR are better indicators for ASCVD risk than BMI and, therefore, implement measuring both in clinical practice. Additionally, thresholds are needed for BMI, WC, and WHR that identify increased risk by sex and ethnicity. Although BMI is useful for an initial screening for many patients, the International Atherosclerosis Society and International Chair on Cardiometabolic Risk Working Group on Visceral Obesity released a consensus statement with the recommendation that measurement of WC be used to augment BMI measures in clinical settings given BMI alone is not sufficient to assess cardio-metabolic risk in some patients [118].

The available evidence for the relationship between body weight, adiposity, and ASCVD outcomes suggests that obesity, especially in the presence of excess abdominal fat, is associated with an increased risk of ASCVD events and mortality

[113, 114, 117]. Although BMI is a useful tool to use in the clinical setting as the initial step in body weight assessment, healthcare professionals should include WC measurement as part of their assessment to better assess the cardiometabolic risk of patients with increased BMI. Furthermore, healthcare professionals should facilitate evidence-based strategies, including ILI, pharmacotherapy, and bariatric surgery when indicated, to reduce excess adiposity in patients with obesity to reduce the risk of ASCVD.

5 Sleep Hygiene and ASCVD Outcomes

It is becoming increasingly evident that adequate sleep is important for both CV health and general health. Sleep impacts health and the potential for disease in multiple ways, and untreated sleep disorders can negatively affect mental health and mood, as well as physical health, including ASCVD risk [119, 120]. Despite the importance of quality sleep for several health outcomes, poor sleep is a concern for many individuals with up to 18% of U.S. adults reporting difficulty falling asleep or staying asleep most days or every day in the past 30 days [121], ~35% are categorized as short sleepers (<7 h), ~20% report excessive daytime sleepiness, and <50% report having a good night of sleep every night [122]. Based on the evidence on the potential influence of sleep patterns on ASCVD risk and that incorporation of sleep as a CV health metric predicts CVD risk [122], the AHA added sleep health to its Life's Simple 7 CV metric, which is now Life's Essential 8 [12]. Although evidence for the effect of adequate sleep on CV health is increasing [12], more research is needed, especially RCTs, to understand how the various mechanisms of sleep impact ASCVD risk. However, research on how sleep impacts ASCVD is difficult given that it is intertwined with other lifestyle factors, such as nutrition, physical activity, body weight, and various chronic diseases [120].

The primary focus of the available research base on sleep and ASCVD risk has been examination of the influence of sleep duration. The American Academy of Sleep Medicine, the Sleep Research Society, and the National Sleep Foundation recommend that adults should strive to achieve between 7 and 9 h of sleep per night for optimal health [120]. This recommendation is supported by results of observational evidence that suggested a J-shaped curve association between sleep duration and CVD and stroke. Each 1 h of sleep less than or more than 7 h each night was associated with a significant 7–11% increased risk of CVD and 12–13% increased risk for fatal and nonfatal stroke [123–125]. The results of Mendelian randomization studies suggested that genetically predicted short sleep duration (<7 h/day) was associated with a significant 20–24% increased risk of CAD and MI, but not stroke; however, genetically predicted long sleep duration (>7 h/day) was not significantly associated with any CVDs [125]. Additionally, a systematic review of seven small studies (4 RCTs, 1 nonrandomized crossover trial, 2 observational studies) that examined the effect of interventions to extend sleep duration on cardiometabolic risk factors reported that increasing sleep duration (between 21 and 177 min) was associated with an improved risk factor profile [126].

Irregular sleep patterns (variability in day-to-day duration or timing) may also be associated with an increased risk of CVD. The pooled analysis results from a systematic review and meta-analysis of 21 observational studies (15 cohort studies, 7 case-control studies; $N = 362,591$) suggested that shift work exposure (i.e., permanent night shift or rotational shift, or a combination of terms indicating shift work hours differ from standard work hours) was associated with a 17% increased risk of any CVD event; however, in subgroup analyses, there was only a significant association between shift work exposure and CHD morbidity and no significant association for other CVD morbidity or CVD mortality [127]. Huang et al. examined the association between sleep regularity, a marker for chronic circadian disruption and intermittent sleep deprivation, with incident CVD events in 1992 participants without CVD from the Multi-Ethnic Study of Atherosclerosis (MESA) cohort who were invited to participate in the MESA Sleep Ancillary Study [128]. The study results showed that the most irregular sleep duration or timing was associated with a >2-fold risk of developing CVD over a median follow-up of 4.9 years compared with the most regular sleep patterns [128]. Additionally, self-reported poor sleep quality has been associated with CHD, but not mortality [124].

The currently available evidence suggests that the recommended 7–9 h of habitual sleep per night for adults is associated with a reduced risk of ASCVD. However, more research is needed to understand the possible connection between irregular sleep patterns and sleep disturbances with poor CV health, as well as to understand the J-shaped association for sleep duration and ASCVD to identify factors that may contribute to the relationship between sleep duration less than or greater than 7–9 h/ night and suboptimal CV health [6].

6 Psychosocial Health, Stress, and ASCVD Outcomes

Similar to sleep health, it is increasingly recognized that psychological health and well-being can both positively and negatively impact CV health and ASCVD outcomes, as well as health in general [12]. Stressors that people experience, such as life events, chronic daily stressors, challenges related to work, financial hardships, discrimination, and lack of social support, as well as traumatic stress, can impact psychological health and well-being [129]. The World Health Organization (WHO) defined *mental health* as "a state of *wellbeing* in which an individual realizes his or her own potential, can cope with the normal stresses of life, can work productively and fruitfully, and is able to make a contribution to her or his community" [130]. The WHO recognized that a variety of individual factors (e.g., genetics, emotional skills, and substance use) and circumstances (e.g., unfavorable social, economic, geopolitical and environmental situations, including poverty, violence, and inequality) increase a person's risk of experiencing mental health conditions, which can negatively impact health [130]. In a scientific statement that examined the relationship between psychological health and CVD, the AHA described *well-being* as a quantifiable state of being that comprises the "cognitive and affective evaluation and assessment of one's life, including physical health, satisfaction, happiness, and a sense of fulfillment," and encompasses the "valuations people make about their lives, including their physical and mental health, their financial position, their social supports and connectedness to community, their opportunities for growth and ability to achieve their goals, and a general sense of purpose and satisfaction with their life course" [129].

Given the relationship between psychological health and CV health, researchers have examined the potential impact of chronic stress on ASCVD risk factors. Meng and colleagues conducted a systematic review to examine the influence of chronic stress on risk factors that contribute to the development of atherosclerosis and proposed biological mechanisms by which chronic stress exacerbates atherosclerosis, such as the presence of low-grade inflammation triggering endothelial dysfunction, plaque instability, dyslipidemia, and hypertension, with ferroptosis, autophagy, and cholesterol efflux presenting as aggravating factors [131]. Hinterdobler et al. extended this hypothesis in a narrative review and discussed the implications of the proinflammatory potential of stress on both the innate and adaptive immune systems [132]. They connected the impact of both chronic and acute stress on release and maintenance of higher levels of clinical inflammatory markers, such as CRP, IL-6, and tumor necrosis factor α. Hinterdobler et al. suggested that systemic inflammation, triggered by both acute and chronic stress, is linked to vascular inflammation and, thereby, the increased risk of ASCVD [132]. Additionally, Sher et al. emphasized the complexity of stress and related mental health conditions and recommended a more precise model of the elements of chronic stress, as well as standardization of criteria to better tease apart mechanisms underpinning the relationship to ASCVD [133].

In preparation for the AHA Scientific Statement on psychological health and CVD mentioned above, Levine et al. conducted a systematic review to identify the available evidence on the relationship between both negative psychological factors (e.g., chronic stress and social stressors, anger and hostility, anxiety, and depression and pessimism) and positive psychological factors (e.g., optimism, sense of purpose, happiness and positive affect, and mindfulness) and CV health. The majority of the evidence was observational studies with self-reported data. Despite these limitations, Levine et al. reported that the available evidence supported associations between poor psychological functioning, psychological stress, trauma, anger and hostility, mental health disorders, and CV health. They also stated that most, but not all, studies were largely consistent and strongly suggestive of positive psychological attributes being independent risk factors for CV health [129]. The European Society for Cardiology Guidelines on CVD Prevention also highlight the association between a number of factors related to mental health and a lower risk of ASCVD and emphasized both biological and environmental factors, e.g., socioeconomic status and smoking, as mediators for these associations [6].

Since the publication of the AHA Scientific Statement on psychological health and CVD, additional studies have been published that examined the relationship between psychological health and CV health. Barger and Struve conducted a cross-sectional analysis of data from the 2005–2018 National Health and Nutrition Examination Survey (NHANES) to examine the association between mild and major depression and 10-year ASCVD risk in participants aged 40–79 years and lifetime ASCVD risk in participants aged 20–39 years (who are not eligible for the 10-year ASCVD risk assessment) [134]. The researchers found a significantly higher 10-year ASCVD risk score in persons aged 40–79 years with mild (6.9%) and major (7.6%) depression compared with those with no depression (6%). They also reported a significantly higher lifetime CVD risk prevalence for women aged 20–39 years with mild (53.2%) and major depression (66.5%) compared to those with no depression (41.9%) with a similar increased prevalence in men aged 20–39 years with mild (64.8%) and major (74.4%) depression compared with those without depression (53.3%) [134]. Additionally, a higher level of perceived stress, measured by the Cumulative Stress Score, which measures generalized, psychosocial, financial, and neighborhood stressors, was associated with an increased BMI, WC, systolic and diastolic blood pressures, HbA1c, and hs-CRP, as well as an increased risk of ASCVD and global CVD (ASCVD, heart failure, and atrial fibrillation) among participants without CVD in the Dallas Heart Study [135]. The results of these studies suggest that both depression and perceived stress are modifiable ASCVD risk factors. Furthermore, psychosocial factors contribute to perceived stress and can negatively impact CV health and ASCVD risk [135, 136].

The results of large cohort studies suggest that, in a healthy population, stress during adulthood has a modest role in the etiology of ASCVD, but adulthood stress is a powerful risk factor for prognosis and outcomes in those with pre-existing CVDs, including stroke. Researchers have recommended that the role of stress in disease progression be the emphasis of future studies, as well as in the development of ASCVD prevention and treatment strategies [137]. In contemporary ASCVD prevention guidelines, scientific organizations and health authorities recognize that stress symptoms and psychosocial stressors modify CVD risk and recommend screening of ASCVD patients for high levels of stress and other mental health concerns [6, 12, 129]. Furthermore, ASCVD prevention guidelines and scientific statements on CV health include recommendations to refer patients with ASCVD who are experiencing stress to stress management programs, including psychotherapy, positive psychology-based programs, and meditation, as well as medical interventions, such as antidepressants to reduce stress symptoms and improve ASCVD outcomes [6, 129]. However, scientific organizations and researchers also caution that more research is needed with higher quality studies, larger sample sizes, and a wider array of biomarker measures in order to ensure direct benefit with the reduction of ASCVD morbidity and mortality. In the AHA Scientific Statement on psychological health and CV health, Levine et al. acknowledged the need for improved methodological tools and consensus on the best tools for assessing positive psychological attributes of interest and measurement of change over time [129]. Because of the limitations with the current evidence, the AHA Presidential Advisory Committee for Life's Essential 8 highlighted the importance of psychological health and well-being, but did not include psychological health and well-being in the updated CV metric because the best methods to represent, measure, and quantify psychological health and well-being have not yet been developed, and the most important factors for improving or optimizing CV health have yet to be identified [12]. Despite these limitations, psychological health is now considered a contributing factor to ASCVD risk and healthcare professionals are encouraged to screen patients for excessive perceived stress and mental health concerns, and refer those who would benefit from stress management interventions to improve CV health and prevent ASCVD.

7 Tobacco Use and Cessation and ASCVD Outcomes

In 2019, tobacco use, including smoking, secondhand smoke, and chewing tobacco, was a leading risk factor globally for attributable deaths, only second to elevated blood pressure [138]. Smoking is considered a major risk factor for ASCVD [4–7, 10] and contributes to atherosclerosis through various mechanisms (Fig. 2). Secondhand smoke also contributes to an increased risk for ASCVD [6, 7, 12].

Evidence from both RCTs and observational studies suggests that smoking cessation can reduce the risk of ASCVD morbidity and mortality, including in secondary prevention patients [140]. In RCTs, intensive smoking cessation programs in patients with CVD [141] or airway obstruction [142] contributed to significantly increased rates of long-term abstinence from smoking and a significantly reduced rate of hospitalization from CVD and all-cause mortality compared to usual care participants [141, 142].

The observational evidence supports the benefits of smoking cessation on ASCVD outcomes. A systematic review and meta-analysis examined the impact of smoking cessation on death from CVD, MACE, nonfatal MI, nonfatal stroke, and

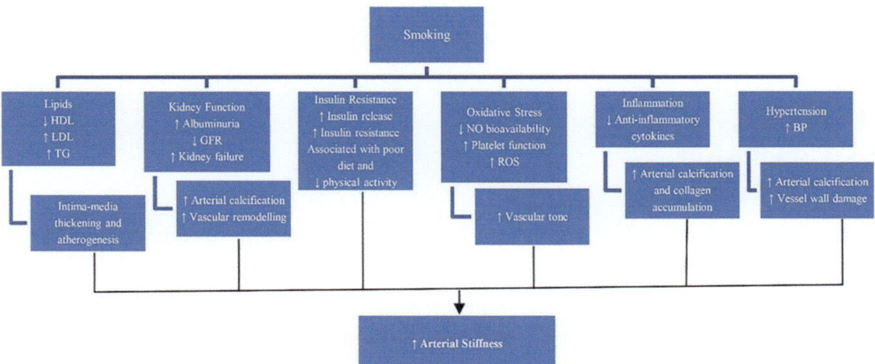

Fig. 2 Potential mechanisms of smoking-induced atherosclerosis [139]. **Note:** Permission to use this figure was obtained from the author of the original article and the editor of the publishing journal, *Journal of Lifestyle Medicine*. **Abbreviations:** *BP* blood pressure, *GFR* glomerular filtration rate, *HDL* high-density lipoprotein, *LDL* low-density lipoprotein, *NO* nitric oxide, *ROS* reactive oxygen species, *TG* triglycerides

Table 6 Recommendations for addressing tobacco use/smoking for ASCVD risk reduction and prevention [6, 7, 12]

All adults should be assessed at every healthcare visit for tobacco use and their tobacco use status recorded as a vital sign to facilitate tobacco cessation
In adults who use tobacco, tobacco cessation is recommended to reduce ASCVD risk
To achieve tobacco cessation, all adults who use tobacco should be firmly advised to quit
In adults who use tobacco, a combination of behavioral interventions plus appropriate pharmacotherapy (e.g., nicotine replacement therapy, varenicline, and bupropion) that is provided by a trained healthcare team is recommended to increase the likelihood of successful cessation
All adults and adolescents should avoid secondhand smoke exposure to reduce ASCVD risk
Smoking cessation is recommended regardless of weight gain, as weight gain does not reduce the ASCVD benefits of cessation
Federal and state regulation of tobacco products and implementation of strategies for tobacco cessation is recommended to reduce the likelihood of tobacco use and to increase the likelihood of successful cessation

all-cause mortality in people with CHD [140]. Based on meta-analyses of the results from 68 prospective cohort studies ($N = 80{,}702$), smoking cessation was associated with a significant reduction in CVD death, MACE, nonfatal MI, and stroke, as well as all-cause mortality in patients with CHD who stopped smoking compared to those who continued to smoke [140]. These results are consistent with a previous systematic review and meta-analysis of 20 prospective cohort studies that found a significant reduction in repeat MI and all-cause mortality in participants with CHD who quit smoking compared to those who continued to smoke [143].

Based on the evidence from RCTs and observational studies, all of the ASCVD prevention guidelines, as well as the guidelines for dyslipidemia management, recommend smoking cessation for the primary prevention of ASCVD and to reduce future risk in secondary prevention patients [4–7, 9, 10, 12]. Table 6 illustrates treatment recommendations and strategies for addressing tobacco use and smoking cessation.

8 Conclusion

A healthy lifestyle across the lifespan is the foundation for the prevention of ASCVD. Although international scientific organizations and health authorities recommend lifestyle interventions to promote CV health and reduce the risk of ASCVD, there is limited RCT evidence for the effects of lifestyle interventions on CV outcomes. There is a large body of evidence from RCTs that demonstrates improved ASCVD risk markers, such as lipids and lipoproteins, glucose, and blood pressures, with the lifestyle interventions discussed in this chapter. Results from observational studies support associations between the recommended health behaviors (e.g., healthy dietary pattern, physical activity, adequate sleep quantity and quality, and abstinence from tobacco) and metrics (body weight/adiposity, blood pressure, lipoprotein lipids, glycemia) and favorable CV outcomes. Thus, the totality of the evidence for the relationship between lifestyle interventions and ASCVD outcomes discussed in this chapter supports the following lifestyle intervention recommendations to reduce the risk of ASCVD: (1) consuming a high-quality dietary pattern, such as the Mediterranean, DASH, or plant-based patterns; (2) limiting the intake of SFAs and replacement with unsaturated fatty acids; (3) limiting the intake of foods and beverages with added sugars; (4) abstaining from alcohol for those who do not currently drink and limiting alcohol intake to ≤1 drink/day for men and women who choose to drink; (5) participating in recommended levels of physical activity; (6) reducing excess adiposity and waist circumference; (7) maintaining healthy sleep habits; (8) managing stressors to improve psychological health; and (9) abstaining from tobacco use, including cessation for those who currently use tobacco.

References

1. World Health Organization. Cardiovascular diseases (CVDs) [Internet]. World Health Organization; 2023. [Updated 2021, June 11; Cited 2023, July 5]. https://www.who.int/news-room/fact-sheets/detail/cardiovascular-diseases-(cvds).
2. Kwak BR, Bäck M, Bochaton-Piallat ML, Caligiuri G, Daemen MJ, Davies PF, et al. Biomechanical factors in atherosclerosis: mechanisms and clinical implications. Eur Heart J. 2014;35(43):3013–20, 3020a–20d. https://doi.org/10.1093/eurheartj/ehu353.
3. American Heart Association. Atherosclerotic cardiovascular disease (ASCVD) [Internet]. Dallas: American Heart Association; 2023. [Cited 2023, July 5]. https://www.heart.org/en/professional/quality-improvement/ascvd.
4. Grundy SM, Stone NJ, Bailey AL, Beam C, Birtcher KK, Blumenthal RS, et al. 2018 AHA/ACC/AACVPR/AAPA/ABC/ACPM/ADA/AGS/APhA/ASPC/NLA/PCNA guideline on the management of blood cholesterol: a report of the American College of Cardiology/American Heart Association Task Force on clinical practice guidelines. J Am Coll Cardiol. 2019;73(24):e285–350. https://doi.org/10.1016/j.jacc.2018.11.003. Erratum in: J Am Coll Cardiol. 2019;73(24):3237–41.
5. Pearson GJ, Thanassoulis G, Anderson TJ, Barry AR, Couture P, Dayan N, et al. 2021 Canadian cardiovascular society guidelines for the management of dyslipidemia for the prevention of cardiovascular disease in adults. Can J Cardiol. 2021;37(8):1129–50. https://doi.org/10.1016/j.cjca.2021.03.016.
6. Visseren FLJ, Mach F, Smulders YM, Carballo D, Koskinas KC, Bäck M, et al. 2021 ESC guidelines on cardiovascular disease prevention in clinical practice. Eur Heart J. 2021;42(34):3227–37. https://doi.org/10.1093/eurheartj/ehab484.
7. Arnett DK, Blumenthal RS, Albert MA, Buroker AB, Goldberger ZD, Hahn EJ, et al. 2019 ACC/AHA guideline on the primary prevention of cardiovascular disease: a report of the American College of Cardiology/American Heart Association Task Force on clinical practice guidelines. Circulation. 2019;140(11):e596–646. https://doi.org/10.1161/CIR.0000000000000678. Erratum in: Circulation. 2019;140(11):e649–50. Erratum in: Circulation. 2020;141(4):e60. Erratum in: Circulation. 2020;141(16):e774.
8. American College of Cardiology, American Heart Association. ASCVD risk estimator [Internet]. [Cited 2023, July 5]. https://tools.acc.org/LDL/ascvd_risk_estimator/index.html#!/calulate/estimator/.

9. Whelton PK, Carey RM, Aronow WS, Casey DE Jr, Collins KJ, Himmelfarb CD, et al. 2017 ACC/AHA/AAPA/ABC/ACPM/AGS/APhA/ASH/ASPC/NMA/PCNA guideline for the prevention, detection, evaluation, and management of high blood pressure in adults: a report of the American College of Cardiology/American Heart Association Task Force on clinical practice guidelines. J Am Coll Cardiol. 2018;71(19):e127–248. https://doi.org/10.1016/j.jacc.2017.11.006. Erratum in: J Am Coll Cardiol. 2018;71(19):2275–79.

10. Mach F, Baigent C, Catapano AL, Koskinas KC, Casula M, Badimon L, et al. 2019 ESC/EAS guidelines for the management of dyslipidaemias: lipid modification to reduce cardiovascular risk. Eur Heart J. 2020;41(1):111–88. https://doi.org/10.1093/eurheartj/ehz455. Erratum in: Eur Heart J. 2020;41(44):4255.

11. Lichtenstein AH, Appel LJ, Vadiveloo M, Hu FB, Kris-Etherton PM, Rebholz CM, et al. 2021 dietary guidance to improve cardiovascular health: a scientific statement from the American Heart Association. Circulation. 2021;2:CIR0000000000001031. https://doi.org/10.1161/CIR.0000000000001031.

12. Lloyd-Jones DM, Allen NB, Anderson CAM, Black T, Brewer LC, Foraker RE, et al. Life's Essential 8: updating and enhancing the American Heart Association's construct of cardiovascular health: a presidential advisory from the American Heart Association. Circulation. 2022;146(5):e18–43. https://doi.org/10.1161/CIR.0000000000001078.

13. Kirkpatrick CF, Sikand G, Petersen KS, Anderson CAM, Aspry KE, Bolick JP, et al. Nutrition interventions for adults with dyslipidemia: a clinical perspective from the National Lipid Association. J Clin Lipidol. 2023;17(4):428–51. S1933-2874(23)00185-X. https://doi.org/10.1016/j.jacl.2023.05.099.

14. Dietary Guidelines Advisory Committee. Scientific report of the 2020 dietary guidelines advisory committee: advisory report to the secretary of agriculture and the secretary of health and human services. Washington, DC: U.S. Department of Agriculture, Agricultural Research Service; 2020.

15. U.S. Department of Agriculture and U.S. Department of Health and Human Services. Dietary guidelines for Americans, 2020–2025. 9th ed. December 2020. DietaryGuidelines.gov.

16. Dinu M, Pagliai G, Casini A, Sofi F. Mediterranean diet and multiple health outcomes: an umbrella review of meta-analyses of observational studies and randomised trials. Eur J Clin Nutr. 2018;72(1):30–43. https://doi.org/10.1038/ejcn.2017.58.

17. Rees K, Takeda A, Martin N, Ellis L, Wijesekara D, Vepa A, et al. Mediterranean-style diet for the primary and secondary prevention of cardiovascular disease. Cochrane Database Syst Rev. 2019;3(3):CD009825. https://doi.org/10.1002/14651858.CD009825.pub3.

18. Estruch R, Ros E, Salas-Salvadó J, Covas MI, Corella D, Arós F, et al. Primary prevention of cardiovascular disease with a Mediterranean diet supplemented with extra-virgin olive oil or nuts. N Engl J Med. 2018;378(25):e34. https://doi.org/10.1056/NEJMoa1800389.

19. de Lorgeril M, Renaud S, Mamelle N, Salen P, Martin JL, Monjaud I, et al. Mediterranean alpha-linolenic acid-rich diet in secondary prevention of coronary heart disease. Lancet. 1994;343(8911):1454–9. https://doi.org/10.1016/s0140-6736(94)92580-1. Erratum in: Lancet. 1995;345(8951):738.

20. Delgado-Lista J, Alcala-Diaz JF, Torres-Peña JD, Quintana-Navarro GM, Fuentes F, Garcia-Rios A, et al. Long-term secondary prevention of cardiovascular disease with a Mediterranean diet and a low-fat diet (CORDIOPREV): a randomised controlled trial. Lancet. 2022;399(10338):1876–85. https://doi.org/10.1016/S0140-6736(22)00122-2.

21. Becerra-Tomás N, Blanco Mejía S, Viguiliouk E, Khan T, Kendall CWC, Kahleova H, et al. Mediterranean diet, cardiovascular disease and mortality in diabetes: a systematic review and meta-analysis of prospective cohort studies and randomized clinical trials. Crit Rev Food Sci Nutr. 2020;60(7):1207–27. https://doi.org/10.1080/10408398.2019.1565281.

22. Rosato V, Temple NJ, La Vecchia C, Castellan G, Tavani A, Guercio V. Mediterranean diet and cardiovascular disease: a systematic review and meta-analysis of observational studies. Eur J Nutr. 2019;58(1):173–91. https://doi.org/10.1007/s00394-017-1582-0.

23. Chiavaroli L, Viguiliouk E, Nishi SK, Blanco Mejia S, Rahelić D, Kahleová H, et al. DASH dietary pattern and cardiometabolic outcomes: an umbrella review of systematic reviews and meta-analyses. Nutrients. 2019;11(2):338. https://doi.org/10.3390/nu11020338.
24. Yokoyama Y, Levin SM, Barnard ND. Association between plant-based diets and plasma lipids: a systematic review and meta-analysis. Nutr Rev. 2017;75(9):683–98. https://doi.org/10.1093/nutrit/nux030.
25. Rees K, Al-Khudairy L, Takeda A, Stranges S. Vegan dietary pattern for the primary and secondary prevention of cardiovascular diseases. Cochrane Database Syst Rev. 2021;2(2):CD013501. https://doi.org/10.1002/14651858.CD013501.pub2.
26. Elliott PS, Kharaty SS, Phillips CM. Plant-based diets and lipid, lipoprotein, and inflammatory biomarkers of cardiovascular disease: a review of observational and interventional studies. Nutrients. 2022;14(24):5371. https://doi.org/10.3390/nu14245371.
27. Jabri A, Kumar A, Verghese E, Alameh A, Kumar A, Khan MS, et al. Meta-analysis of effect of vegetarian diet on ischemic heart disease and all-cause mortality. Am J Prev Cardiol. 2021;7:100182. https://doi.org/10.1016/j.ajpc.2021.100182.
28. Dybvik JS, Svendsen M, Aune D. Vegetarian and vegan diets and the risk of cardiovascular disease, ischemic heart disease and stroke: a systematic review and meta-analysis of prospective cohort studies. Eur J Nutr. 2023;62(1):51–69. https://doi.org/10.1007/s00394-022-02942-8.
29. Petersen KS, Kris-Etherton PM. Diet quality assessment and the relationship between diet quality and cardiovascular disease risk. Nutrients. 2021;13(12):4305. https://doi.org/10.3390/nu13124305.
30. Hu EA, Steffen LM, Coresh J, Appel LJ, Rebholz CM. Adherence to the Healthy Eating Index-2015 and other dietary patterns may reduce risk of cardiovascular disease, cardiovascular mortality, and all-cause mortality. J Nutr. 2020;150(2):312–21. https://doi.org/10.1093/jn/nxz218.
31. Shan Z, Li Y, Baden MY, Bhupathiraju SN, Wang DD, Sun Q, et al. Association between healthy eating patterns and risk of cardiovascular disease. JAMA Intern Med. 2020;180(8):1090–100. https://doi.org/10.1001/jamainternmed.2020.2176.
32. Morze J, Danielewicz A, Hoffmann G, Schwingshackl L. Diet quality as assessed by the healthy eating index, alternate healthy eating index, dietary approaches to stop hypertension score, and health outcomes: a second update of a systematic review and meta-analysis of cohort studies. J Acad Nutr Diet. 2020;120(12):1998–2031.e15. https://doi.org/10.1016/j.jand.2020.08.076.
33. Mente A, Dehghan M, Rangarajan S, O'Donnell M, Hu W, Dagenais G, et al. Diet, cardiovascular disease, and mortality in 80 countries. Eur Heart J. 2023;44(28):2560–79. https://doi.org/10.1093/eurheartj/ehad269.
34. Hooper L, Martin N, Jimoh OF, Kirk C, Foster E, Abdelhamid AS. Reduction in saturated fat intake for cardiovascular disease. Cochrane Database Syst Rev. 2020;8(8):CD011737. https://doi.org/10.1002/14651858.CD011737.pub3.
35. Maki KC, Dicklin MR, Kirkpatrick CF. Saturated fats and cardiovascular health: current evidence and controversies. J Clin Lipidol. 2021;15(6):765–72. https://doi.org/10.1016/j.jacl.2021.09.049.
36. Sacks FM, Lichtenstein AH, Wu JHY, Appel LJ, Creager MA, Kris-Etherton PM, et al. Dietary fats and cardiovascular disease: a presidential advisory from the American Heart Association. Circulation. 2017;136(3):e1–e23. https://doi.org/10.1161/CIR.0000000000000510. Erratum in: Circulation. 2017;136(10):e195.
37. Li Y, Hruby A, Bernstein AM, Ley SH, Wang DD, Chiuve SE, et al. Saturated fats compared with unsaturated fats and sources of carbohydrates in relation to risk of coronary heart disease: a prospective cohort study. J Am Coll Cardiol. 2015;66(14):1538–48. https://doi.org/10.1016/j.jacc.2015.07.055.
38. Farvid MS, Ding M, Pan A, Sun Q, Chiuve SE, Steffen LM, et al. Dietary linoleic acid and risk of coronary heart disease: a systematic review and meta-analysis of pro-

spective cohort studies. Circulation. 2014;130(18):1568–78. https://doi.org/10.1161/CIRCULATIONAHA.114.010236.

39. Bergwall S, Johansson A, Sonestedt E, Acosta S. High versus low-added sugar consumption for the primary prevention of cardiovascular disease. Cochrane Database Syst Rev. 2022;1(1):CD013320. https://doi.org/10.1002/14651858.CD013320.pub2.

40. Te Morenga LA, Howatson AJ, Jones RM, Mann J. Dietary sugars and cardiometabolic risk: systematic review and meta-analyses of randomized controlled trials of the effects on blood pressure and lipids. Am J Clin Nutr. 2014;100(1):65–79. https://doi.org/10.3945/ajcn.113.081521.

41. Chiavaroli L, de Souza RJ, Ha V, Cozma AI, Mirrahimi A, Wang DD, et al. Effect of fructose on established lipid targets: a systematic review and meta-analysis of controlled feeding trials. J Am Heart Assoc. 2015;4(9):e001700. https://doi.org/10.1161/JAHA.114.001700.

42. Ter Horst KW, Schene MR, Holman R, Romijn JA, Serlie MJ. Effect of fructose consumption on insulin sensitivity in nondiabetic subjects: a systematic review and meta-analysis of diet-intervention trials. Am J Clin Nutr. 2016;104(6):1562–76. https://doi.org/10.3945/ajcn.116.137786.

43. Huang Y, Chen Z, Chen B, Li J, Yuan X, Li J, et al. Dietary sugar consumption and health: umbrella review. BMJ. 2023;381:e071609. https://doi.org/10.1136/bmj-2022-071609.

44. Narain A, Kwok CS, Mamas MA. Soft drinks and sweetened beverages and the risk of cardiovascular disease and mortality: a systematic review and meta-analysis. Int J Clin Pract. 2016;70(10):791–805. https://doi.org/10.1111/ijcp.12841.

45. Bechthold A, Boeing H, Schwedhelm C, Hoffmann G, Knüppel S, Iqbal K, et al. Food groups and risk of coronary heart disease, stroke and heart failure: a systematic review and dose-response meta-analysis of prospective studies. Crit Rev Food Sci Nutr. 2019;59(7):1071–90. https://doi.org/10.1080/10408398.2017.1392288.

46. Yin J, Zhu Y, Malik V, Li X, Peng X, Zhang FF, et al. Intake of sugar-sweetened and low-calorie sweetened beverages and risk of cardiovascular disease: a meta-analysis and systematic review. Adv Nutr. 2021;12(1):89–101. https://doi.org/10.1093/advances/nmaa084.

47. Zhang YB, Jiang YW, Chen JX, Xia PF, Pan A. Association of consumption of sugar-sweetened beverages or artificially sweetened beverages with mortality: a systematic review and dose-response meta-analysis of prospective cohort studies. Adv Nutr. 2021;12(2):374–83. https://doi.org/10.1093/advances/nmaa110.

48. Sun T, Zhang Y, Ding L, Zhang Y, Li T, Li Q. The relationship between major food sources of fructose and cardiovascular outcomes: a systematic review and dose-response meta-analysis of prospective studies. Adv Nutr. 2023;14(2):256–69. https://doi.org/10.1016/j.advnut.2022.12.002.

49. Vos MB, Kaar JL, Welsh JA, Van Horn LV, Feig DI, Anderson CAM, et al. Added sugars and cardiovascular disease risk in children: a scientific statement from the American Heart Association. Circulation. 2017;135(19):e1017–34. https://doi.org/10.1161/CIR.0000000000000439.

50. Johnson RK, Appel LJ, Brands M, Howard BV, Lefevre M, Lustig RH, et al. Dietary sugars intake and cardiovascular health: a scientific statement from the American Heart Association. Circulation. 2009;120(11):1011–20. https://doi.org/10.1161/CIRCULATIONAHA.109.192627.

51. Brien SE, Ronksley PE, Turner BJ, Mukamal KJ, Ghali WA. Effect of alcohol consumption on biological markers associated with risk of coronary heart disease: systematic review and meta-analysis of interventional studies. BMJ. 2011;342:d636. https://doi.org/10.1136/bmj.d636.

52. Huang Y, Li Y, Zheng S, Yang X, Wang T, Zeng J. Moderate alcohol consumption and atherosclerosis : meta-analysis of effects on lipids and inflammation. Wien Klin Wochenschr. 2017;129(21–22):835–43. https://doi.org/10.1007/s00508-017-1235-6.

53. Ricci C, Schutte AE, Schutte R, Smuts CM, Pieters M. Trends in alcohol consumption in relation to cause-specific and all-cause mortality in the United States: a report from the

NHANES linked to the US mortality registry. Am J Clin Nutr. 2020;111(3):580–9. https://doi.org/10.1093/ajcn/nqaa008.

54. Tian Y, Liu J, Zhao Y, Jiang N, Liu X, Zhao G, et al. Alcohol consumption and all-cause and cause-specific mortality among US adults: prospective cohort study. BMC Med. 2023;21(1):208. https://doi.org/10.1186/s12916-023-02907-6.

55. Ronksley PE, Brien SE, Turner BJ, Mukamal KJ, Ghali WA. Association of alcohol consumption with selected cardiovascular disease outcomes: a systematic review and meta-analysis. BMJ. 2011;342:d671. https://doi.org/10.1136/bmj.d671.

56. Wood AM, Kaptoge S, Butterworth AS, Willeit P, Warnakula S, Bolton T, et al. Risk thresholds for alcohol consumption: combined analysis of individual-participant data for 599 912 current drinkers in 83 prospective studies. Lancet. 2018;391(10129):1513–23. https://doi.org/10.1016/S0140-6736(18)30134-X. Erratum in: Lancet. 2018;391(10136):2212.

57. Biddinger KJ, Emdin CA, Haas ME, Wang M, Hindy G, Ellinor PT, et al. Association of habitual alcohol intake with risk of cardiovascular disease. JAMA Netw Open. 2022;5(3):e223849. https://doi.org/10.1001/jamanetworkopen.2022.3849. Erratum in: JAMA Netw Open. 2022;5(4):e2212024.

58. National Institute on Alcohol Abuse and Alcoholism. What is a standard drink? [Internet]. National Institutes of Health; n.d. [Cited 2023, July 3]. https://www.niaaa.nih.gov/alcohols-effects-health/overview-alcohol-consumption/what-standard-drink.

59. U.S. Department of Health and Human Services. Physical activity guidelines for Americans. 2nd ed. Washington, DC: U.S. Department of Health and Human Services; 2018. https://health.gov/paguidelines/second-edition/pdf/Physical_Activity_Guidelines_2nd_edition.pdf.

60. World Health Organization. WHO guidelines on physical activity and sedentary behaviour. Geneva: World Health Organization; 2020. https://apps.who.int/iris/rest/bitstreams/1315866/retrieve.

61. MacIntosh BR, Murias JM, Keir DA, Weir JM. What is moderate to vigorous exercise intensity? Front Physiol. 2021;12:682233. https://doi.org/10.3389/fphys.2021.682233.

62. Ainsworth BE, Haskell WL, Herrmann SD, Meckes N, Bassett DR Jr, Tudor-Locke C, et al. 2011 Compendium of Physical Activities: a second update of codes and MET values. Med Sci Sports Exerc. 2011;43(8):1575–81. https://doi.org/10.1249/MSS.0b013e31821ece12.

63. Mann S, Beedie C, Jimenez A. Differential effects of aerobic exercise, resistance training and combined exercise modalities on cholesterol and the lipid profile: review, synthesis and recommendations. Sports Med. 2014;44(2):211–21. https://doi.org/10.1007/s40279-013-0110-5.

64. Wang Y, Xu D. Effects of aerobic exercise on lipids and lipoproteins. Lipids Health Dis. 2017;16(1):132. https://doi.org/10.1186/s12944-017-0515-5.

65. Whelton SP, Chin A, Xin X, He J. Effect of aerobic exercise on blood pressure: a meta-analysis of randomized, controlled trials. Ann Intern Med. 2002;136(7):493–503. https://doi.org/10.7326/0003-4819-136-7-200204020-00006.

66. Diaz KM, Shimbo D. Physical activity and the prevention of hypertension. Curr Hypertens Rep. 2013;15(6):659–68. https://doi.org/10.1007/s11906-013-0386-8.

67. de Castro QJT, Tomaz FSC, Watai PY, Grabe-Guimarães A. Physical exercise combined with antihypertensive drug therapy on left ventricular hypertrophy: systematic review and meta-analysis. High Blood Press Cardiovasc Prev. 2020;27(6):493–503. https://doi.org/10.1007/s40292-020-00403-z.

68. Huang L, Fang Y, Tang L. Comparisons of different exercise interventions on glycemic control and insulin resistance in prediabetes: a network meta-analysis. BMC Endocr Disord. 2021;21(1):181. https://doi.org/10.1186/s12902-021-00846-y.

69. Mannucci E, Bonifazi A, Monami M. Comparison between different types of exercise training in patients with type 2 diabetes mellitus: a systematic review and network metanalysis of randomized controlled trials. Nutr Metab Cardiovasc Dis. 2021;31(7):1985–92. https://doi.org/10.1016/j.numecd.2021.02.030.

70. Dawson LP, Lum M, Nerleker N, Nicholls SJ, Layland J. Coronary atherosclerotic plaque regression: JACC State-of-the-Art Review. J Am Coll Cardiol. 2022;79(1):66–82. https://doi.org/10.1016/j.jacc.2021.10.035.

71. Nishitani-Yokoyama M, Miyauchi K, Shimada K, Miyazaki T, Ogita M, Okazaki S, et al. Effects of phase II comprehensive cardiac rehabilitation on coronary plaque volume after acute coronary syndrome. Int Heart J. 2015;56(6):597–604. https://doi.org/10.1536/ihj.15-049.

72. Nishitani-Yokoyama M, Miyauchi K, Shimada K, Yokoyama T, Ouchi S, Aikawa T, et al. Impact of physical activity on coronary plaque volume and components in acute coronary syndrome patients after early phase II cardiac rehabilitation. Circ J. 2019;83(1):101–9. https://doi.org/10.1253/circj.CJ-18-0738.

73. Vesterbekkmo EK, Aamot Aksetøy IL, Follestad T, Nilsen HO, Hegbom K, Wisløff U, et al. High intensity interval training induces beneficial effects on coronary atheromatous plaques—a randomized trial. Eur J Prev Cardiol. 2023;30(5):384–92. https://doi.org/10.1093/eurjpc/zwac309.

74. Dempsey PC, Strain T, Khaw KT, Wareham NJ, Brage S, Wijndaele K. Prospective associations of accelerometer-measured physical activity and sedentary time with incident cardiovascular disease, cancer, and all-cause mortality. Circulation. 2020;141(13):1113–5. https://doi.org/10.1161/CIRCULATIONAHA.119.043030.

75. Ramakrishnan R, Doherty A, Smith-Byrne K, Rahimi K, Bennett D, Woodward M, et al. Accelerometer measured physical activity and the incidence of cardiovascular disease: evidence from the UK Biobank cohort study. PLoS Med. 2021;18(1):e1003487. https://doi.org/10.1371/journal.pmed.1003487. Erratum in: PLoS Med. 2021;18(9):e1003809.

76. Yerramalla MS, McGregor DE, van Hees VT, Fayosse A, Dugravot A, Tabak AG, et al. Association of daily composition of physical activity and sedentary behaviour with incidence of cardiovascular disease in older adults. Int J Behav Nutr Phys Act. 2021;18(1):83. https://doi.org/10.1186/s12966-021-01157-0.

77. Khurshid S, Al-Alusi MA, Churchill TW, Guseh JS, Ellinor PT. Accelerometer-derived "weekend warrior" physical activity and incident cardiovascular disease. JAMA. 2023;330(3):247–52. https://doi.org/10.1001/jama.2023.10875.

78. Kraus WE, Powell KE, Haskell WL, Janz KF, Campbell WW, Jakicic JM, et al. Physical activity, all-cause and cardiovascular mortality, and cardiovascular disease. Med Sci Sports Exerc. 2019;51(6):1270–81. https://doi.org/10.1249/MSS.0000000000001939.

79. Kubota Y, Evenson KR, Maclehose RF, Roetker NS, Joshu CE, Folsom AR. Physical activity and lifetime risk of cardiovascular disease and cancer. Med Sci Sports Exerc. 2017;49(8):1599–605. https://doi.org/10.1249/MSS.0000000000001274.

80. Park S, Han K, Lee S, Kim Y, Lee Y, Kang MW, et al. Association between moderate-to-vigorous physical activity and the risk of major adverse cardiovascular events or mortality in people with various metabolic syndrome status: a nationwide population-based cohort study including 6 million people. J Am Heart Assoc. 2020;9(22):e016806. https://doi.org/10.1161/JAHA.120.016806.

81. Dhana K, Koolhaas CM, Berghout MA, Peeters A, Ikram MA, Tiemeier H, et al. Physical activity types and life expectancy with and without cardiovascular disease: the Rotterdam Study. J Public Health (Oxf). 2017;39(4):e209–18. https://doi.org/10.1093/pubmed/fdw110.

82. Stefanick ML, King AC, Mackey S, Tinker LF, Hlatky MA, LaMonte MJ, et al. Women's Health Initiative strong and healthy pragmatic physical activity intervention trial for cardiovascular disease prevention: design and baseline characteristics. J Gerontol A Biol Sci Med Sci. 2021;76(4):725–34. https://doi.org/10.1093/gerona/glaa325.

83. Elliott EG, Laden F, James P, Rimm EB, Rexrode KM, Hart JE. Interaction between long-term exposure to fine particulate matter and physical activity, and risk of cardiovascular disease and overall mortality in U.S. women. Environ Health Perspect. 2020;128(12):127012. https://doi.org/10.1289/EHP7402.

84. Florido R, Zhao D, Ndumele CE, Lutsey PL, McEvoy JW, Windham BG, et al. Physical activity, parental history of premature coronary heart disease, and incident atherosclerotic cardiovascular disease in the Atherosclerosis Risk in Communities (ARIC) study. J Am Heart Assoc. 2016;5(9):e003505. https://doi.org/10.1161/JAHA.116.003505.

85. de Souto Barreto P, Cesari M, Andrieu S, Vellas B, Rolland Y. Physical activity and incident chronic diseases: a longitudinal observational study in 16 European countries. Am J Prev Med. 2017;52(3):373–8. https://doi.org/10.1016/j.amepre.2016.08.028.

86. Banach M, Lewek J, Surma S, Penson PE, Sahebkar A, Martin SS, et al. The association between daily step count and all-cause and cardiovascular mortality: a meta-analysis. Eur J Prev Cardiol. 2023;30(18):1975–85. https://doi.org/10.1093/eurjpc/zwad229. Erratum in: Eur J Prev Cardiol. 2023.

87. Shailendra P, Baldock KL, Li LSK, Bennie JA, Boyle T. Resistance training and mortality risk: a systematic review and meta-analysis. Am J Prev Med. 2022;63(2):277–85. https://doi.org/10.1016/j.amepre.2022.03.020.

88. U.S. Department of Health and Human Services, Centers for Disease Control and Prevention. Body mass index: considerations for practitioners [Pamphlet]. Atlanta: Centers for Disease Control and Prevention. [Cited 2023 July 20]. https://www.cdc.gov/obesity/downloads/bmi-forpractitioners.pdf.

89. Khan SS, Ning H, Wilkins JT, Allen N, Carnethon M, Berry JD, et al. Association of body mass index with lifetime risk of cardiovascular disease and compression of morbidity. JAMA Cardiol. 2018;3(4):280–7. https://doi.org/10.1001/jamacardio.2018.0022.

90. Mestre LM, Lartey ST, Ejima K, Mehta T, Keith S, Maki KC, et al. Body mass index, obesity, and mortality—part 1. Nutr Today. 2023;58(3):92–9. https://doi.org/10.1097/NT.0000000000000609.

91. De Paola L, Mehta A, Pana TA, Carter B, Soiza RL, Kafri MW, et al. Body mass index and mortality, recurrence and readmission after myocardial infarction: systematic review and meta-analysis. J Clin Med. 2022;11(9):2581. https://doi.org/10.3390/jcm11092581.

92. Xia JY, Lloyd-Jones DM, Khan SS. Association of body mass index with mortality in cardiovascular disease: new insights into the obesity paradox from multiple perspectives. Trends Cardiovasc Med. 2019;29(4):220–5. https://doi.org/10.1016/j.tcm.2018.08.006.

93. Ortega FB, Sui X, Lavie CJ, Blair SN. Body mass index, the most widely used but also widely criticized index: would a criterion standard measure of total body fat be a better predictor of cardiovascular disease mortality? Mayo Clin Proc. 2016;91(4):443–55. https://doi.org/10.1016/j.mayocp.2016.01.008.

94. Iyen B, Weng S, Vinogradova Y, Akyea RK, Qureshi N, Kai J. Long-term body mass index changes in overweight and obese adults and the risk of heart failure, cardiovascular disease and mortality: a cohort study of over 260,000 adults in the UK. BMC Public Health. 2021;21(1):576. https://doi.org/10.1186/s12889-021-10606-1.

95. Yang Y, Song L, Wang L, Li D, Chen S, Wu S, et al. Effect of body mass index trajectory on lifetime risk of cardiovascular disease in a Chinese population: a cohort study. Nutr Metab Cardiovasc Dis. 2023;33(3):523–31. https://doi.org/10.1016/j.numecd.2022.11.025.

96. Knowler WC, Barrett-Connor E, Fowler SE, Hamman RF, Lachin JM, Walker EA, et al. Reduction in the incidence of type 2 diabetes with lifestyle intervention or metformin. N Engl J Med. 2002;346(6):393–403. https://doi.org/10.1056/NEJMoa012512.

97. Look AHEAD Research Group, Wing RR, Bolin P, Brancati FL, Bray GA, Clark JM, Coday M, et al. Cardiovascular effects of intensive lifestyle intervention in type 2 diabetes. N Engl J Med. 2013;369(2):145–54. https://doi.org/10.1056/NEJMoa1212914. Erratum in: N Engl J Med. 2014;370(19):1866.

98. Schwingshackl L, Dias S, Hoffmann G. Impact of long-term lifestyle programmes on weight loss and cardiovascular risk factors in overweight/obese participants: a systematic review and network meta-analysis. Syst Rev. 2014;3:130. https://doi.org/10.1186/2046-4053-3-130.

99. Goldberg RB, Orchard TJ, Crandall JP, Boyko EJ, Budoff M, Dabelea D, et al. Effects of long-term metformin and lifestyle interventions on cardiovascular events in the Diabetes

Prevention Program and its outcome study. Circulation. 2022;145(22):1632–41. https://doi.org/10.1161/CIRCULATIONAHA.121.056756.

100. Maki KC, Kirkpatrick CF, Allison DB, Gadde KM. Pharmacotherapy for obesity: recent evolution and implications for cardiovascular risk reduction. Expert Rev Endocrinol Metab. 2023;18(4):307–19. https://doi.org/10.1080/17446651.2023.2209176.

101. Ma C, Avenell A, Bolland M, Hudson J, Stewart F, Robertson C, et al. Effects of weight loss interventions for adults who are obese on mortality, cardiovascular disease, and cancer: systematic review and meta-analysis. BMJ. 2017;359:j4849. https://doi.org/10.1136/bmj.j4849.

102. Novo Nordisk. Company announcement. Novo Nordisk A/S: semaglutide 2.4 mg reduces the risk of major adverse cardiovascular events by 20% in adults with overweight or obesity in the SELECT trial [Internet]. Bagsværd: Novo Nordisk A/S; 2023 August 8 [Cited 2023, September 4]. https://www.novonordisk.com/news-and-media/news-and-ir-materials/news-details.html?id=166301.

103. Cesaro A, De Michele G, Fimiani F, Acerbo V, Scherillo G, Signore G, et al. Visceral adipose tissue and residual cardiovascular risk: a pathological link and new therapeutic options. Front Cardiovasc Med. 2023;10:1187735. https://doi.org/10.3389/fcvm.2023.1187735.

104. Ibrahim MM. Subcutaneous and visceral adipose tissue: structural and functional differences. Obes Rev. 2010;11(1):11–8. https://doi.org/10.1111/j.1467-789X.2009.00623.x.

105. Roever LS, Resende ES, Diniz ALD, Penha-Silva N, Veloso FC, Casella-Filho A, et al. Abdominal obesity and association with atherosclerosis risk factors: the Uberlândia Heart Study. Medicine (Baltimore). 2016;95(11):e1357. https://doi.org/10.1097/MD.0000000000001357.

106. Hiuge-Shimizu A, Kishida K, Funahashi T, Ishizaka Y, Oka R, Okada M, et al. Absolute value of visceral fat area measured on computed tomography scans and obesity-related cardiovascular risk factors in large-scale Japanese general population (the VACATION-J study). Ann Med. 2012;44(1):82–92. https://doi.org/10.3109/07853890.2010.526138.

107. Vasan SK, Osmond C, Canoy D, Christodoulides C, Neville MJ, Di Gravio C, et al. Comparison of regional fat measurements by dual-energy X-ray absorptiometry and conventional anthropometry and their association with markers of diabetes and cardiovascular disease risk. Int J Obes (Lond). 2018;42(4):850–7. https://doi.org/10.1038/ijo.2017.289.

108. Gowri SM, Antonisamy B, Geethanjali FS, Thomas N, Jebasingh F, Paul TV, et al. Distinct opposing associations of upper and lower body fat depots with metabolic and cardiovascular disease risk markers. Int J Obes (Lond). 2021;45(11):2490–8. https://doi.org/10.1038/s41366-021-00923-1.

109. Silva RFD, Iwamoto JM, Filho DMP, Monteiro HL, Villar R, Zago AS. A cross-sectional analysis of risk factors for cardiovascular diseases in older females: association between body fat distribution and physical fitness. J Women Aging. 2022;34(2):181–93. https://doi.org/10.1080/08952841.2021.1877098.

110. Ruder K. Mounting evidence suggests that BMI isn't the only measure needed to predict mortality risk. JAMA. 2023;330(6):490–1. https://doi.org/10.1001/jama.2023.13602.

111. Sanguankeo A, Lazo M, Upala S, Brancati FL, Bonekamp S, Pownall HJ, et al. Effects of visceral adipose tissue reduction on CVD risk factors independent of weight loss: the Look AHEAD Study. Endocr Res. 2017;42(2):86–95. https://doi.org/10.1080/07435800.2016.1194856.

112. Barzi F, Woodward M, Czernichow S, Lee CM, Kang JH, Janus E, et al. The discrimination of dyslipidaemia using anthropometric measures in ethnically diverse populations of the Asia-Pacific Region: the Obesity in Asia Collaboration. Obes Rev. 2010;11(2):127–36. https://doi.org/10.1111/j.1467-789X.2009.00605.x.

113. Li M, Zhu P, Wang SX. Risk for cardiovascular death associated with waist circumference and diabetes: a 9-year prospective study in the Wan Shou Lu cohort. Front Cardiovasc Med. 2022;9:856517. https://doi.org/10.3389/fcvm.2022.856517.

114. Sahakyan KR, Somers VK, Rodriguez-Escudero JP, Hodge DO, Carter RE, Sochor O, et al. Normal-weight central obesity: implications for total and cardiovascular mortality. Ann Intern Med. 2015;163(11):827–35. https://doi.org/10.7326/M14-2525.
115. Bigaard J, Frederiksen K, Tjønneland A, Thomsen BL, Overvad K, Heitmann BL, et al. Waist circumference and body composition in relation to all-cause mortality in middle-aged men and women. Int J Obes (Lond). 2005;29(7):778–84. https://doi.org/10.1038/sj.ijo.0802976.
116. Bigaard J, Christensen J, Tjønneland A, Thomsen BL, Overvad K, Sørensen TIA. Influence of lifestyle aspects on the association of body size and shape with all-cause mortality in middle-aged men and women. Obes Facts. 2010;3(4):252–60. https://doi.org/10.1159/000319579.
117. Cao Q, Yu S, Xiong W, Li Y, Li H, Li J, et al. Waist-hip ratio as a predictor of myocardial infarction risk: a systematic review and meta-analysis. Medicine (Baltimore). 2018;97(30):e11639. https://doi.org/10.1097/MD.0000000000011639.
118. Ross R, Neeland IJ, Yamashita S, Shai I, Seidell J, Magni P, et al. Waist circumference as a vital sign in clinical practice: a consensus statement from the IAS and ICCR Working Group on Visceral Obesity. Nat Rev Endocrinol. 2020;16(3):177–89. https://doi.org/10.1038/s41574-019-0310-7.
119. St-Onge MP, Grandner MA, Brown D, Conroy MB, Jean-Louis G, Coons M, et al. Sleep duration and quality: impact on lifestyle behaviors and cardiometabolic health: a scientific statement from the American Heart Association. Circulation. 2016;134(18):e367–86. https://doi.org/10.1161/CIR.0000000000000444.
120. Ramar K, Malhotra RK, Carden KA, Martin JL, Abbasi-Feinberg F, Aurora RN, et al. Sleep is essential to health: an American Academy of Sleep Medicine position statement. J Clin Sleep Med. 2021;17(10):2115–9. https://doi.org/10.5664/jcsm.9476.
121. Adjaye-Gbewonyo D, Ng AE, Black LI. Sleep difficulties in adults: United States, 2020. NCHS Data Brief. 2022;(436):1–8.
122. Makarem N, Castro-Diehl C, St-Onge MP, Redline S, Shea S, Lloyd-Jones D, et al. Redefining cardiovascular health to include sleep: prospective associations with cardiovascular disease in the MESA Sleep Study. J Am Heart Assoc. 2022;11(21):e025252. https://doi.org/10.1161/JAHA.122.025252.
123. Yin J, Jin X, Shan Z, Li S, Huang H, Li P, et al. Relationship of sleep duration with all-cause mortality and cardiovascular events: a systematic review and dose-response meta-analysis of prospective cohort studies. J Am Heart Assoc. 2017;6(9):e005947. https://doi.org/10.1161/JAHA.117.005947.
124. Kwok CS, Kontopantelis E, Kuligowski G, Gray M, Muhyaldeen A, Gale CP, et al. Self-reported sleep duration and quality and cardiovascular disease and mortality: a dose-response meta-analysis. J Am Heart Assoc. 2018;7(15):e008552. https://doi.org/10.1161/JAHA.118.008552.
125. Wang S, Li Z, Wang X, Guo S, Sun Y, Li G, et al. Associations between sleep duration and cardiovascular diseases: a meta-review and meta-analysis of observational and Mendelian randomization studies. Front Cardiovasc Med. 2022;9:930000. https://doi.org/10.3389/fcvm.2022.930000.
126. Henst RHP, Pienaar PR, Roden LC, Rae DE. The effects of sleep extension on cardiometabolic risk factors: a systematic review. J Sleep Res. 2019;28(6):e12865. https://doi.org/10.1111/jsr.12865.
127. Torquati L, Mielke GI, Brown WJ, Kolbe-Alexander T. Shift work and the risk of cardiovascular disease. A systematic review and meta-analysis including dose-response relationship. Scand J Work Environ Health. 2018;44(3):229–38. https://doi.org/10.5271/sjweh.3700.
128. Huang T, Mariani S, Redline S. Sleep irregularity and risk of cardiovascular events: the Multi-Ethnic Study of Atherosclerosis. J Am Coll Cardiol. 2020;75(9):991–9. https://doi.org/10.1016/j.jacc.2019.12.054.
129. Levine GN, Cohen BE, Commodore-Mensah Y, Fleury J, Huffman JC, Khalid U, et al. Psychological health, well-being, and the mind-heart-body connection: a scientific state-

ment from the American Heart Association. Circulation. 2021;143(10):e763–83. https://doi.org/10.1161/CIR.0000000000000947.
130. World Health Organization. Mental health [Internet]. World Health Organization; 2023. [Updated 2022, June 17; Cited 2023, July 17]. https://www.who.int/news-room/fact-sheets/detail/mental-health-strengthening-our-response.
131. Meng LB, Zhang YM, Luo Y, Gong T, Liu DP. Chronic stress a potential suspect zero of atherosclerosis: a systematic review. Front Cardiovasc Med. 2021;8:738654. https://doi.org/10.3389/fcvm.2021.738654.
132. Hinterdobler J, Schunkert H, Kessler T, Sager HB. Impact of acute and chronic psychosocial stress on vascular inflammation. Antioxid Redox Signal. 2021;35(18):1531–50. https://doi.org/10.1089/ars.2021.0153.
133. Sher LD, Geddie H, Olivier L, Cairns M, Truter N, Beselaar L, et al. Chronic stress and endothelial dysfunction: mechanisms, experimental challenges, and the way ahead. Am J Physiol Heart Circ Physiol. 2020;319(2):H488–506. https://doi.org/10.1152/ajpheart.00244.2020.
134. Barger SD, Struve GC. Association of depression with 10-year and lifetime cardiovascular disease risk among US adults, National Health and Nutrition Examination Survey, 2005-2018. Prev Chronic Dis. 2022;19:E28. https://doi.org/10.5888/pcd19.210418.
135. Eleazu I, Ayers C, Navar AM, Salhadar K, Albert M, Carnethon M, et al. Associations of cumulative perceived stress with cardiovascular risk factors and outcomes: findings from the Dallas Heart Study. medRxiv [Preprint]. 2023:2023.06.15.23291460. https://doi.org/10.1101/2023.06.15.23291460.
136. Shen R, Zhao N, Wang J, Guo P, Shen S, Liu D, et al. Association between socioeconomic status and arteriosclerotic cardiovascular disease risk and cause-specific and all-cause mortality: data from the 2005-2018 National Health and Nutrition Examination Survey. Front Public Health. 2022;10:1017271. https://doi.org/10.3389/fpubh.2022.1017271.
137. Kivimäki M, Steptoe A. Effects of stress on the development and progression of cardiovascular disease. Nat Rev Cardiol. 2018;15(4):215–29. https://doi.org/10.1038/nrcardio.2017.189.
138. GBD 2019 Risk Factors Collaborators. Global burden of 87 risk factors in 204 countries and territories, 1990–2019: a systematic analysis for the Global Burden of Disease Study 2019. Lancet. 2020;396(10258):1223–49. https://doi.org/10.1016/S0140-6736(20)30752-2.
139. Kapoor G. Association of physical, psychological and psychosocial attributes with arterial stiffness in cardiovascular disorders: a systematic literature review. J Lifestyle Med. 2023;13(1):27–43. https://doi.org/10.15280/jlm.2023.13.1.27.
140. Wu AD, Lindson N, Hartmann-Boyce J, Wahedi A, Hajizadeh A, Theodoulou A, et al. Smoking cessation for secondary prevention of cardiovascular disease. Cochrane Database Syst Rev. 2022;8(8):CD014936. https://doi.org/10.1002/14651858.CD014936.pub2.
141. Mohiuddin SM, Mooss AN, Hunter CB, Grollmes TL, Cloutier DA, Hilleman DE. Intensive smoking cessation intervention reduces mortality in high-risk smokers with cardiovascular disease. Chest. 2007;131(2):446–52. https://doi.org/10.1378/chest.06-1587.
142. Anthonisen NR, Skeans MA, Wise RA, Manfreda J, Kanner RE, Connett JE, et al. The effects of a smoking cessation intervention on 14.5-year mortality: a randomized clinical trial. Ann Intern Med. 2005;142(4):233–9. https://doi.org/10.7326/0003-4819-142-4-200502150-00005.
143. Critchley JA, Capewell S. Mortality risk reduction associated with smoking cessation in patients with coronary heart disease: a systematic review. JAMA. 2003;290(1):86–97. https://doi.org/10.1001/jama.290.1.86.

Lipids, Lipoproteins, and Cardiovascular Outcomes

Alexander Sakers, Reed Mszar, and Daniel Soffer

Key Points
- Dyslipidemia is common, caused by environmental and genetic variability in lipid/lipoprotein production, metabolism, and clearance, and is a major modifiable risk factor for the development of atherosclerotic cardiovascular disease (ASCVD).
- Cholesterol and triglyceride (TG) are the main clinically measured lipids; they play key physiological roles in cell membranes, steroid hormone synthesis, and energy metabolism, and their trafficking throughout the body is essential for metabolic homeostasis.
- The predominant atherogenic lipoprotein is low-density lipoprotein (LDL); however, all apolipoprotein (Apo)B-containing lipoproteins, including lipoprotein(a) [Lp(a)], TG-rich lipoproteins, and their remnants also contribute to the development of ASCVD.
- LDL cholesterol (LDL-C) is the most widely used metric to assess the contribution of lipids/lipoproteins to atherogenesis, since it approximates the contribu-

Alexander Sakers and Reed Mszar contributed equally to this work.

A. Sakers
Perelman School of Medicine, University of Pennsylvania, Philadelphia, PA, USA

Department of Medicine, Massachusetts General Hospital, Boston, MA, USA

R. Mszar
Department of Physiology, Georgetown University, Washington, DC, USA

D. Soffer (✉)
Perelman School of Medicine, University of Pennsylvania, Philadelphia, PA, USA

Perelman Center for Advanced Medicine, University of Pennsylvania Health System, Philadelphia, PA, USA
e-mail: Daniel.soffer@pennmedicine.upenn.edu

© The Author(s), under exclusive license to Springer Nature Switzerland AG 2024
K. C. Maki, D. P. Wilson (eds.), *Cardiovascular Outcomes Research*, Contemporary Cardiology, https://doi.org/10.1007/978-3-031-54960-1_9

201

tion of most atherogenic cholesterol to atherosclerosis. Alternative measures, including more accurate formulas for estimating LDL-C, and more robust metrics, such as non-high-density lipoprotein cholesterol (non-HDL-C) and ApoB, better capture atherogenic risk and should replace reliance on the Friedewald estimate of LDL-C in clinical decision-making.

- Despite their different primary mechanisms of action and potency, several medications, including statins, the cholesterol absorption inhibitor ezetimibe, and proprotein convertase subtilisin/kexin type 9 (PCSK9) monoclonal antibodies yield similar proportional reductions in relative ASCVD risk per unit of LDL-C lowering achieved.
- Hypertriglyceridemia (HTG), which affects nearly one in four adults, is commonly caused by the interaction of environmental factors with the cumulative effect of multiple genetic variants; HTG is associated with elevated ASCVD risk proportional to the accompanying elevation in ApoB.
- ASCVD risk reduction from TG-lowering therapies has been mixed, and novel TG-lowering therapies are being actively investigated.
- HDL-C levels in the normal range are inversely associated with ASCVD risk. However, targeting HDL-C has not been effective in reducing ASCVD risk.
- Novel Lp(a)-lowering therapeutics are in late-stage development, and results from these clinical trials will demonstrate whether this approach has a role in clinical care.

1 Introduction

Cardiovascular disease (CVD) is the leading cause of morbidity and mortality in the United States and worldwide [1, 2]. In addition to familial predisposition and conventional risk factors—hypertension, obesity, smoking, and diabetes mellitus (DM)—dyslipidemia represents a major modifiable factor causally implicated in increased CVD risk. Over the past several decades, advances in the fields of clinical lipidology, metabolism, and genetics have yielded greater insight into the heritable and environmental causes of lipid and lipoprotein derangements, leading to the development of pharmacotherapies to optimize lipid levels and reduce CVD risk.

In this chapter, we will review the fundamental role of lipids and lipoproteins in physiology, describe commonly used risk estimation strategies in the clinic, and provide a contemporary overview of the evidence linking apolipoprotein (Apo) B-containing lipoproteins [low-density (LDL), very low-density (VLDL), triglyceride (TG)-rich remnant lipoproteins (TRL), and lipoprotein(a) (Lp(a))] and high-density lipoproteins (HDL) with CVD risk, emphasizing their fundamental role as the building blocks of atheroma. Moreover, we will discuss effective lipid/lipoprotein-directed therapies developed to manage atherosclerotic cardiovascular disease (ASCVD) risk. We will review a select group of inherited disorders as a model for the impact of lipid/lipoprotein derangements on ASCVD risk, as well as evidence from recent randomized controlled trials (RCT), meta-analyses, and

Mendelian randomization studies that assess the relationship between lipids/lipoproteins and CVD risk.

2   Overview of Lipid and Lipoprotein Physiology

Lipids play a vital role in myriad biological processes. Cholesterol and TG are fundamental clinical lipids. They function as the primary constituent of cell membranes (phospholipids and cholesterol), the building block for bile acids and steroid hormones (cholesterol), and a major source of fuel for cellular metabolism (fatty acids and TG) [3] (Fig. 1). Since lipids are not soluble in water, they are incorporated within specialized particles called lipoproteins to facilitate being transported in the bloodstream. The exterior surface of lipoproteins is hydrophilic and composed of amphipathic phospholipids and free cholesterol [4]. This hydrophilic surface conceals the hydrophobic TG and cholesteryl esters (CE) contained within the core of the particle and enables solubility in the blood (Fig. 2).

The body produces several types of lipoproteins, which have distinct functions and lifecycles (Table 1). The identity of a lipoprotein is dictated by its permanent protein scaffold (e.g., ApoB-100, ApoB-48, or Apo-A1) and relative lipid concentrations, which together influence its density or buoyancy. ApoB-containing lipoproteins (e.g., chylomicrons [CM], VLDL, LDL, and their remnants) are the principal vehicles by which TG is transported from their origin (liver and intestines) to the rest of the body. Apo-A1 is the core structural protein for HDL, which has pleiotropic roles in atherogenesis, many of which are protective, including promotion of reverse cholesterol transport, modulation of inflammation, and inhibition of oxidative stress [5].

ApoB is among the largest proteins in the human body (515 kD mass); it is so large that each lipoprotein in which it is found only contains a single molecule of ApoB [6, 7]. ApoB is found in two forms: (1) full-length ApoB-100 protein that is secreted by the liver and (2) ApoB-48, a truncated form expressed selectively in enterocytes that contains the first 48% of the full-length protein and excludes the LDL receptor (LDL-R) binding domain.

ApoB-containing lipoproteins undergo a three-stage lifecycle consisting of (1) production, (2) metabolism, and (3) clearance [8] (Fig. 3). ApoB-48-containing CM are synthesized by enterocytes from mostly exogenous (dietary) and intestinally derived lipids, while endogenous lipids are synthesized and packaged by the liver into ApoB-100-containing VLDL. Increased lipid availability, resulting from a high-fat meal or elevated liver fat stores, promotes the secretion of larger and more TG-rich CM and VLDL, respectively [9, 10].

After secretion, CM and VLDL undergo extensive metabolism and modification, including (1) lipolysis of TG in peripheral tissues via lipoprotein lipase (LPL), (2) interaction with hepatic lipase, (3) exchange of TG for CE (from HDL and other lipoproteins) via the action of cholesteryl ester transfer protein (CETP), and (4) apolipoprotein exchange [7, 11]. These processes yield successively smaller, denser,

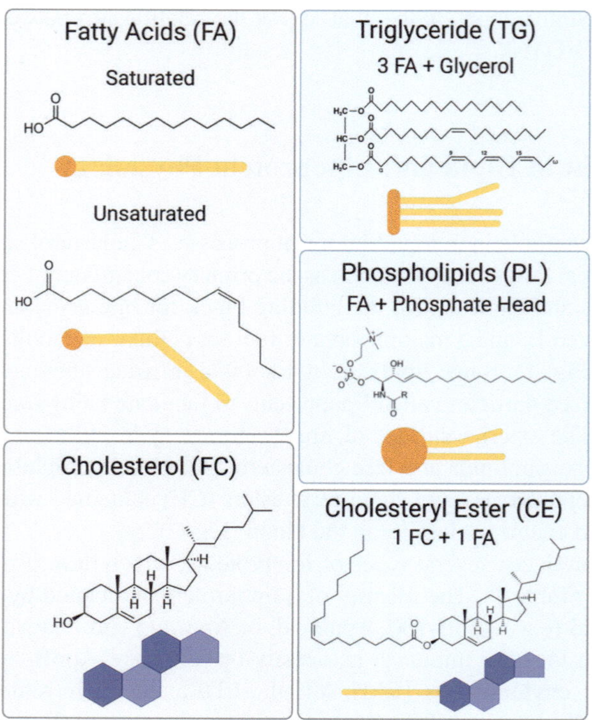

Fig. 1 Lipids. Lipids are a diverse class of biological molecules which are defined by their solubility in nonpolar solvents and poor solubility in water. In each panel, chemical structures are depicted above with cartoon representations below. Fatty acids (FA) contain a hydrophilic carboxylic acid head attached to a hydrocarbon tail. Saturated fatty acids contain a hydrocarbon tail with no carbon-carbon double bonds. Unsaturated fatty acids have one (monounsaturated FA) or more (polyunsaturated FA) carbon-carbon double bonds in their hydrocarbon tails. Free cholesterol (FC) is an amphipathic molecule, with a hydrophilic hydroxyl group at one end and an otherwise hydrophobic structure. Triglycerides are hydrophobic molecules generated by combining glycerol with three fatty acids. Phospholipids (PL) are critical cell membrane components which contain a hydrophilic phosphate-containing head group and two hydrophobic hydrocarbon tails, typically derived from one or more FAs. Cholesteryl esters (CE) are formed by combining the carboxylic acid head of FA with the hydroxyl group of FC, generating a highly hydrophobic molecule. *Created with* BioRender.com

more TG-depleted/cholesterol-enriched particles. In this way, after hepatic secretion, VLDL is metabolized to VLDL remnants, then to intermediate-density lipoprotein (IDL), and finally to LDL, while intestinally derived CM are metabolized to CM remnants (which may become as small and dense as IDL) [12].

At any stage of their lifecycle, lipoproteins may be cleared from the circulation by hepatic lipoprotein receptors, especially the LDL-R, and, in the case of TRL, by the LDL receptor-related protein 1 (LRP1) [13, 14]. ApoB and ApoE are the primary and secondary ligands that directly bind to the LDL-R via protein-protein interactions, facilitating uptake by hepatocytes. ApoE has a primary role in

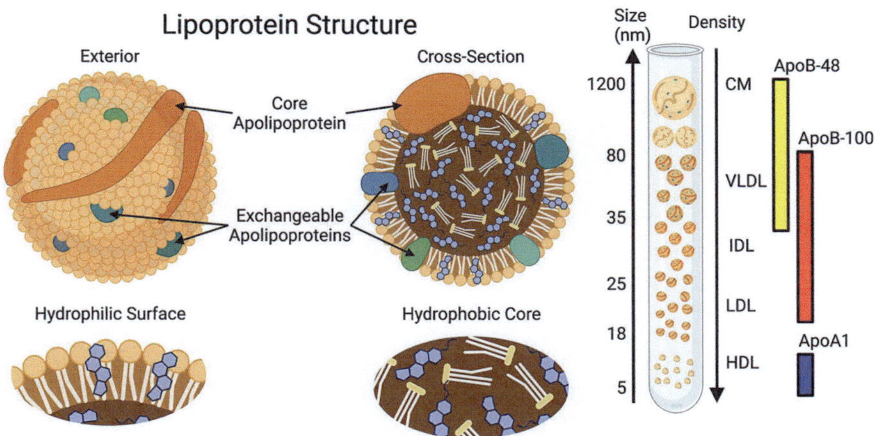

Fig. 2 Lipoproteins: structure and physical properties. *Left:* Lipoproteins share general structural characteristics, including a hydrophilic surface composed of phospholipids and free cholesterol and a hydrophobic core containing triglyceride (TG) and cholesteryl esters. Apolipoprotein (Apo) B-containing lipoproteins have ApoB as a scaffold and include chylomicrons (CM), very low-density lipoprotein (VLDL), intermediate-density lipoprotein (IDL), and low-density lipoprotein (LDL), as well as their remnants. ApoA1 is the scaffold for high-density lipoprotein (HDL). Lipoproteins additionally contain numerous other apolipoproteins which confer functionality on the particles, for example, by enabling receptor binding (e.g., ApoE) or modulating enzyme activation (e.g., ApoC). *Right:* In general, as lipoprotein size decreases, TG content decreases and density increases. *Far right*: Bars depicting the size/density ranges of lipoproteins based around the core apolipoproteins ApoB48, ApoB100, and ApoA1. *Created with* BioRender.com

Table 1 Composition of major lipoproteins. Data adapted from [158]

Lipoprotein	Size (nm)	Density (g/mL)	Scaffold protein	Triglyceride %	Cholesterol %
Chylomicron	75–1200	<0.930	ApoB-48	80–95	3–7
VLDL	30–80	0.930–1.006	ApoB-100	45–65	20–30
IDL	25–35	1.006–1.019	ApoB-100	–	–
LDL	18–25	1.019–1.063	ApoB-100	4–8	51–58
HDL	5–12	1.063–1.210	ApoA1	2–7	18–25
Lp(a)	30	1.045–1.080	ApoB-100	–	–

Note: Triglyceride and cholesterol percentages are not included for IDL and Lp(a)
Abbreviations. *Apo* apolipoprotein, *HDL* high-density lipoprotein, *IDL* intermediate-density lipoprotein, *LDL* low-density lipoprotein, *Lp(a)* lipoprotein(a), *VLDL* very low-density lipoprotein

mediating the uptake of TRL by LRP. The steady-state serum levels of lipoproteins are dictated by the relative rates of production, metabolism, and clearance. For individuals with normal TG levels, the metabolism of VLDL and CM is rapid, while LDL, which has the longest serum residence time, is the most abundant lipoprotein in circulation. Under physiologic circumstances, for every 1 particle of CM or CM remnant, there are approximately 10 VLDL particles and 90 LDL particles [15].

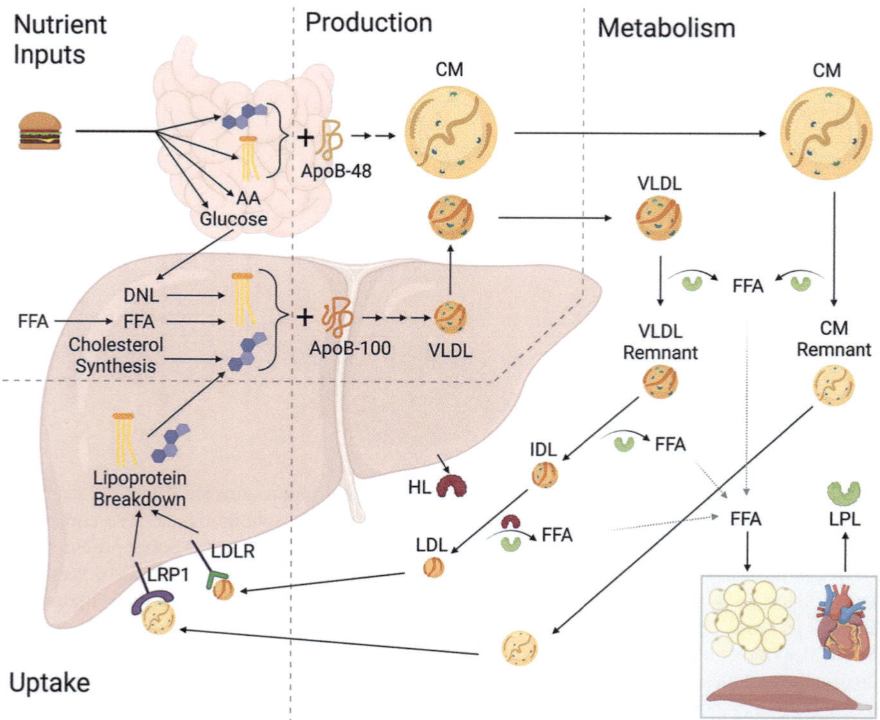

Fig. 3 Lipoprotein lifecycle: production, metabolism, and uptake. *Production:* Lipoprotein production relies on inputs from exogenous and endogenous sources. Exogenous: Dietary fat and cholesterol from digested food are packaged into ApoB48-containing chylomicrons. Endogenous: The hepatic triglyceride (TG) pool is derived from (1) circulating FFA, (2) recycled lipoproteins, and (3) DNL (which uses excess nutrients, including proteins and dietary sugars such as glucose and fructose, to make lipids). TG and cholesterol are then packaged with ApoB100 into VLDL and secreted by the liver. *Metabolism*: Once secreted, VLDL and CM are metabolized through serial rounds of lipolysis by LPL. LPL is generated by adipose tissue, muscle, and cardiac muscle, and liberates FFA from VLDL/CM TGs, enabling FFA delivery into the underlying tissues. Processing by LPL, HL, and other enzymes leads to the formation of CM remnants, VLDL remnants, IDL, and eventually LDL. *Uptake:* Specific receptors, especially the LDL-R, are required to clear lipoproteins from the circulation. Abbreviations. *AA* amino acids, *Apo* apolipoprotein, *CM* chylomicron, *DNL* de novo lipogenesis, *FFA* free fatty acids, *IDL* intermediate-density lipoprotein, *LDL-R* LDL receptor, *LRP1* LDL-R-related protein 1, *HL* hepatic lipase, *LPL* lipoprotein lipase, *VLDL* very low-density lipoprotein. *Created with* BioRender.com

3 Lipoproteins and the Development of ASCVD

Elevated levels of low-density lipoproteins sustained over a relatively long period of time promote atherosclerosis [16]; this conclusion is supported by a large body of evidence from genetic, epidemiologic, animal, and clinical intervention studies [17]. Furthermore, recent evidence strongly suggests that all ApoB-containing lipoproteins, except large CM, which are >70 nm in diameter, are similarly atherogenic on a particle-for-particle basis [15, 18]. However, individuals with smaller LDL particles are more prone to having accompanying hypertriglyceridemia (HTG) and/or low HDL-C and other features of insulin resistance/metabolic syndrome, and a higher number of atherogenic particles (higher ApoB) for a given LDL-C concentration.

The fundamental driver of atherosclerosis is the entry and subsequent retention of ApoB-containing lipoproteins within the subendothelial glycoprotein matrix of the arterial wall (Fig. 4) [19]. This process is driven by the concentration gradient between the lumen and subendothelium, specific lipoprotein properties, endothelium permeability, and features of the subendothelial matrix. Atherogenic lipoproteins can become trapped within the subendothelial space due to the interaction of ApoB and other components of the lipoprotein with arterial extracellular matrix proteins. The extracellular matrix composition of the subendothelial space varies in different vascular beds, partially explaining the increased susceptibility of certain

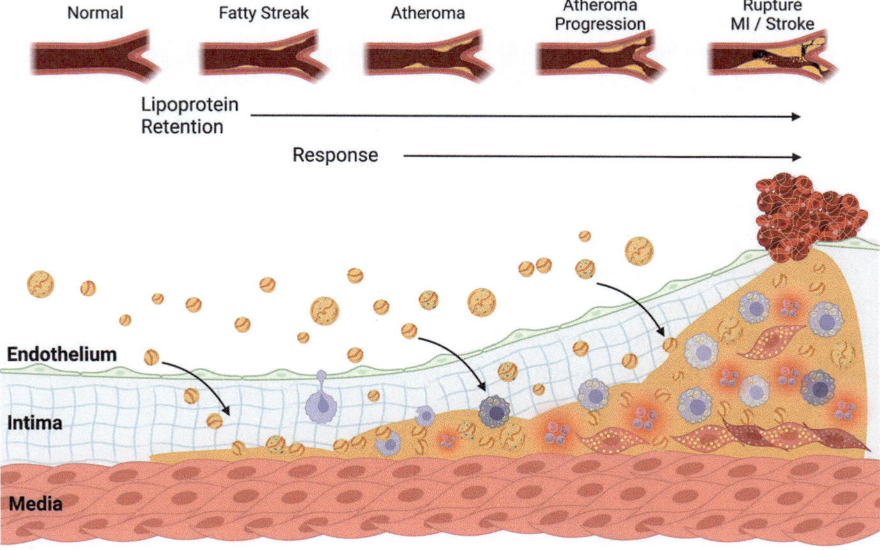

Fig. 4 Atherosclerosis mechanisms: lipoprotein retention and response to retention. Atherosclerosis starts with the formation of fatty streaks and accumulations of cholesterol within the subendothelial space of arteries, due to the retention of apolipoprotein (Apo)B-containing lipoproteins. The interaction of ApoB-lipoproteins with the extracellular matrix (grid) favors retention. Over time, ApoB-containing lipoproteins continue to accumulate, leading to macrophage and other immune cell infiltration and the formation of an atheroma. With continued deposition of ApoB-containing lipoproteins, the atheroma grows in size and there is continued immune cell infiltration and inflammation. Additionally, macrophages and smooth muscle cells become filled with cholesterol, leading to the characteristic "foam cell" phenotype. Eventually, atheroma may become so large that they impinge upon the lumen of the artery, restricting blood flow and leading to stable angina. They may also rupture, leading to exposure of the atheroma to blood, which causes an acute thrombosis and an acute ischemic event. Abbreviation: *MI* myocardial infarction. *Created with* BioRender.com

vessels to lipoprotein retention and atherosclerosis [20]. Once lipoproteins are retained, a series of maladaptive changes occur, especially lipoprotein oxidation, inflammation, and infiltration of T cells, macrophages, and neutrophils. This immunologic response creates a microenvironment that further promotes lipoprotein retention and recruitment and maturation of cholesterol-laden macrophages (also known as foam cells) [19].

In general, the TG and protein components of lipoproteins can be metabolized, but the sterol/cholesterol content accumulates in the growing atheroma [21]. Over the course of years, the continued retention of lipoproteins results in the accumulation of foam cells along with the consequences of their inflammatory actions. Advanced atherosclerotic plaques contain cholesterol both within foam cells and as extracellular cholesterol crystals [22]. The atheroma expands outward initially in a process known as Glagov remodeling, which spares encroachment upon the lumen. Eventually, the atheroma can become large enough to partially occlude the arterial lumen and affect blood flow. During periods of increased oxygen demand, lumen stenosis can cause a stable pattern of ischemia. Endothelial rupture or erosion of the plaque, as a consequence of secreted proteases and inflammatory cytokines, exposes the atheroma contents to the blood (especially tissue factor), triggering localized blood clotting which may completely obstruct the lumen, resulting in an acute ischemic event such as a heart attack or stroke, or may result in auto-thrombolysis, repair, and remodeling (progressive disease).

Atheroma formation begins early, starting in childhood, and proceeds continuously over time at rates that depend on multiple factors. Atherogenesis accelerates around 20 years of age and, by middle age, approximately 70% of men and almost 50% of women have evidence of subclinical atherosclerosis [23]. The principal modifiable determinant of atheroma formation is circulating LDL/ApoB-containing lipoprotein concentrations (Fig. 5). The degree of atherosclerosis is proportional to cumulative exposure to atherogenic lipoproteins (i.e., the concentration of

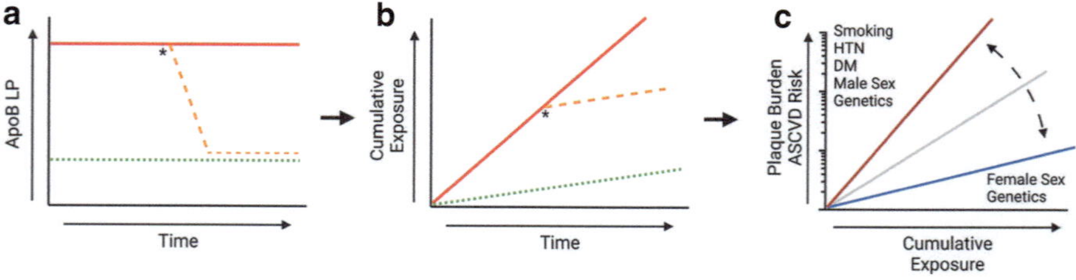

Fig. 5 ApoB lipoprotein exposure and ASCVD risk. (**a**) Higher plasma levels of ApoB-containing lipoproteins over time lead to (**b**) increased cumulative exposure over time. Cumulative exposure = level × time = area under the curve (AUC). (*) Represents initiation of ApoB lipoprotein-lowering therapy. Lipid-lowering therapy reduces the rate of increase in cumulative exposure moving forward. Atherosclerotic plaque burden correlates with atherosclerotic cardiovascular disease (ASCVD) risk. (**c**) Plaque burden is directly related to cumulative exposure, although there is substantial inter-individual variation in the relationship between plaque burden and cumulative exposure. Protective or predisposing factors alter the relationship between level of cumulative exposure and degree of plaque burden (exaggerated for visibility). *Created with* BioRender.com

circulating atherogenic lipoproteins), and duration of exposure (time), although numerous modulating factors can accelerate or decelerate atheroma development. Atheroma formation follows a log-linear relationship with exposure, such that linear increases/decreases in exposure lead to exponential increases/decreases in ASCVD [24]. LDL has a long-circulating residence time and is the predominant ApoB-containing lipoprotein under almost all physiologic conditions, even in individuals with HTG and/or elevated Lp(a) levels [15]. LDL is therefore central to the pathogenesis of atherosclerosis, and targeting LDL is a cornerstone of ASCVD prevention. Finally, multiple clinical risk-enhancing and risk-reducing factors accelerate (e.g., smoking, DM, hypertension, genetics) or decelerate (e.g., female sex, genetics) the rate of atheroma formation at any given circulating lipoprotein concentration [25]; many additional factors that are not generally measured play a role as well (e.g., variation in endothelial or vascular structure and inflammatory proteins).

4 Risk Estimation and Laboratory Measurements

4.1 Laboratory Measurements

ApoB-containing lipoproteins, especially LDL, are the "building blocks" of the atheroma and foam cell formation. As such, measurement of lipoprotein concentrations (which dictates the vessel lumen vs subendothelium concentration gradient) is a vital tool for estimating the risk of ASCVD, monitoring response to lipid/lipoprotein-lowering therapies, and guiding shared decision-making.

Historically and in most clinical settings, treatment of dyslipidemia is directed by estimated or measured levels of LDL-C as a surrogate for the concentration of LDL particles present in circulation. Direct measurement of LDL-C and other lipoprotein cholesterol levels with beta-quantification requires ultracentrifugation to separate lipoproteins into subfractions [26]; this method is expensive, time-consuming, and no longer available for clinical use. Automated approaches are now the standard in clinical practice and involve measurement of the concentrations of total cholesterol (TC), TG, and HDL-C directly via inexpensive enzymatic assays, after which LDL-C and VLDL-C are estimated using a mathematical formula or multivariable table. In the past, the Friedewald calculation (LDL-C = TC—HDL-C—VLDL-C/5) was the most widely used method of estimating LDL-C [27]. This formula is reliable enough when (1) nearly all cholesterol is contained in LDL, HDL, and VLDL, (2) the ratio of VLDL-C to TG is ~5:1 (in mg/dL), (3) IDL and Lp(a) do not contribute significantly to circulating cholesterol concentrations, and (4) lipoprotein X (LpX) is not present [28].

However, many lipid profiles encountered in routine clinical practice do not conform to the Friedewald equation's assumptions, for example, in the cases of HTG (TG >150 mg/dL) and low LDL-C. HTG is common, affecting approximately 25%

of the general population in the United States and a greater proportion of those with overweight/obesity, insulin resistance, and prediabetes/DM [29, 30]. Advances in lipid-targeting therapies such as proprotein convertase subtilisin/kexin type-9 inhibitors (PCSK9i) enable the lowering of LDL-C to levels well below 70 mg/dL [31]. To limit inaccuracies without increasing cost in LDL-C reporting, alternative formulas have been developed. Notable validated examples include the Martin/Hopkins calculator derived from the Very Large Database of Lipids, which accounts for the variable TG/VDL-C ratio across a range of TG levels [32], and the Sampson/National Institutes of Health (NIH) formula, which is derived from multiple large databases [33]. Both methods perform better than the Friedewald equation across a wide range of TGs, especially in the ranges of 150–400 mg/dL [26]. The Sampson formula is especially useful for patients with TG levels as high as 800 mg/dL [26, 33], and the Martin/Hopkins formula is particularly useful for the assessment of LDL-C at levels around or below the treatment threshold of 70 mg/dL [34, 35].

When using LDL-C for clinical decision-making, the Friedewald calculation should be replaced by all clinical laboratories with better-performing alternatives. Web-based calculators employing the Martin/Hopkins and Sampson/NIH formulas are available and some commercial laboratories have already made the change. Since both are validated, they are preferred over less well-validated approaches, such as the use of direct LDL-C measurements [36], which add to the cost of testing without evidence of improved accuracy. Alternatively, targeting non-HDL-C or ApoB is preferred since they are both direct measurements, outperform LDL-C as a metric to assess response to therapy, and represent complete atherogenic potential from lipoproteins rather than limited potential from LDL alone.

4.2 Risk Estimation

A variety of ASCVD risk prediction methods incorporate lipid/lipoprotein measurements. In general, these methods correlate a measurement of lipoproteins with ASCVD outcomes, while incorporating information from conventional risk factors such as age, sex, hypertension, smoking, and DM. Early calculators were developed using data from ~5000 White participants in the Framingham Heart Study and performed well for White, middle-aged populations [37]. Newer calculators, which perform better in diverse general populations, incorporate data from a much larger number of individuals across a broader range of races and comorbidities. The Pooled Cohort Equations (PCE) predict 10-year ASCVD risk for people aged 40–75 years and were developed using data from non-Hispanic White and non-Hispanic Black populations [38]. It is recommended by the 2019 American College of Cardiology (ACC)/American Heart Association (AHA) Guideline on the Primary Prevention of Cardiovascular Disease and can be accessed via web calculators [35, 39]. There are similar risk calculators available for European populations that take into consideration regional differences in ASCVD outcomes [40].

Improving ASCVD risk prediction is an active area of research, and novel methods that estimate risk more accurately and in wider populations are published frequently. For example, the ACC offers an enhanced and updated PCE-based risk calculator [39], which incorporates additional data from the Million Hearts Initiative [41]. These and other enhanced risk calculators are very useful for describing populations but can fail to accurately capture individual risk, especially in younger patients. Atherosclerosis imaging, especially coronary artery calcium scoring (CACS) by electrocardiogram (ECG)-gated computed tomography, is a superior tool for the identification of atherosclerosis, the obligatory precursor to atherosclerosis events but requires testing that cannot be performed at the clinic bedside.

The optimal tool for population study may not be ideal for individual patient-based clinical care, and the best lipid/lipoprotein measurement has been a source of ongoing debate [42]. For example, non-HDL-C and ApoB have a high degree of correlation with LDL-C in populations. However, non-HDL-C alone may be insufficient in certain clinical scenarios; for example, the measurement of ApoB is required to make the diagnosis of remnant disease (formerly known as type III hyperlipoproteinemia) unless the clinician has access to beta-quantification, and ApoB is helpful in the differential management of hyperchylomicronemia (familial vs multifactorial chylomicronemia syndromes) and moderate HTG syndromes (familial combined hyperlipidemia vs familial HTG). There may also be significant discordance between ApoB and LDL-C (or non-HDL-C), especially in individuals with high TG and/or low HDL-C, which may result in undertreatment based on lipoprotein concentration; conversely, individuals with high LDL-C and high HDL-C may have discordance that results in overtreatment. In these cases, measuring ApoB allows for more precise risk stratification and determination of which patients are more likely to benefit from initiation or intensification of lipid-lowering therapy. Given the high correlation between non-HDL-C and ApoB in populations, some have argued that the additional cost of ApoB is not justified despite these exceptions [15]. We believe the use of ApoB measurement has the potential to significantly enhance individualized care and represents a single standardized measure that optimizes lipoprotein management for ASCVD risk [15, 43].

4.3 Practical Considerations: Fasting vs Non-Fasting Measurements

Lipoprotein measurements are often performed when the patient is fasting, although non-fasting lipoprotein measurements are sufficient for estimating risk from ApoB-containing lipoproteins, especially in initial screening [36]. Although TG may be higher in the non-fasting state, they are typically only modestly elevated (10–20%) compared with the fasting state. The remainder of the lipid profile is even less affected [44]. Furthermore, non-fasting HTG may inform susceptibility to postprandial HTG and, when found, should trigger measurement of a fasting lipid profile and the investigation into the underlying causes. Lastly, methods that measure ApoB are not affected by food intake and may therefore be performed in the fasting or non-fasting state [44].

5 LDL-C and CVD Risk

Approximately 28 million adults in the United States (12%) have TC levels >240 mg/dL and more than 94 million have levels >200 mg/dL [1]. Recent estimates indicate that nearly one-third of the deaths caused by ischemic heart disease or stroke are attributable to elevated plasma LDL-C levels [45] and LDL is the principal building block for atherosclerosis in every affected patient regardless of their LDL-C level. Therefore, in addition to a heart-healthy lifestyle (detailed elsewhere [46]), excellent blood pressure control, and appropriate use of antiplatelet therapy, lipid-lowering pharmacotherapy has a key role in reducing ASCVD risk. Because of a wealth of clinical data and ease of use, statin drugs are the foundation of care for ASCVD risk reduction.

5.1 Targeting LDL-C/ApoB-Lipoproteins with Pharmacotherapy to Manage CVD Risk

5.1.1 Statins

Statins are safe, effective, evidence-based, well-tolerated, convenient, and affordable [47]. As such, they are the cornerstone of pharmacotherapy for lowering ASCVD risk (See Table 2 for a comparison of lipid-lowering therapies) [35]. Statins work primarily by inhibiting hepatic 3-hydroxy-3-methylglutaryl coenzyme A (HMG-CoA) reductase, the rate-limiting enzyme in de novo cholesterol synthesis. Decreased hepatic cholesterol leads to compensatory upregulation of the LDL-R and increased holoparticle clearance of circulating lipoproteins, which restores intrahepatic cholesterol levels while reducing circulating LDL [48]. The efficacy of statins in preventing ASCVD is largely due to their ability to reduce plasma levels of LDL and other ApoB-containing lipoproteins [49], although other proposed beneficial non-lipid effects on thrombosis, inflammation, plaque stability, and endothelial function may also play a role and may not be present in other medicines that lower LDL-C [50].

Guidelines on cholesterol management in the United States and other countries rely heavily on the findings from relatively short-term RCTs to assess the role of lipid therapy in ASCVD risk reduction. Although atherosclerosis is a lifelong process, RCTs have been conducted mostly in individuals with advanced ASCVD over study periods of <5 years. Nonetheless, in RCTs, statins consistently reduce ASCVD events across a wide range of baseline risk and atherosclerosis burden, with benefits

Table 2 Different classes of lipid-lowering therapies with their respective mechanisms of action, effects on lipid levels, evidence of cardiovascular benefits, and other clinically relevant parameters including safety, cost, and ease of administration

Lipid-Lowering Therapies	Mechanism of Action	LDL-C Lowering	CV Outcomes Benefit	Safety / Tolerability	Ease of Administration	Cost
Statins	Inhibits HMG-CoA reductase	+++	+++	+++ / ++	+++	low
Ezetimibe	Inhibits cholesterol absorption	+	++	+++ / +++	+++	low
PCSK9 Monoclonal Antibodies	Facilitates clearance of PCSK9	+++	++	+++ / +++	++	high
Bile Acid Sequestrants	Disrupts enterohepatic circulation of bile acids	+	+ (monotherapy)	+++ +	+	variable
Fibric Acid Derivatives	Decreases hepatic ApoC-III production and increases lipoprotein lipase via PPAR-alpha	+	+ ++ (monotherapy)	++	+++	low
Icosapent Ethyl	Multiple: decreases VLDL-TG synthesis / secretion and increases TG clearance	n/a	++	++ / ++	++	high
Niacin	Inhibits hormone-sensitive lipase	+	+	+/+	+	high
Bempedoic Acid	Inhibits ATP-citrate lyase	+	n/a	+/? ++	+++	high
Inclisiran	Disrupts mRNA in synthesis of PCSK9	+++	n/a	+? +++	+++	high

Abbreviations: *HMG-CoA* 3-hydroxy-3-methyl-glutaryl-coenzyme A, *ApoC-III* apolipoprotein C-III, *CV* cardiovascular, *LDL-C* low-density lipoprotein cholesterol, *PPAR* peroxisome proliferator-activated receptor, *PCSK9* proprotein convertase subtilisin/kexin type 9, *TG* triglyceride, *ATP* adenosine triphosphate, and *mRNA* messenger ribonucleic acid

proportional to LDL-C reduction. The Cholesterol Treatment Trialists' (CTT) Collaboration was founded in 1994 to analyze data from large ($\geq$1000 participants), "long-term" ($\geq$2 years), and high-quality blinded placebo-controlled RCTs of statins using individual patient-level data [51]. CTT analyses, especially of "statin vs placebo" and "more vs less intensive" statin trials strongly support the use of statins in contemporary management of ASCVD risk in many patient population subgroups and suggest the primary benefit is proportional to LDL-C reduction [35].

CTT meta-analyses have examined the effects of LDL-C lowering with statins on major vascular events, major coronary events, stroke, coronary revascularization, and mortality. Major adverse cardiovascular events (MACE) are defined as a composite outcome of major coronary events (nonfatal myocardial infarction (MI) or coronary death), nonfatal stroke, fatal stroke, or coronary revascularization. All outcomes are reported as event rate ratios, weighted per 1.0 mmol/L (39 mg/dL) reduction in LDL-C. This weighting allows comparison across a wider range of baseline risks/LDL-C levels and normalizes the different strengths of various statins in lowering LDL-C.

The first CTT meta-analysis was published in 2005 and examined the effect of statin vs placebo in 90,056 individuals across 14 statin trials [52]. The trials analyzed included predominantly nondiabetic (79%) and male (76%) participants ranging from 18 to 90 years old, with established vascular disease (54%) or a history of MI (32%). This meta-analysis found a significant 21% decrease in major vascular events for every 1.0 mmol/L reduction in LDL-C. These results corresponded with significantly reduced MI (23%), need for coronary revascularization (24%), and fatal or nonfatal stroke (17%), along with a 12% reduction in all-cause mortality for each 1.0 mmol/L LDL-C reduction. Mortality reduction was predominantly driven by a significant 19% reduction in coronary deaths, with nonsignificant reductions in noncoronary (7%) and nonvascular (5%) mortality. There was no effect on overall or site-specific cancer incidence (relative risk [RR] = 1.0). The benefits of statins were statistically and clinically significant within the first year of treatment (RR = 0.9 for major vascular event in year 0–1) and the benefit increased with increasing duration of treatment (RR = 0.74 for major vascular event in year 5+).

A follow-up analysis in 2010 extended the results of the 2005 study to examine the safety and efficacy of more vs less intensive LDL-C lowering with statins [53]. This analysis was important, as it was unclear at the time whether high potency statins like atorvastatin and rosuvastatin, which may reduce LDL-C >50%, offered additional benefit (without additional harm) over widely prescribed moderate-intensity statins (e.g., pravastatin, simvastatin). The 2010 CTT meta-analysis included 21 statins vs placebo trials (129,526 individuals) and 5 more vs less intensive statin trials (39,612 individuals) with similar baseline characteristics to the 2005 CTT analysis (73% male, 81% nondiabetic, 59% with established vascular disease). In the 5 more vs less intensive trials, more intensive regimens reduced LDL-C by an additional 0.51 mmol/L, leading to significantly reduced major vascular events (15%), coronary death/nonfatal MI (13%), and coronary revascularization (19%). These benefits were comparable per 1.0 mmol/L LDL-C reduction to what was observed in statin vs control trials. Importantly, there was no apparent threshold LDL-C level beyond which further LDL-C reductions did not yield a benefit, though most RCTs did not achieve LDL-C levels much below 70 mg/dL. Notably, subjects with baseline LDL-C <2.0 mmol/L (~77 mg/dL) had similar proportional reductions per mmol/L LDL-C lowering as those with higher baseline LDL-C. Furthermore, when statin vs control and more vs less intensive statin trials were analyzed together, a 22% reduction in major vascular events per 1.0 mmol/L LDL-C reduction was observed, which was remarkably consistent across all subgroups studied (age, smoking status, sex, previous vascular disease, DM, hypertension, etc.). In a novel approach to assessing the impact of care, Bangalore et al. [54] demonstrated that targeting LDL-C levels (i.e., specific threshold LDL-C mg/dL) did not enhance outcomes once >50% LDL-C reduction had been achieved. In contrast, targeting >50% LDL-C reduction in addition to absolute LDL-C level achieved did show improved CVD risk reduction. These findings together provided major support for the high-intensity statin treatment approach for high-risk individuals recommended by cholesterol management guidelines (rather than targeting particular LDL-C goals) [35, 40].

5.1.2 Statins in Select Populations

Several additional CTT analyses have examined the safety and efficacy of LDL-C lowering with statins in select populations. These analyses are especially valuable for patient populations whose representation in any individual statin trial is too small to draw definitive conclusions. In general, these studies have confirmed that the ~20% major vascular event reduction per mmol/L LDL-C lowering found in earlier trials applies broadly across a range of patient populations.

A 2012 CTT analysis (27 statin RCTs; 174,149 patients) evaluated whether statin therapy conferred similar benefits across varying levels of baseline CVD risk [55]. Individual patient data were analyzed to separate patients into five categories of baseline "5-year major vascular event risk" (<5%, 5–10%, 10–20%, 20–30%, ≥30%). In people at low CVD risk, lowering cholesterol with a statin yielded highly significant reductions in the relative risk of major vascular events, with benefits per mmol/L LDL-C lowering comparable to or better than the relative benefit observed in higher-risk groups (RR per mmol/L LDL-C lowering overall = 0.79. All results were significant; 0.62, 0.69, 0.79, 0.81, and 0.79 from lowest to highest risk groups). Importantly, for the lowest risk categories, this translated to an absolute risk reduction of 11/1000 over 5 years of treatment, which outweighs any known risks associated with statin therapy [55].

A CTT analysis from 2015 examined the same trials (27 statin RCTs; 174,149 patients; 27% women) to compare the efficacy of statins in men vs women [56]. In general, women were at lower risk of major vascular events than men. Both men and women benefitted from statin therapy (RR per mmol/L LDL-C reduction; major vascular events: women = 0.84 and men = 0.78; mortality: women = 0.91 and men = 0.9; all results significant), although there was a nonsignificant trend toward less benefit in women per unit of LDL-C lowering. Statins were safe in both sexes, with no observed increases in cancer or nonvascular mortality.

Evidence is limited supporting the benefits and safety of statins across underserved groups. This observation has been quantified in a recent systematic review, which demonstrates severe underreporting and underrepresentation of non-Hispanic Blacks in major statin trials and in more recent, non-statin RCTs [57]. Until such inequities and exclusions are corrected in the design and funding of future studies, it is unreasonable to assume that the next generation of care will be improved for these vulnerable populations.

5.1.3 Statins in High-Risk Groups

Separate CTT analyses have evaluated the safety and efficacy of statins in three groups at high risk for ASCVD: older individuals [58], patients with DM [59], and patients with chronic kidney disease (CKD) [60]. The most recent CTT analysis, published in 2019, examined 186,854 patients across 28 RCTs of statins, including 14,483 (8%) aged ≥75 years [58]. This study showed that statins significantly reduced major vascular events and mortality in all age brackets, including those over 75. There was an observable but nonsignificant trend toward less benefit per mmol/L LDL-C reduction with increasing age (RR per mmol/L LDL-C reduction: all participants = 0.79, ≥75 years old = 0.87), which was diminished when trials that exclusively included patients with established heart failure or dialysis were excluded (RR per mmol/L LDL-C reduction: all participants = 0.77, ≥75 years old = 0.82). When patients were subdivided into those with established vascular disease and those without, statins were not found to yield statistically significant benefits in those ≥70 years of age without vascular disease, although there was no trend toward harm. In those with vascular disease, there was a nonsignificant trend toward less relative risk reduction per mmol/L LDL-C reduction after age 75 (RR per mmol/L LDL-C reduction: all participants = 0.80, ≥75 years old = 0.85). Of note, concern about loss of efficacy in relative risk reduction is overcome by the increase in absolute risk of major vascular events that occur with age. Overall, this analysis demonstrated that statins are beneficial for major vascular event risk reduction regardless of age, especially in those with established ASCVD, although their value in primary prevention in those aged 70–75 years is less clear.

A 2008 CTT meta-analysis examined data from 18,686 patients with DM (T1DM [n = 1466], T2DM [n = 17,220]) across 14 RCTs of statin vs placebo control [59]. It found an identical 21% proportional reduction in major vascular events per 1.0 mmol/L LDL-C reduction for those with and without DM. The reduction in major vascular events was driven by significant reductions in MI/coronary death (22%), coronary revascularization (25%), and stroke (21%). The mortality reduction per mmol/L LDL-C reduction was significant, although smaller, in patients with DM (9%) compared to those without DM (13%). This was driven by significant reductions in vascular mortality (13%), without a significant effect on nonvascular mortality. These results were comparable between patients with T1DM and T2DM. Overall, this study indicated that patients with DM receive a similar relative benefit from statin therapy per mmol/L LDL-C reduction compared to those without DM. Since DM is a risk equivalent for ASCVD [61], this relative risk reduction translates to a clinically significant absolute risk reduction (even for those without established vascular disease). Accordingly, moderate-intensity statins are recommended for the primary prevention of ASCVD in adults 40–75 with DM and LDL-C ≥70 mg/dL, while high-intensity statins are suggested for those with additional risk-enhancing characteristics [35].

Finally, a CTT analysis from 2016 examined the role of statin therapy in those with CKD [60]. Previous studies were limited by less-than-expected LDL-C reductions on statin therapy in these patients, potentially due to medication adherence or disease effects. Overall, statin therapy reduced the risk of major vascular events by 21% per 1.0 mmol/L LDL-C reduction; this effect declined significantly as the estimated glomerular filtration rate (eGFR) declined, although statins showed significant benefit in all patients with eGFR ≥30 (RR = 0.85). Even patients in the lowest eGFR group (eGFR <30; RR = 0.85) and on dialysis (RR = 0.94) showed a nonsignificant trend toward benefit. Current guidelines recommend considering statin initiation in intermediate-risk patients with CKD, given the role of CKD as an ASCVD risk-enhancing factor. Guidelines additionally suggest that it may be reasonable for patients already on statins to continue treatment as they transition to dialysis, but recommend against statin initiation in this group [35]. Of note, statins with little or no renal excretion/metabolism should be selected (e.g., atorvastatin) whenever possible.

5.1.4 Non-Statin Therapies for LDL-C Lowering

Several non-statin therapies are available for patients who require additional LDL-C lowering despite maximally tolerated statin therapy (Table 2), but of these, only PCSK9 monoclonal antibodies and ezetimibe have RCT evidence of ASCVD risk reduction when added to statin therapy. Despite their different mechanisms of action, therapies that enhance LDL clearance by upregulating the LDL-R, which improves LDL/ApoB clearance, produce consistent results in cardiovascular outcomes trials. Specifically, in a recent meta-regression analysis (49 clinical trials; 312,175 participants), each 1 mmol/L reduction in LDL-C level was associated with a significant 23% decreased RR of major vascular events for statins and 25% decreased RR for the non-statin interventions [49].

5.1.5 Ezetimibe

Ezetimibe is a small-molecule inhibitor of intestinal sterol absorption [62]. Reduced intestinal CM cholesterol results in less delivery of exogenous cholesterol to the liver, leading to upregulation of the LDL-R and enhanced LDL clearance from the circulation [63]. Ezetimibe is a once-daily, well-tolerated oral tablet that selectively inhibits the sterol transporter Niemann-Pick C1-Like-1 (NPC1L1) and does not increase bile acid secretion or inhibit hepatic cholesterol synthesis [64, 65].

Ezetimibe was initially approved in 2002, although for several years it was not widely prescribed due to its relatively modest (15–25% on average) reduction in LDL-C, lack of cardiovascular outcomes data, and high price to the consumer as a branded product. The Improved Reduction of Outcomes: Vytorin Efficacy International Trial (IMPROVE-IT, 2015) (18,144 patients) assessed whether further reduction of LDL-C with ezetimibe in combination with moderate-intensity statin therapy improved cardiovascular outcomes in those with acute coronary syndrome (ACS), compared to moderate-intensity statin therapy alone [66]. The primary endpoint was a composite of major vascular events, including nonfatal MI, unstable angina requiring hospitalization, coronary revascularization, or nonfatal stroke. The primary endpoint event rate was very high in both groups but was significantly reduced in the simvastatin-ezetimibe group (32.7%) compared to the simvastatin monotherapy group (34.7%) over 7 years of follow-up (hazard ratio [HR] = 0.936, 95% confidence interval [CI] 0.89–0.99). This correlated with lower time-weighted LDL-C levels in the simvastatin-ezetimibe group of 53.7 mg/dL vs 69.5 mg/dL in the monotherapy group. Ezetimibe is recommended by current guidelines as a reasonable additional therapeutic option for patients who require further LDL-C lowering despite maximally tolerated statin therapy; it is most strongly recommended for those with established ASCVD (especially recent ACS) who have LDL-C ≥70 mg/dL despite maximally tolerated statin [35].

5.1.6 PCSK9 Inhibitors

PCSK9 is a serine protease, primarily produced in the liver, which binds to and promotes intracellular degradation of the LDL-R in hepatocytes [67]. Genetic variants leading to gain- or loss-of-function mutations in *PCSK9* have been discovered that lead to increased or decreased LDL-C and risk of ASCVD, respectively [68]. Using insights from this genetic research, several therapeutics were developed to reduce PCSK9 levels. Mechanistically, these medications promote enhanced LDL-R recycling, resulting in increased hepatocyte LDL-R expression and improved LDL clearance. The three PCSK9i available in the United States are the monoclonal antibodies, evolocumab and alirocumab (both FDA-approved in 2015), and the small interfering RNA, inclisiran (FDA-approved December 2021); all are administered as subcutaneous injections.

The safety and efficacy of PCSK9i have been examined in several cardiovascular outcomes trials. As a class, PCSK9i are among the most effective therapies for lowering LDL-C, with typical reductions of 50–70% from baseline. The Further Cardiovascular Outcomes Research With PCSK9 Inhibition in Subjects With Elevated Risk (FOURIER) trial examined the efficacy of evolocumab in 27,564 patients with stable ASCVD and LDL-C/non-HDL-C levels $\geq 70/100$ mg/dL who were receiving high-intensity statin therapy [31]. At 48 weeks, evolocumab reduced LDL-C levels by an additional 59% compared with placebo (least-squares mean percentage reduction), correlating with significantly lower risk of the primary endpoint (composite of cardiovascular death, MI, stroke, hospitalization for unstable angina, and coronary revascularization) over 2.2 years follow-up (HR, 0.85 [95% CI, 0.79, 0.92]; $p < 0.001$).

The ODYSSEY OUTCOMES trial examined the efficacy and safety of another anti-PCSK9 antibody, alirocumab, in 18,924 high-risk patients who (1) experienced an ACS within the previous 12 months, (2) had LDL-C levels ≥ 70 mg/dL, or non-HDL-C ≥ 100 mg/dL, or ApoB ≥ 80 mg/dL, and (3) were receiving high-intensity or maximally tolerated statin therapy [69]. Like the FOURIER trial, over a median follow-up period of 2.8 years, ODYSSEY OUTCOMES found a lower risk of the primary composite endpoint (death from coronary heart disease, nonfatal MI, fatal or nonfatal ischemic stroke, or unstable angina requiring hospitalization) in the alirocumab group (9.5%) compared with placebo (11.1%) (HR, 0.85 [95% CI, 0.78, 0.93]; $p < 0.001$).

Cardiovascular outcomes trials for inclisiran [70] are ongoing, and the results will clarify its role in clinical care.

Targeting PCSK9 is a promising strategy for safely producing sustained and potentially lifelong reductions in LDL-C and other ApoB-containing lipoproteins. As such, the development of novel methods to inhibit PCSK9 is an active area of research, and the "standard of care" is likely to change over the coming decade as novel therapeutic technologies, including small interfering RNAs (inclisiran) [70], oral PCSK9 inhibitors [71], antisense oligonucleotides (ASO), PCSK9 vaccines [72], and even gene editing [73], mature and reach clinical practice.

5.1.7 Bempedoic Acid

Like statins, bempedoic acid targets the hepatic cholesterol biosynthesis pathway to reduce intrahepatic cholesterol levels, leading to upregulation of the LDL-R and enhanced clearance of circulating LDL [74]. Bempedoic acid is a prodrug that requires enzymatic activation by very long-chain acyl-CoA synthetase 1 (ACSVL1) to generate the active metabolite bempedoyl-CoA [75]. Bempedoyl-CoA then inhibits ATP citrate lyase (ACL), an enzyme multiple steps upstream of HMG-CoA reductase in cholesterol biosynthesis. ACSVL1 is highly expressed in the liver, but not in muscle, leading to hepatocyte selective inhibition of cholesterol synthesis [76]; therefore, bempedoic acid represents a promising therapeutic option for those who experience statin-associated muscle symptoms. Ongoing research is examining whether daily bempedoic acid reduces the risk of adverse cardiovascular events in stable patients with high vascular risk, inadequate LDL-C reduction with standard therapy, and documented statin intolerance [77]. The results of this study will likely guide future adoption of this drug in clinical practice.

5.1.8 Bile Acid Sequestrants

Bile acid sequestrants (BAS) are an older class of drugs that were used prior to the availability of statins. BAS—including cholestyramine, colestipol, and colesevelam—reduce LDL-C levels by altering enterohepatic bile acid exchange, limiting intestinal bile acid reabsorption, which promotes enhanced secretion of cholesterol in the bile and increase expression of hepatic LDL-R [78]. They are effective in reducing serum LDL-C concentrations by 5–30% in a dose-dependent manner and are likely effective in reducing ASCVD, although large cardiovascular outcomes studies are lacking in the post-statin era [78]. Their widespread adoption has been limited by high rates of gastrointestinal side effects, less potent LDL-C lowering compared to other available therapies, TG-raising in susceptible patients, and cost. However, they remain an option for patients who need additional LDL-C lowering despite maximally tolerated doses of other medications.

6 Lp(a) and CVD Risk

Elevated levels of Lp(a) are an independent causal factor associated with an increased risk of ASCVD and aortic valve stenosis [79]. Lp(a) is formed by the covalent attachment of apolipoprotein(a) [apo(a)] by a disulfide bond to ApoB, which generates an LDL-like particle with enhanced atherogenic potential [80]. The precise mechanisms by which Lp(a) promotes atherogenesis are incompletely understood, but likely involve (1) increased propensity for subendothelial retention due to interactions of apo(a) with the extracellular matrix, (2) enrichment with oxidized phospholipids, which promote inflammation and calcification, (3) contribution to endothelial dysfunction, and (4) interference with thrombolysis [81].

Lp(a) was discovered in the 1960s and early studies through the 1970–1980s linked elevated levels to increased risk of coronary heart disease [81]. Recent genetic studies [82], meta-analyses [83], and Mendelian randomization studies [84], as well as sub-analyses of PCSK9i outcomes trials examining the effects of Lp(a) reduction [85], have confirmed and extended these findings. There is now strong evidence of an independent association between Lp(a) levels and the risk of MI, stroke, peripheral artery disease, and aortic valve stenosis among individuals with or without established ASCVD at baseline.

Lp(a) levels are highly genetically determined (~70–90%) and remarkably stable across the lifespan within a given person [86]. Between individuals, however, Lp(a) levels vary widely in a "left-shifted" Gaussian curve, from <0.1 mg/dL to >200 mg/dL, with notable differences across self-reported racial and ethnic groups [86]. For example, mean Lp(a) levels in Black and South-Asian populations are nearly two-fold greater than those in White and East-Asian populations [87]. It is estimated that approximately one in every five adults, corresponding to more than 1.5 billion people worldwide, have elevated Lp(a) levels >50 mg/dL (~125 nmol/L) and may therefore benefit from dedicated Lp(a) lowering therapy [88, 89]. Measuring Lp(a) is complicated because of variability in the LDL and apo(a) moieties. Recent scientific statements from the AHA, National Lipid Association (NLA), and European Atherosclerosis Society (EAS) broadly agree, recommending that clinicians use assays that are (1) insensitive to apo(a) isoforms, (2) traceable to the internationally accepted calibrator (World Health Organization/International Federation of Clinical Chemistry Reference Material SRM-2B), and (3) reported in nmol/L [81, 90, 91].

6.1 Current and Future Pharmacological Interventions

Common strategies to reduce lipid and lipoprotein levels and improve cardiovascular health, including healthy lifestyle behaviors and modifications, have not been shown to have a significant impact on Lp(a) levels [91]. Furthermore, conventional methods to lower LDL-C have minimal/mixed (statins) or modest (PCSK9i) impact on Lp(a). Niacin has been shown to decrease Lp(a) levels by 30–40%, but it does not have a role in the contemporary care of patients at risk for ASCVD except under very unique circumstances [91, 92].

Mixed evidence exists on the association between statin therapy and changes in Lp(a). Preliminary studies showed no significant statin-induced changes in Lp(a), with some even showing increases. A recent meta-analysis of 39 studies including 24,448 participants indicated that statin therapy produces no change in Lp(a) (0.1% mean increase; 95% CI −3.6 to 4.0%) [93]. Similarly, no specific statins or statin intensities were found to significantly reduce Lp(a). In light of these data, it is unlikely that statins produce clinically meaningful changes in Lp(a), especially when weighed against the expected CVD risk reduction of lowering

LDL-C. Accordingly, current guidelines treat elevated Lp(a) as a risk-enhancing factor for ASCVD, which favors the initiation of statin therapy in individuals at intermediate risk [35]. However, statin therapy does not fully mitigate ASCVD risk from elevated Lp(a). Independent of improvements in LDL-C, when Lp(a) levels remain elevated, individuals experience higher ASCVD risk [93, 94].

While RCTs have yet to directly examine whether pharmacologically lowering Lp(a) results in long-term improvements in cardiovascular outcomes, recent post hoc analyses of PCSK9i trials support the viability of this approach. Analysis of the FOURIER trial found that evolocumab treatment in patients with established ASCVD led to significant reductions in Lp(a) levels and that participants with higher Lp(a) levels at baseline experienced greater absolute improvements [95]. Similarly, post hoc analysis of ODYSSEY OUTCOMES showed that Lp(a) lowering with PCSK9i therapy was associated with significant reductions in cardiovascular events among patients with recent ACS. Specifically, each 5 mg/dL reduction in Lp(a) corresponded with a 2.5% relative risk reduction in cardiovascular events [96]. Other studies have generated similar estimates, finding that lowering Lp(a) by 50 mg/dL would be needed to produce a 20% risk reduction in secondary prevention trials [97]; lowering Lp(a) by 100 mg/dL would be necessary to yield an equivalent risk reduction to lowering LDL-C by 39 mg/dL (1 mmol/L) [98]. With mounting evidence showing moderate improvements in Lp(a) levels with PCSK9i pharmacotherapies, additional investigations are needed before updating current guidelines and informing clinical decision-making practices.

In patients with elevated Lp(a) and LDL-C who continue to have progressive ASCVD despite optimal medical therapy, lipoprotein apheresis may also be considered in individuals with LDL-C >100 mg/dL and Lp(a) >60 mg/dL. A recent retrospective cohort study found a 63% reduction in Lp(a) levels with lipoprotein apheresis therapy and a 94% decrease in major cardiovascular events on treatment compared to pretreatment over a mean period of 4 years [99]. Despite its potential utility, however, barriers to apheresis use include its high cost, discomfort and duration, and potential negative impact on the patients' quality of life. Further, it may not be available close enough to a patient's home to be accessible on a regular basis [100].

Novel pharmacotherapies are currently being investigated that directly or indirectly target Lp(a). One phase 2 trial conducted in nearly 300 patients with Lp(a) levels ≥60 mg/dL found that pelacarsen (formerly known as AKCEA-APO(a)-L$_{Rx}$), an ASO targeting the mRNA *LPA* gene product, produced a greater than 80% reduction in Lp(a) levels at its highest dose. Moreover, 98% of patients achieved Lp(a) levels ≤50 mg/dL at the highest cumulative dose regimen [101]. Further research is ongoing to test whether this and small interfering mRNA therapeutic interventions [102] will reduce ASCVD events in a safe, well-tolerated regimen. The CETP inhibitor, obicetrapib, has demonstrated significant Lp(a) reductions as well and may prove to be effective for ASCVD risk reduction (see HDL section below).

7 Triglyceride-Rich Lipoproteins, Triglycerides, and CVD Risk

HTG, defined by national organizations and in multiple scientific statements as a 12-h fasting lipid profile with TG $\geq$150 mg/dL, is present in approximately one in every four individuals in the United States and is an independent risk factor/risk-enhancing factor for the development of ASCVD [21, 103] and a component of the metabolic syndrome indicating the presence of insulin resistance. Compared to those with non-fasting TG of ~70 mg/dL, individuals with TG of 580 mg/dL have a >5-fold risk for MI, >3-fold risk for ischemic heart disease and ischemic stroke, and >2-fold risk for all-cause mortality [21]. Individuals with TG $\geq$500 mg/dL are also at increased risk for acute pancreatitis.

TG is predominantly carried by lipoproteins in the circulation within TRL. Therefore, TG levels serve as a nonlinear proxy for TRL levels. As a class, TRLs constitute a heterogenous pool of lipoproteins, including VLDL, IDL, and CM, as well as their remnants [21, 104]. The relationship between TG levels and TRL abundance is complex, since both the number of TRL particles and the amount of TGs contained within each particle vary. Importantly, TRLs (which are ApoB-containing lipoproteins) smaller than 70 nm can cross the endothelial barrier and directly contribute to atherosclerosis [15]. Supporting this, ApoB48 has been found in human atherosclerotic plaques [105] and TG levels are causally associated with ASCVD in epidemiologic [106] and Mendelian randomization studies [107]. TRLs may contribute to atherosclerosis by several mechanisms including (1) directly, by subendothelial glycoprotein matrix entrapment followed by macrophage uptake and foam cell formation, (2) indirectly, by fatty acid-induced endothelial dysfunction/injury, and (3) as a bystander in individuals where HTG is a strong signal of accompanying insulin resistance and other metabolic derangements that by themselves contribute to ASCVD risk (e.g., hypertension, hyperglycemia, and conditions characterized by inflammation and increased coagulation) [15].

7.1 Common Causes of Hypertriglyceridemia and Treatment Approaches

Most forms of HTG develop due to a combination of genetic and environmental causes [108]. HTG is generally multifactorial and polygenic, occurring in individuals with susceptibility due to the cumulative effect of multiple genes and exposure to a permissive environment, such as the calorie-rich, highly processed, and nutrient-poor foods found in a "Western" diet. Furthermore, there are strong overlaps between factors associated with HTG and insulin resistance/metabolic syndrome [10].

HTG is caused by increased production or impaired clearance of TRLs or often both [109]. Accordingly, there are several therapies that modulate TRL production and metabolism to reduce TG levels, including fibrates, omega-3 fatty acids, and recent novel therapies targeting angiopoietin-like protein 3 (ANGPTL3) and ApoC-III. The data on decreasing TGs to reduce ASCVD risk are complicated by several key failures in cardiovascular outcomes trials of fibrates and other TG-lowering therapeutics. Nordestgaard reviewed multiple lipid management guidelines published between 1984 and 2014 and found all contained recommendations to treat HTG when the TG level is ≥500 mg/dL to prevent episodes of acute pancreatitis. However, they found that guidelines were inconsistent with respect to HTG treatment for moderate elevations to reduce ASCVD risk [21]. In addition, Marston et al. concluded from a systematic review that TG-lowering results in improved ASCVD outcomes, but to a lesser extent than from lowering LDL-C or non-HDL-C [110] suggesting that ASCVD risk is reduced by clearance of atherogenic particles, while acute pancreatitis risk is reduced by improved hydrolysis of TRL fatty acids (i.e., TG lowering).

7.1.1 Fibrates

Fibrates are agonists of the hormone receptor peroxisome proliferator-activated receptor (PPAR)-alpha; they reduce LDL-C by ~6–12% and TG by ~20–40% [111, 112]. A major meta-analysis conducted in 2010, including data from 18 fibrate trials and 45,058 participants, found that while fibrates did significantly reduce coronary events (~13%), they did not lead to significant reductions in stroke risk, vascular mortality, or all-cause mortality [112]. Furthermore, the Action to Control Cardiovascular Risk in Diabetes (ACCORD) trial, conducted in 2010, examined the role of adding fenofibrate to simvastatin in 5518 patients with type 2 diabetes [113]. It found no additional benefit of fenofibrate compared to simvastatin alone on fatal cardiovascular events, nonfatal cardiovascular events, or stroke. Considering these results, in 2016, the FDA withdrew approvals it had previously given for the use of fenofibrate with statins for the treatment of hypercholesterolemia.

Findings from a subgroup analysis of fibrate trials indicated that patients with higher TGs may derive more benefit than those with normal or only modestly elevated TGs. The Pemafibrate to Reduce Cardiovascular OutcoMes by Reducing Triglycerides IN patiENTs With Diabetes (PROMINENT) trial was conducted to investigate this approach, but it was stopped early (2022) due to futility [114]. These results support a reasonable conclusion that fibrates do not reduce ASCVD risk when added to statins despite evidence of benefit as monotherapy in the pre-statin era.

7.1.2 Omega-3 Fatty Acids

Omega-3 fatty acids are a class of long-chain polyunsaturated fatty acids (PUFA), including eicosapentaenoic acid (EPA) and docosahexaenoic acid (DHA), which are the major bioactive lipids found in fish oils. Interest in fish oils in general, and

EPA and DHA in particular, for the prevention of ASCVD began in the 1970s, with the observation that indigenous residents of Greenland had a diet rich in fat due to consumption of fatty fish, yet experienced lower rates of cardiovascular disease than Western populations with comparable fat intake [115]. This triggered a wave of research examining the effects of a variety of different fish oil products or purified EPA and DHA on cardiovascular outcomes. Despite initial promise in early trials, by 2012, larger meta-analyses revealed a mixed picture, with evidence of beneficial effects on vascular death, but not on total mortality, sudden death, stroke, or arrhythmia [116].

Two trials, the Reduction of Cardiovascular Events with Icosapent Ethyl-Intervention Trial (REDUCE-IT) [117] and the Outcomes Study to Assess STatin Residual Risk Reduction with EpaNova in HiGh CV Risk PatienTs with Hypertriglyceridemia (STRENGTH) [118], have attempted to clarify the role of pharmaceutical grade high-dose EPA alone or EPA/DHA in ASCVD prevention. REDUCE-IT examined the effect of high-dose EPA ethyl ester (icosapent ethyl) vs mineral oil placebo in 8179 patients at high risk for ASCVD (70% secondary prevention, 30% primary prevention) with elevated TG (median 216 mg/dL) and well-controlled LDL-C on statin therapy (range 41–100 mg/dL, mean 75). Over 4.9 years of follow-up, treatment with 4 g/day EPA significantly reduced major cardiovascular events (cardiovascular death, nonfatal MI, coronary revascularization, or unstable angina) by 25% compared to placebo, achieving an absolute risk reduction of 4.8% (17.2% vs 22.0% event rates in EPA-treated vs placebo). These effects corresponded to 19.7% and 6.6% greater median reductions in TGs and LDL-C, respectively, in treatment compared to placebo, though the differences in LDL-C were mostly driven by increases from the mineral oil placebo. However, the event reduction is more than expected based on the lipid differences alone. Adverse effects were notable for a nonsignificant trend toward increased serious bleeding events (2.7% EPA vs 2.1% placebo) and a significantly increased rate of hospitalization for atrial fibrillation or flutter (3.1% EPA vs 2.1% placebo).

STRENGTH examined the effects of high doses of a mixed carboxylic acid preparation of EPA/DHA (EPA 0.55 g, DHA 0.2 g per capsule) vs corn oil control on cardiovascular events in a population similar to the one studied in REDUCE-IT [118]. STRENGTH included 13,078 patients at high CVD risk (55% with established ASCVD), with elevated TG (median 239 mg/dL) and controlled LDL-C (median 75 mg/dL) on statin therapy, with a mean follow-up of 42 months. The trial was stopped early for futility, with a HR of 0.99 for the primary composite endpoint of cardiovascular death, nonfatal MI, nonfatal stroke, coronary revascularization, or hospitalization for unstable angina. The reasons for the large difference between STRENGTH and REDUCE-IT remain unclear, with proposed mechanisms including (1) the lower EPA content in the STRENGTH study drug, (2) a potential deleterious effect of the mineral oil placebo in REDUCE-IT, or (3) potential deleterious effects of DHA which counterbalance the favorable properties of EPA [119]. Future studies will likely provide more clarity on these issues. For now, multiple organizations recommend that clinicians consider icosapent ethyl as an adjunct to statin therapy in adult patients with elevated TG and high risk of ASCVD who have characteristics of those enrolled in REDUCE-IT (NLA Statement [120]; ACC Expert Consensus Decision Pathway [121]; and EAS/European Society of Cardiology [122]).

7.2 ApoC-III and ANGPTL3 Inhibition Development

ApoC-III (found on TRLs) and ANGPTL3 (circulating) are two proteins that elevate circulating TG/TRL and atherogenic lipoprotein levels. They do so through various mechanisms, including by inhibiting LPL and suppressing hepatic uptake of lipoproteins (VLDL remnants in the case of ApoC-III and LDL in the case of ANGPTL3), among others [123]. Novel therapies targeting these proteins are currently under development, which promise to reduce residual ASCVD risk for patients with elevated TGs despite optimal LDL-C-lowering therapy.

7.2.1 ApoC-III

In 2019, the first-in-human study investigating volanesorsen, an ASO that inhibits hepatic ApoC-III production, was published, showing significant reductions in TG among 66 patients with familial chylomicronemia syndrome (FCS). Volanesorsen lowered TG levels by 77%, from a baseline mean of 2267 down to 590 mg/dL [124]. Despite these results, this therapy has not received approval in the United States due to drug-induced side effects including a reduction in platelets, injection site reactions, and flu-like symptoms [125]. A phase 1/2a dose-escalation trial of the next-generation N-acetylgalactosamine (GalNAc)-conjugated ASO olezarsen (formerly AKCEA-APOCIII-L$_{Rx}$) was completed in 40 healthy volunteers with variable elevation of TG levels (either ≥90 or ≥200 mg/dL). In addition to finding a favorable safety profile, the study also showed significant lipid profile improvements including decreased TC, ApoB, VLDL-C, and non-HDL-C, as well as increased HDL-C [126]. To better understand the efficacy of olezarsen in patients with, or at high risk for, established CVD, a phase 2b dose-ranging study was conducted in 114 patients with HTG (TG 200–500 mg/dL). Treatment with olezarsen significantly decreased ApoC-III, TGs, and atherogenic lipoproteins compared to placebo [127]. Cardiovascular outcomes trials are still needed to determine whether inhibition of ApoC-III produces the expected reduction in ASCVD suggested by its favorable effects on lipids and ApoB levels.

7.2.2 ANGPTL3

Several pharmacotherapies have been developed to specifically target ANGPTL3 for TG lowering, including vupanorsen, a GalNAc-conjugated ASO (development discontinued as of 2022), and evinacumab, a fully human monoclonal antibody. For the former, a phase 1 study of 44 healthy volunteers showed a significant reduction in atherogenic lipoproteins including TG, VLDL-C, ApoC-III, and LDL-C [128]. The latter, evinacumab, was shown to decrease TG and other lipid levels in a dose-dependent manner in both a single ascending dose study ($n = 83$) and a multiple ascending dose study ($n = 56$). These phase 1 studies, conducted among individuals with mixed dyslipidemia and borderline high TG, found that the highest dose of evinacumab lowered TGs by ~80% while also lowering LDL-C levels [129]. Evinacumab does not effectively lower TG in individuals with FCS who do not express LPL. However, it does have clinical utility and FDA approval for the treatment of individuals who have homozygous familial hypercholesterolemia (HoFH), in which there are defects in both copies of the *LDL-R* gene, and for whom there are limited available therapeutic options [130].

7.3 *Less Common Causes of HTG and Treatment Approaches*

HTG may be severe and in those cases is almost always due to environmental factors and polygenic influences. Polygenic and multifactorial HTG syndromes include familial combined hyperlipidemia (FCHL), familial hypertriglyceridemia (FHTG), and multifactorial chylomicronemia syndrome (MCS), while familial chylomicronemia syndrome (FCS), familial dysbetalipoproteinemia (FDBL), and inherited lipodystrophy (LD) are monogenic disorders [131].

FCHL and FHTG represent comparatively common conditions with prevalence rates of 1:100 and 1:100–200, respectively. Multiple cardiometabolic risk factors and comorbidities are closely associated with FCHL including insulin resistance/ DM, abdominal obesity, and hepatic steatosis. Given its clinical presentation, characterized by moderate-to-severe HTG and severe hypercholesterolemia with elevated ApoB levels, this condition carries a very high ASCVD risk and is an indication for high-intensity statin as foundational therapy [132]. Patients with FHTG experience moderate-to-severe HTG as a result of excess VLDL; their lifetime risk of acute pancreatitis and ASCVD is proportional to their TG and ApoB levels, respectively [107].

FCS and inherited LD are both rare conditions that affect approximately 1 in every 1 million individuals. FCS is an autosomal recessive disorder predominantly caused by biallelic mutations in the genes that encode LPL (*LPL*) or LPL helper proteins (*APOC2, APOA5, GPIHBP1, LMF1*), leading to impaired CM-TG lipolysis and prolonged CM circulating residence time. Generally presenting in childhood, FCS is characterized by persistent fasting serum TG levels >880 mg/dL, eruptive xanthomas, and increased risk for recurrent episodes of acute pancreatitis [133]. Moreover, FCS may be initially suspected in asymptomatic infants with lipemic plasma. Symptoms and avoidance of pancreatitis can generally be achieved with strict dietary fat restriction and avoidance of alcohol, although not in all cases. Additionally, adherence is difficult to sustain and adversely affects quality of life. While current pharmacologic interventions are ineffective in patients with minimal or no LPL activity, novel therapies that target ApoC-III may hold promise in the long-term care for patients with FCS [134]. ANGPTL3-targeting therapies are being investigated in others with severe HTG (but not FCS) [135]. Additionally, lomitapide, a small-molecule inhibitor of microsomal TG transfer protein (MTTP), which is FDA-approved for the treatment of HoFH, has been studied in FCS. However, side effects, including steatorrhea and accumulated hepatic fat, and other factors have precluded its use in FCS [136].

Those affected by inherited LD have a diminished capacity to store excess lipids in peripheral adipose tissue [137], which, depending on the severity, can lead to variable degrees of insulin resistance and hepatic steatosis. The impairments in fatty acid mobilization and peripheral lipolysis observed in LD syndromes, which stem from alterations in adipose tissue function, can cause elevated serum TG levels [138]. There are a wide range of LD syndromes, and the reader is encouraged to review the impact of LD on lipids and ASCVD from the work by Hussain, Patni, and Garg [139] for further clarification. In individuals who are leptin-deficient, replacement therapy may help manage insulin resistance, hyperglycemia, hepatic steatosis, and insatiable hunger [131] and is being investigated as a potential therapy in partial LD [140].

8   HDL and CVD Risk

HDLs are the smallest and densest class of lipoproteins produced. HDLs are a heterogenous group of particles with distinct sizes, densities, and protein and lipid contents, which share the common feature of an ApoA1 protein scaffold [141]. While commonly used terms for HDL (or what is clinically measured, HDL-C) such as "good cholesterol" do reflect a general scientific consensus that HDL has important anti-atherogenic properties, the actual relationship between HDL and the development of ASCVD is complex and incompletely understood. Therapeutics that raise HDL-C have failed to improve ASCVD outcomes and dampened enthusiasm for HDL-altering drugs; however, targeting HDL function may prove a more promising strategy for future therapeutics.

8.1   HDL-C and ASCVD

Early reports, beginning in the 1970s [142, 143] and confirmed by numerous epidemiological studies over the subsequent decades [144], linked low levels of plasma HDL-C to an elevated risk of ASCVD, while higher levels of HDL-C (up to ~75 mg/dL) were associated with protection from ASCVD. Consistent with this, HDL-C levels are useful in ASCVD risk prediction and commonly used risk estimators, such as the PCE, include HDL-C levels in their models [38]. Furthermore, several rare genetic conditions, including Tangier disease (*ABCA1* mutation) and ApoA1 deficiency (*APOA1* mutation), are characterized by very low HDL levels and (likely) accelerated development of ASCVD [145, 146].

Despite compelling epidemiology, additional evidence sheds a different light on the nature of the relationship between HDL-C and ASCVD. First, HDL-C levels exhibit a curvilinear and possibly even U-shaped relationship with ASCVD risk, with increased risk observed at both extreme highs ($\geq$100 mg/dL) and lows of HDL-C [147]. In particular, a recent multicenter prospective cohort study conducted in nearly 20,000 patients with HDL-C levels >80 mg/dL found that very high HDL-C levels were associated with an increased risk of all-cause mortality (HR, 1.96; 95% CI, 1.42–2.71; $p < 0.001$) and cardiovascular death (HR, 1.71; 95% CI, 1.09–2.68; $p = 0.02$) when compared to individuals with HDL-C levels of 40–60 mg/dL [148]. Moreover, several Mendelian randomization studies have cast doubt on whether HDL-C levels are causally related to ASCVD development, since single-nucleotide polymorphisms leading to genetically elevated or decreased levels of HDL-C did not appear to confer protection or susceptibility to ASCVD in these studies [149–151]. Lastly, therapies designed to increase HDL-C levels, such as CETP inhibitors, have yielded mixed results in cardiovascular outcomes studies, despite markedly increasing HDL-C; additionally, when ASCVD risk reduction was achieved, it was felt to be due to the LDL-C lowering rather than HDL-C raising effects of these medications [152]. These observations suggest that the pleiotropic functions that HDL serves in health and disease cannot be estimated directly by HDL-C or HDL particle levels alone [5]. Furthermore, in many individuals, the level of HDL-C likely reflects secondary effects from HTG-associated CETP activity and thus is a better indicator of the negative impact of insulin resistance/HTG rather than the direct impact of low levels of HDL.

Several aspects of HDL functionality have been proposed to contribute to its anti-atherosclerotic effects, including its antioxidative and anti-inflammatory properties and its central role in the efflux of cholesterol from atheroma [5]. The recognition that HDL function or "quality" may be more important than the quantity of HDL-C has led to the development of several assays measuring HDL functionality, which may find their way into clinical practice [153]. Assays of cholesterol efflux capacity, a proxy for reverse cholesterol transport that predicts ASCVD risk, represent one notable example [154].

8.2 Targeting HDL

Targeting HDL to reduce ASCVD risk remains largely experimental, as no therapies to date have been FDA-approved for this purpose. CETP inhibitors increase HDL-C and reduce LDL-C by preventing the exchange of HDL-C for ApoB-TG. The three earliest CETP inhibitors, torcetrapib, dalcetrapib, and evacetrapib, had phase 3 cardiovascular outcomes studies resulting in either harm (torcetrapib) or futility despite potent HDL-C increases.

More recently, however, a phase 3 study of anacetrapib in 30,499 patients with established ASCVD on high-intensity atorvastatin therapy showed a significant reduction in major coronary events (RR = 0.91), along with an increase in HDL-C of 104% and a decrease in non-HDL-C of 18% (17 mg/dL) [155]. Notably, this reduction in major coronary events was in line with what would be expected from a 17 mg/dL reduction in LDL-C over a similar timeframe, casting doubt on whether increased HDL-C levels played any beneficial role in this trial [156]. Ultimately, despite the success of this trial, further development of anacetrapib and FDA approval were not pursued. One additional CETP inhibitor, obicetrapib, is currently in phase 3 trials and has properties that suggest it will be useful in reducing ASCVD by lowering LDL-C and Lp(a) by >40% each and raising HDL-C by >100% [157].

9 Conclusion

We have reviewed both the physiological and pathological roles of lipids and lipoproteins, as well as potential causes for their derangements and strategies for their management. Despite specific areas with a large evidence base, future basic science, clinical, and epidemiological research is still needed to understand the complex relationship between lipids, lipoproteins, and ASCVD risk. Moreover, ongoing clinical trials investigating new targets, especially Lp(a) and TRLs, show promise in helping to reduce residual ASCVD risk in those for whom LDL-C is already well-controlled. Looking forward, novel targeting strategies, including monoclonal antibodies, ASO, small interfering RNA therapeutics, vaccinations, and gene editing tools may broaden the therapeutic options available to patients affected by dyslipidemia.

A bigger challenge than managing complex dyslipidemias may be broader adherence to, acceptance of, and availability of therapeutics for those in need. Contemporary guideline adherence rates are greatly hampered by gaps in payor coverage, widespread skepticism about statin therapy despite overwhelming evidence of benefit and low risk, and severe underrepresentation and underreporting affecting underserved groups in our society. It is our hope that this review provides useful information that will help clinicians, investigators, and organizations to reverse this divergence and to ensure that high-quality and timely care is delivered to those who need it the most.

Disclosures and Conflicts of Interests DS acts as a consultant for Amgen, Novartis, Ionis, and Akcea and as an investigator for Akcea, Amgen, Amryt, Astra-Zeneca, Ionis, Novartis, Regeneron, RegenXBio, and Verve Therapeutics.

References

1. Tsao CW, et al. Heart disease and stroke statistics-2022 update: a report from the American Heart Association. Circulation. 2022;145:e153–639.
2. World Health Organization. Vol. 2022. World Health Organization; 2022. www.who.int.

3. Dowhan W, Bogdanov M, Mileykovskaya E. Biochemistry of lipids, lipoproteins and membranes. Elsevier; 2016. p. 1–40.

4. Litwack G. In: Litwack G, editor. Human biochemistry. Boston: Academic; 2022. p. 227–85.

5. Rohatgi A, Westerterp M, von Eckardstein A, Remaley A, Rye KA. HDL in the 21st century: a multifunctional roadmap for future HDL research. Circulation. 2021;143:2293–309.

6. Phillips ML, et al. A single copy of apolipoprotein B-48 is present on the human chylomicron remnant. J Lipid Res. 1997;38:1170–7.

7. Uhlen M, et al. Proteomics. Tissue-based map of the human proteome. Science. 2015;347:1260419.

8. Ference BA, Kastelein JJP, Catapano AL. Lipids and lipoproteins in 2020. JAMA. 2020;324:595–6.

9. Dash S, Xiao C, Morgantini C, Lewis GF. New insights into the regulation of chylomicron production. Annu Rev Nutr. 2015;35:265–94.

10. Heeren J, Scheja L. Metabolic-associated fatty liver disease and lipoprotein metabolism. Mol Metab. 2021;50:101238.

11. Gin P, et al. The acidic domain of GPIHBP1 is important for the binding of lipoprotein lipase and chylomicrons. J Biol Chem. 2008;283:29554–62.

12. Chait A, et al. Remnants of the triglyceride-rich lipoproteins, diabetes, and cardiovascular disease. Diabetes. 2020;69:508–16.

13. Willnow TE. Mechanisms of hepatic chylomicron remnant clearance. Diabet Med. 1997;14(Suppl 3):S75–80.

14. Goldstein JL, Brown MS. The LDL receptor. Arterioscler Thromb Vasc Biol. 2009;29:431–8.

15. Sniderman AD, et al. Apolipoprotein B particles and cardiovascular disease: a narrative review. JAMA Cardiol. 2019;4:1287–95.

16. Ference BA, et al. Low-density lipoproteins cause atherosclerotic cardiovascular disease. 1. Evidence from genetic, epidemiologic, and clinical studies. A consensus statement from the European Atherosclerosis Society Consensus Panel. Eur Heart J. 2017;38:2459–72.

17. Boren J, et al. Low-density lipoproteins cause atherosclerotic cardiovascular disease: pathophysiological, genetic, and therapeutic insights: a consensus statement from the European Atherosclerosis Society Consensus Panel. Eur Heart J. 2020;41:2313–30.

18. Salinas CAA, Chapman MJ. Remnant lipoproteins: are they equal to or more atherogenic than LDL? Curr Opin Lipidol. 2020;31:132–9.

19. Boren J, Williams KJ. The central role of arterial retention of cholesterol-rich apolipoprotein-B-containing lipoproteins in the pathogenesis of atherosclerosis: a triumph of simplicity. Curr Opin Lipidol. 2016;27:473–83.

20. Nakashima Y, Wight TN, Sueishi K. Early atherosclerosis in humans: role of diffuse intimal thickening and extracellular matrix proteoglycans. Cardiovasc Res. 2008;79:14–23.

21. Nordestgaard BG. Triglyceride-rich lipoproteins and atherosclerotic cardiovascular disease: new insights from epidemiology, genetics, and biology. Circ Res. 2016;118:547–63.

22. Libby P, et al. Atherosclerosis. Nat Rev Dis Primers. 2019;5:56.

23. Fernández-Friera L, et al. Prevalence, vascular distribution, and multiterritorial extent of subclinical atherosclerosis in a middle-aged cohort. Circulation. 2015;131:2104–13.

24. Ference BA, et al. Effect of long-term exposure to lower low-density lipoprotein cholesterol beginning early in life on the risk of coronary heart disease: a Mendelian randomization analysis. J Am Coll Cardiol. 2012;60:2631–9.

25. Goldstein JL, Brown MS. A century of cholesterol and coronaries: from plaques to genes to statins. Cell. 2015;161:161–72.

26. Ginsberg HN, et al. LDL-C calculated by Friedewald, Martin-Hopkins, or NIH equation 2 versus beta-quantification: pooled alirocumab trials. J Lipid Res. 2022;63:100148.

27. Friedewald WT, Levy RI, Fredrickson DS. Estimation of the concentration of low-density lipoprotein cholesterol in plasma, without use of the preparative ultracentrifuge. Clin Chem. 1972;18:499–502.

28. Martin SS, et al. Friedewald-estimated versus directly measured low-density lipoprotein cholesterol and treatment implications. J Am Coll Cardiol. 2013;62:732–9.
29. Fan W, Philip S, Granowitz C, Toth PP, Wong ND. Prevalence of US adults with triglycerides >/= 150 mg/dl: NHANES 2007-2014. Cardiol Ther. 2020;9:207–13.
30. Xiao C, Dash S, Morgantini C, Hegele RA, Lewis GF. Pharmacological targeting of the atherogenic dyslipidemia complex: the next frontier in CVD prevention beyond lowering LDL cholesterol. Diabetes. 2016;65:1767–78.
31. Sabatine MS, et al. Evolocumab and clinical outcomes in patients with cardiovascular disease. N Engl J Med. 2017;376:1713–22.
32. Martin SS, et al. Comparison of a novel method vs the Friedewald equation for estimating low-density lipoprotein cholesterol levels from the standard lipid profile. JAMA. 2013;310:2061–8.
33. Sampson M, et al. A new equation for calculation of low-density lipoprotein cholesterol in patients with normolipidemia and/or hypertriglyceridemia. JAMA Cardiol. 2020;5:540–8.
34. Maki KC, Grant JK, Orringer CE. LDL-C estimation: the perils of living with imperfection. J Am Coll Cardiol. 2022;79:542–4.
35. Grundy SM, et al. 2018 AHA/ACC/AACVPR/AAPA/ABC/ACPM/ADA/AGS/APhA/ASPC/ NLA/PCNA guideline on the management of blood cholesterol: a report of the American College of Cardiology/American Heart Association Task Force on clinical practice guidelines. Circulation. 2019;139:e1082–143.
36. Wilson PWF, et al. Lipid measurements in the management of cardiovascular diseases: practical recommendations a scientific statement from the national lipid association writing group. J Clin Lipidol. 2021;15:629–48.
37. Wilson PW, et al. Prediction of coronary heart disease using risk factor categories. Circulation. 1998;97:1837–47.
38. Stone NJ, et al. 2013 ACC/AHA guideline on the treatment of blood cholesterol to reduce atherosclerotic cardiovascular risk in adults: a report of the American College of Cardiology/ American Heart Association Task Force on practice guidelines. Circulation. 2014;129:S1–45.
39. ACC/AHS. Vol. 2022. 2022. tools.acc.org.
40. Mach F, et al. 2019 ESC/EAS guidelines for the management of dyslipidaemias: lipid modification to reduce cardiovascular risk. Eur Heart J. 2020;41:111–88.
41. Lloyd-Jones DM, et al. Estimating longitudinal risks and benefits from cardiovascular preventive therapies among Medicare patients. J Am Coll Cardiol. 2017;69:1617–36.
42. Nordestgaard BG, et al. Quantifying atherogenic lipoproteins for lipid-lowering strategies: consensus-based recommendations from EAS and EFLM. Atherosclerosis. 2020;294:46–61.
43. Langlois MR, et al. Quantifying atherogenic lipoproteins: current and future challenges in the era of personalized medicine and very low concentrations of LDL cholesterol. A consensus statement from EAS and EFLM. Clin Chem. 2018;64:1006–33.
44. Nordestgaard BG, et al. Fasting is not routinely required for determination of a lipid profile: clinical and laboratory implications including flagging at desirable concentration cutpoints—a joint consensus statement from the European Atherosclerosis Society and European Federation. Eur Heart J. 2016;37:1944–58.
45. World Health Organization. Global health risks: mortality and burden of disease attributable to selected major risks. World Health Organization; 2009.
46. Arnett DK, et al. 2019 ACC/AHA guideline on the primary prevention of cardiovascular disease: a report of the American College of Cardiology/American Heart Association Task Force on clinical practice guidelines. Circulation. 2019;140:e596–646.
47. Newman CB, et al. Statin safety and associated adverse events: a scientific statement from the American Heart Association. Arterioscler Thromb Vasc Biol. 2019;39:e38–81.
48. Ness GC, Zhao Z, Lopez D. Inhibitors of cholesterol biosynthesis increase hepatic low-density lipoprotein receptor protein degradation. Arch Biochem Biophys. 1996;325:242–8.
49. Silverman MG, et al. Association between lowering LDL-C and cardiovascular risk reduction among different therapeutic interventions: a systematic review and meta-analysis. JAMA. 2016;316:1289–97.

50. Davignon J. Beneficial cardiovascular pleiotropic effects of statins. Circulation. 2004;109:III39–43.
51. Cholesterol Treatment Trialists' (CTT) Collaboration. Protocol for a prospective collaborative overview of all current and planned randomized trials of cholesterol treatment regimens. Cholesterol Treatment Trialists' (CTT) Collaboration. Am J Cardiol. 1995;75:1130–4.
52. Baigent C, et al. Efficacy and safety of cholesterol-lowering treatment: prospective meta-analysis of data from 90,056 participants in 14 randomised trials of statins. Lancet. 2005;366:1267–78.
53. Cholesterol Treatment Trialists' (CTT) Collaboration, et al. Efficacy and safety of more intensive lowering of LDL cholesterol: a meta-analysis of data from 170,000 participants in 26 randomised trials. Lancet. 2010;376:1670–81.
54. Bangalore S, et al. 2013 cholesterol guidelines revisited: percent LDL cholesterol reduction or attained LDL cholesterol level or both for prognosis? Am J Med. 2016;129:384–91.
55. Cholesterol Treatment Trialists' (CTT) Collaborators. The effects of lowering LDL cholesterol with statin therapy in people at low risk of vascular disease: meta-analysis of individual data from 27 randomised trials. Lancet. 2012;380:581–90.
56. Cholesterol Treatment Trialists' (CTT) Collaborators. Efficacy and safety of LDL-lowering therapy among men and women: meta-analysis of individual data from 174 000 participants in 27 randomised trials. Lancet. 2015;385:1397–405.
57. Grant JK, et al. Under-reporting and under-representation of non-Hispanic black subjects in lipid-lowering atherosclerotic cardiovascular disease outcomes trials: a systematic review. J Clin Lipidol. 2022;16:608.
58. Armitage J, et al. Efficacy and safety of statin therapy in older people: a meta-analysis of individual participant data from 28 randomised controlled trials. Lancet. 2019;393:407–15.
59. Cholesterol Treatment Trialists' (CTT) Collaborators, et al. Efficacy of cholesterol-lowering therapy in 18,686 people with diabetes in 14 randomised trials of statins: a meta-analysis. Lancet. 2008;371:117–25.
60. Cholesterol Treatment Trialists' (CTT) Collaborators, et al. Impact of renal function on the effects of LDL cholesterol lowering with statin-based regimens: a meta-analysis of individual participant data from 28 randomised trials. Lancet Diabetes Endocrinol. 2016;4:829–39.
61. Low Wang CC, Hess CN, Hiatt WR, Goldfine AB. Clinical update: cardiovascular disease in diabetes mellitus: atherosclerotic cardiovascular disease and heart failure in type 2 diabetes mellitus—mechanisms, management, and clinical considerations. Circulation. 2016;133:2459–502.
62. Toth P, Phan B, Dayspring T. Ezetimibe therapy: mechanism of action and clinical update. Vasc Health Risk Manag. 2012;8:415.
63. Jia L, Betters JL, Yu L. Niemann-pick C1-like 1 (NPC1L1) protein in intestinal and hepatic cholesterol transport. Annu Rev Physiol. 2011;73:239–59.
64. Garcia-Calvo M, et al. The target of ezetimibe is Niemann-Pick C1-Like 1 (NPC1L1). Proc Natl Acad Sci USA. 2005;102:8132–7.
65. Sudhop T, et al. Changes in cholesterol absorption and cholesterol synthesis caused by ezetimibe and/or simvastatin in men. J Lipid Res. 2009;50:2117–23.
66. Cannon CP, et al. Ezetimibe added to statin therapy after acute coronary syndromes. N Engl J Med. 2015;372:2387–97.
67. Ferri N, et al. Proprotein convertase subtilisin kexin type 9 (PCSK9) secreted by cultured smooth muscle cells reduces macrophages LDLR levels. Atherosclerosis. 2012;220:381–6.
68. Shapiro MD, Tavori H, Fazio S. PCSK9. Circ Res. 2018;122:1420–38.
69. Schwartz GG, et al. Alirocumab and cardiovascular outcomes after acute coronary syndrome. N Engl J Med. 2018;379:2097–107.
70. Ray KK, et al. Two phase 3 trials of Inclisiran in patients with elevated LDL cholesterol. N Engl J Med. 2020;382:1507–19.
71. ClinicalTrials.gov, A Study of the Efficacy and Safety of MK-0616 (Oral PCSK9 inhibitor) in Adults with Hypercholesterolemia (MK-0616-008);

NCT05261126. https://clinicaltrials.gov/ct2/show/NCT05261126?term=oral+ pcsk9&draw=2&rank=1.

72. Sahebkar A, Momtazi-Borojeni AA, Banach M. PCSK9 vaccine: so near, yet so far! Eur Heart J. 2021;42:4007–10.

73. Musunuru K, et al. In vivo CRISPR base editing of PCSK9 durably lowers cholesterol in primates. Nature. 2021;593:429–34.

74. Ballantyne CM, et al. Role of bempedoic acid in clinical practice. Cardiovasc Drugs Ther. 2021;35:853–64.

75. Pinkosky SL, et al. Liver-specific ATP-citrate lyase inhibition by bempedoic acid decreases LDL-C and attenuates atherosclerosis. Nat Commun. 2016;7:13457.

76. Agarwala A, Goldberg AC. Bempedoic acid: a promising novel agent for LDL-C lowering. Futur Cardiol. 2020;16:361–71.

77. Nicholls S, et al. Rationale and design of the CLEAR-outcomes trial: evaluating the effect of bempedoic acid on cardiovascular events in patients with statin intolerance. Am Heart J. 2021;235:104–12.

78. Ross S, et al. Effect of bile acid sequestrants on the risk of cardiovascular events: a Mendelian randomization analysis. Circ Cardiovasc Genet. 2015;8:618–27.

79. Koschinsky ML, Marcovina SM, May LF, Gabel BR. Analysis of the mechanism of lipoprotein(a) assembly. Clin Genet. 1997;52:338–46.

80. Tsimikas S. A test in context: lipoprotein(a): diagnosis, prognosis, controversies, and emerging therapies. J Am Coll Cardiol. 2017;69:692–711.

81. Reyes-Soffer G, et al. Lipoprotein(a): a genetically determined, causal, and prevalent risk factor for atherosclerotic cardiovascular disease: a scientific statement from the American Heart Association. Arterioscler Thromb Vasc Biol. 2022;42:e48–60.

82. Kamstrup PR, Tybjaerg-Hansen A, Steffensen R, Nordestgaard BG. Genetically elevated lipoprotein(a) and increased risk of myocardial infarction. JAMA. 2009;301:2331–9.

83. Erqou S, et al. Emerging Risk Factors Collaboration. Lipoprotein(a) concentration and the risk of coronary heart disease, stroke, and nonvascular mortality. JAMA. 2009;302:412–23.

84. Kamstrup PR, Tybjaerg-Hansen A, Nordestgaard BG. Extreme lipoprotein(a) levels and improved cardiovascular risk prediction. J Am Coll Cardiol. 2013;61:1146–56.

85. Tsimikas S, Narula J. Lipoprotein(a) and CT angiography: novel insights into high-risk plaque progression. J Am Coll Cardiol. 2022;79:234–7.

86. Schmidt K, Noureen A, Kronenberg F, Utermann G. Structure, function, and genetics of lipoprotein (a). J Lipid Res. 2016;57:1339–59.

87. Enkhmaa B, Anuurad E, Berglund L. Lipoprotein (a): impact by ethnicity and environmental and medical conditions. J Lipid Res. 2016;57:1111–25.

88. Wilkinson MJ, et al. The prevalence of lipoprotein(a) measurement and degree of elevation among 2710 patients with calcific aortic valve stenosis in an academic echocardiography laboratory setting. Angiology. 2017;68:795–8.

89. Tsimikas S, Stroes ESG. The dedicated "Lp(a) clinic": a concept whose time has arrived? Atherosclerosis. 2020;300:1–9.

90. Kronenberg F, et al. Lipoprotein(a) in atherosclerotic cardiovascular disease and aortic stenosis: a European Atherosclerosis Society consensus statement. Eur Heart J. 2022;43:3925.

91. Wilson DP, et al. Use of Lipoprotein(a) in clinical practice: a biomarker whose time has come. A scientific statement from the National Lipid Association. J Clin Lipidol. 2019;13:374–92.

92. Banach M. Lipoprotein (a)—we know so much yet still have much to learn. J Am Heart Assoc. 2016;5:e003597.

93. de Boer LM, et al. Statin therapy and lipoprotein(a) levels: a systematic review and meta-analysis. Eur J Prev Cardiol. 2022;29:779–92.

94. Willeit P, et al. Baseline and on-statin treatment lipoprotein(a) levels for prediction of cardiovascular events: individual patient-data meta-analysis of statin outcome trials. Lancet. 2018;392:1311–20.

95. O'Donoghue ML, et al. Lipoprotein(a), PCSK9 inhibition, and cardiovascular risk. Circulation. 2019;139:1483–92.

96. Szarek M, et al. Lipoprotein(a) lowering by alirocumab reduces the total burden of cardiovascular events independent of low-density lipoprotein cholesterol lowering: ODYSSEY OUTCOMES trial. Eur Heart J. 2020;41:4245–55.

97. Madsen CM, Kamstrup PR, Langsted A, Varbo A, Nordestgaard BG. Lipoprotein(a)-lowering by 50 mg/dL (105 nmol/L) may be needed to reduce cardiovascular disease 20% in secondary prevention: a population-based study. Arterioscler Thromb Vasc Biol. 2020;40:255–66.

98. Burgess S, et al. Association of LPA variants with risk of coronary disease and the implications for lipoprotein(a)-lowering therapies: a Mendelian randomization analysis. JAMA Cardiol. 2018;3:619–27.

99. Moriarty PM, Gray JV, Gorby LK. Lipoprotein apheresis for lipoprotein(a) and cardiovascular disease. J Clin Lipidol. 2019;13:894–900.

100. Wang A, et al. Systematic review of low-density lipoprotein cholesterol apheresis for the treatment of familial hypercholesterolemia. J Am Heart Assoc. 2016;5:e003294.

101. Fernández-Ruiz I. AKCEA-APO(a)-LRx is an antisense oligonucleotide targeting LPA mRNA. Nat Rev Cardiol. 2020;17:132.

102. Nissen SE, et al. Single ascending dose study of a short interfering RNA targeting lipoprotein(a) production in individuals with elevated plasma lipoprotein(a) levels. JAMA. 2022;327:1679–87.

103. Carroll MD, Kit BK, Lacher DA. Trends in elevated triglyceride in adults: United States, 2001–2012. NCHS data brief, no 198. Hyattsville: National Center for Health Statistics; 2015.

104. Ginsberg HN, et al. Triglyceride-rich lipoproteins and their remnants: metabolic insights, role in atherosclerotic cardiovascular disease, and emerging therapeutic strategies-a consensus statement from the European Atherosclerosis Society. Eur Heart J. 2021;42:4791–806.

105. Nakano T, et al. Detection of apolipoproteins B-48 and B-100 carrying particles in lipoprotein fractions extracted from human aortic atherosclerotic plaques in sudden cardiac death cases. Clin Chim Acta. 2008;390:38–43.

106. Nordestgaard BG, Benn M, Schnohr P, Tybjærg-Hansen A. Nonfasting triglycerides and risk of myocardial infarction, ischemic heart disease, and death in men and women. JAMA. 2007;298:299.

107. Laufs U, Parhofer KG, Ginsberg HN, Hegele RA. Clinical review on triglycerides. Eur Heart J. 2020;41:99–109c.

108. Lewis GF, Xiao C, Hegele RA. Hypertriglyceridemia in the genomic era: a new paradigm. Endocr Rev. 2015;36:131–47.

109. Taskinen MR, et al. Dual metabolic defects are required to produce hypertriglyceridemia in obese subjects. Arterioscler Thromb Vasc Biol. 2011;31:2144–50.

110. Marston NA, et al. Association between triglyceride lowering and reduction of cardiovascular risk across multiple lipid-lowering therapeutic classes. Circulation. 2019;140:1308–17.

111. Bougarne N, et al. Molecular actions of PPARα in lipid metabolism and inflammation. Endocr Rev. 2018;39:760–802.

112. Jun M, et al. Effects of fibrates on cardiovascular outcomes: a systematic review and meta-analysis. Lancet. 2010;375:1875–84.

113. ACCORD Study Group, et al. Effects of combination lipid therapy in type 2 diabetes mellitus. N Engl J Med. 2010;362:1563–74.

114. Pradhan AD, et al. Rationale and design of the Pemafibrate to Reduce Cardiovascular Outcomes by Reducing Triglycerides in Patients with Diabetes (PROMINENT) study. Am Heart J. 2018;206:80–93.

115. Leaf A. Historical overview of n−3 fatty acids and coronary heart disease. Am J Clin Nutr. 2008;87:1978S–80S.

116. Kotwal S, Jun M, Sullivan D, Perkovic V, Neal B. Omega 3 fatty acids and cardiovascular outcomes. Circ Cardiovasc Qual Outcomes. 2012;5:808–18.

117. Bhatt DL, et al. Cardiovascular risk reduction with Icosapent ethyl for hypertriglyceridemia. N Engl J Med. 2019;380:11–22.
118. Nicholls SJ, et al. Effect of high-dose omega-3 fatty acids vs corn oil on major adverse cardiovascular events in patients at high cardiovascular risk: the STRENGTH randomized clinical trial. JAMA. 2020;324:2268–80.
119. Khan SU, et al. Effect of omega-3 fatty acids on cardiovascular outcomes: a systematic review and meta-analysis. EClinicalMedicine. 2021;38:100997.
120. Orringer CE, Jacobson TA, Maki KC. National Lipid Association Scientific Statement on the use of icosapent ethyl in statin-treated patients with elevated triglycerides and high or very-high ASCVD risk. J Clin Lipidol. 2019;13:860–72.
121. Virani SS, et al. 2021 ACC expert consensus decision pathway on the management of ASCVD risk reduction in patients with persistent hypertriglyceridemia. J Am Coll Cardiol. 2021;78:960–93.
122. Visseren FLJ, et al. 2021 ESC Guidelines on cardiovascular disease prevention in clinical practice. Eur Heart J. 2021;42:3227–337.
123. Tall AR, Thomas DG, Gonzalez-Cabodevilla AG, Goldberg IJ. Addressing dyslipidemic risk beyond LDL-cholesterol. J Clin Invest. 2022;132:e148559.
124. Witztum JL, et al. Volanesorsen and triglyceride levels in familial chylomicronemia syndrome. N Engl J Med. 2019;381:531–42.
125. Reeskamp LF, Tromp TR, Stroes ESG. The next generation of triglyceride-lowering drugs: will reducing apolipoprotein C-III or angiopoietin like protein 3 reduce cardiovascular disease? Curr Opin Lipidol. 2020;31:140–6.
126. Alexander VJ, et al. N-acetyl galactosamine-conjugated antisense drug to APOC3 mRNA, triglycerides and atherogenic lipoprotein levels. Eur Heart J. 2019;40:2785–96.
127. Tardif J-C, et al. Apolipoprotein C-III reduction in subjects with moderate hypertriglyceridaemia and at high cardiovascular risk. Eur Heart J. 2022;43:1401–12.
128. Graham MJ, et al. Cardiovascular and metabolic effects of ANGPTL3 antisense oligonucleotides. N Engl J Med. 2017;377:222–32.
129. Ahmad Z, et al. Inhibition of angiopoietin-like protein 3 with a monoclonal antibody reduces triglycerides in hypertriglyceridemia. Circulation. 2019;140:470–86.
130. Gaudet D, et al. ANGPTL3 inhibition in homozygous familial hypercholesterolemia. N Engl J Med. 2017;377:296–7.
131. Mszar R, Webb GB, Kulkarni VT, Ahmad Z, Soffer D. Genetic lipid disorders associated with atherosclerotic cardiovascular disease: molecular basis to clinical diagnosis and epidemiologic burden. Med Clin North Am. 2022;106:325–48.
132. van Greevenbroek MM, Stalenhoef AF, de Graaf J, Brouwers MC. Familial combined hyperlipidemia: from molecular insights to tailored therapy. Curr Opin Lipidol. 2014;25:176–82.
133. Valdivielso P, Ramirez-Bueno A, Ewald N. Current knowledge of hypertriglyceridemic pancreatitis. Eur J Intern Med. 2014;25:689–94.
134. Boren J, Packard CJ, Taskinen MR. The roles of ApoC-III on the metabolism of triglyceride-rich lipoproteins in humans. Front Endocrinol (Lausanne). 2020;11:474.
135. Vol. 2022. 2021. ClinicalTrials.gov, https://clinicaltrials.gov/ct2/show/NCT04863014?term=angptl3&draw=3&rank=14.
136. Williams L, et al. Familial chylomicronemia syndrome: bringing to life dietary recommendations throughout the life span. J Clin Lipidol. 2018;12:908–19.
137. Sakers A, De Siqueira MK, Seale P, Villanueva CJ. Adipose-tissue plasticity in health and disease. Cell. 2022;185:419–46.
138. Akinci B, Sahinoz M, Oral E. Lipodystrophy syndromes: presentation and treatment. [Updated 2018 Apr 24]. In: Feingold KR, Anawalt B, Boyce A, et al., editors. Endotext [Internet]. South Dartmouth: MDText.com, Inc.; 2000. https://www.ncbi.nlm.nih.gov/books/NBK513130/.
139. Hussain I, Patni N, Garg A. Lipodystrophies, dyslipidaemias and atherosclerotic cardiovascular disease. Pathology. 2019;51:202–12.

140. Vol. 2022. 2021. ClinicalTrials.gov. https://clinicaltrials.gov/ct2/show/NCT05164341?term=metreleptin&draw=2&rank=1.
141. Rosenson RS, et al. HDL measures, particle heterogeneity, proposed nomenclature, and relation to atherosclerotic cardiovascular events. Clin Chem. 2011;57:392–410.
142. Miller GJ, Miller NE. Plasma-high-density-lipoprotein concentration and development of ischaemic heart-disease. Lancet. 1975;1:16–9.
143. Castelli WP, et al. HDL cholesterol and other lipids in coronary heart disease. The cooperative lipoprotein phenotyping study. Circulation. 1977;55:767–72.
144. Emerging Risk Factors Collaboration, et al. Major lipids, apolipoproteins, and risk of vascular disease. JAMA. 2009;302:1993–2000.
145. Geller AS, et al. Genetic and secondary causes of severe HDL deficiency and cardiovascular disease. J Lipid Res. 2018;59:2421–35.
146. Hooper AJ, Hegele RA, Burnett JR. Tangier disease: update for 2020. Curr Opin Lipidol. 2020;31:80–4.
147. Madsen CM, Varbo A, Nordestgaard BG. Extreme high high-density lipoprotein cholesterol is paradoxically associated with high mortality in men and women: two prospective cohort studies. Eur Heart J. 2017;38:2478–86.
148. Liu C, et al. Association between high-density lipoprotein cholesterol levels and adverse cardiovascular outcomes in high-risk populations. JAMA Cardiol. 2022;7:672.
149. Voight BF, et al. Plasma HDL cholesterol and risk of myocardial infarction: a mendelian randomisation study. Lancet. 2012;380:572–80.
150. Varbo A, et al. Remnant cholesterol as a causal risk factor for ischemic heart disease. J Am Coll Cardiol. 2013;61:427–36.
151. Holmes MV, et al. Mendelian randomization of blood lipids for coronary heart disease. Eur Heart J. 2015;36:539–50.
152. Lincoff AM, et al. Evacetrapib and cardiovascular outcomes in high-risk vascular disease. N Engl J Med. 2017;376:1933–42.
153. Allard-Ratick MP, et al. HDL: fact, fiction, or function? HDL cholesterol and cardiovascular risk. Eur J Prev Cardiol. 2021;28:166–73.
154. Rohatgi A, et al. HDL cholesterol efflux capacity and incident cardiovascular events. N Engl J Med. 2014;371:2383–93.
155. HPS3/TIMI55–REVEAL Collaborative Group, et al. Effects of anacetrapib in patients with atherosclerotic vascular disease. N Engl J Med. 2017;377:1217–27.
156. Tall AR, Rader DJ. Trials and tribulations of CETP inhibitors. Circ Res. 2018;122:106–12.
157. Vol. 2022. 2022. ClinicalTrials.gov. https://clinicaltrials.gov/ct2/show/NCT05202509?term=obicetrapib&draw=2&rank=7.
158. Bredefeld CL, Lau R, Hussain MM. In: Richard M, McPherson A, Matthew M, Pincus R, editors. Henry's clinical diagnosis and management by laboratory methods. Elsevier; 2022. Chap. 18.

Inflammation and Cardiovascular Outcomes

Priyanka Satish and Anandita Agarwala

Key Points

- Chronic inflammation plays a key role in the development and progression of atherosclerotic cardiovascular disease (ASCVD).
- Endothelial dysfunction leads to the activation of cytokines that give rise to pro-atherogenic changes in the vascular walls.
- Inflammation also plays a role in degrading the fibrous cap of atheromatous plaque and activating prothrombotic pathways that lead to acute coronary syndrome.
- High-sensitivity C-reactive protein (hs-CRP) is commonly used as a downstream biomarker of inflammatory pathway activation. Elevated hs-CRP levels are associated with an increased cardiovascular risk.
- Inflammation plays an important role in the interplay between traditional risk factors and cardiovascular risk. Medications like statins and sodium-glucose cotransporter-2 (SGLT2) inhibitors that reduce cardiovascular risk also have effects on inflammation.
- Chronic inflammatory diseases like rheumatoid arthritis, psoriasis, and systemic lupus erythematosus (SLE) are associated with a higher risk of cardiovascular disease. These diseases are considered risk enhancers in the 2019 American College of Cardiology (ACC)/American Heart Association (AHA) Guideline on the Primary Prevention of Cardiovascular Disease.

P. Satish
Department of Cardiology, Houston Methodist DeBakey Heart and Vascular Center, Houston, TX, USA

A. Agarwala (✉)
Division of Cardiology, Center for Cardiovascular Disease Prevention, Baylor Scott & White Heart Hospital Baylor Plano, Plano, TX, USA
e-mail: Anandita.Kulkarni@bswhealth.org

K. C. Maki, D. P. Wilson (eds.), *Cardiovascular Outcomes Research*, Contemporary Cardiology, https://doi.org/10.1007/978-3-031-54960-1_10

- Drugs that specifically target inflammation as an ASCVD prevention strategy have shown promise in reducing cardiovascular events. Drugs being studied include canakinumab and colchicine.
- Targeting inflammatory and immune mechanisms has the potential to further reduce residual risk in patients optimally treated with traditional risk-lowering therapies.

# 1	Introduction

Atherosclerosis is the leading cause of cardiovascular disease and is associated with significant morbidity and mortality worldwide [1]. While the etiology of atherosclerotic cardiovascular disease (ASCVD) is multifactorial, there is increasing recognition of the role played by chronic inflammation in its development and progression. Inflammation also acts mechanistically as a common link between risk factors and the development of atherosclerosis.

Acute inflammation is an important mechanism of tissue response to microbial infection and injury. This highly coordinated response is facilitated by a complex interplay between inflammatory cells and cytokines produced by the host. Cytokines are secreted proteins that exert a multitude of biological effects necessary for the host immune response to injury. They also play a vital role in the systemic response associated with acute inflammation. With persistence of tissue injury, the development of specific adaptive changes in both cellular and humoral immune responses leads to chronic inflammation. The mechanisms involved in the chronic inflammatory pathway have crucial implications in chronic disease processes such as atherosclerosis. This chapter will review the role of inflammation in atherosclerosis, discuss ASCVD risk in chronic inflammatory states, describe the role of inflammatory biomarkers, and highlight the use of therapeutics that target inflammation.

# 2	Molecular Mechanisms of Inflammation in Atherosclerosis

The inflammatory response involves a complex interplay between the arterial wall, blood cells, and both the innate and adaptive immune systems. The endothelial layer of the vessel wall plays a central role in the development and progression of atherosclerosis [2, 3]. The endothelial lining mediates vasodilation and constriction in response to a number of different influences (metabolic, mechanical, neurohormonal, etc.), thereby regulating the amount of blood flow to various tissues (Fig. 1).

Endothelial dysfunction develops at areas of metabolic stress, for example, from hypertension, diabetes, dyslipidemia, and metabolic syndrome (Fig. 2).

Endothelial injury and dysfunction are mediated by a variety of cardiovascular risk factors including hypertension, hyperlipidemia, and diabetes mellitus, which will be discussed in more detail later in the chapter. Cardiovascular risk factors

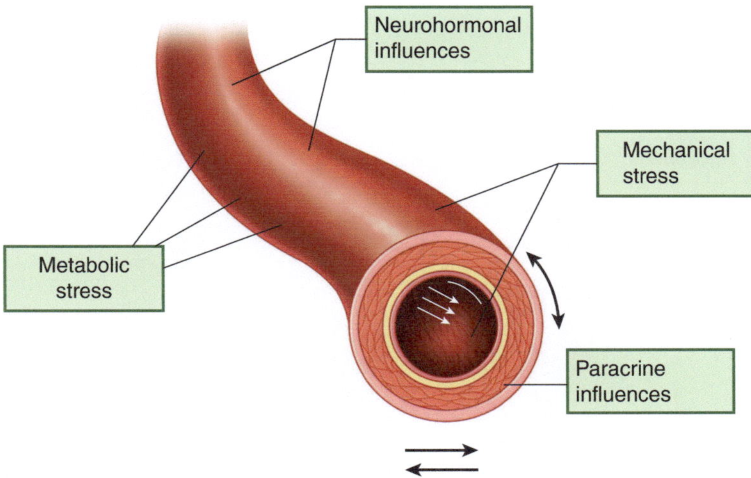

Fig. 1 Endothelial lining mediates vasodilation and constriction and exerts a variety of effects to regulate blood flow. **Adapted from:** Zipes DP, Libby P, Bonow RO, Mann DL, Tomaselli GF. (2018). *Braunwald's Heart Disease: A Textbook of Cardiovascular Medicine, 11th edition.* Elsevier. ISBN 0275970922

upregulate the production of pro-inflammatory cytokines, such as interleukin 1 beta (IL-1 β), tumor necrosis factor-alpha (TNF-α), and C-reactive protein (CRP), that bind to their receptors and activate nuclear transcription factor kappa beta (NF-kB). This, in turn, stimulates the production of vascular cell adhesion molecule-1 (VCAM-1), intercellular adhesion molecule-1 (ICAM-1), and E-selectin. This process leads to trans-endothelial migration of monocytes toward the intimal layer, which differentiate into macrophages that further amplify the inflammatory cascade. CRP downregulates the transcription of endothelial nitric oxide synthase (eNOS) at sites of endothelial dysfunction, thereby resulting in decreased nitric oxide availability and vasoconstriction.

The inflammatory cascade facilitates the development and progression of atherosclerosis. Elevated levels of circulating low-density lipoproteins (LDL) lead to their accumulation in the vessel wall [4–6]. In these areas, reactive oxygen species interact with LDL particles to form oxidized LDL (Ox-LDL) [7, 8]. Macrophages take up LDL particles to transform into foam cells (Fig. 3).

Apoptosis of these macrophages leads to formation of the lipid-rich plaque core, initially called the "fatty streak." Vascular smooth muscle cells migrate from the tunica media (middle layer of the arterial wall) to the intimal layer and have pleiotropic effects in producing collagens, elastins, and proteoglycans, which together form the fibrous cap of the atherosclerotic plaque [9, 10]. The fibrous cap lends stability to the atherosclerotic plaque and can be degraded under inflammatory conditions leading to thrombotic events like myocardial infarction (MI) and stroke. This will be discussed in a subsequent section of this chapter.

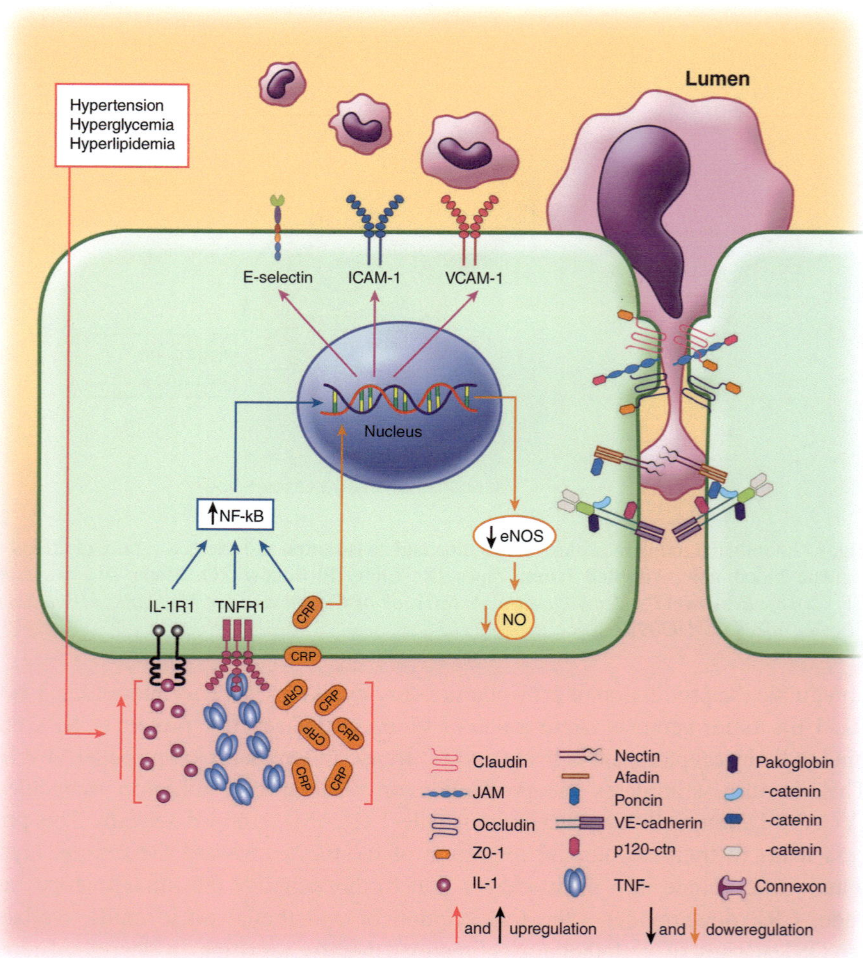

Fig. 2 Pro-inflammatory cytokines are upregulated by cardiovascular risk factors (i.e., hypertension, hyperglycemia, and hyperlipidemia) that trigger a cascade of events resulting in endothelial dysfunction. **From:** Medina-Leyte, DJ, et al. Int J Mol Sci. 2021;22 (8):3850. This is an open access article distributed under the terms and conditions of the Creative Commons Attribution (CC BY) license https://creativecommons.org/licenses/by/4.0/. Abbreviations: *CRP* C-reactive protein, *eNOS* endothelial nitric oxide synthase, *ICAM-1* intercellular adhesion molecule-1, *IL-1R1* interleukin 1 receptor 1, *NF-kB* nuclear factor kappa beta, *NO* nitric oxide, *TNFR1* tumor necrosis factor receptor 1, *VCAM-1* vascular cell adhesion molecule-1

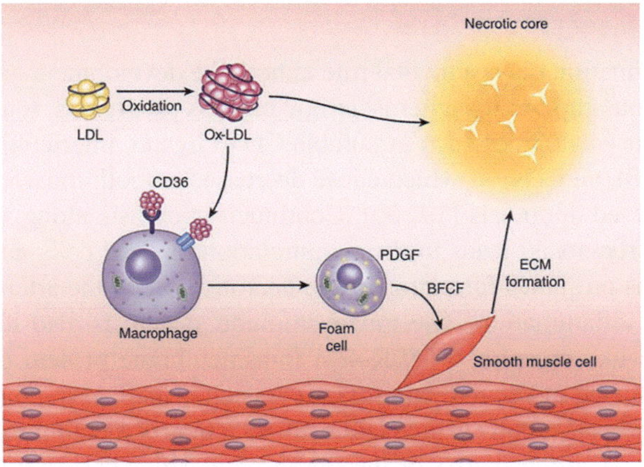

Fig. 3 Pivotal role of LDL particles in formation of the necrotic core. Abbreviations: *BFCF* basic fibroblast growth factor, *CD36* cluster of differentiation 36, *ECM* extracellular matrix, *LDL* low-density lipoprotein, *OX-LDL* oxidized LDL, *PDGF* platelet-derived growth factor. **Adapted from:** Leiva E, Wehinger S, Guzman L, Orrego R. (2015). Role of oxidized LDL in atherosclerosis. In Kumar SA (Ed.), *Hypercholesterolemia*. IntechOpen. https://www.intechopen.com/chapters/47808

2.1 Inflammatory Cytokines and the Inflammasome

The inflammasome is a protein complex that activates the inflammatory response. It facilitates the maturation of pro-inflammatory cytokines produced by macrophages, endothelial cells, and smooth muscle cells. The nucleotide-binding oligomerization domain (NOD)-like receptor protein (NLRP) 3 inflammasome has been closely linked to atherosclerosis [11].

Cholesterol crystals and Ox-LDL activate the NLRP3 inflammasome which leads to the cleavage and secretion of pro-inflammatory cytokines IL-1 β and interleukin 18 (IL-18) [12]. IL-1 β, along with other pro-inflammatory cytokines, such as interferon gamma (IFN-γ) and TNF-α, are expressed in excess within atherosclerotic plaques [13]. TNF-α causes differentiation of vascular smooth muscle cells into osteoblast-like cells which produce microcalcifications associated with vulnerable plaque that is prone to rupture [14–16]. These cytokines also increase the expression of adhesion molecules and stimulate the production of interleukin 6 (IL-6). IL-6, in turn, induces the production of acute-phase proteins like CRP and acts as a chemokine for neutrophils [17, 18]. Serum IL-6 and high-sensitivity C-reactive protein (hs-CRP) levels are hence clinically measured reflections of the downstream pathways of IL-1β activation. Over the course of years, the balance between pro- and anti-inflammatory cytokines, cell proliferation, and apoptosis determines the development and progression of atherosclerotic plaque.

3 Inflammation and Acute Thrombotic Syndromes

Chronic inflammation plays a pivotal role in both the development and the degradation of the fibrous cap. As the atherosclerotic process progresses, foam cells release pro-inflammatory cytokines such as soluble CD40 ligand, interleukins (IL-1, IL-3, IL-8, and IL-18), and TNF-α which cause decreased smooth muscle cell proliferation and increased apoptosis [19, 20]. Continued apoptosis along with inefficient clearance (efferocytosis) leads to the accumulation of dead cells and extracellular lipids [21]. This promotes formation of the necrotic core in the arterial wall, which begets further inflammation. The innate immune system is also involved in this process as toll-like receptor 4 (TLR-4; a transmembrane protein that recognizes pathogen-associated molecular patterns) expression is increased in unstable plaque. Macrophages and other cells in the plaque produce matrix metalloproteinases which degrade the extracellular matrix of the fibrous cap. This leads to a thinning of the fibrous cap and increased vulnerability for plaque rupture (Fig. 4) [22].

Once plaque rupture has occurred, exposure of the endothelial layer to extracellular lipids promotes platelet recruitment, adhesion, aggregation, and activation leading to the formation of an intravascular thrombus. Tissue factor plays an important role in the events leading to thrombus formation after endothelial injury

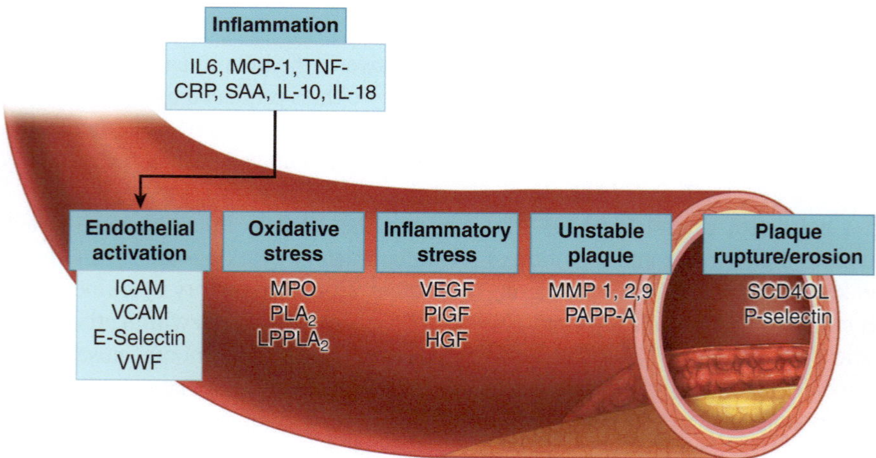

Fig. 4 Interplay of inflammation and endothelial activation in acute coronary syndrome. Abbreviations: *CRP* C-reactive protein, *HGF* hepatocyte growth factor, *ICAM* intercellular adhesion molecule, *IL* interleukin, *LPPLA₂* lipoprotein-associated phospholipase A₂, *MCP* monocyte chemotactic protein, *MMP* matrix metalloproteinases, *MPO* myeloperoxidase, *PAPP-A* pregnancy-associated plasma peptide A, *PLA₂* phospholipase A1, *TNF* tumor necrosis factor, *PIGF* placental growth factor, *SAA* serum amyloid A, *SCD40L* soluble CD40L, *VCAM* vascular cell adhesion molecule, *vWF* von Willebrand factor. **Adapted from:** Armstrong E. Inflammatory biomarkers in acute coronary syndrome. Circulation. 2006; 113:372–e75 and Libby P. Current concepts of the pathogenesis of acute coronary syndromes. Circulation. 2001;104:365–372

[23–25]. Intravascular thrombus formation then occludes the vessel lumen causing the clinical manifestations of acute coronary syndrome (ACS) and acute ischemic stroke. It is important to note that while inflammation plays an important role in a majority of patients, it may not be the inciting mechanism in all cases of ACS [26]. Plaque erosion may occur without rupture and is suspected to be a distinct entity that is increasingly recognized by optical coherence tomography as a cause for ACS.

4   Biomarkers of Inflammation and Cardiovascular Disease

CRP, hs-CRP, IL-6, and IL-1β: CRP is an annular glycoprotein produced in the liver. The IL-1β signaling pathway and the NLRP3 inflammasome produce IL-6 which stimulates CRP production. Ridker et al. pioneered findings on the association of CRP levels with future risk of MI or stroke in men from the Physicians' Health Study [27]. Early epidemiological studies established the association of CRP with outcomes after ACS [28–30]. CRP is likely a downstream mediator of the inflammatory cascade, and IL-1β and IL-6 may be better clinical markers of the inflammatory pathway activation [31–33]. Indeed, elevated IL-6 and IL-1β levels were associated with a greater than twofold increased cardiovascular risk in the Physicians' Health and Women's Health studies [34]. However, clinical assays have traditionally measured hs-CRP to assess cardiovascular risk. While both CRP and hs-CRP measure the same protein in the blood, the hs-CRP test has a much lower range (0.5–10 mg/dL), making it useful in detecting low-grade, long-term inflammation, which increases the risk of cardiovascular disease. In contrast, the CRP test (range from 10 to 1000 mg/dL) is generally used to evaluate people who have signs and symptoms of a serious bacterial infection or in the evaluation of chronic systemic inflammatory diseases such as rheumatoid arthritis (RA). There is a large body of evidence supporting the use of hs-CRP in tailoring primary prevention strategies [35]. The Emerging Risk Factors Collaboration found that an increase in log normalized hs-CRP was associated with an increase in the risk of coronary artery disease (CAD), ischemic stroke, and vascular mortality [36]. Indeed, hs-CRP offered a modestly better risk stratification of subjects at low or intermediate ASCVD risk when compared to the Framingham risk score alone [37]. This was confirmed with data from randomized controlled trials (RCTs). The Justification for the Use of Statins in Prevention: An Intervention Trial Evaluating Rosuvastatin (JUPITER) demonstrated that patients with a residual hs-CRP >2 mg/L had a significantly decreased risk of a first cardiovascular event with statin use, even when LDL cholesterol (LDL-C) levels were <130 mg/dL [38]. The 2019 American College of Cardiology (ACC)/American Heart Association (AHA) Guideline on the Primary Prevention of Cardiovascular Disease recommends considering an elevated hs-CRP concentration as a risk enhancer if the 10-year ASCVD risk is borderline (5% to <7.5%) or intermediate (7.5% to <20%) [39].

While hs-CRP has mainly been used in primary prevention settings, there is also a large body of evidence showing the association of hs-CRP with cardiovascular events in patients with established ASCVD [40]. Both the Pravastatin or Atorvastatin Evaluation and Infection Therapy-Thrombolysis In Myocardial Infarction 22 (PROVE-IT-TIMI 22) trial and the Improved Reduction of Outcomes: Vytorin Efficacy International Trial (IMPROVE-IT) showed that residual hs-CRP elevation was associated with an increased risk of cardiovascular events in patients after an ACS [41, 42]. This has led to the concept of "dual targets" (i.e., LDL-C <70 mg/dL and hs-CRP <2 mg/L) for secondary prevention. In the Canakinumab Anti-Inflammatory Thrombosis Outcome Study (CANTOS) investigating canakinumab, an IL-1β inhibitor, patients with the greatest on-treatment reduction in hs-CRP had a 27% reduction in the composite endpoint of MI, stroke, and cardiovascular death. Conversely, patients in the highest tertile of residual hs-CRP derived no benefit in the primary outcome from canakinumab [43]. This would suggest that hs-CRP levels may be used as a surrogate to gauge adequacy of treatment in individual patients.

Homocysteine: Homocysteine is thought to be causally associated with atherosclerosis by inducing oxidative stress [44, 45]. Folic acid is involved in homocysteine metabolism, and a number of RCTs have studied folic acid supplementation as an inexpensive method to reduce ASCVD risk [46–48]. Meta-analyses of these RCTs have shown variable results without a benefit in reducing the risk of MI, but with a potential benefit in the primary prevention of stroke [49, 50]. Widespread dietary fortification with folate makes it challenging to study the additional benefit of folic acid supplementation, but there has been potential benefit in areas with less fortification of foods [51].

Myeloperoxidase (MPO): MPO catalyzes the formation of reactive oxygen species thereby contributing to tissue damage during inflammation. Observational studies have shown an association between elevated MPO levels and the risk of CAD, heart failure, and all-cause mortality [52]. Further studies are needed to determine if MPO may be a viable therapeutic target.

Lipoprotein-Associated Phospholipase-A2 (LpPLA$_2$): LpPLA$_2$ is produced by macrophages and metabolizes oxidized phospholipids to release pro-inflammatory products that have a role in the development of endothelial dysfunction and plaque inflammation. Higher plasma levels of LpPLA$_2$ are associated with an increased risk of CAD and stroke; however, therapies that inhibit LpPLA$_2$ have not shown a reduction in cardiovascular outcomes [53].

Serum Amyloid A (SAA): SAA is an acute-phase reactant that binds high-density lipoprotein (HDL) and attenuates its anti-oxidative function. Prolonged inflammatory stimulus leads to persistent elevations in SAA levels and the deposition of pathological amyloid fibrils [54]. Epidemiological studies have shown an association between SAA levels and cardiovascular disease, as well as obesity [55].

5   Cardiovascular Risk Factors and Inflammation

Many traditional risk factors such as dyslipidemia, hypertension, diabetes mellitus, and obesity exert their influence on cardiovascular risk through inflammatory pathways. This section reviews common cardiovascular risk factors and their effects on vascular inflammation.

5.1   Dyslipidemia

LDL-C: Accumulation of LDL particles in the subendothelial layer contributes to both endothelial injury and atherosclerosis [56]. The pathophysiology of LDL uptake and foam cell formation in atherosclerosis has been previously described. Apart from total LDL content, the size of LDL particles also contributes to atherogenic risk. Small dense LDL particles are inherently more prone to oxidation and entrapment in the arterial wall, and may be more commonly seen in "metabolic dyslipidemia" associated with obesity [57].

Despite the advances made in lowering LDL-C, the treatment of other dyslipidemias has yielded mixed results. Atherogenic dyslipidemia is the triad of small dense LDL particles, high triglyceride levels, and low HDL-C levels, often seen in patients with metabolic syndrome. HDL is responsible for removing cholesterol from cholesterol-rich macrophages and peripheral tissues and transporting cholesterol esters back to the liver, a process known as reverse cholesterol transport. HDL also participates in exchanging cholesterol esters for triglycerides. HDL has, for many years, been thought to have anti-inflammatory and anti-oxidant functions [58]. Cholesteryl ester transfer protein (CETP), a protein involved in the reverse cholesterol transport pathway, is now speculated to also participate in the immune response to bacterial infections [59]. However, treatment to increase HDL levels has not been shown to reduce ASCVD events [60]. It is now recognized that there are multiple types of HDL particles and the quality of these particles is likely more important than their quantity. Pro-inflammatory HDL has a higher level of ceruloplasmin and SAA, as well as decreased apolipoprotein-A1 levels. This phenotype is associated with increased risk of developing atherosclerosis [61].

Lipoprotein(a) [Lp(a)]: An elevated Lp(a) level is an independent causal risk factor for cardiovascular disease. Lp(a) promotes monocyte extravasation and increases expression of pro-inflammatory cytokines such as IL-1 and TNF-α, which recruit more macrophages to form foam cells. The treatment of elevated Lp(a) remains a challenge due to its poor response to conventional lipid-lowering therapy. Proprotein convertase subtilisin/kexin type 9 (PCSK9) inhibitors reduce Lp(a) levels by 30%. Newer therapies, including small interfering RNA (siRNA) and antisense oligonucleotides to reduce Lp(a) levels, are under evaluation [62].

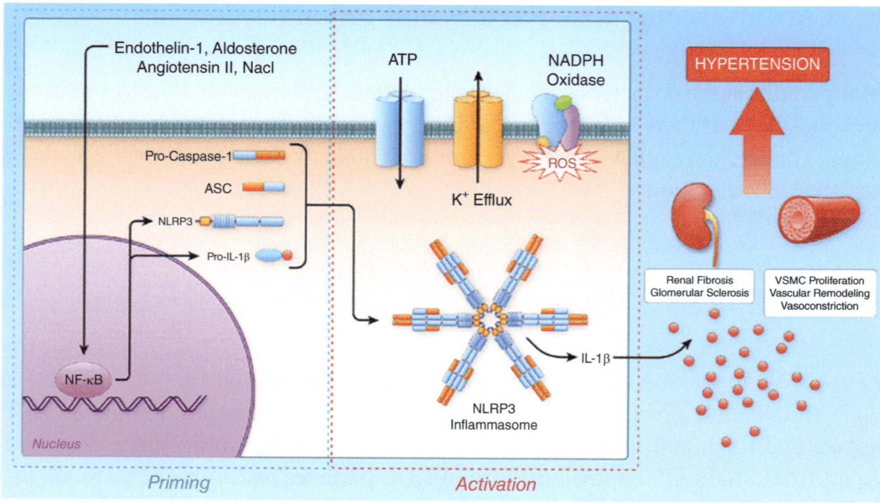

Fig. 5 Endogenous and exogenous inflammatory pathways in the pathogenesis of hypertension. **From:** Madhur MS, et al. Circulation Research. 2021;128:908–933, a PubMed Central (PMC) Open Access, HHS Public Access article. Abbreviations: *ASC* apoptosis-associated speck-like adaptor protein, *ATP* adenosine triphosphate, *IL-1β* interleukin 1β, *K+* potassium, *NaCl* sodium chloride, *NADPH* nicotinamide adenine dinucleotide phosphate, *NF-kB* nuclear factor-kappa beta, *NLRP3* NOD-like receptor family pyrin domain containing 3, *ROS* reactive oxygen species, *VSMC* vascular smooth muscle

5.2 Hypertension

Hypertension is a primary risk factor for CAD, stroke, and kidney disease. The relationship between inflammation and hypertension is complex and involves components of both innate and adaptive immunity [63]. Mechanical wall stress and circulating mediators like angiotensin II promote the formation of reactive oxygen species in endothelial cells within the vascular wall [64]. Increased oxidative stress releases inflammatory cytokines which then promote extracellular matrix deposition and cell death (Fig. 5) [65]. Indeed, early vascular aging is a key feature of hypertension with pathological remodeling, stiffening, and loss of vascular reactivity [66]. This phenomenon occurs in both the macro- and micro-circulation and correlates with cardiovascular events [67, 68].

5.3 Diabetes

Diabetes is a metabolic disorder with numerous etiologies and biological mechanisms. Chronic inflammation plays an important role in the pathophysiology of diabetes and its complications. A recent study evaluated 76 different biomarkers of inflammation in 414 patients with recent onset diabetes. These patients were divided into five categories including autoimmune diabetes, insulin-deficient diabetes, insulin-resistant diabetes, mild obesity-related diabetes, and mild age-related diabetes. The highest levels of inflammation were seen in patients with severe insulin-resistant diabetes [69]. O-linked-N-acetylglucosaminylation (O-GlcNAcylation) appears to be an important molecular mechanism by which hyperglycemia induces inflammation via the NF-kB pathway [70]. A second mechanism of target organ damage in patients with diabetes is through advanced glycosylation end products (AGE). AGE interact with their receptors causing endothelial apoptosis and failure of endothelium-dependent vasodilation [71]. Thirdly, oxidative stress and free fatty acids activate the NLRP3 inflammasome resulting in increased IL-1β levels that directly lead to pancreatic beta cell destruction [72].

Therapeutics used to treat diabetes also have anti-inflammatory effects that may influence cardiovascular risk. Metformin, an agent commonly used to reduce insulin resistance in type 2 diabetes, has been shown to reduce CRP, monocyte chemoattractant protein-1 (MCP-1), AGE, and NF-κB activity [73–75]. Glucagon-like peptide-1 (GLP-1) agonists mimic the anorexic and glucose-lowering effects of endogenous GLP-1 [76]. These agents reduce ICAM-1 levels in animal models and epicardial white adipose tissue in humans, thereby promoting weight loss and improving cardiovascular risk [77, 78]. Inhibitors of the sodium-glucose cotransporter 2 (SGLT-2i) have far-reaching benefits beyond glucose-lowering, in terms of prevention of ASCVD, heart failure, and kidney disease [79]. This class of drugs has been found to decrease pro-inflammatory cytokines, such as IL-1β, by inhibiting the NLRP3 inflammasome. They change the polarity of immune cells from secreting pro-inflammatory to anti-inflammatory cytokines, and decrease the accumulation of T cells in adipose tissue [80, 81]. The full mechanisms of action of these drugs on kidney function and heart muscle metabolism are incompletely understood and constitute an area of active study.

5.4 Metabolic Syndrome

Chronic low-grade inflammation is a common feature of patients with various components of metabolic syndrome, including obesity. Adipose tissue is metabolically active and contributes to the chronic inflammatory state through several mechanisms. It promotes local inflammation, increases the production of acute-phase reactants, and secretes multiple pro-inflammatory cytokines, such as IL-1, IL-6, and TNF-α, leading to a systemic inflammatory state [82]. Hypoxia from growing adipose tissue leads to adipose cell death and fibrosis. This leads to upregulation of pro-inflammatory mediators and downregulation of anti-inflammatory mediators such as adiponectin [83].

The clinical consequences of obesity extend beyond the risk of ASCVD and include an increased risk of heart failure, pulmonary hypertension, and atrial fibrillation, among other chronic medical comorbidities. The distribution of adipose tissue matters more than its total volume. Studies have shown increased glucose and triglyceride levels, as well as higher ASCVD event rates, in patients with higher levels of visceral obesity [84, 85]. The potential benefit of quantifying visceral fat (i.e., perivascular or pericardial fat) using imaging techniques is an area of active research [86]. Metabolic inflammation is a dynamic state, and the treatment of obesity may improve these markers. Studies with both the Mediterranean diet and bariatric surgery have shown an improvement in inflammatory markers with weight loss [87, 88].

5.5 Genetic Risk Factors

An individual's ASCVD risk is determined by the interplay between modifiable risk factors and genetic predisposition, a non-modifiable risk factor. Individuals with a family history of heart disease have a 1.5 times greater risk of CAD than those without [89]. Genome-wide association studies have identified many variations in genes, such as *APOA5, NOS3, PCSK9, LPL,* and *LPA,* which provide a link between inflammation and ASCVD. These genes are associated with lipid metabolism, inflammation, and endothelial function [90]. Other polymorphisms confer a benefit. For example, IL-6 polymorphisms have been associated with a lower hs-CRP level and lower vascular risk.

5.6 Additional Risk Factors

Tobacco use: There is overwhelming evidence that demonstrates a strong association between tobacco use and ASCVD, which is thought to be at least partly mediated by inflammation. People who smoke tobacco have a higher T lymphocyte count as well as increased levels of TNF-α, IL-1, and IL-6 [91–93]. In the Multi-Ethnic Study of Atherosclerosis (MESA) cohort, smoking was associated with higher levels of hs-CRP suggesting higher levels of systemic inflammation [94]. Tobacco cessation is associated with decreased hs-CRP and leukocyte count as well as decreased ASCVD risk.

Pollution: Air pollution has increasingly been recognized as a leading cause of morbidity and mortality globally. A meta-analysis showed a 10% increase in cardiovascular mortality in populations living in areas with chronically elevated air pollution levels [95]. The adaptive responses to air pollution include activation of the sympathetic nervous system, endothelial dysfunction, systemic and adipose tissue inflammation, and oxidative stress, as well as changes in adipokine expression [96]. Noise pollution, for example, from aircraft noise during the night, is associated with worsening endothelial function, increased stress hormone levels, and decreased sleep quality [97, 98].

Psychological Stress: Chronic psychological stress increases glucocorticoid and catecholamine levels and activates a stress-sensitive neuro-immune axis postulated to affect cardiovascular health [99].

6 Rheumatological Disease and Cardiovascular Risk

Patients with chronic inflammatory conditions are at increased ASCVD risk when compared to the general population. For example, in patients with systemic lupus erythematosus (SLE), premature ASCVD is a leading cause of morbidity and mortality. This risk, although well-known, is not captured by traditional risk calculators [100]. Patients with underlying chronic inflammatory conditions are more likely to develop atherogenic dyslipidemia, higher blood pressure, and endothelial dysfunction [101]. Similarly, increased cardiovascular risk has been noted in patients with other inflammatory conditions such as RA, psoriasis, and inflammatory bowel disease [102–104]. The increased risk associated with chronic rheumatological diseases is not fully explained by traditional cardiovascular risk factors, and chronic inflammation is thought to play a role. These conditions are hence considered "risk enhancers" for persons at an intermediate ASCVD risk (10-year risk 7.5% to $\leq$20%) in the 2018 ACC/AHA/Multisociety Guideline on the Management of Blood Cholesterol [39].

6.1 Mechanisms of Increased Risk in Patients with Chronic Inflammatory Conditions

Multiple pathways of immune dysfunction have been implicated in the increased ASCVD risk demonstrated in individuals with chronic rheumatological conditions. Atherogenic dyslipidemia in these patients is characterized by alterations in HDL function due to oxidative stress. The HDL particles develop abnormalities in cholesterol efflux capacity and become pro-inflammatory, a process that is potentially reversible with treatment. These patients also show an increase in circulating myeloid cells and platelets, as well as a higher scavenger-mediated uptake of Ox-LDL leading to formation of foam cells [105]. The levels of pro-inflammatory cytokines are also increased leading to endothelial dysfunction [106, 107]. Concomitantly, a high concentration of arginine dimethylarginine (ADMA), an endogenous nitric oxide inhibitor, leads to a decrease in circulating nitric oxide-mediated vasodilation [108]. Many other pathways including abnormalities in hematopoiesis have been described linking inflammatory diseases with ASCVD. These are outside the scope of the chapter.

6.2 Cardiometabolic Effects of Anti-Inflammatory Therapies Used for Rheumatological Diseases

A significant number of patients with rheumatologic disease are treated with anti-inflammatory therapies. These pharmacologic agents act by modifying different components of inflammatory pathways and may affect the patient's cardiovascular risk. The cardiovascular effects of commonly used anti-rheumatic drugs will be discussed in greater detail below.

Methotrexate: Methotrexate is used for the treatment of many autoimmune diseases including RA, psoriasis, and SLE. It inhibits dihydrofolate reductase, thereby inhibiting the synthesis of purines and pyrimidines needed for DNA and RNA synthesis. It also lowers the levels of NF-κB which further contributes to its anti-inflammatory activity [109]. Observational studies have suggested a reduction in cardiovascular risk with methotrexate use in patients with rheumatological disease. Methotrexate was also studied in a secondary prevention cohort of patients without rheumatological disease, but was not found to be beneficial [110, 111].

Hydroxychloroquine: Hydroxychloroquine (HCQ) is an anti-malarial agent that is used for the treatment of RA, SLE, and other rheumatologic diseases. In the early 2000s, it was noted that patients taking HCQ for at least 4 years had a 77% reduced risk of developing diabetes [112]. Observational data also showed that HCQ use for RA for 3 months was associated with better lipid profiles, irrespective of disease activity or statin use [113]. With regard to cardiovascular outcomes, a retrospective study evaluated the association between HCQ use and incident ASCVD in patients with RA. The authors found a 70% reduction in the primary composite outcome of CAD, stroke, transient ischemic attack, sudden cardiac death, and peripheral artery disease with arterial revascularization procedure (hazard ratio 0.30, 95% confidence interval 0.13–0.68, $P = 0.004$) [114]. An RCT in patients with SLE compared the use of HCQ combined with aspirin to HCQ alone or aspirin alone. The combination was found to confer a greater reduction in cardiovascular risk when compared to either drug alone [115]. Purported mechanisms of cardiovascular benefit of HCQ include an inhibition of phospholipid antibody binding and inhibition of platelet aggregation [116]. It is important to note that HCQ is not recommended for cardiovascular prevention in the absence of a rheumatological or other appropriate clinical indication for its use. Side effects of HCQ include gastrointestinal side effects, hypoglycemia, and cardiovascular toxicity in the form of prolonged QT interval at higher doses.

TNF-α Inhibitors: TNF-α inhibitors are biological disease-modifying anti-rheumatic drugs (DMARDS) used in the treatment of RA. In an early observational study, the use of TNF-α inhibitors in patients with RA was associated with a 35% decrease in total mortality [117]. A retrospective cohort study found a reduction in MI with TNF-α inhibitors when compared to synthetic DMARDs [118]. Another meta-analysis of 28 studies showed superiority of TNF-α inhibitors to methotrexate in the reduction of cardiovascular events [119]. These benefits are possibly from an improvement in endothelial function, a shift from a pro- to an anti-atherogenic lipoprotein profile, and antagonism of the effects of inflammation on coagulation [111].

IL-6 Inhibitors: The IL-6 inhibitor, tocilizumab, is another biological DMARD that is approved for the treatment of RA, juvenile idiopathic arthritis, and giant cell arteritis. It has also been used in the treatment of cytokine storm in patients with cytokine release syndrome after chimeric antigens receptor (CAR) T-cell therapy and in patients with SARS-CoV-2 infection (COVID-19) [120]. A significant concern with the chronic use of IL-6 inhibitor therapy for inflammatory conditions has been the increased levels of LDL-C and triglycerides seen immediately after therapy initiation. These levels tend to improve with time and appear to not translate into higher cardiovascular risk [111]. A meta-analysis found a decreased risk of cardiovascular events with tocilizumab compared with TNF-α inhibitors; the benefit was seen mainly in patients with prior CAD [121].

7 Targeting the Inflammatory Pathway for Primary and Secondary Prevention of Cardiovascular Disease

Given the ubiquitous role of inflammation in ASCVD, efforts have been made to target inflammation primarily as a means to reduce cardiovascular risk. In a retrospective cohort, 34% of patients post-percutaneous coronary intervention (PCI) had an elevated residual inflammatory risk (hs-CRP >2 mg/dL) despite existing secondary prevention therapies. Persistent inflammation strongly correlated with a risk for major adverse cardiovascular events within 1 year of hs-CRP measurement [122]. Existing and newer therapeutic agents are being studied that affect the inflammatory pathway.

7.1 Statins

Statins, which are 3-hydroxy-3-methylglutaryl coenzyme A (HMG Co-A) reductase inhibitors, have changed the landscape of ASCVD prevention. They have well-known effects in lowering LDL-C levels but also help reduce inflammation in part by inhibiting production of IL-1β, TNF-α, and other pro-inflammatory cytokines, as well as by upregulating endothelial nitric oxide synthase [123–125]. Multiple RCTs have shown the significant cardiovascular benefits of statins. JUPITER enrolled over 11,000 men and 6500 women with LDL-C <130 mg/dL but elevated hs-CRP (>2 mg/dL) to either rosuvastatin 20 mg daily or placebo. The trial was stopped early at 1.9 years for a significant 44% reduction in the primary outcome of first-ever MI, stroke, hospitalization for unstable angina, arterial revascularization, or cardiovascular death. The lowest event rates in the study were seen in patients achieving an LDL-C goal of <70 mg/dL and an hs-CRP level of <2 mg/dL [126].

The Air Force/Texas Coronary Atherosclerosis Prevention Study (AFCAPS/TEXCAPS) investigators evaluated the effect of lovastatin in a primary prevention cohort with average LDL-C levels and below-average HDL-C levels. They found a significant decrease in the incidence of first major coronary event with lovastatin use [127]. Interestingly, this effect was seen in persons with a high total-C/non-HDL-C ratio and a low hs-CRP level, but not in persons with a low ratio and low hs-CRP level [128]. Similar results were noted in the PROVE-IT-TIMI 22 trial; patients who achieved a low on-treatment hs-CRP level had the greatest reduction in cardiovascular risk, irrespective of LDL-C level [129].

7.2 Colchicine

Colchicine inhibits microtubule polymerization of immune cells and inhibits the inflammasome [130]. The Low Dose Colchicine for Secondary Prevention of Cardiovascular Disease (LoDoCo) trial was an open-label trial that randomized 532 patients with stable CAD on statin and antiplatelet therapy to either 0.5 mg colchicine daily or no colchicine. At the 3-year follow-up, patients on colchicine had a 67% relative reduction in the composite primary endpoint of incident ACS, cardiac arrest, and non-cardioembolic ischemic stroke [131]. The Colchicine Cardiovascular Outcomes Trial (COLCOT) enrolled 4745 patients who had an MI within the last 30 days and randomized them to 0.5 mg of colchicine daily or placebo. This trial also showed that patients randomized to colchicine had a 33% reduction in the composite of death from cardiovascular causes, resuscitated cardiac arrest, MI, stroke, or urgent hospitalization for angina leading to coronary revascularization. The results were driven mainly by a reduction in stroke. It is worth noting that there was a significant increase in the incidence of pneumonia in the colchicine arm of this trial [132]. The Low Dose Colchicine for Secondary Prevention of Cardiovascular Disease 2 (LoDoCo2) trial enrolled 5522 patients with stable CAD to colchicine or placebo. At a median follow-up of 28.6 months, the colchicine arm had a 31% reduction in risk of the primary composite endpoint of cardiovascular death, spontaneous (nonprocedural) MI, ischemic stroke, or ischemia-driven coronary revascularization. However, there was an increase in death from any cause in the colchicine arm, driven by non-cardiovascular deaths [133]. Several trials are ongoing to study the effect of colchicine in preventing CAD and stroke, which should shed light on its role in primary and secondary ASCVD prevention.

7.3 Canakinumab

Canakinumab is an anti-IL-1β human monoclonal antibody that was initially approved for IL-1β over-expression disorders. The CANTOS trial enrolled individuals with a prior MI and with an hs-CRP ≥2 mg/dL to either various doses of canakinumab (50 mg, 150 mg, or 300 mg) or placebo. At a median follow-up of 3.7 years, canakinumab produced robust reductions in IL-6, hs-CRP, and fibrinogen levels. The 150 mg dose met the primary endpoint of nonfatal MI, nonfatal stroke, or cardiovascular death, with a 15% relative risk reduction [134]. There was no difference in all-cause mortality, and canakinumab was associated with a higher incidence of fatal infection when compared to placebo. The US Food and Drug Administration did not give regulatory approval for canakinumab citing minimal benefits and high cost of the drug.

8 Conclusion

Inflammation plays a fundamental role in the pathophysiology of atherosclerosis and its downstream complications such as MI and stroke. An increasing understanding of this complex and interdependent relationship has led to the development of novel therapeutic agents targeting inflammation. At its most basic level, a healthy lifestyle with a Mediterranean-style diet and regular exercise are fundamentally important to reduce inflammation and cardiovascular risk. Newer therapeutic agents are associated with exciting opportunities for reducing cardiovascular risk, but this enthusiasm needs to be carefully balanced against the risk of side effects. Given the magnitude of cardiovascular disease burden worldwide, there is an urgent need for safe and effective agents that reduce cardiovascular disease risk by targeting inflammation.

References

1. Chan YH, Ramji DP. Atherosclerosis: pathogenesis and key cellular processes, current and emerging therapies, key challenges, and future research directions. In: Ramji D, editor. Atherosclerosis: methods and protocols [Internet]. New York: Springer US; 2022. [Cited 2022 Mar 13]. p. 3–19. (Methods in molecular biology). https://doi.org/10.1007/978-1-0716-1924-7_1.
2. Ross R. Atherosclerosis: the role of endothelial injury, smooth muscle proliferation and platelet factors. Triangle Sandoz J Med Sci. 1976;15(2–3):45–51.
3. Ross R. The pathogenesis of atherosclerosis—an update. N Engl J Med. 1986;314(8):488–500.
4. Huang L, Chambliss KL, Gao X, Yuhanna IS, Behling-Kelly E, Bergaya S, et al. SR-B1 drives endothelial cell LDL transcytosis via DOCK4 to promote atherosclerosis. Nature. 2019;569(7757):565–9.
5. Tabas I, Williams KJ, Borén J. Subendothelial lipoprotein retention as the initiating process in atherosclerosis: update and therapeutic implications. Circulation. 2007;116(16):1832–44.
6. Chatzizisis YS, Coskun AU, Jonas M, Edelman ER, Feldman CL, Stone PH. Role of endothelial shear stress in the natural history of coronary atherosclerosis and vascular remodeling: molecular, cellular, and vascular behavior. J Am Coll Cardiol. 2007;49(25):2379–93.
7. Buckley ML, Ramji DP. The influence of dysfunctional signaling and lipid homeostasis in mediating the inflammatory responses during atherosclerosis. Biochim Biophys Acta (BBA) Mol Basis Dis. 2015;1852(7):1498–510.

8. Berliner JA, Leitinger N, Tsimikas S. The role of oxidized phospholipids in atherosclerosis. J Lipid Res. 2009;50:S207–12.

9. Adiguzel E, Ahmad PJ, Franco C, Bendeck M. Collagens in the progression and complications of atherosclerosis. Vasc Med. 2009;14:73.

10. Basatemur GL, Jørgensen HF, Clarke MCH, Bennett MR, Mallat Z. Vascular smooth muscle cells in atherosclerosis. Nat Rev Cardiol. 2019;16(12):727–44.

11. Libby P. Targeting inflammatory pathways in cardiovascular disease: the inflammasome, interleukin-1, interleukin-6 and beyond. Cells. 2021;10(4):951.

12. Duewell P, Kono H, Rayner KJ, Sirois CM, Vladimer G, Bauernfeind FG, et al. NLRP3 inflammasomes are required for atherogenesis and activated by cholesterol crystals. Nature. 2010;464(7293):1357–61.

13. Tousoulis D, Oikonomou E, Economou EK, Crea F, Kaski JC. Inflammatory cytokines in atherosclerosis: current therapeutic approaches. Eur Heart J. 2016;37(22):1723–32.

14. Tintut Y, Patel J, Parhami F, Demer LL. Tumor necrosis factor-α promotes in vitro calcification of vascular cells via the cAMP pathway. Circulation. 2000;102(21):2636–42.

15. Dweck MR, Aikawa E, Newby DE, Tarkin JM, Rudd JHF, Narula J, et al. Noninvasive molecular imaging of disease activity in atherosclerosis. Circ Res. 2016;119(2):330–40.

16. Hutcheson JD, Goettsch C, Bertazzo S, Maldonado N, Ruiz JL, Goh W, et al. Genesis and growth of extracellular-vesicle-derived microcalcification in atherosclerotic plaques. Nat Mater. 2016;15(3):335–43.

17. Kaplanski G, Marin V, Montero-Julian F, Mantovani A, Farnarier C. IL-6: a regulator of the transition from neutrophil to monocyte recruitment during inflammation. Trends Immunol. 2003;24(1):25–9.

18. Reiss AB, Siegart NM, De Leon J. Interleukin-6 in atherosclerosis: atherogenic or atheroprotective? Clin Lipidol. 2017;12(1):14–23.

19. Libby P, Ridker PM. Inflammation and atherothrombosis. J Am Coll Cardiol. 2006;48(9 Suppl):A33–46.

20. Beck-Joseph J, Lehoux S. Molecular interactions between vascular smooth muscle cells and macrophages in atherosclerosis. Front Cardiovasc Med [Internet]. 2021. [Cited 2022 Mar 13];8. https://www.frontiersin.org/article/10.3389/fcvm.2021.737934.

21. Tabas I. Macrophage death and defective inflammation resolution in atherosclerosis. Nat Rev Immunol. 2010;10(1):36–46.

22. Silvestre-Roig C, de Winther MP, Weber C, Daemen MJ, Lutgens E, Soehnlein O. Atherosclerotic plaque destabilization: mechanisms, models, and therapeutic strategies. Circ Res. 2014;114(1):214–26.

23. Grover SP, Mackman N. Tissue factor in atherosclerosis and atherothrombosis. Atherosclerosis. 2020;307:80–6.

24. Iacoviello L, Di Castelnuovo A, de Curtis A, Agnoli C, Frasca G, Mattiello A, et al. Circulating tissue factor levels and risk of stroke. Stroke. 2015;46(6):1501–7.

25. Liang W, Fan Y, Lu H, Chang Z, Hu W, Sun J, et al. KLF11 (Krüppel-like factor 11) inhibits arterial thrombosis via suppression of tissue factor in the vascular wall. Arterioscler Thromb Vasc Biol. 2019;39(3):402–12.

26. Crea F, Libby P. Acute coronary syndromes: the way forward from mechanisms to precision treatment. Circulation. 2017;136(12):1155–66.

27. Ridker PM, Cushman M, Stampfer MJ, Tracy RP, Hennekens CH. Inflammation, aspirin, and the risk of cardiovascular disease in apparently healthy men. N Engl J Med. 1997;336(14):973–9.

28. Calabrò P, Golia E, Yeh ETH. Role of C-reactive protein in acute myocardial infarction and stroke: possible therapeutic approaches. Curr Pharm Biotechnol. 2012;13(1):4–16.

29. Liuzzo G, Biasucci LM, Gallimore JR, Grillo RL, Rebuzzi AG, Pepys MB, et al. The prognostic value of C-reactive protein and serum amyloid a protein in severe unstable angina. N Engl J Med. 1994;331(7):417–24.

30. Ridker PM, Rifai N, Pfeffer MA, Sacks FM, Moye LA, Goldman S, et al. Inflammation, pravastatin, and the risk of coronary events after myocardial infarction in patients with average cholesterol levels. Circulation. 1998;98(9):839–44.

31. Elliott P, Chambers JC, Zhang W, Clarke R, Hopewell JC, Peden JF, et al. Genetic loci associated with C-reactive protein levels and risk of coronary heart disease. JAMA. 2009;302(1):37–48.

32. Wyss CA, Neidhart M, Altwegg L, Spanaus KS, Yonekawa K, Wischnewsky MB, et al. Cellular actors, Toll-like receptors, and local cytokine profile in acute coronary syndromes. Eur Heart J. 2010;31(12):1457–69.

33. Maier W, Altwegg LA, Corti R, Gay S, Hersberger M, Maly FE, et al. Inflammatory markers at the site of ruptured plaque in acute myocardial infarction. Circulation. 2005;111(11):1355–61.

34. Ridker PM, Rifai N, Stampfer MJ, Hennekens CH. Plasma concentration of interleukin-6 and the risk of future myocardial infarction among apparently healthy men. Circulation. 2000;101(15):1767–72.

35. Ridker PM. A test in context: high-sensitivity C-reactive protein. J Am Coll Cardiol. 2016;67(6):712–23.

36. Emerging Risk Factors Collaboration, Kaptoge S, Di Angelantonio E, Lowe G, Pepys MB, Thompson SG, et al. C-reactive protein concentration and risk of coronary heart disease, stroke, and mortality: an individual participant meta-analysis. Lancet Lond Engl. 2010;375(9709):132–40.

37. Emerging Risk Factors Collaboration, Kaptoge S, Di Angelantonio E, Pennells L, Wood AM, White IR, et al. C-reactive protein, fibrinogen, and cardiovascular disease prediction. N Engl J Med. 2012;367(14):1310–20.

38. Ridker PM, Danielson E, Fonseca FA, Genest J, Gotto AM, Kastelein JJ, et al. Reduction in C-reactive protein and LDL cholesterol and cardiovascular event rates after initiation of rosuvastatin: a prospective study of the JUPITER trial. Lancet Lond Engl. 2009;373(9670):1175–82.

39. Arnett DK, Blumenthal RS, Albert MA, Buroker AB, Goldberger ZD, Hahn EJ, et al. 2019 ACC/AHA guideline on the primary prevention of cardiovascular disease: a report of the American College of Cardiology/American Heart Association Task Force on clinical practice guidelines. Circulation. 2019;140(11):e596–646.

40. Lawler PR, Bhatt DL, Godoy LC, Lüscher TF, Bonow RO, Verma S, et al. Targeting cardiovascular inflammation: next steps in clinical translation. Eur Heart J. 2021;42(1):113–31.

41. Bohula EA, Giugliano RP, Cannon CP, Zhou J, Murphy SA, White JA, et al. Achievement of dual Low-density lipoprotein cholesterol and high-sensitivity C-reactive protein targets more frequent with the addition of ezetimibe to simvastatin and associated with better outcomes in IMPROVE-IT. Circulation. 2015;132(13):1224–33.

42. Ridker PM, Morrow DA, Rose LM, Rifai N, Cannon CP, Braunwald E. Relative efficacy of atorvastatin 80 mg and pravastatin 40 mg in achieving the dual goals of low-density lipoprotein cholesterol <70 mg/dl and C-reactive protein <2 mg/l: an analysis of the PROVE-IT TIMI-22 trial. J Am Coll Cardiol. 2005;45(10):1644–8.

43. Ridker PM, Libby P, MacFadyen JG, Thuren T, Ballantyne C, Fonseca F, et al. Modulation of the interleukin-6 signalling pathway and incidence rates of atherosclerotic events and all-cause mortality: analyses from the Canakinumab Anti-Inflammatory Thrombosis Outcomes Study (CANTOS). Eur Heart J. 2018;39(38):3499–507.

44. Karger AB, Steffen BT, Nomura SO, Guan W, Garg PK, Szklo M, et al. Association between homocysteine and vascular calcification incidence, prevalence, and progression in the MESA cohort. J Am Heart Assoc. 2020;9(3):e013934.

45. Wong ND, Zhao Y, Quek RGW, Blumenthal RS, Budoff MJ, Cushman M, et al. Residual atherosclerotic cardiovascular disease risk in statin-treated adults: the Multi-Ethnic Study of Atherosclerosis. J Clin Lipidol. 2017;11(5):1223–33.

46. Albert CM, Cook NR, Gaziano JM, Zaharris E, MacFadyen J, Danielson E, et al. Effect of folic acid and B vitamins on risk of cardiovascular events and total mortality among women at high risk for cardiovascular disease: a randomized trial. JAMA. 2008;299(17):2027–36.

47. Bostom AG, Carpenter MA, Kusek JW, Levey AS, Hunsicker L, Pfeffer MA, et al. Homocysteine-lowering and cardiovascular disease outcomes in kidney transplant recipients. Circulation. 2011;123(16):1763–70.

48. Galan P, Kesse-Guyot E, Czernichow S, Briancon S, Blacher J, Hercberg S. Effects of B vitamins and omega 3 fatty acids on cardiovascular diseases: a randomised placebo controlled trial. BMJ. 2010;341:c6273.

49. Li Y, Huang T, Zheng Y, Muka T, Troup J, Hu FB. Folic acid supplementation and the risk of cardiovascular diseases: a meta-analysis of randomized controlled trials. J Am Heart Assoc. 2016;5(8):e003768.

50. Yang HT, Lee M, Hong KS, Ovbiagele B, Saver JL. Efficacy of folic acid supplementation in cardiovascular disease prevention: an updated meta-analysis of randomized controlled trials. Eur J Intern Med. 2012;23(8):745–54.

51. Zeng R, Xu CH, Xu YN, Wang YL, Wang M. The effect of folate fortification on folic acid-based homocysteine-lowering intervention and stroke risk: a meta-analysis. Public Health Nutr. 2015;18(8):1514–21.

52. Nicholls SJ, Hazen SL. Myeloperoxidase and cardiovascular disease. Arterioscler Thromb Vasc Biol. 2005;25(6):1102–11.

53. STABILITY Investigators. Darapladib for preventing ischemic events in stable coronary heart disease. N Engl J Med. 2014;370(18):1702–11.

54. Sack GH. Serum Amyloid A (SAA) proteins. In: Hoeger U, Harris JR, editors. Vertebrate and invertebrate respiratory proteins, lipoproteins and other body fluid proteins [Internet]. Cham: Springer International Publishing; 2020. [Cited 2022 Feb 27]. p. 421–36. (Subcellular biochemistry). https://doi.org/10.1007/978-3-030-41769-7_17.

55. Getz GS, Krishack PA, Reardon CA. Serum amyloid A and atherosclerosis. Curr Opin Lipidol. 2016;27(5):531–5.

56. Borén J, Chapman MJ, Krauss RM, Packard CJ, Bentzon JF, Binder CJ, et al. Low-density lipoproteins cause atherosclerotic cardiovascular disease: pathophysiological, genetic, and therapeutic insights: a consensus statement from the European Atherosclerosis Society Consensus Panel. Eur Heart J. 2020;41(24):2313–30.

57. Ikezaki H, Lim E, Cupples LA, Liu C, Asztalos BF, Schaefer EJ. Small dense low-density lipoprotein cholesterol is the most atherogenic lipoprotein parameter in the prospective Framingham offspring study. J Am Heart Assoc. 2021;10(5):e019140.

58. Helkin A, Stein JJ, Lin S, Siddiqui S, Maier KG, Gahtan V. Dyslipidemia part 1—review of lipid metabolism and vascular cell physiology. Vasc Endovasc Surg. 2016;50(2):107–18.

59. Bonacina F, Pirillo A, Catapano AL, Norata GD. HDL in immune-inflammatory responses: implications beyond cardiovascular diseases. Cells. 2021;10(5):1061.

60. Siddiqi HK, Kiss D, Rader D. HDL-cholesterol and cardiovascular disease: rethinking our approach. Curr Opin Cardiol. 2015;30(5):536–42.

61. Rosenson RS, Brewer HB, Ansell BJ, Barter P, Chapman MJ, Heinecke JW, et al. Dysfunctional HDL and atherosclerotic cardiovascular disease. Nat Rev Cardiol. 2016;13(1):48–60.

62. Tsimikas S. A test in context: lipoprotein(a): diagnosis, prognosis, controversies, and emerging therapies. J Am Coll Cardiol. 2017;69(6):692–711.

63. Xiao L, Harrison DG. Inflammation in hypertension. Can J Cardiol. 2020;36(5):635–47.

64. Loperena R, Harrison DG. Oxidative stress and hypertensive diseases. Med Clin North Am. 2017;101(1):169–93.

65. Wu J, Saleh MA, Kirabo A, Itani HA, Montaniel KRC, Xiao L, et al. Immune activation caused by vascular oxidation promotes fibrosis and hypertension. J Clin Invest. 2016;126(1):50–67.

66. Guzik TJ, Touyz RM. Oxidative stress, inflammation, and vascular aging in hypertension. Hypertension. 2017;70(4):660–7.

67. Laurent S, Briet M, Boutouyrie P. Large and small artery cross-talk and recent morbidity-mortality trials in hypertension. Hypertension. 2009;54(2):388–92.

68. Bruno RM, Nilsson PM, Engström G, Wadström BN, Empana JP, Boutouyrie P, et al. Early and supernormal vascular aging: clinical characteristics and association with incident cardiovascular events. Hypertension (Dallas Tex 1979). 2020;76(5):1616–24.
69. Herder C, Maalmi H, Strassburger K, Zaharia OP, Ratter JM, Karusheva Y, et al. Differences in biomarkers of inflammation between novel subgroups of recent-onset diabetes. Diabetes. 2021;70(5):1198–208.
70. Bolanle IO, Palmer TM. Targeting protein O-GlcNAcylation, a link between type 2 diabetes mellitus and inflammatory disease. Cells. 2022;11(4):705.
71. Garay-Sevilla ME, Gomez-Ojeda A, González I, Luévano-Contreras C, Rojas A. Contribution of RAGE axis activation to the association between metabolic syndrome and cancer. Mol Cell Biochem. 2021;476(3):1555–73.
72. Grant R, Dixit V. Mechanisms of disease: inflammasome activation and the development of type 2 diabetes. Front Immunol [Internet]. 2013. [Cited 2022 Jun 23];4. https://www.frontiersin.org/article/10.3389/fimmu.2013.00050.
73. Adeshirlarijaney A, Zou J, Tran HQ, Chassaing B, Gewirtz AT. Amelioration of metabolic syndrome by metformin associates with reduced indices of low-grade inflammation independently of the gut microbiota. Am J Physiol Endocrinol Metab. 2019;317(6):E1121–30.
74. Li SN, Wang X, Zeng QT, Feng YB, Cheng X, Mao XB, et al. Metformin inhibits nuclear factor κB activation and decreases serum high-sensitivity C-reactive protein level in experimental atherogenesis of rabbits. Heart Vessels. 2009;24(6):446–53.
75. Saisho Y. Metformin and inflammation: its potential beyond glucose-lowering effect. Endocr Metab Immune Disord Drug Targets. 2015;15(3):196–205.
76. Wilding JPH, Batterham RL, Calanna S, Davies M, Van Gaal LF, Lingvay I, et al. Once-weekly semaglutide in adults with overweight or obesity. N Engl J Med. 2021;384(11):989–1002.
77. Iacobellis G, Mohseni M, Bianco SD, Banga PK. Liraglutide causes large and rapid epicardial fat reduction. Obesity. 2017;25(2):311–6.
78. Chait A, den Hartigh LJ. Adipose tissue distribution, inflammation and its metabolic consequences, including diabetes and cardiovascular disease. Front Cardiovasc Med [Internet]. 2020. [Cited 2022 Mar 25];7. https://www.frontiersin.org/article/10.3389/fcvm.2020.00022.
79. Brown E, Heerspink HJL, Cuthbertson DJ, Wilding JPH. SGLT2 inhibitors and GLP-1 receptor agonists: established and emerging indications. Lancet. 2021;398(10296):262–76.
80. D'Marco L, Morillo V, Gorriz JL, Suarez MK, Nava M, Ortega Á, et al. SGLT2i and GLP-1RA in cardiometabolic and renal diseases: from glycemic control to adipose tissue inflammation and senescence. J Diabetes Res. 2021;2021:e9032378.
81. Cowie MR, Fisher M. SGLT2 inhibitors: mechanisms of cardiovascular benefit beyond glycaemic control. Nat Rev Cardiol. 2020;17(12):761–72.
82. Rana MN, Neeland IJ. Adipose tissue inflammation and cardiovascular disease: an update. Curr Diab Rep. 2022;22(1):27–37.
83. Hosogai N, Fukuhara A, Oshima K, Miyata Y, Tanaka S, Segawa K, et al. Adipose tissue hypoxia in obesity and its impact on adipocytokine dysregulation. Diabetes. 2007;56(4):901–11.
84. Liu J, Fox CS, Hickson DA, May WD, Hairston KG, Carr JJ, et al. Impact of abdominal visceral and subcutaneous adipose tissue on cardiometabolic risk factors: the Jackson Heart Study. J Clin Endocrinol Metab. 2010;95(12):5419–26.
85. Neeland IJ, Turer AT, Ayers CR, Berry JD, Rohatgi A, Das SR, et al. Body fat distribution and incident cardiovascular disease in obese adults. J Am Coll Cardiol. 2015;65(19):2150–1.
86. Mancio J, Oikonomou EK, Antoniades C. Perivascular adipose tissue and coronary atherosclerosis. Heart. 2018;104(20):1654–62.
87. Esposito K, Pontillo A, Di Palo C, Giugliano G, Masella M, Marfella R, et al. Effect of weight loss and lifestyle changes on vascular inflammatory markers in obese women: a randomized trial. JAMA. 2003;289(14):1799–804.
88. Askarpour M, Khani D, Sheikhi A, Ghaedi E, Alizadeh S. Effect of bariatric surgery on serum inflammatory factors of obese patients: a systematic review and meta-analysis. Obes Surg. 2019;29(8):2631–47.

89. Krarup NT, Borglykke A, Allin KH, Sandholt CH, Justesen JM, Andersson EA, et al. A genetic risk score of 45 coronary artery disease risk variants associates with increased risk of myocardial infarction in 6041 Danish individuals. Atherosclerosis. 2015;240(2):305–10.

90. Wang H, Liu Z, Shao J, Jiang M, Lu X, Lin L, et al. Pathogenesis of premature coronary artery disease: focus on risk factors and genetic variants. Genes Dis. 2020;9(2):370–80.

91. Smith MR, Kinmonth AL, Luben RN, Bingham S, Day NE, Wareham NJ, et al. Smoking status and differential white cell count in men and women in the EPIC-Norfolk population. Atherosclerosis. 2003;169(2):331–7.

92. Aicher A, Heeschen C, Mohaupt M, Cooke JP, Zeiher AM, Dimmeler S. Nicotine strongly activates dendritic cell–mediated adaptive immunity. Circulation. 2003;107(4):604–11.

93. Nizri E, Irony-Tur-Sinai M, Lory O, Orr-Urtreger A, Lavi E, Brenner T. Activation of the cholinergic anti-inflammatory system by nicotine attenuates neuroinflammation via suppression of Th1 and Th17 responses. J Immunol. 2009;183(10):6681–8.

94. Al Rifai M, DeFilippis AP, McEvoy JW, Hall ME, Acien AN, Jones MR, et al. The relationship between smoking intensity and subclinical cardiovascular injury: the Multi-Ethnic Study of Atherosclerosis (MESA). Atherosclerosis. 2017;258:119–30.

95. Hoek G, Krishnan RM, Beelen R, Peters A, Ostro B, Brunekreef B, et al. Long-term air pollution exposure and cardio- respiratory mortality: a review. Environ Health. 2013;12(1):43.

96. Brook RD, Newby DE, Rajagopalan S. Air pollution and cardiometabolic disease: an update and call for clinical trials. Am J Hypertens. 2017;31(1):1–10.

97. Schmidt FP, Basner M, Kröger G, Weck S, Schnorbus B, Muttray A, et al. Effect of nighttime aircraft noise exposure on endothelial function and stress hormone release in healthy adults. Eur Heart J. 2013;34(45):3508–14.

98. Schmidt F, Kolle K, Kreuder K, Schnorbus B, Wild P, Hechtner M, et al. Nighttime aircraft noise impairs endothelial function and increases blood pressure in patients with or at high risk for coronary artery disease. Clin Res Cardiol. 2015;104(1):23–30.

99. Schloss MJ, Swirski FK, Nahrendorf M. Modifiable cardiovascular risk, hematopoiesis, and innate immunity. Circ Res. 2020;126(9):1242–59.

100. Drosos GC, Vedder D, Houben E, Boekel L, Atzeni F, Badreh S, et al. EULAR recommendations for cardiovascular risk management in rheumatic and musculoskeletal diseases, including systemic lupus erythematosus and antiphospholipid syndrome. Ann Rheum Dis [Internet]. 2022 Feb 1. [Cited 2022 Mar 27]. https://ard.bmj.com/content/early/2022/02/01/annrheumdis-2021-221733.

101. Reiss AB, Jacob B, Ahmed S, Carsons SE, DeLeon J. Understanding accelerated atherosclerosis in systemic lupus erythematosus: toward better treatment and prevention. Inflammation. 2021;44(5):1663–82.

102. Avina-Zubieta JA, Thomas J, Sadatsafavi M, Lehman AJ, Lacaille D. Risk of incident cardiovascular events in patients with rheumatoid arthritis: a meta-analysis of observational studies. Ann Rheum Dis. 2012;71(9):1524–9.

103. Cainzos-Achirica M, Glassner K, Zawahir HS, Dey AK, Agrawal T, Quigley EMM, et al. Inflammatory bowel disease and atherosclerotic cardiovascular disease: JACC review topic of the week. J Am Coll Cardiol. 2020;76(24):2895–905.

104. Choi H, Uceda DE, Dey AK, Abdelrahman KM, Aksentijevich M, Rodante JA, et al. Treatment of psoriasis with biologic therapy is associated with improvement of coronary artery plaque lipid-rich necrotic core. Circ Cardiovasc Imaging. 2020;13(9):e011199.

105. Dragoljevic D, Kraakman MJ, Nagareddy PR, Ngo D, Shihata W, Kammoun HL, et al. Defective cholesterol metabolism in haematopoietic stem cells promotes monocyte-driven atherosclerosis in rheumatoid arthritis. Eur Heart J. 2018;39(23):2158–67.

106. Davies R, Williams J, Sime K, Jin HS, Thompson C, Jordan L, et al. The role of interleukin-6 trans-signalling on cardiovascular dysfunction in inflammatory arthritis. Rheumatology. 2021;60(6):2852–61.

107. Akhmedov A, Crucet M, Simic B, Kraler S, Bonetti NR, Ospelt C, et al. TNFα induces endothelial dysfunction in rheumatoid arthritis via LOX-1 and arginase 2: reversal by monoclonal TNFα antibodies. Cardiovasc Res. 2022;118(1):254–66.
108. Erre GL, Mangoni AA, Castagna F, Paliogiannis P, Carru C, Passiu G, et al. Meta-analysis of asymmetric dimethylarginine concentrations in rheumatic diseases. Sci Rep. 2019;9(1):5426.
109. Ahmed S, Jacob B, Carsons SE, De Leon J, Reiss AB. Treatment of cardiovascular disease in rheumatoid arthritis: a complex challenge with increased atherosclerotic risk. Pharmaceuticals (Basel). 2021;15(1):11.
110. Westlake SL, Colebatch AN, Baird J, Kiely P, Quinn M, Choy E, et al. The effect of methotrexate on cardiovascular disease in patients with rheumatoid arthritis: a systematic literature review. Rheumatology (Oxford). 2010;49(2):295–307.
111. Atzeni F, Rodríguez-Carrio J, Popa CD, Nurmohamed MT, Szűcs G, Szekanecz Z. Cardiovascular effects of approved drugs for rheumatoid arthritis. Nat Rev Rheumatol. 2021;17(5):270–90.
112. Wasko MCM, Hubert HB, Lingala VB, Elliott JR, Luggen ME, Fries JF, et al. Hydroxychloroquine and risk of diabetes in patients with rheumatoid arthritis. JAMA. 2007;298(2):187–93.
113. Kerr G, Aujero M, Richards J, Sayles H, Davis L, Cannon G, et al. Associations of hydroxychloroquine use with lipid profiles in rheumatoid arthritis: pharmacologic implications. Arthritis Care Res. 2014;66(11):1619–26.
114. Sharma TS, Wasko MCM, Tang X, Vedamurthy D, Yan X, Cote J, et al. Hydroxychloroquine use is associated with decreased incident cardiovascular events in rheumatoid arthritis patients. J Am Heart Assoc. 2016;5(1):e002867.
115. Fasano S, Pierro L, Pantano I, Iudici M, Valentini G. Long term hydroxychloroquine therapy and low-dose aspirin may have an additive effectiveness in the primary prevention of cardiovascular events in patients with systemic lupus erythematosus. J Rheumatol. 2017;44(7):1032–8.
116. Schrezenmeier E, Dörner T. Mechanisms of action of hydroxychloroquine and chloroquine: implications for rheumatology. Nat Rev Rheumatol. 2020;16(3):155–66.
117. Jacobsson LTH, Turesson C, Nilsson JÅ, Petersson IF, Lindqvist E, Saxne T, et al. Treatment with TNF blockers and mortality risk in patients with rheumatoid arthritis. Ann Rheum Dis. 2007;66(5):670–5.
118. Low ASL, Symmons DPM, Lunt M, Mercer LK, Gale CP, Watson KD, et al. Relationship between exposure to tumour necrosis factor inhibitor therapy and incidence and severity of myocardial infarction in patients with rheumatoid arthritis. Ann Rheum Dis. 2017;76(4):654–60.
119. Roubille C, Richer V, Starnino T, McCourt C, McFarlane A, Fleming P, et al. The effects of tumour necrosis factor inhibitors, methotrexate, non-steroidal anti-inflammatory drugs and corticosteroids on cardiovascular events in rheumatoid arthritis, psoriasis and psoriatic arthritis: a systematic review and meta-analysis. Ann Rheum Dis. 2015;74(3):480–9.
120. Albuquerque AM, Tramujas L, Sewanan LR, Williams DR, Brophy JM. Mortality rates among hospitalized patients with COVID-19 infection treated with tocilizumab and corticosteroids: a Bayesian reanalysis of a previous meta-analysis. JAMA Netw Open. 2022;5(2):e220548.
121. Singh S, Fumery M, Singh AG, Singh N, Prokop LJ, Dulai PS, et al. Comparative risk of cardiovascular events with biologic and synthetic disease-modifying antirheumatic drugs in patients with rheumatoid arthritis: a systematic review and meta-analysis. Arthritis Care Res. 2020;72(4):561–76.
122. Guedeney P, Claessen BE, Kalkman DN, Aquino M, Sorrentino S, Giustino G, et al. Residual inflammatory risk in patients with Low LDL cholesterol levels undergoing percutaneous coronary intervention. J Am Coll Cardiol. 2019;73(19):2401–9.

123. Collins R, Reith C, Emberson J, Armitage J, Baigent C, Blackwell L, et al. Interpretation of the evidence for the efficacy and safety of statin therapy. Lancet (Lond Engl). 2016;388(10059):2532–61.

124. Antonopoulos AS, Margaritis M, Lee R, Channon K, Antoniades C. Statins as anti-inflammatory agents in atherogenesis: molecular mechanisms and lessons from the recent clinical trials. Curr Pharm Des. 2012;18(11):1519–30.

125. Mason RP, Dawoud H, Sherratt SCR, Wagner MR, Malinski T. Progressive LDL reduction to very low levels improves dimeric nitric oxide synthase, nitric oxide bioavailability and reduces peroxynitrite in endothelial cells during hyperglycemia. Am J Pharmacol Toxicol. 2019;14(1):7–16.

126. Ridker PM, Danielson E, Fonseca FAH, Genest J, Gotto AM, Kastelein JJP, et al. Rosuvastatin to prevent vascular events in men and women with elevated C-reactive protein. N Engl J Med. 2008;359(21):2195–207.

127. Downs JR, Clearfield M, Weis S, Whitney E, Shapiro DR, Beere PA, et al. Primary prevention of acute coronary events with lovastatin in men and women with average cholesterol levels: results of AFCAPS/TexCAPS. JAMA. 1998;279(20):1615–22.

128. Ridker PM, Rifai N, Clearfield M, Downs JR, Weis SE, Miles JS, et al. Measurement of C-reactive protein for the targeting of statin therapy in the primary prevention of acute coronary events. N Engl J Med. 2001;344(26):1959–65.

129. Ridker PM, Cannon CP, Morrow D, Rifai N, Rose LM, McCabe CH, et al. C-reactive protein levels and outcomes after statin therapy. N Engl J Med. 2005;352(1):20–8.

130. Hansson GK, Klareskog L. Pulling down the plug on atherosclerosis: cooling down the inflammasome. Nat Med. 2011;17(7):790–1.

131. Nidorf SM, Eikelboom JW, Budgeon CA, Thompson PL. Low-dose colchicine for secondary prevention of cardiovascular disease. J Am Coll Cardiol. 2013;61(4):404–10.

132. Tardif JC, Kouz S, Waters DD, Bertrand OF, Diaz R, Maggioni AP, et al. Efficacy and safety of low-dose colchicine after myocardial infarction. N Engl J Med. 2019;381(26):2497–505.

133. Nidorf SM, Fiolet ATL, Mosterd A, Eikelboom JW, Schut A, Opstal TSJ, et al. Colchicine in patients with chronic coronary disease. N Engl J Med. 2020;383(19):1838–47.

134. Ridker PM, Everett BM, Thuren T, MacFadyen JG, Chang WH, Ballantyne C, et al. Antiinflammatory therapy with canakinumab for atherosclerotic disease. N Engl J Med. 2017;377(12):1119–31.

Thrombosis, Hemostasis, and Cardiovascular Outcomes

Agastya D. Belur, Shengnan Zheng, Munis Raza, and Dinesh K. Kalra

Key Points

- Hemostasis is the prevention of blood loss due to vessel injury; efficient and effective hemostasis is critical to survival and to the overall success rate of all invasive procedures. A fine and orchestrated balance exists between clotting and bleeding to maintain blood vessel wall integrity and prevent either thrombosis or bleeding.
- Venous and arterial thromboembolism carries one of the highest burdens of morbidity and mortality worldwide with significant healthcare costs.
- Endothelial injury, stasis or turbulent blood flow, and hypercoagulability are essential to thrombogenesis; the risk of thrombogenesis is increased in patients with infection, inflammation, malignancy, and inherited or acquired hypercoagulable states.
- Over time, thrombi may undergo propagation, embolization, dissolution, or organization. Rarely, thrombi may become infected, regardless of chronicity.
- The composition of thrombi changes over time as does their embolic potential—thus, chronicity of thrombi is one of the factors considered before choosing any pharmacological or mechanical treatment options.
- A wide variety of oral and parenteral anticoagulant and antiplatelet drugs are available; they have variable potency with regard to their efficacy and adverse effects, i.e., bleeding risk.

A. D. Belur · S. Zheng · M. Raza
Division of Cardiology, University of Louisville, Louisville, KY, USA

D. K. Kalra (✉)
Division of Cardiology, University of Louisville, Louisville, KY, USA

Division of Cardiology, Department of Medicine, Rudd Heart and Lung Center, University of Louisville School of Medicine, Louisville, KY, USA
e-mail: dinesh.kalra@louisville.edu

© The Author(s), under exclusive license to Springer Nature Switzerland AG 2024

K. C. Maki, D. P. Wilson (eds.), *Cardiovascular Outcomes Research*, Contemporary Cardiology, https://doi.org/10.1007/978-3-031-54960-1_11

- Catheter-directed thrombolytic therapy and mechanical thrombectomy are increasingly used to treat massive and submassive pulmonary emboli and reduce the incidence of right-sided heart failure leading to cardiogenic shock, cardiac arrest, and respiratory failure when compared to anticoagulation alone.

1 Introduction: A History of Thrombosis

The first description of a case most likely to be a deep vein thrombus (DVT) comes from the Middle Ages [1, 2] in an account of a 20-year-old cobbler named Raoul in a manuscript by Guillaume de Saint Pathus entitled "La vie et les miracles de Saint Louis." In 1784, well before Virchow demonstrated the relationship between DVT and fatal pulmonary embolism (PE), Hunter performed venous ligations above thromboses to prevent the extension of clots [3, 4]. This became the standard of treatment until the nineteenth century. A cornerstone in our understanding of thrombosis came in the nineteenth century when physicians noticed an association between DVT and infection, pregnancy, and prolonged bedrest for a febrile illness. Until this discovery, and the proven efficacy of anticoagulants such as heparin in the mid-twentieth century [5–7], the treatment of DVT relied on bed rest to fix the thrombus in place, elevation of the affected extremity to favor venous return, application of heat with warm compresses to reduce vasospasm and increase collateral circulation, and venous ligation [2, 4, 8]. The prophylaxis and treatment of thromboembolism have come a long way since Raoul the cobbler, and our understanding of the complex pathophysiology of these conditions and their effects on cardiovascular outcomes has evolved in the last few centuries. We now know that hemostasis and thromboembolism are intricately linked, both pathways being innate responses of the vascular system to various insults.

2 Epidemiology and Pathobiology of Thrombus Formation

In 2017, approximately 695,000 people in the United States were estimated to have experienced a new coronary arterial thrombotic event and more than 325,000 people had recurrent thrombotic events [9]. Approximately 795,000 strokes from a thrombotic event within the cerebral circulation also occurred that year [9]. Currently, there are 300,000–600,000 new cases of venous thromboembolism (VTE) each year, approximately 30% of which result in death within 30 days of diagnosis; the majority of the deaths are sudden and due to PE [9–11]. In fact, thromboembolism is the cause of one in four deaths worldwide [9, 10]. There is a substantial economic burden from VTE as well, and 2016 statistics show direct medical costs of an acute VTE in the United States as high as $15,000 within 1 year after the event, and subsequent per incidence complication costs average as high as $23,000 [12]. The incidence of thromboembolism increases sharply after approximately 45 years of age, with rates being slightly higher in males.

Three major pathologic mechanisms trigger the coagulation cascade and lead to thrombus formation as first described by Rudolf Virchow in 1856; these include (1) endothelial injury, (2) stasis or turbulent blood flow, and (3) hypercoagulability of blood. Common risk factors for VTE include age, exogenous factors such as smoking, surgery, hospitalization, immobility, trauma, pregnancy, and hormone use, and endogenous factors such as malignancy, metabolic syndrome, pro-inflammatory states, and inherited and acquired disorders of hypercoagulation [11, 13]. The most common inherited cause of a hypercoagulable state is the factor V Leiden mutation, which is present in approximately 5% of the Caucasian population and 15–20% of all patients presenting with VTE [14–16]. Studies in the last decade have identified several other gene variants associated with VTEs in certain loci and genes that were previously not known to be associated with thrombosis [17, 18].

Arterial thromboembolism accounts for the highest burden of cardiovascular morbidity and mortality in the world [10] and is almost always associated with underlying atherosclerosis of the involved artery [19]. Compared to veins, arteries are characterized by high rates of blood flow, higher blood pressure, and more streamlined laminar flow of blood, all of which naturally prevent blood stasis, platelet aggregation, and activation of the coagulation cascade. Thus, endothelial injury and any factors that induce turbulent flow of blood are of particular significance in thrombus formation in the arterial circulation. Physical loss of endothelium (as occurs with rupture of an arterial plaque) can precipitate platelet adhesion and endothelial activation, which lead to the release of platelet and coagulation pathway-mediated procoagulant factors and eventual thrombus formation and myocardial infarction (MI). Risk factors include any insult that could predispose to endothelial injury and disrupt laminar flow directly (e.g., smoking, hypertension, bacterial endotoxins, systemic inflammation, radiation injury, and metabolic conditions such as homocysteinemia) or indirectly via promotion of cholesterol plaque formation (e.g., hyperlipidemia and diabetes) [10, 20]. Local arterial dilation from aneurysm formation also causes local stasis and turbulent flow, predisposing patients to thrombus formation within the aneurysm. Atrial fibrillation is a well-recognized major risk factor for stroke and systemic arterial thromboembolism [21].

In a study of patients with acute ST elevation MI (STEMI), Silvain et al. used aspiration thrombectomy to extract occlusive thrombi from the culprit vessels ($n = 45$) at the time of primary percutaneous coronary intervention (PCI). Using scanning electron microscopy, they observed that the major component in these thrombi was fibrin (60%), with the remainder of the ~40% comprised variably of platelets, cholesterol crystals, red blood cells, and leukocytes [22, 23]. They also noted that patients who had suffered longer periods of ischemia had thrombi with higher amounts of fibrin and fewer red blood cells, leukocytes, and platelets [22–24]. Thus, ischemic time and clot composition may impact the choice of therapies, such as fibrinolytic therapy or mechanical thrombectomy as discussed in further detail below.

3 Infection, Inflammation, and Thrombosis

Inflammation creates a prothrombotic state and is a risk factor for arterial and venous thrombosis and the development and progression of atherosclerosis [25]. Briefly, inflammation triggers the activation of platelets, which may accompany damage to the endothelium, resulting in fibrin deposition and thrombus formation. The clinical significance of this heightened risk has been validated in recent years; systemic inflammation is associated with early adverse cardiovascular outcomes, especially among patients who suffer from autoimmune inflammatory conditions such as psoriasis and psoriatic arthritis [26], rheumatoid arthritis [26, 27], and systemic lupus erythematosus [28]. Several large trials in the last 5 years [29–32] have shown that reducing inflammation leads to improved cardiovascular outcomes, in terms of reduced major adverse cardiovascular events (MACE) such as MI and stroke.

Systemic or localized infections increase the risk of thrombosis by ~2- to 20-fold and are independent risk factors for VTE and MACE [33–35]. Unfortunately, the mechanisms by which infection-associated thrombosis is induced, maintained, and resolved are poorly understood, as is the contribution thrombosis makes to host control of infection and pathogen spread [33]. It is believed that the presence of the pathogen and its products, along with an appropriate response from the host immune system, create an inflammation-mediated prothrombotic state such as described above. This suggests the ultimate risk of thrombosis after infection is influenced by both host- and pathogen-derived factors. In some cases of severe infections and sepsis, there can be diffuse activation of the immune system and coagulation cascade leading to disseminated intravascular coagulation, which carries a risk of mortality as high as 20–25% [36].

4 SARS-CoV-2: The Novel Coronavirus and Thromboembolism

Infection with the novel coronavirus (COVID-19 infection) has been associated with an increased risk of arterial and venous thromboembolism [37]. A meta-analysis reported on the incidence of VTE among hospitalized COVID-19 patients from 26 studies with 34 patient cohorts [38]. The overall incidence of all VTE events in COVID-19 infection was ~28.3%, with a higher incidence of VTE (close to 40%) in patients with severe infection. Furthermore, about a fifth of all patients with COVID-19 infection were found to have some form of DVT, as reported in 17 studies with 21 patient cohorts. Similar numbers were reported for the incidence of PE (17.6% among all patients and 21.7% among patients with severe infection) described in 19 studies with 24 patient cohorts. This study also reported the association between increased mortality and VTE in COVID-19 infection described in eight studies, with five severe and four general COVID-19 cohorts. Patients with severe infection who had VTE were found to have a significantly greater mortality rate (38.1%; 95% confidence interval [CI], 24.7–52.4%) compared to those with severe COVID-19 without VTE (22.0%; 95% CI, 9.4–37.5%) with an odds ratio of 2.02 (95% CI, 1.15–3.53%; $p = 0.014$). A similar association was not found among patients with less severe infection, with no statistically significant mortality difference between patients with and without VTE in this population. Another review and meta-analysis reported similar findings; the overall prevalence of VTE in hospitalized patients with COVID-19 was approximately 30% but with considerable heterogeneity. VTE prevalence was high, even in patients receiving standard dose thromboprophylaxis, although it was lower when patients were on full-dose or therapeutic anticoagulation. Not surprisingly, patients with COVID-19 who had VTE had higher mortality than those who did not develop VTE [39]. All critically ill patients admitted to intensive care units (ICUs) are at very high VTE risk because of circumstances and procedures commonly utilized in the ICU (immobilization, sedation, vasopressors, or central venous catheters) irrespective of etiology, all of which may contribute to the higher incidence of VTE and the higher mortality in patients with severe COVID-19 infection. This novel virus is also thought to induce a prothrombotic state via mechanisms similar to those of other infections; there is an induction of an excessive inflammatory state via a cytokine storm combined with endothelial injury and pulmonary vascular microthrombosis, which could considerably increase the risk for VTE, mainly PE [40–42]. The association between VTE and COVID-19 infection is not limited to acute illness; studies have shown conflicting data on the post-discharge incidence of arterial and venous thrombosis in these patients. It is generally agreed that the incidence of thrombosis and bleeding in patients discharged after COVID-19 hospitalization are comparable to those of medically ill patients without COVID-19 [43–45]. At this time, guidelines recommend routine DVT/PE prophylaxis with pharmacologic thromboprophylaxis (e.g., with the usual prophylactic dose of low molecular weight heparin [LMWH]), unless contraindicated due to high bleeding risk or other factors, for patients admitted for COVID-19 infection, with continuation of outpatient anticoagulants if the patient was already taking them for a preexisting condition (such as atrial fibrillation). Treatment with full-strength anticoagulation with heparin products or other anticoagulants is recommended only if there is evidence of VTE, with consideration of thrombolytic therapy recommended if the patient has life- or limb-threatening ischemia from arterial or venous thromboembolism [46]. Individuals with documented VTE require a minimum of 3 months of anticoagulation after discharge; based on the low incidence of VTE despite the infrequent use of post-discharge prophylactic anticoagulation, routine post-discharge thromboprophylaxis is not used [46]. Post-discharge thromboprophylaxis can be considered in patients with major prothrombotic risk factors such as a history of VTE or recent major surgery or trauma, as long as they are not at high bleeding risk. Options for post-discharge prophylaxis include those used in recent clinical trials, such as rivaroxaban 10 mg daily for 31–39 days [46, 47].

The role of pharmacological agents in the prevention and treatment of thrombosis in COVID-19 infections is being explored in placebo-controlled and head-to-head trials (especially comparing heparin products, aspirin, direct oral anti-coagulants such as apixaban, direct thrombin inhibitors such as bivalirudin and argatroban, and thrombolytic agents such as tenecteplase) [48–53]. Another facet being explored is the dose of such pharmacological agents (DVT prophylaxis dose versus VTE treatment dose) [54–58].

5   Cardiovascular Outcomes of Thrombosis

In patients who survive the initial insult without antithrombotic treatment, over a period of days to weeks, all thrombi undergo a combination of four outcomes: (1) propagation; (2) embolization; (3) dissolution; and (4) organization and recanalization.

The thrombus may recruit additional platelets, fibrin, and other components of the coagulation cascade, a phenomenon known as *propagation.*

The thrombus may *embolize*, a term first used by Virchow in 1848 to describe the process of thrombus dislodgement and migration to other sites in the vasculature. More than 50% of all DVTs will embolize to the pulmonary vasculature [59], leading to significant short- and long-term morbidity and mortality. The Centers for Disease Control and Prevention (CDC) estimates that 10–30% of patients with acute PE will die within 1 month of diagnosis. Sudden death from PE is the first symptom in 25% of patients who suffer VTE. Furthermore, among patients who experience a DVT, 33–50% will have long-term complications such as swelling, pain, discoloration, and scaling of the affected limb; approximately 33% of patients suffer recurrent VTE within 10 years [60, 61].

The third possible outcome of a thrombus is *dissolution*. This is more common in relatively newer and smaller thrombi and occurs as a result of fibrinolysis, leading to shrinkage and, in certain cases, even disappearance of the thrombus. In contrast, large and old thrombi have higher amounts of fibrin, as previously discussed, and these thrombi tend not to dissolve spontaneously. Thrombus composition may change over time after the initial vessel occlusion in STEMI. Such changes in thrombus composition may have important implications for mechanical thrombectomy, aspiration, and thrombolysis, explaining why thrombolytic therapy is generally effective only when administered within the first few hours of the thrombotic episode. Further research is required to understand the mechanisms through which thrombi change in structure and composition [22].

The fourth possible fate, especially in older thrombi, is *organization and recanalization*. There is ingrowth of endothelial cells, smooth muscle cells, and fibroblasts, with the eventual formation of capillary channels through the thrombus that re-establish the flow of blood, to some degree, through the original vessel lumen. Over time, the thrombus may organize into a smaller mass of connective tissue that becomes incorporated into the vessel wall. Thrombus organization is more likely when anticoagulant therapy is not administered acutely or started early after thrombus development, and the thrombus has weeks to months to evolve, fibrose, and organize. It occurs more often with bulkier clots such as those seen in the iliofemoral veins [62].

Infection is a worrisome complication of long-standing thrombi irrespective of their location and treatment status, clinically referred to as septic thrombophlebitis. Patients with bacteremia from any source of infection may seed preexisting thrombi, and these infected thrombi may become a nidus for recurrent infection and persistent bacteremia. Infective endocarditis, a dreaded cardiovascular complication of septic thrombophlebitis, may lead to persistent bacteremia, especially in patients with congenital or valvular heart disease, valve repair or replacement procedures, and implanted cardiac devices. Over time, an infected thrombus, especially those in arteries, may erode and weaken the vessel wall and, if left untreated, can lead to the formation of a mycotic aneurysm that may rupture acutely with high morbidity and mortality.

6 Outcomes Studies of VTE and MACE

The Worcester VTE Trial was one of the first studies exploring the clinical outcomes of VTE [63]. In this study, 1567 persons with first-time VTE were identified and followed over a mean period of 1216 days. In three cohorts of patients who were followed after their first VTE in 1999, 2001, and 2003, long-term rates of recurrent VTE were approximately 17%. After controlling for potentially confounding demographic and clinical differences in the three groups, there was a trend toward reduced VTE recurrence in the 2003 cohort (odds ratio 0.75; 95% CI 0.54, 1.04), likely due to more widespread use of heparin as time progressed. Rates of major bleeding were approximately 12–13% for the three study cohorts and did not differ significantly by cohort year. Long-term mortality decreased slightly between the initial study cohort of 1999 (43.3%) and the 2003 cohort (37.7%), but this difference was not statistically significant. No significant changes in the rates of recurrent PE were detected over this period. As time progressed, our ability to detect and safely treat VTE has improved, with subsequent improvement in long-term outcomes in these patients. A study by Huang et al. from the population-based Worcester VTE Study (1999–2009) showed that while PE patients were consistently admitted to the hospital for treatment during the time of the study, the proportion of patients diagnosed with DVT-alone who were hospitalized decreased from 67% in 1999 to 37% in 2009 (p-value for trend <0.001). Among hospitalized patients, the mean length of stay decreased from 5.6 to 4.8 days (p-value for trend <0.001). Between 1999 and 2009, treatment of VTE shifted from warfarin and unfractionated heparin toward the use of LMWH and newer anticoagulants; also, 3-year cumulative event rates decreased for all-cause mortality (from 41% to 26%, $p < 0.001$), major bleeding (from 12% to 6%, $p = 0.002$), and recurrent VTE (from 17% to 9%, $p < 0.001$) [64]. Outcomes of VTE and the evolution and treatment of post-thrombotic syndrome among survivors of VTE are topics of ongoing clinical investigation [65–67]. Another topic of interest and ongoing investigation is the use of novel oral drugs for pharmacological prophylaxis against VTE among hospitalized patients and postoperative patients [68, 69], both independent predisposing factors for DVT, especially among patients with risk factors for VTE, as described previously.

7 Hemostasis

Hemostasis is the prevention of blood loss due to vessel injury. It comprises several processes including vascular constriction, formation of a platelet plug, blood coagulation leading to physiological clot formation and eventual growth of fibrous tissue to permanently heal the vessel wall. Vascular constriction, mediated by the contraction of smooth muscles in the vessel wall, instantaneously reduces the flow of blood to minimize blood loss. The intensity of vascular constriction depends on the severity of the injury to the vessel wall. This vascular spasm lasts from a few minutes to hours and can be problematic in a few cases of cardiac catheterization utilizing the radial artery.

Platelets formed from the fragmentation of megakaryocytes are essential to hemostasis. The normal platelet count is 150,000–300,000 per microliter, with a half-life of 8–12 days. Platelets become activated by exposed collagen in the injured vessel wall, after which they attach to the vessel wall and begin secreting adenosine diphosphate (ADP) and thromboxane A2 (TxA2), which in turn activate more platelets. In this way, platelets are recruited to the injured vessel wall and begin to form a platelet plug. A complex interplay between the platelet plug, prothrombotic proteins, and clotting factors leads to the formation of a thrombus, which seals the defect in the vessel wall.

Early hemostasis at the arterial access site used in the invasive management of acute coronary syndromes (ACS) is essential because bleeding complications are an important predictor of outcomes in ACS. Several mechanisms have been proposed to explain this association. Hemodynamic effects associated with massive bleeding might result in higher mortality. Bleeding at distant sites such as intracranial hemorrhage due to fibrinogen would cause a higher incidence of morbidity and mortality. Even minor bleeding may lead to a physiologic increase in levels of neurohormones such as epinephrine, angiotensin, endothelin-1, and vasopressin, all of which are associated with adverse cardiac events.

During invasive coronary procedures, patients are given systemic antiplatelet and anticoagulant medications to help prevent the formation of thrombus in the coronary circulation related to the presence of catheters and interventional wires in the coronary arteries. As there is a minor iatrogenic vascular injury during coronary intervention, inadequate antiplatelet/anticoagulant medication can lead to new thrombus formation within or near the stent. However, this understandably comes with an increased risk of bleeding at the vascular access site. These bleeding complications are associated with increased hospitalization, increased hospital costs, patient dissatisfaction, morbidity, and higher 1-year mortality [70]. Various strategies can be adopted to reduce the burden of bleeding complications. Pharmacological advances, including the use of LMWH, abciximab, or fondaparinux, have led to decreased rates of bleeding complications [71, 72]. Procedural (vascular access) and technological (vascular closure devices) approaches to improve bleeding complications are discussed below.

7.1 Femoral Artery Access

Femoral artery access and the use of intravascular sheaths heralded the modern era of interventional cardiology, replacing the cutdown of the brachial artery as the predominant arterial access site. The femoral artery is punctured at the site of the common femoral artery. The Femoral Arterial Access with Ultrasound Trial (FAUST) [73] showed that the use of ultrasound to obtain vascular access decreased the rate of vascular complications and the number of attempts to gain access in the femoral artery. Micropuncture to safely and accurately access the femoral artery is essential for reducing the complications of vascular access.

There are many options to achieve hemostasis at the site of femoral artery access including manual pressure, closure devices, such as sutures, clips, and collagen plugs, and femoral compression systems. The location of the common femoral artery over the femoral head allows hemostasis to be achieved by manual compression using the femoral head as a pressure point against which the femoral artery can be compressed. Vascular closure devices can only be used for common femoral artery access at the level of the femoral head. Studies have shown a difference in bleeding complications with the use of vascular closure devices [74–76]. These devices may have a slightly higher risk of infection but shorter times for hemostasis, earlier ambulation, and enhanced patient comfort. As there are no definitive data showing that one device is superior to another regarding safety and efficacy, the choice of a vascular closure device depends on operator preference and expertise. Patients being considered for vascular closure devices should undergo a femoral angiogram to ensure their arterial anatomy and location of puncture are suitable. The routine use of vascular closure devices is not recommended for the purpose of decreasing vascular complications, including bleeding. Following an interventional procedure with systemic anticoagulation, failure of the device can lead to immediate, and potentially life-threatening, bleeding. Failed closure has been associated with an increased risk of vascular complications. Immediate hemostasis is required with manual compression and may require endovascular rescue with contralateral access and balloon tamponade or covered stent placement of the access site in these situations.

7.2 Radial Artery Access

Trans-radial access is facilitated with the palm of the patient's hand secured in the supine position, slightly hyperextended at the wrist, and parallel to the floor. Arterial access may be obtained via either a single- or a double-wall puncture technique.

Both techniques are safe and effective and are associated with low rates of radial artery occlusion and other bleeding complications [77]. Multiple trials have shown that, when compared to femoral access in patients with ACS, radial artery access was associated with a lower risk of vascular complications, decreased overall risk of fatal and non-fatal bleeding, and even lower incidence of a composite endpoint of death, MI, stroke, or non-coronary artery bypass graft bleeding [78–82]. Furthermore, there is a subjective benefit with improved patient comfort in transradial access compared to femoral artery access. There are a few limitations with radial artery access including the smaller diameter of the radial artery, which limits the sheath size that can be used to only 6 or 7 French. Furthermore, there is a steeper learning curve and more operator expertise is required for successful cardiac catheterization via radial artery access compared to femoral artery access. Most importantly, however, is the possibility of vascular constriction, which can lead to arterial spasms. This decreases the ability to manipulate catheters easily and, in some cases, might lead to catheter entrapment, a serious complication of radial artery access. This can be overcome using a cocktail of antispasmodic drugs in different dosages, most commonly verapamil and nitroglycerin. There may be a higher rate of procedure failure with the radial approach, necessitating crossover to femoral access [83]. Devices that use air to compress the arteriotomy site are used to achieve hemostasis. The device is deflated slowly to allow enough time for hemostasis to occur, with the minimal amount of air required for hemostasis left in an inflatable band across the skin overlying the arteriotomy, until hemostasis is achieved.

8 Pharmacological Agents in the Prevention and Treatment of Thrombosis

8.1 Parenteral Anticoagulant Drugs

8.1.1 General Use and Clinical Experience

Common clinical indications for the parenteral anticoagulants described below include prophylaxis of VTE in acutely ill patients or patients at high risk of thromboembolism, prophylaxis of VTE after surgical procedures, such as hip or knee replacement surgery, and treatment of ACS. Selected circumstances, such as periprocedural anticoagulation and bridging anticoagulant therapy in the setting of chronic anticoagulation for conditions such as atrial fibrillation, benefit from the use of unfractionated heparin (UFH) given its ease of reversibility and short dose-dependent half-life. Heparin is also commonly used as a bridging therapy while initiating warfarin.

Heparins

Unfractionated Heparin (UFH)

UFH represents one of the most frequently used agents in the prevention and treatment of thrombosis. Discovered in the 1920s, the use of UFH as an anticoagulant in clinical practice became routine after the publication of several seminal papers in the early 1970s showing it prevented VTE and PE in patients following surgery. UFH exerts its effect through an interaction with antithrombin (AT) III, which, once bound to the UFH molecule, enhances its anticoagulant effect 1000-fold [84, 85]. This inactivates (1) thrombin, thus preventing the conversion of fibrin to fibrinogen, and (2) activated coagulation factors IX, X, XI, and XII. Other mechanisms through which heparin acts are by inactivation of thrombin by heparin cofactor II and, to a lesser extent, through direct modulation of factors Xa (FXa) and IXa. Following intravenous (IV) administration, UFH binds to several plasma proteins, endothelial cells, and macrophages, explaining the wide variability in the anticoagulant effect previously shown for a given dose. The most cost-effective and widely used tests to check for therapeutic levels in patients receiving UFH are activated partial thromboplastin time (aPTT) and activated coagulation time (ACT).

Use of UFH

Previous clinical trials compared the benefits of UFH and aspirin among patients with unstable angina and non-STEMI (NSTEMI) [86]. Since the 1980s, these individual trials and pooled analyses have shown a reduced incidence of a combined endpoint of death/MI in favor of combination therapy, which now forms the mainstay of management of ACS in patients without bleeding complications.

Acute MI: During acute MI, UFH can be administered concomitantly with thrombolytic therapy or during primary PCI. In ACS, UFH can be used and is most beneficial in the setting of elevated troponin, irrespective of ECG changes.

Elective PCI: During elective PCI, a standard heparin regimen consists of 70–100 U/kg body weight, with additional weight-adjusted boluses to achieve and maintain an ACT of 200–250 s [87–89]. If a glycoprotein (GP) IIb/IIIa inhibitor is also given, the initial heparin dosage is reduced to 70 U/kg, followed by additional boluses as needed to maintain an ACT of 200 s. Heparin should be discontinued immediately following the PCI.

Mechanical Circulatory Support (MCS) and Extracorporeal Membrane Oxygenation (ECMO): MCS can provide short-term partial or total cardiac support for a wide spectrum of patients including those with severe cardiogenic shock and select individuals who require cardiac procedures. Furthermore, ECMO is also capable of providing oxygenation through an artificial lung. Blood exposure to the intravascular components of MCS and the large surface area of ECMO circuits disrupt normal hemostasis and can also induce an inflammatory response, which might precipitate thrombosis. In the absence of heparin-induced thrombocytopenia (HIT), anticoagulation with UFH is necessary to prevent clotting of the ECMO circuit with a goal aPTT level of 1.5–2 times the upper limit of normal. As with other MCS devices that require anticoagulation, thrombotic and bleeding complications are common and occur in up to 50% of patients on ECMO [90]. Anticoagulation therapy can be withheld during MCS or ECMO support if life-threatening bleeding occurs.

Left Ventricular Assist Device (LVAD) Thrombosis: The standard treatment for suspected or confirmed pump thrombosis in LVAD patients is anticoagulation with IV UFH and the addition of antiplatelet therapy. Direct thrombin inhibitors, such as bivalirudin, have been used as an alternative anticoagulant to UFH; however, they are more expensive and not clearly proven to be superior to UFH. The only clear indication for these drugs is in patients with HIT. Dual antiplatelet therapy (DAPT) with aspirin plus clopidogrel or dipyridamole to enhance the antiplatelet effect can be considered. Confirmed LVAD thrombosis not responsive to medical therapy is usually treated with pump exchange, especially in patients with hemodynamic compromise or end-organ hypoperfusion. Heart transplantation is another option if a donor heart is available. Thrombolytic therapy is not recommended for either suspected or confirmed pump thrombosis in patients eligible for surgical pump exchange due to the high risk of intracranial hemorrhage [91].

Structural Heart Interventions: Structural heart procedures including transcatheter aortic valve replacement are associated with a significant risk of both thromboembolic and bleeding complications. Most of these procedures have been associated with successful outcomes; however, thromboembolic complications such as stroke are always a concern. In the Placement of Aortic Transcatheter Valves (PARTNER) trial, the incidence of stroke was higher in the transcatheter aortic valve replacement group compared with the surgical replacement group at 1-year follow-up [92]. The clinical significance of valve thrombosis and the role of oral anticoagulation in these patients are the subject of ongoing investigations.

Adverse Effects

Bleeding is the most common complication of UFH administration. The rarest, albeit most feared, complication is the development of HIT. Other adverse effects include hypersensitivity reactions, adrenal hemorrhage with shock, and, with long-term administration, osteopenia.

Reversal

Major or life-threatening hemorrhage is a serious complication among patients receiving parenteral anticoagulants. For the reversal of the effects of UFH, protamine sulfate is the drug of choice. Protamine neutralizes approximately 40–50% of LMWHs, as discussed below. Prothrombin complex concentrate or recombinant factor VII infusion can be used in initial attempts at hemostasis in individuals with refractory bleeding secondary to parenteral anticoagulants.

LMWHs

LMWHs are derived from UFH by chemical depolymerization. This process creates fragments that are approximately one-third the molecular weight of UFH. LMWHs work via catalyzing AT-mediated inhibition of coagulation factors, promoting FXa inhibition. This makes LMWHs more selective in the inhibition of FXa as compared to UFH. Other favorable features of LMWHs include reduced protein binding that improves pharmacokinetic properties, resulting in a more predictable anticoagulant response and reduced interaction with platelets, which reduces the likelihood of HIT. Skin and soft tissue necrosis at the site of subcutaneous injections is a rare complication that may represent a form of local HIT. The presence of renal insufficiency should be considered before prescribing LMWH.

Direct Thrombin Inhibitors (DTIs)

DTIs interact directly with thrombin and do not require AT or heparin cofactors to achieve an anticoagulant effect. They specifically and reversibly inhibit free and clot-bound thrombin by binding to the active site of thrombin. Bivalirudin is a bivalent thrombin inhibitor that binds to both the catalytic and substrate recognition sites of thrombin. Argatroban is a univalent DTI, binding only to the catalytic (active) site of thrombin as a competitive inhibitor of the same.

Bivalirudin is FDA-approved for use in patients with NSTEMI ACS undergoing PCI. The Randomized Evaluation of PCI Linking Angiomax to Reduced Clinical Events (REPLACE)-1 [93] and REPLACE-2 [94] trials showed that bivalirudin was associated with a reduction in the composite clinical endpoint of death, MI, or urgent revascularization, as well as bleeding complications, when compared to UFH and urgent or elective PCI, respectively. Bivalirudin should be used with caution in patients with moderate-to-severe renal dysfunction.

Argatroban is another DTI that is approved for use in patients with HIT, including those with current HIT, previous HIT, and/or those with heparin-dependent antibodies.

Selective FXa Inhibitors

Fondaparinux, the first drug in this class, is a chemically synthesized sulfated pentasaccharide that specifically targets AT. After binding to AT, a permanent conformational change occurs in the molecule that causes an increased affinity for FXa. Fondaparinux does not inhibit thrombin directly, but inactivation of FXa by AT causes strong inhibition of thrombin generation.

Fondaparinux is approved for the prophylaxis of DVT in patients undergoing abdominal surgery, traumatic hip surgery, hip replacement, and knee replacement. The Organization to Assess Strategies in Acute Ischemic Syndromes (OASIS)-5 study [95] compared patients with ACS receiving fondaparinux or enoxaparin and found that the incidence of death, MI, and refractory ischemia was similar in both groups, satisfying noninferiority criteria. However, the rate of major bleeding at 9 days was markedly lowered with fondaparinux compared to enoxaparin. The OASIS-6 study [96] compared fondaparinux to placebo in patients with STEMI. Death or reinfarction at 30 days was significantly reduced from 11.2% in the control group to 9.7% in patients receiving fondaparinux. In the comparison of patients receiving fondaparinux versus those given UFH, fondaparinux was found to be superior in preventing death or reinfarction at 30 days and at the end of the study. The use of a single fixed dose (2.5 mg once daily subcutaneously) of fondaparinux without monitoring across a broad range of kidney function, coupled with its simplicity, safety, and efficacy in ACS, may facilitate its use. However, it is an expensive drug when compared to both UFH and LMWH.

8.2 Oral Anticoagulant Drugs

8.2.1 General Use and Clinical Experience

Common clinical indications for oral anticoagulant drugs include (1) stroke prophylaxis in patients with atrial flutter and atrial fibrillation; (2) thrombosis prophylaxis in patients with mechanical heart valves; and (3) treatment and secondary prevention of VTE and VTE prophylaxis in certain patients, such as those with known inherited or acquired thrombophilia.

Warfarin

Until the introduction of direct oral anticoagulants (DOACs), vitamin K antagonists such as warfarin were the only available oral anticoagulants. Initially developed as a rodenticide, warfarin is a vitamin K antagonist that interferes with the synthesis of vitamin K-dependent clotting factors, namely factors II (prothrombin), VII, IX, and X. The synthesis of vitamin K-dependent anticoagulant proteins C and S is also inhibited by warfarin [97]. Warfarin inhibits vitamin K epoxide reductase and blocks the gamma-carboxylation of vitamin K-dependent clotting factors, a process essential for the expression of the activity of these factors through calcium-dependent binding to anionic phospholipid surfaces. Warfarin results in the synthesis of partially gamma-carboxylated clotting proteins with reduced activity, which gradually replace their fully active counterparts. The half-lives of factor X and prothrombin are 24 and 72 h, respectively, which delays the initial effect of warfarin. Thus, patients at high risk for thrombosis or those with established VTE initially require concomitant treatment with the rapidly acting parenteral anticoagulants discussed above until the target international normalized ratio (INR) is reached on warfarin. Warfarin is rapidly and almost completely absorbed in the gastrointestinal tract. Peak levels occur at about 90 min after administration with a half-life of 36–42 h. Ninety-seven percent of circulating warfarin is bound to albumin, and only a small fraction of unbound warfarin is biologically active [97].

Monitoring

Because warfarin inhibits the synthesis of factors VII (a component of the extrinsic coagulation pathway), X, and II (components of the combined clotting pathway), it causes prolongation of the prothrombin time. This test can be used to monitor the therapeutic action of warfarin. Prothrombin time testing involves the addition of thromboplastin to citrated plasma and determining the time until clot formation. Thromboplastins vary in their sensitivity with less sensitive thromboplastins triggering the administration of higher doses of warfarin to achieve target prothrombin time, thereby increasing the risk of bleeding. The INR was developed to circumvent these problems. INR can be calculated by dividing the patient's prothrombin time by the mean normal prothrombin time and then multiplying this ratio by the international sensitivity index, a predetermined index of the sensitivity of the thromboplastin being used for the test. Although it has limitations, the use of the INR has helped standardize the monitoring of anticoagulant activity in patients on warfarin and is the standard of care for the same.

For most indications, warfarin is administered to maintain a target INR of 2.0–3.0. Patients with mechanical mitral valves and patients with any mechanical heart valve who have additional risk factors for stroke, such as atrial fibrillation, need more robust anticoagulation to a target INR of 2.5–3.5. Patients are at an increased risk for ischemic stroke when the INR falls below 1.7, and bleeding events increase with INR values higher than 4.5. Furthermore, a study in patients receiving long-term warfarin therapy for unprovoked VTE demonstrated a higher rate of recurrent VTE with a target INR of 1.5–1.9 compared to a target INR of 2.0–3.0 [98]. This highlights the narrow therapeutic window of warfarin and other vitamin K antagonists.

Side Effects

Bleeding is a major side effect of warfarin, as is expected of all anticoagulants. A rare complication of warfarin is skin necrosis. Warfarin crosses the placenta and is teratogenic; therefore, it should be avoided during pregnancy.

More than 50% of bleeding complications occur when the INR exceeds the therapeutic range. In asymptomatic patients whose INR is between 3.5 and 9.0, the drug should be withheld until the INR returns to the therapeutic range. Oral or sublingual vitamin K can be administered if the patient is at high risk of bleeding and has an INR between 4.9 and 9.0 but no overt evidence of bleeding. Higher doses of vitamin K produce a more rapid reversal of the INR and can be used if the INR is excessively elevated. Patients with evidence of bleeding require vitamin K by slow IV infusion with additional doses of oral vitamin K until the INR is within the therapeutic range. Patients with serious bleeding can be treated with prothrombin complex concentrate, which is preferred over fresh frozen plasma because it normalizes the INR more rapidly and because the volume of administration is smaller. Patients who experience bleeding when their INR is in therapeutic range require further investigation of the source of bleeding, such as peptic ulcer disease or a tumor of the gastrointestinal or genitourinary tract.

Skin necrosis is a rare complication of warfarin that usually occurs 2–5 days after the initiation of therapy. This occurs in patients with congenital or acquired deficiencies of protein C or protein S, or in patients with HIT who are not receiving an alternate parenteral anticoagulant. The resultant procoagulant state triggers thrombosis in the microvasculature of subcutaneous adipose tissue via unknown mechanisms, leading to skin necrosis. Treatment involves discontinuation of warfarin and administration of vitamin K if needed. An alternative anticoagulant such as heparin or LMWH, or fondaparinux or rivaroxaban for patients with HIT, should be immediately administered. Protein C concentrates may be administered to accelerate the healing of skin lesions. Patients with extensive skin loss may need skin grafting.

Periprocedural Management

Warfarin must be stopped 5 days before elective invasive procedures that are associated with moderate or high risk of bleeding. Only patients at high risk of thrombosis, such as those with mechanical heart valves or atrial fibrillation with a history of stroke, require bridging with a heparin drip or subcutaneous LMWH when the INR falls below 2.0. A heparin drip can be stopped a few hours prior to the procedure, but the last dose of LMWH should be given no later than 12 h before the procedure. Once hemostasis is restored, treatment with warfarin can be resumed. Thromboprophylaxis with parenteral anticoagulants (most commonly LMWH) can be started the day after surgery and should be continued until the INR is within therapeutic range. In contrast, there is no need to stop warfarin prior to procedures associated with low risk for bleeding including dental cleaning or extractions, cataract surgery, or skin biopsy [97].

Direct Oral Anticoagulants (DOACs)

DOACs are small molecules that bind reversibly to the active site of their target enzyme to produce an anticoagulant effect. Table 1 outlines the broad uses of DOACs, and Table 2 highlights landmark trials and studies comparing various DOACs to warfarin. Table 3 lists the collective advantages of DOACs over warfarin.

Uses of DOACs

All DOACs can be used for the prevention of stroke in patients with nonvalvular atrial fibrillation. Dose adjustment is required for patients with at least two of the following criteria: age over 80 years, body weight under 60 kg, and creatinine over 1.5 g/dL. All commercially available DOACs are also approved for the treatment of

Table 1 DOACs and indications [101, 130–134]

DOAC	FDA-approved indications
Dabigatran	Stroke prevention in NVAF
	Treatment of deep vein thrombosis and pulmonary embolism
	Prevention of recurrent deep vein thrombosis and pulmonary embolism
	Prevention of thromboembolism after total hip replacement
Rivaroxaban	Stroke prevention in NVAF
	Treatment of deep vein thrombosis and pulmonary embolism
	Prevention of recurrent deep vein thrombosis and pulmonary embolism
	Prevention of thromboembolism after total knee replacement and after total hip replacement
	Prevention of thromboembolism in hospitalized acutely ill medical patients
	Prevention of major cardiovascular events in patients with chronic CAD/peripheral artery disease
Apixaban	Stroke prevention in NVAF
	Prevention of thromboembolism after total knee replacement and after total hip replacement
	Treatment of deep vein thrombosis and pulmonary embolism
	Prevention of recurrent deep vein thrombosis and pulmonary embolism
Edoxaban	Stroke prevention in NVAF
	Treatment of deep vein thrombosis and pulmonary embolism
Betrixaban	Prevention of deep vein thrombosis and pulmonary embolism in adults hospitalized for an acute medical illness

Legend: *CAD* coronary artery disease, *DOAC* direct oral anticoagulant, *FDA* US Food and Drug Administration, *NVAF* nonvalvular atrial fibrillation

patients with VTE. As shown in Table 3, dabigatran and edoxaban are started after a 5-day course of treatment with a parenteral anticoagulant, such as LMWH. In contrast, rivaroxaban and apixaban can be given in all oral regimens, with a higher starting dose that is reduced to a lower maintenance dose for the indicated duration of therapy. Furthermore, DOACs have been studied and approved for stroke prevention in patients undergoing catheter ablation of atrial fibrillation. Dabigatran, rivaroxaban, and apixaban are approved for VTE prophylaxis after elective hip or knee surgery. Outside of Japan, edoxaban is not licensed for this indication.

Side Effects

Bleeding is the most common side effect of DOACs. When compared to warfarin, all DOACs are associated with a lower risk of intracranial bleeding, but dabigatran is associated with a higher risk of gastrointestinal bleeding [99–102]. An acidic coating essential to the absorption of dabigatran etexilate may be associated with an increased incidence of dyspepsia and acid reflux associated with this drug. These may be minimized by taking the drug with food.

Table 2 Major trials of DOACs in nonvalvular atrial fibrillation (NVAF)

Trial	No of pts, % on ASA, mean CHADS2-VASC score	Major bleeding (event rate in %/year)			Stroke or systemic embolic event (event rate in %/year)			Hemorrhagic stroke (event rate in %/year)			Death (event rate in %/year)		
		DOAC	Warfarin	Relative effect (95% CI)	DOAC	Warfarin	Relative effect (95% CI)	DOAC	Warfarin	Relative effect (95% CI)	DOAC	Warfarin	Relative effect (95% CI)
RE-LY [101] (dabigatran 110 mg twice daily or 150 mg twice daily vs. warfarin with target INR 2.0–3.0)	18,113, 40, 2.1	2.71	3.36	RR 0.80 (0.69–0.93)	1.53	1.69	RR 0.91 (0.74–1.11)	0.12	0.38	RR 0.31 (0.17–0.56)	3.75	4.13	RR 0.91 (0.8–1.03)
		3.11	3.36	RR 0.93 (0.81–1.07)	1.11	1.69	RR 0.66 (0.53–0.82)	0.1	0.38	RR 0.26 (0.14–0.49)	3.64	4.13	RR 0.88 (0.77–1.00)
ROCKET-AF [130] (rivaroxaban 20 mg once daily vs. warfarin with target INR 2.0–3.0)	14,264, 36, 3.5	3.6	3.4	2.1	2.4	HR 0.88 (0.75–1.03)	0.26	0.44	HR 0.59 (0.37–0.93)	4.5	4.9	HR 0.92 (0.82–1.03)	–
ARISTOTLE [131] (apixaban 5 mg twice daily vs. warfarin with target INR 2.0–3.0)	18,201, 31, 2.1	2.13	3.09	HR 0.69 (0.6–0.8)	1.27	1.6	HR 0.79 (0.66–0.95)	0.24	0.47	HR 0.51 (0.35–0.75)	3.52	3.94	HR 0.89 (0.80–0.998)

ENGAGE AF-TIMI 48 [132] (edoxaban 30 mg once daily or 60 mg once daily vs. warfarin with target INR 2.0–3.0)	21,105, 29, 2.8	1.61	3.43	HR 0.47 (0.41–0.55)	2.04	1.8	HR 1.13 (0.96–1.34)	0.16	0.47	HR 0.33 (0.22–0.50)	3.8	4.35	HR 0.87 (0.79–0.96)
		2.75	3.43	HR 0.80 (0.71–0.91)	1.57	1.8	HR 0.87 (0.73–1.04)	0.26	0.47	HR 0.54 (0.38–0.77)	3.99	4.35	HR 0.92 (0.83–1.01)

ARISTOTLE Apixaban for Reduction in Stroke and Other Thromboembolic Events in Atrial Fibrillation, *ASA* acetylsalicylic acid, *CAD* coronary artery disease, *CI* confidence interval, *DOAC* direct oral anticoagulant, *ENGAGE AF-TIMI 48* Effective Anticoagulation with Factor Xa Next Generation in Atrial Fibrillation-Thrombolysis in Myocardial Infarction 48, *FDA* Food and Drug Administration, *HR* hazard ratio, *INR* international normalized ratio, *PCI* percutaneous coronary intervention, *RE-LY* Randomized Evaluation of Long-term Anticoagulation Therapy, *ROCKET-AF* Rivaroxaban Once Daily Oral Direct Factor Xa Inhibition Compared with Vitamin K Antagonism for Prevention of Stroke and Embolism Trial in Atrial Fibrillation, *RR* relative risk

Table 3 Advantages of DOACs vs. warfarin and clinical benefits

Advantage of DOAC	Clinical benefit
Rapid onset of action and shorter half-life	Once or twice daily administration, less peri-procedural bleeding events
More predictable level of anticoagulation Fixed doses produce the same level of anticoagulation	More convenient to administer with no need for monitoring with INR checks No need for frequent dose adjustments or risk of unpredictable response
Safer than warfarin	Less incidence of serious bleeding, especially intracranial hemorrhage as compared to warfarin
More rapid onset of action compared to warfarin Do not inhibit protein C and protein S	No need for bridging therapy with heparin while starting an anticoagulant-naïve patient on DOAC[a]

DOAC direct oral anticoagulant, *INR* international normalized ratio

[a] Except dabigatran and edoxaban that need a 5-day course of low molecular weight heparin prior to initiation

Periprocedural Management

Similar to warfarin, DOACs must be discontinued before surgical procedures associated with a moderate to high risk of bleeding. DOACs should be withheld for a minimum of 1–2 days prior to the procedure, or longer in patients with renal impairment. Assessment of residual anticoagulant activity with prothrombin time for FXa inhibitors, aPTT for dabigatran, and anti-FXa assays for apixaban may be needed prior to high-risk procedures [103]. After surgery, patients should receive thromboprophylaxis with parenteral anticoagulants, such as heparin, until hemostasis is restored after which DOACs can be resumed. Some cardiac procedures, such as catheter ablation of arrhythmias or pacemaker implantation, can be performed without interruption of DOACs; however, the decision to withhold anticoagulation prior to the procedure depends upon the bleeding risk and operator experience. In many cases, it may be prudent to withhold anticoagulation at least on the day of the procedure to avoid such invasive interventions being performed during peak drug levels.

Management of Bleeding

Withholding one or two doses of the DOAC drug is usually sufficient to control minor bleeding [104]. The approach to severe bleeding is similar to that with warfarin, with the exception that vitamin K administration is of no benefit in patients receiving DOACs. Supportive measures including appropriate resuscitation with fluids and blood products as necessary should be immediately initiated. Coagulation testing (described above) and renal function should be checked to determine the extent of anticoagulation and the half-life of the drug, respectively. Timing of the last dose is important, and oral activated charcoal may prevent absorption if the drug was administered in the last 4 h. Indications to reverse anticoagulation include life-threatening bleeding, bleeding in a critical organ, such as the eye, or bleeding into a closed space, such as the pericardium or retroperitoneum.

Reversal

Idarucizumab, a humanized antibody fragment, is indicated for dabigatran reversal in patients with serious bleeding or those requiring urgent surgical procedures. Idarucizumab works by binding to dabigatran with a 350-fold higher affinity than that of dabigatran for thrombin, to form an irreversible complex that is subsequently cleared by the kidneys. This rapidly reverses the anticoagulant effect of dabigatran, normalizing the aPTT, diluted thrombin time, or ecarin clot time [104–106].

Andexanet alfa and ciraparantag are under development for reversal of rivaroxaban, apixaban, and edoxaban, but neither drug is licensed for use. Pending approval of these agents, current guidelines recommend a four-factor prothrombin complex concentrate to reverse these anticoagulant drugs. If there is continued bleeding, activated prothrombin complex concentrate or recombinant factor VIIa can be used [104].

Novel Anticoagulants in Development

While DOACs represent a major advance in oral anticoagulation therapy compared to warfarin, safer and more effective anticoagulants are needed. Factor XII and factor XI have been shown to be important components in thrombus stabilization and propagation, creating interest in developing anticoagulants that target these factors.

A phase II, proof-of-concept study revealed that lowering factor XI levels with an antisense oligonucleotide prior to elective knee replacement surgery was more effective than enoxaparin in preventing postoperative VTE without increasing the risk of bleeding [107]. Although promising, more studies involving inhibitors of factor XI and factor XII are needed to identify a better target and to assess the efficacy and safety of these anticoagulants.

8.3 Antiplatelet Drugs

Table 4 outlines the mechanisms of action, side effects, and limitations of various FDA-approved antiplatelet agents.

8.3.1 Aspirin

Aspirin is one of the oldest and most widely used medications in the world that acts by causing irreversible acetylation and subsequent inhibition of cyclooxygenase (COX)-1. This is an essential enzyme in the synthesis of thromboxane A2, a protein produced by activated platelets during hemostasis that stimulates the activation of new platelets and increases platelet aggregation. Given its efficacy and affordability, aspirin forms the foundation of many antiplatelet regimens and can even be used as monotherapy for primary and secondary prevention of MACE.

Table 4 FDA-approved antiplatelet agents

Class with reference	Antiplatelet drug	Route of administration	Year FDA approved	Mechanism of action	Side effects	Limitations
Salicylates [135, 136]	Aspirin	PO	1982	Irreversible acetylation of cyclooxygenase-1	Bleeding, GI toxicity	Weak antiplatelet drug
Glycoprotein IIb/IIIa inhibitors [137]	Abciximab	IV	1994	Integrin αIIbβ3 antagonist	Bleeding, thrombocytopenia	Only IV administration
	Eptifibatide	IV	1998	Integrin αIIbβ3 antagonist	Bleeding, thrombocytopenia	Only IV administration
	Tirofiban	IV	1999	Integrin αIIbβ3 antagonist	Bleeding, thrombocytopenia	Only IV administration
Cyto-pentyl-triazolopyrimidine [116]	Ticagrelor	PO	2011	Reversible inhibition of P2Y$_{12}$	Bleeding, dyspnea	High incidence of dyspnea
Thienopyridines [138–140]	Ticlopidine (first generation)	PO	1991	Irreversible inhibition of P2Y$_{12}$	Bleeding, GI toxicity, rash, neutropenia, TTP	Severe neutropenia rarely
	Clopidogrel (second generation)	PO	2002	Irreversible inhibition of P2Y$_{12}$	Bleeding, GI toxicity, rash, neutropenia, TTP	Variable response to drug dependent on CY2C19 polymorphisms
	Prasugrel (third generation)	PO	2009	Irreversible inhibition of P2Y$_{12}$	Bleeding	High bleeding risk, expensive, limited to age <75 years and weight >60 kg with no prior stroke
Phosphodiesterase and ADA inhibitor [141]	Dipyridamole	PO	1997	Inhibition of cyclic nucleotide phosphodiesterase and adenosine uptake	Bleeding, headache, hypotension, flushing, GI toxicity, rash	Limited use, must be combined with aspirin
Phosphodiesterase III inhibitor [142]	Cilostazol	PO	2005	Inhibition of cyclic nucleotide phosphodiesterase and adenosine uptake	Bleeding, headache, rash, pancytopenia, palpitations	15% of users stop due to side effects
PAR-1 antagonists [121, 122]	Vorapaxar	PO	2014	Inhibition of thrombin-related platelet aggregation	Bleeding	Higher bleeding risk, long half-life, no reversal agent

ADA adenosine deaminase, *CYP2C19* cytochrome P450 2C19, *FDA* Food and Drug Administration, *GI* gastrointestinal, *IV* intravenous, *PAR-1* protease-activated receptor-1, *PO* by mouth, *TTP* thrombotic thrombocytopenic purpura

Uses

Although aspirin has a wide variety of uses including analgesic and antipyretic effects, anti-inflammatory uses in patients with rheumatic disease, treatment of pericarditis, prevention of arterial and venous thrombosis, prevention of pre-eclampsia, and off-label use for primary prevention of colorectal cancer, in this section we will focus on its use in the prevention of thromboembolism. The cardiovascular effects of aspirin pertaining to its use in the prevention of thromboembolism will be focused on in this chapter. Aspirin can lower the risk of MACE, including MI and stroke, by up to 20% [108]. Thus, it is widely used for secondary prevention of MACE in patients with established coronary, cerebrovascular, and peripheral artery disease. There are clear benefits of using aspirin for primary prevention of MACE, especially in relatively younger, moderate- to high-risk individuals. However, the use of aspirin for primary prevention in older, low-risk patients who are at increased risk for bleeding has been an active topic of debate in recent times [109, 110]. While meta-analyses suggest that daily aspirin use may produce a 20–25% reduction in the risk of a first cardiovascular event in patients at moderate to high risk for cardiovascular disease, recent studies have challenged these benefits due to higher risk for gastrointestinal and intracerebral hemorrhage from aspirin [111]. Consequently, aspirin is no longer recommended for primary prevention unless the patient's baseline risk for developing MACE is at least 1% per year or 10% at 10 years, after shared decision-making between the prescriber and the patient based on a detailed discussion of risks and benefits [112].

There is a class I indication for the use of aspirin in combination with heparin, as discussed above, for the initial treatment of all ACS, including unstable angina, NSTEMI, and STEMI in the absence of bleeding risk. Aspirin is also used as initial with continued maintenance therapy in all patients undergoing PCI, carotid artery stenting, and placement of stents in peripheral arteries.

Patients with bioprosthetic aortic or mitral valve replacement should receive warfarin monotherapy for 3–6 months followed by transition to aspirin monotherapy if they are at low risk of bleeding. For patients at high risk of bleeding, aspirin monotherapy should be initiated within 24 h of surgery with no initial treatment with warfarin [113]. In patients with mechanical aortic or mitral valve replacement, aspirin is required in combination with warfarin indefinitely. Aspirin should also be used either as monotherapy or in combination with clopidogrel for 3–6 months after transcatheter aortic valve replacement and for at least 6 months after transcatheter mitral valve repair with clip device [113].

Aspirin can also be considered for use in select patients to prevent recurrent VTE if unable to take an anticoagulant, VTE prophylaxis in combination with rivaroxaban for total hip or knee arthroplasty, and the prevention of VTE in patients with polycythemia vera (except in patients with concurrently acquired von Willebrand syndrome).

Side Effects

The most common side effects of aspirin occur in the gastrointestinal tract, ranging from dyspepsia to peptic ulcer disease or erosive gastritis that may be complicated by gastrointestinal bleeding and, less frequently, perforation. Unfortunately, the use of enteric-coated aspirin does not reduce the risk of gastrointestinal side effects. The risk of major bleeding among patients taking aspirin is about 1–3% per year; the risk understandably increases with the concomitant use of other anticoagulants such as warfarin. The risk of aspirin-induced upper gastrointestinal bleeding in patients with peptic ulcer disease may be reduced by the administration of proton pump inhibitors and eradication of *Helicobacter pylori* infection, if present.

About 0.3% of the general population have a history of aspirin allergy characterized by bronchospasm. This is more common in patients with chronic urticaria or asthma, especially in those with coexisting chronic rhinitis or nasal polyps. Aspirin should not be used in these patients, and clopidogrel can be used instead.

Periprocedural Management

Aspirin can be safely continued until the day of most cardiovascular surgeries, including coronary artery bypass surgery, carotid endarterectomy, and PCI as discussed above. For patients undergoing noncardiac surgery at high risk of bleeding, clinicians should consider stopping aspirin 5–7 days before surgery after carefully weighing the risks and benefits. Patients with an indication for long-term aspirin use should have their aspirin resumed as soon as possible when the perioperative risk of major bleeding has passed. Aspirin can be safely continued in most patients undergoing surgical procedures with low risk for bleeding including cataract surgery, dental surgery, and dermatologic procedures.

8.3.2 Thienopyridines: Irreversible Blockers of P2Y$_{12}$

The thienopyridine group includes ticlopidine, clopidogrel, and prasugrel. These drugs act by irreversibly binding to and blocking P2Y$_{12}$, an ADP receptor on platelets that is essential for ADP-induced platelet aggregation. Thienopyridines are administered as prodrugs that need metabolic activation by the hepatic cytochrome P450 (CYP450) enzyme. Thus, when given at their usual doses, ticlopidine and clopidogrel have a delayed onset of action. Prasugrel has a more efficient metabolic activation, leading to a more rapid onset of action. Ticlopidine is no longer available for use in the United States and has been largely replaced by clopidogrel.

Uses

In patients with recent ischemic stroke, MI, or peripheral arterial disease, clopidogrel reduced the risk of cardiovascular death, MI, and stroke by 8.7% when compared to aspirin [114], indicating that clopidogrel is slightly more effective than
aspirin. Aspirin and clopidogrel when used in combination exert a synergistic antiplatelet effect by inhibiting complementary pathways of platelet activation and
adhesion; this combination is recommended after PCI.

Thienopyridines, especially clopidogrel, should be used with aspirin and a parenteral anticoagulant in all patients with ACS, especially in those with STEMI. A
higher loading dose achieves rapid ADP receptor blockade, which is sustained by a
lower maintenance dose. Providers should be mindful of the potential need for
urgent surgical revascularization in patients with ACS, as administration of thienopyridines within 5 days of surgical procedures (especially cardiovascular surgeries
that are associated with a high risk of bleeding) increases the incidence of perioperative bleeding. In patients undergoing PCI with bare metal stents, current guidelines recommend DAPT with aspirin and a thienopyridine for a minimum of
1 month, with some experts recommending at least 6 months and up to 12 months
[115]. In patients receiving drug-eluting stents, DAPT is recommended for at least
6 months and up to 12 months; if bleeding occurs or the patient is at high risk of
bleeding, DAPT may be stopped after 3 months. As a general rule, in patients at
high bleeding risk, a shorter duration of treatment may be considered. At the end of
the minimum recommended duration of therapy, providers should assess bleeding
and ischemic risks to determine whether the patient should receive longer therapy.

In patients who have already received IV thrombolytic drugs, the timing of antiplatelet therapy depends on the original indication for thrombolysis. If thrombolytic
therapy is used for ACS, antiplatelet therapy can be started immediately. If it was
used for transient ischemic attack or stroke, antiplatelet therapy is generally delayed
for at least 24 h and should be administered as soon as possible thereafter.

Clopidogrel can be used for secondary prevention of MACE in patients with
coronary artery disease, cerebrovascular disease, symptomatic and asymptomatic
carotid artery atherosclerosis, and peripheral artery disease, especially in patients
who are allergic to aspirin.

Side Effects

Bleeding is the most common side effect of thienopyridine use. A special consideration is clopidogrel resistance that occurs due to genetic polymorphisms in the CYP
enzymes, especially CYP2C19, which is responsible for the metabolic activation of
clopidogrel. Estimates suggest that 25% of Whites, 30% of Blacks, and 50% of
Asians carry the loss-of-function gene, which could render them resistant to
clopidogrel.

When compared to clopidogrel, prasugrel reduced the incidence of a composite endpoint of cardiovascular death, MI, and stroke in patients with ACS scheduled to undergo PCI. The incidence of stent thrombosis was lower in patients on prasugrel as compared to clopidogrel. However, these benefits came at the cost of a higher risk of fatal bleeding in patients taking prasugrel, especially those who were older than 75 years or who had a history of stroke [114]. Thus, prasugrel should be used with caution in the elderly and is contraindicated in patients with a history of cerebrovascular disease. Furthermore, it should be used with caution in patients who weigh less than 60 kg and those who have renal impairment.

Periprocedural Management

Irreversible binding to $P2Y_{12}$ confers a higher bleeding risk in patients taking thienopyridines. To minimize bleeding complications, clopidogrel should be withheld for 5 days, and prasugrel for 7 days, prior to surgical procedures.

8.3.3 Reversible Blockers of $P2Y_{12}$

Ticagrelor is an oral inhibitor of $P2Y_{12}$ that differs from thienopyridines in that it binds reversibly and noncompetitively to the $P2Y_{12}$ receptors at a site distinct from that of the endogenous ADP. Furthermore, ticagrelor does not require metabolic activation. This gives ticagrelor a more rapid onset and offset of action and the ability to produce greater and more predictable inhibition of ADP-induced platelet aggregation when compared to clopidogrel.

Uses

When compared with clopidogrel in patients with ACS, ticagrelor produced a greater reduction in the primary end point of the composite of cardiovascular death, MI, and stroke at 1 year [116]. Furthermore, there was no difference in rates of major bleeding between both drugs. However, when minor bleeding was added to the results, ticagrelor showed an overall increase in the incidence of bleeding compared to clopidogrel. Ticagrelor was also found to be superior to clopidogrel in patients who underwent PCI or cardiac surgery for ACS. Based on these observations, guidelines prefer ticagrelor over clopidogrel, especially in higher-risk patients [117]. Similar to clopidogrel, ticagrelor can be used in combination with aspirin and a parenteral anticoagulant in patients with ACS, especially STEMI. A higher loading dose followed by a maintenance dose is required for patients undergoing PCI [88, 115]. The duration of DAPT with aspirin and ticagrelor is similar to that of aspirin and clopidogrel. In patients who receive fibrinolytic therapy, it is recommended to administer clopidogrel instead of ticagrelor in combination with the fibrinolytic, aspirin, and parenteral anticoagulant as soon as possible. In patients who are less than 75 years of age, clopidogrel may be transitioned to ticagrelor 12 h after fibrinolytics have been administered. Ticagrelor can also be considered for primary prevention in patients with coronary artery disease at high risk for ischemic cardiovascular events. Short-term use of ticagrelor may be considered in select patients with minor ischemic stroke or high-risk transient ischemic attack.

Side Effects

Bleeding is a common side effect of all $P2Y_{12}$ inhibitors, and hemorrhage may occur at virtually any site. The most commonly reported side effect is dyspnea, with an estimated incidence between 14 and 21%. This is usually mild and self-limited, but can persist, necessitating drug discontinuation and switching to clopidogrel. Ticagrelor inhibits the reuptake of adenosine. Dyspnea is thought to be adenosine-mediated, although the exact mechanism responsible is unknown.

Periprocedural Management

Minor surgical and dental procedures usually do not require the cessation of anti-platelet therapy. Ticagrelor should be withheld 3–5 days before surgery, and some experts recommend shorter discontinuation periods for procedures with low bleeding risk.

Cangrelor

Cangrelor is a selective, reversible $P2Y_{12}$ antagonist administered intravenously. It has an immediate onset of action and a half-life of approximately 3–5 min. The offset of action is within an hour. It is approved for use in patients undergoing PCI, and its biggest advantage is its ability to produce rapid ADP receptor blockade in patients who have not received a loading dose of other oral antiplatelet agents. Cangrelor can be discontinued as late as 1–6 h prior to surgical incision in high bleeding risk procedures after careful evaluation of risk for thrombotic complications.

8.3.4 Phosphodiesterase Inhibitors

Dipyridamole acts by synergistically modifying various biochemical pathways, including inhibition of platelet cAMP-phosphodiesterase and potentiation of adenosine inhibition of platelet function by blocking its reuptake. Increased levels of cAMP reduce intracellular calcium and inhibit platelet activation. By itself, dipyridamole is a relatively weak antiplatelet agent; however, an extended-release formulation of dipyridamole combined with low-dose aspirin is also available, which is used for secondary prevention of stroke in patients with transient ischemic attacks.

Uses

When compared to either aspirin or dipyridamole alone and placebo, the combination of aspirin and dipyridamole was found to be superior in reducing the risk for stroke in patients with a transient ischemic attack or an ischemic stroke [118]. However, this combination is not superior to clopidogrel. A large randomized trial showed similar rates of ischemic stroke, vascular death, and MI. The combination of dipyridamole plus aspirin was associated with higher incidences of hemorrhagic stroke and significantly higher incidence of major bleeding events [119]. Dipyridamole can also be used as an adjunctive therapy for VTE prophylaxis in patients with cardiac valve replacement.

Side Effects

Due to its effects on the breakdown of cAMP, dipyridamole has vasodilatory effects. As there is a paucity of data supporting its use in patients with symptomatic coronary artery disease, it is contraindicated in these individuals. Clopidogrel is a better choice for patients with coronary artery disease. Dipyridamole is also associated with transient gastrointestinal symptoms, facial flushing, headaches, dizziness, and hypotension, which often subside with prolonged use of this drug.

Perioperative Management

There are no data on the safety of dipyridamole in the perioperative period. However, if a decision is made to withhold the drug after weighing the risks of bleeding and ischemic events, most experts recommend stopping the drug at least 2 days before surgery. The dipyridamole/low-dose aspirin combination should be withheld 7–10 days prior to surgery because of its aspirin component.

8.3.5 Glycoprotein IIb/IIIa (GPIIb/IIIa) Inhibitors

GPIIb/IIIa is a member of the integrin family of receptors and is the most abundant receptor expressed on the surface of platelets and megakaryocytes. This receptor is inactive on resting platelets. Platelet activation triggers a conformational change of the receptor, which in turn leads to its activation. Activated GPIIb/IIIa promotes platelet aggregation by binding to fibrinogen and, under certain conditions, von Willebrand factor. The three agents that act as parenteral GPIIb/IIIa antagonists are abciximab, eptifibatide, and tirofiban.

Uses

Abciximab, which has been used in patients undergoing PCI, especially for acute MI, is no longer available in the United States. Eptifibatide and tirofiban are not routinely used; however, they may be considered as an IV bolus followed by infusion in certain patients undergoing PCI and in high-risk patients with unstable angina. Due to the limited benefit on ischemic outcomes and more bleeding complications associated with GPIIb/IIIa inhibitors, the combination of aspirin with an oral $P2Y_{12}$ inhibitor discussed previously is preferred, unless patients are at high risk of acute stent thrombosis. GPIIb/IIIa inhibitors may also be used in the absence of pretreatment with a $P2Y_{12}$ inhibitor.

Side Effects

Thrombocytopenia is the most serious complication of GPIIb/IIIa inhibitors. In these patients, platelet destruction is an immune-mediated process with an incidence of approximately 5% with abciximab and approximately 1% with the other two agents [98]. Eptifibatide and tirofiban are cleared renally and require dose adjustment with renal impairment.

8.3.6 Protease-Activated Receptor (PAR)-1 Inhibitor

PAR-1 is a major thrombin receptor on human platelets. Vorapaxar is unique among antiplatelet drugs in its ability to inhibit PAR-1. When compared with placebo for secondary prevention in patients with previous MI, ischemic stroke, or peripheral arterial disease, vorapaxar reduced the risk for cardiovascular death, MI, and stroke by 13% but doubled the risk of intracranial bleeding [120]. The benefit of vorapaxar was highest among patients with prior MI with a reduction in risk of cardiovascular death, subsequent MI, and stroke by 20% in this specific subgroup. Based on this, vorapaxar is now approved for use in adult ($\geq$18 years old) patients younger than 75 years and who weigh more than 60 kg with a history of MI and no history of stroke, transient ischemic attack, or intracranial bleeding [121, 122]. Significant drug interactions exist with vorapaxar, and providers are encouraged to consult a drug interactions database prior to initiation of this drug.

8.4 Fibrinolytic Drugs

Fibrinolytic drugs are used to lyse thrombi and can be administered systemically or locally via catheters directly into a thrombus. This class of drugs acts by converting plasminogen (the proenzyme) to plasmin (the active form) [123], which can trigger a systemic thrombolytic state. Fibrinolytic drugs approved for use in humans include streptokinase, acylated plasminogen streptokinase activator complex (anistreplase), urokinase, recombinant tissue plasminogen activator (rt-PA), which is also called alteplase, and two other recombinant derivatives of t-PA, tenecteplase and reteplase. Plasminogen exists in two forms: free in circulation and bound to fibrin. Fibrinolytic drugs can be either fibrin-specific with preferential activation of fibrin-bound plasminogen (such as alteplase and its derivatives) or non-specific in their mechanism of action (streptokinase, anistreplase, and urokinase).

8.4.1 Streptokinase

Streptokinase is a unique fibrinolytic drug in that it is not an enzyme and acts by directly forming a complex with plasminogen rather than converting plasminogen to plasmin. Streptokinase binding to plasminogen causes a conformational change in the latter, thereby exposing its active site and leading to non-specific activation of both free and fibrin-bound plasminogen. Unopposed plasmin induces a systemic lytic state in addition to degrading fibrin in the culprit thrombus. Streptokinase can be administered in patients with acute MI and has been shown to reduce mortality in these patients. Allergic reactions to this drug may manifest as rash, fevers, chills, and rigors in up to 5% of patients. Anaphylactic reactions are rare. Streptokinase may cause hypotension through the plasmin-mediated release of bradykinin; this is usually transient and responds to leg elevation, administration of fluids, or low-dose norepinephrine or dopamine. Providers should be aware of the possibility of developing antibodies to streptokinase in patients who have received it in the past or patients with a history of streptococcal infection. These antibodies may reduce the efficacy of streptokinase.

8.4.2 Anistreplase

Anistreplase is generated by mixing equimolar amounts of streptokinase and a plasmin-cleaved form of plasminogen called Lys-plasminogen. This allows it to be administered as a single bolus dose, which is more convenient than streptokinase. After administration, the anisoyl group of the mixture is removed by deacetylation, leading to non-specific activation of plasminogen and development of a systemic lytic state similar to streptokinase. The incidence of allergic reactions and hypotension is similar between anistreplase and streptokinase. When compared to anistreplase in patients with acute MI, alteplase brought about more rapid reperfusion [98]. The high cost of anistreplase and only modest improvement in outcomes make it a less popular fibrinolytic drug for use in acute MI.

8.4.3 Alteplase

Alteplase is a recombinant form of single-chain t-PA with a very high affinity for fibrin. As a result, alteplase selectively activates plasminogen in the presence of fibrin. A trial comparing alteplase to streptokinase for the treatment of acute MI demonstrated that, although the absolute difference was small, alteplase had significantly lower mortality rates [98]. The subset of patients who benefitted the most were those who were older than 75 years of age presenting less than 6 h from the onset of symptoms. Alteplase can also be used in the treatment of acute ischemic stroke in the absence of contraindications. Alteplase is not immunogenic and is relatively safe with a lower incidence of allergic reactions and hypotension.

8.4.4 Tenecteplase

Tenecteplase is a genetically engineered form of t-PA that was designed to have a longer half-life than t-PA. Tenecteplase is also more fibrin-specific than t-PA. It can be administered as a single IV bolus in patients with coronary thrombosis. Thirty-day mortality with tenecteplase was similar to that with accelerated-dose t-PA in a large phase III trial that enrolled more than 16,000 patients [98]. Furthermore, rates of non-cerebral bleeding and the need for blood transfusion were lower in patients who received tenecteplase, although the rates of intracranial hemorrhage were similar. These outcomes are probably from its enhanced fibrin specificity.

8.4.5 Urokinase

Urokinase is synthesized using recombinant DNA technology, but was originally isolated from cultured fetal kidney cells. Urokinase directly converts plasminogen to plasmin and has a distinct advantage over streptokinase in that it does not stimulate the production of antibodies, and allergic reactions to urokinase are less frequent. A non-specific fibrinolytic drug, urokinase produces a systemic lytic state. The availability of urokinase is limited due to production problems, making it another rarely used fibrinolytic agent. It may be considered in catheter-directed lysis of thrombi in deep veins or peripheral arteries. There are no data on the use of urokinase in coronary fibrinolysis.

8.4.6 Reteplase

Reteplase is a recombinant t-PA derivative that binds fibrin more weakly than t-PA. Reteplase is not glycosylated as it is produced in *E. coli*, endowing it with a longer half-life than t-PA. Clinical trials showed improved 30-day survival rates with reteplase when compared to streptokinase, but it was non-inferior when compared to alteplase [98].

9 Catheter-Directed Thrombolytic Therapy

Patients with massive [defined as PE with sustained hypotension (systolic blood pressure <90 mm Hg for at least 15 min or requiring inotropic support, not due to a cause other than PE), pulselessness, or persistent profound bradycardia] and submassive PE [defined as PE without systemic hypotension (systolic blood pressure$\geq$90 mm Hg) but with either RV dysfunction or myocardial necrosis] being treated only with anticoagulation are at high risk of developing right-sided heart failure leading to cardiogenic shock, cardiac arrest, and respiratory failure. In these patients, therapeutic options include thrombolysis (systemic or catheter-directed) or mechanical thrombectomy (surgical or catheter-directed). The choice of therapeutic options depends upon the patient's clinical condition and operator preference. Catheter-directed thrombolysis (CDT) has benefits over systemic thrombolysis in terms of decreased rate of bleeding, but it still has a mild risk of major bleeding [124, 125]. There are different catheters available, but there is no evidence to show the superiority of one catheter over any other [126]. CDT uses a specialized catheter placed in the affected pulmonary artery so that TPA (8–24 mg) can be delivered locally over 4–24 h [127].

10 Mechanical Management of Thromboembolic Disease

Percutaneous mechanical thrombectomy refers to the mechanical extraction of thrombus. Thrombectomy is achieved using mechanical aspiration along with systemic anticoagulation with heparin. It is approved for use in pulmonary arteries and peripheral vasculature. Clinical trials have shown that patients with acute submassive PE who underwent mechanical thrombectomy with systemic anticoagulation with heparin had significant improvement in right ventricle-to-left ventricle ratio with lower incidence of bleeding complications when compared to patients who received thrombolytic plus heparin therapy [128, 129]. These trials were single-arm studies, and there are no comparative data for both catheters.

11 Summary

In summary, thrombosis and thromboembolism are important components of contemporary clinical practice, due to their causal role in CVD-related and non-CVD-related morbidity and mortality. Invasive treatment of thromboembolic conditions, such as catheter-based thrombectomy or thrombolysis for PE or PCI for MI, are particularly challenging scenarios that involve cannulation of a vessel (either a vein or an artery depending on the location of the thrombus) and simultaneous use of a combination of parenteral anticoagulants, such as heparin, oral or parenteral antiplatelet drugs, and fibrinolytic agents. Understandably, the use of these drugs increases the risk of iatrogenic bleeding at the venipuncture or arteriotomy site, and these bleeding complications increase morbidity and mortality related to the invasive procedure. Effective and efficient local hemostasis at the site of vessel puncture in these circumstances is imperative to successful outcomes of invasive procedures, and a fine balance must be maintained between the treatment of thromboembolism and achieving hemostasis. Novel drugs and devices to prevent and treat thromboembolism and to achieve hemostasis in safer and more efficient ways are under development with endless room for improvement.

Conflict of Interest Dr. Belur: None.
 Dr. Zheng: None.
 Dr. Raza: None.
 Dr. Kalra: None.

Financial Disclosures None.

References

1. Dexter L. The chair and venous thrombosis. Trans Am Clin Climatol Assoc. 1973;84:1–15.
2. Galanaud JP, Laroche JP, Righini M. The history and historical treatments of deep vein thrombosis. J Thromb Haemost. 2013;11(3):402–11. https://doi.org/10.1111/jth.12127.
3. Bagot CN, Arya R. Virchow and his triad: a question of attribution. Br J Haematol. 2008;143(2):180–90. https://doi.org/10.1111/j.1365-2141.2008.07323.x.
4. Wright IS. Thrombophlebitis. Bull N Y Acad Med. 1941;17(5):348–72.
5. Murray GD, Best CH. The use of heparin in thrombosis. Ann Surg. 1938;108(2):163–77. https://doi.org/10.1097/00000658-193808000-00002.
6. Bauer G. Thrombosis; early diagnosis and abortive treatment with heparin. Lancet. 1946;1(6396):447–54. https://doi.org/10.1016/s0140-6736(46)91429-8.
7. McLean J. The discovery of heparin. Circulation. 1959;19(1):75–8. https://doi.org/10.1161/01.cir.19.1.75.
8. Mannucci PM. Venous thrombosis: the history of knowledge. Pathophysiol Haemost Thromb. 2002;32(5–6):209–12. https://doi.org/10.1159/000073567.
9. Benjamin EJ, Blaha MJ, Chiuve SE, et al. Heart disease and stroke statistics-2017 update: a report from the American Heart Association. Circulation. 2017;135(10):e146–603. https://doi.org/10.1161/CIR.0000000000000485.
10. Wendelboe AM, Raskob GE. Global burden of thrombosis: epidemiologic aspects. Circ Res. 2016;118(9):1340–7. https://doi.org/10.1161/CIRCRESAHA.115.306841.
11. Cushman M. Epidemiology and risk factors for venous thrombosis. Semin Hematol. 2007;44(2):62–9. https://doi.org/10.1053/j.seminhematol.2007.02.004.
12. Grosse SD, Nelson RE, Nyarko KA, Richardson LC, Raskob GE. The economic burden of incident venous thromboembolism in the United States: a review of estimated attributable healthcare costs. Thromb Res. 2016;137:3–10. https://doi.org/10.1016/j.thromres.2015.11.033.
13. Anderson FA, Spencer FA. Risk factors for venous thromboembolism. Circulation. 2003;107(23 Suppl 1):I9–16. https://doi.org/10.1161/01.CIR.0000078469.07362.E6.
14. Cushman M. Inherited risk factors for venous thrombosis. Hematology Am Soc Hematol Educ Program. 2005:452–7. https://doi.org/10.1182/asheducation-2005.1.452.
15. Wolberg AS, Rosendaal FR, Weitz JI, et al. Venous thrombosis. Nat Rev Dis Primers. 2015;1:15006. https://doi.org/10.1038/nrdp.2015.6.
16. Campello E, Spiezia L, Simioni P. Diagnosis and management of factor V Leiden. Expert Rev Hematol. 2016;9(12):1139–49. https://doi.org/10.1080/17474086.2016.1249364.
17. Germain M, Chasman DI, de Haan H, et al. Meta-analysis of 65,734 individuals identifies TSPAN15 and SLC44A2 as two susceptibility loci for venous thromboembolism. Am J Hum Genet. 2015;96(4):532–42. https://doi.org/10.1016/j.ajhg.2015.01.019.

18. Tang W, Teichert M, Chasman DI, et al. A genome-wide association study for venous thromboembolism: the extended cohorts for heart and aging research in genomic epidemiology (CHARGE) consortium. Genet Epidemiol. 2013;37(5):512–21. https://doi.org/10.1002/gepi.21731.

19. Palasubramaniam J, Wang X, Peter K. Myocardial infarction-from atherosclerosis to thrombosis. Arterioscler Thromb Vasc Biol. 2019;39(8):e176–85. https://doi.org/10.1161/ATVBAHA.119.312578.

20. Previtali E, Bucciarelli P, Passamonti SM, Martinelli I. Risk factors for venous and arterial thrombosis. Blood Transfus. 2011;9(2):120–38. https://doi.org/10.2450/2010.0066-10.

21. Watson T, Shantsila E, Lip GYH. Mechanisms of thrombogenesis in atrial fibrillation: Virchow's triad revisited. Lancet. 2009;373(9658):155–66. https://doi.org/10.1016/S0140-6736(09)60040-4.

22. Alkarithi G, Duval C, Shi Y, Macrae FL, Ariëns RAS. Thrombus structural composition in cardiovascular disease. Arterioscler Thromb Vasc Biol. 2021;41(9):2370–83. https://doi.org/10.1161/ATVBAHA.120.315754.

23. Silvain J, Collet JP, Nagaswami C, et al. Composition of coronary thrombus in acute myocardial infarction. J Am Coll Cardiol. 2011;57(12):1359–67. https://doi.org/10.1016/j.jacc.2010.09.077.

24. Sadowski M, Ząbczyk M, Undas A. Coronary thrombus composition: links with inflammation, platelet and endothelial markers. Atherosclerosis. 2014;237(2):555–61. https://doi.org/10.1016/j.atherosclerosis.2014.10.020.

25. Riva N, Donadini MP, Ageno W. Epidemiology and pathophysiology of venous thromboembolism: similarities with atherothrombosis and the role of inflammation. Thromb Haemost. 2015;113(6):1176–83. https://doi.org/10.1160/TH14-06-0563.

26. Ogdie A, Yu Y, Haynes K, et al. Risk of major cardiovascular events in patients with psoriatic arthritis, psoriasis and rheumatoid arthritis: a population-based cohort study. Ann Rheum Dis. 2015;74(2):326–32. https://doi.org/10.1136/annrheumdis-2014-205675.

27. Nikiphorou E, de Lusignan S, Mallen CD, et al. Cardiovascular risk factors and outcomes in early rheumatoid arthritis: a population-based study. Heart. 2020;106(20):1566–72. https://doi.org/10.1136/heartjnl-2019-316193.

28. Zeller CB, Appenzeller S. Cardiovascular disease in systemic lupus erythematosus: the role of traditional and lupus related risk factors. Curr Cardiol Rev. 2008;4(2):116–22. https://doi.org/10.2174/157340308784245775.

29. Ridker PM, Everett BM, Thuren T, et al. Antiinflammatory therapy with canakinumab for atherosclerotic disease. N Engl J Med. 2017;377(12):1119–31. https://doi.org/10.1056/NEJMoa1707914.

30. Tardif JC, Kouz S, Waters DD, et al. Efficacy and safety of low-dose colchicine after myocardial infarction. N Engl J Med. 2019;381(26):2497–505. https://doi.org/10.1056/NEJMoa1912388.

31. Hennessy T, Soh L, Bowman M, et al. The Low Dose Colchicine after Myocardial Infarction (LoDoCo-MI) study: a pilot randomized placebo controlled trial of colchicine following acute myocardial infarction. Am Heart J. 2019;215:62–9. https://doi.org/10.1016/j.ahj.2019.06.003.

32. Bouabdallaoui N, Tardif JC, Waters DD, et al. Time-to-treatment initiation of colchicine and cardiovascular outcomes after myocardial infarction in the Colchicine Cardiovascular Outcomes Trial (COLCOT). Eur Heart J. 2020;41(42):4092–9. https://doi.org/10.1093/eurheartj/ehaa659.

33. Beristain-Covarrubias N, Perez-Toledo M, Thomas MR, Henderson IR, Watson SP, Cunningham AF. Understanding infection-induced thrombosis: lessons learned from animal models. Front Immunol. 2019;10:2569. https://doi.org/10.3389/fimmu.2019.02569.

34. Dalager-Pedersen M, Søgaard M, Schønheyder HC, Nielsen H, Thomsen RW. Risk for myocardial infarction and stroke after community-acquired bacteremia: a 20-year

population-based cohort study. Circulation. 2014;129(13):1387–96. https://doi.org/10.1161/CIRCULATIONAHA.113.006699.

35. Smeeth L, Cook C, Thomas S, Hall AJ, Hubbard R, Vallance P. Risk of deep vein thrombosis and pulmonary embolism after acute infection in a community setting. Lancet. 2006;367(9516):1075–9. https://doi.org/10.1016/S0140-6736(06)68474-2.

36. Iba T, Levy JH, Warkentin TE, et al. Diagnosis and management of sepsis-induced coagulopathy and disseminated intravascular coagulation. J Thromb Haemost. 2019;17(11):1989–94. https://doi.org/10.1111/jth.14578.

37. Kunutsor SK, Laukkanen JA. Incidence of venous and arterial thromboembolic complications in COVID-19: a systematic review and meta-analysis. Thromb Res. 2020;196:27–30. https://doi.org/10.1016/j.thromres.2020.08.022.

38. Liu Y, Cai J, Wang C, Jin J, Qu L. A systematic review and meta-analysis of incidence, prognosis, and laboratory indicators of venous thromboembolism in hospitalized patients with coronavirus disease 2019. J Vasc Surg Venous Lymphat Disord. 2021;9(5):1099–1111.e6. https://doi.org/10.1016/j.jvsv.2021.01.012.

39. Kollias A, Kyriakoulis KG, Lagou S, Kontopantelis E, Stergiou GS, Syrigos K. Venous thromboembolism in COVID-19: a systematic review and meta-analysis. Vasc Med. 2021;26(4):415–25. https://doi.org/10.1177/1358863X21995566.

40. Nadkarni GN, Lala A, Bagiella E, et al. Anticoagulation, bleeding, mortality, and pathology in hospitalized patients with COVID-19. J Am Coll Cardiol. 2020;76(16):1815–26. https://doi.org/10.1016/j.jacc.2020.08.041.

41. Joly BS, Siguret V, Veyradier A. Understanding pathophysiology of hemostasis disorders in critically ill patients with COVID-19. Intensive Care Med. 2020;46(8):1603–6. https://doi.org/10.1007/s00134-020-06088-1.

42. Gerotziafas GT, Catalano M, Colgan MP, et al. Guidance for the management of patients with vascular disease or cardiovascular risk factors and COVID-19: position paper from VAS-European Independent Foundation in Angiology/Vascular Medicine. Thromb Haemost. 2020;120(12):1597–628. https://doi.org/10.1055/s-0040-1715798.

43. Rungjirajittranon T, Owattanapanich W, Leelakanok N, et al. Thrombotic and hemorrhagic incidences in patients after discharge from COVID-19 infection: a systematic review and meta-analysis. Clin Appl Thromb Hemost. 2021;27:10760296211069082. https://doi.org/10.1177/10760296211069082.

44. Doyle AJ, Thomas W, Retter A, et al. Updated hospital associated venous thromboembolism outcomes with 90-days follow-up after hospitalisation for severe COVID-19 in two UK critical care units. Thromb Res. 2020;196:454–6. https://doi.org/10.1016/j.thromres.2020.10.007.

45. Patell R, Bogue T, Koshy A, et al. Postdischarge thrombosis and hemorrhage in patients with COVID-19. Blood. 2020;136(11):1342–6. https://doi.org/10.1182/blood.2020007938.

46. Cuker A, Peyvandi F. COVID-19: hypercoagulability. In: Leung LL, editor. UpToDate. UpToDate; 2021.

47. Kreuziger LB. COVID-19 and VTE/anticoagulation: frequently asked questions. https://www.hematology.org/covid-19/covid-19-and-vte-anticoagulation.

48. Fuster V. FREEDOM COVID-19 anticoagulation strategy (FREEDOM COVID): NCT04512079. https://clinicaltrials.gov/ct2/show/NCT04512079?cond=covid+anticoagulation&draw=2&rank=1. Accessed 20 Jan 2022. https://clinicaltrials.gov/ct2/show/NCT04512079?cond=covid+anticoagulation&draw=2&rank=1.

49. Anticoagulation in critically ill patients with COVID-19 (The IMPACT Trial) (IMPACT): NCT04406389. https://clinicaltrials.gov/ct2/show/NCT04406389?cond=covid+anticoagulation&draw=2&rank=4. Accessed 20 Jan 2022. https://clinicaltrials.gov/ct2/show/NCT04406389?cond=covid+anticoagulation&draw=2&rank=4.

50. Poor H. Tenecteplase in patients with COVID-19: NCT04505592. https://clinicaltrials.gov/ct2/show/NCT04505592?cond=covid+anticoagulation&draw=2&rank=22. Accessed 20 Jan 2022. https://clinicaltrials.gov/ct2/show/NCT04505592?cond=covid+anticoagulation&draw=2&rank=22.

51. Apixaban for PrOphyLaxis of thromboemboLic Outcomes in COVID-19 (APOLLO): NCT04746339. https://clinicaltrials.gov/ct2/show/NCT04746339?cond=covid+anticoagulation&draw=2&rank=26. Accessed 20 Jan 2022. https://clinicaltrials.gov/ct2/show/NCT04746339?cond=covid+anticoagulation&draw=2&rank=26.
52. Geraldo Rocha V. Hemostasis in COVID-19: an adaptive clinical trial: NCT04466670. https://clinicaltrials.gov/ct2/show/NCT04466670?cond=covid+anticoagulation&draw=2&rank=27. Accessed 20 Jan 2022. https://clinicaltrials.gov/ct2/show/NCT04466670?cond=covid+anticoagulation&draw=2&rank=27.
53. Lance MD. Anticoagulation in patients suffering from COVID-19 disease the ANTI-CO trial: NCT04445935. https://clinicaltrials.gov/ct2/show/NCT04445935?cond=covid+anticoagulation&draw=3&rank=2. Accessed 20 Jan 2022. https://clinicaltrials.gov/ct2/show/NCT04445935?cond=covid+anticoagulation&draw=3&rank=2.
54. ANTIcoagulation in Severe COVID-19 Patients (ANTICOVID): NCT04808882. https://clinicaltrials.gov/ct2/show/NCT04808882?cond=covid+anticoagulation&draw=2&rank=3. Accessed 20 Jan 2022. https://clinicaltrials.gov/ct2/show/NCT04808882?cond=covid+anticoagulation&draw=2&rank=3.
55. Coagulopathy of COVID-19: a pragmatic randomized controlled trial of therapeutic anticoagulation versus standard care: NCT04362085. https://clinicaltrials.gov/ct2/show/NCT04362085?cond=covid+anticoagulation&draw=2&rank=6. Accessed 20 Jan 2022. https://clinicaltrials.gov/ct2/show/NCT04362085?cond=covid+anticoagulation&draw=2&rank=6.
56. Musa F. Prophylactic versus therapeutic dose anticoagulation in COVID-19 infection at the time of admission to critical care units: NCT04829552. https://clinicaltrials.gov/ct2/show/NCT04829552?cond=covid+anticoagulation&draw=2&rank=8. Accessed 20 Jan 2022. https://clinicaltrials.gov/ct2/show/NCT04829552?cond=covid+anticoagulation&draw=2&rank=8.
57. Parikh SA. Intermediate or prophylactic-dose anticoagulation for venous or arterial thromboembolism in severe COVID-19 (IMPROVE): NCT04367831. https://clinicaltrials.gov/ct2/show/NCT04367831?cond=covid+anticoagulation&draw=2&rank=13. Accessed 20 Jan 2022. https://clinicaltrials.gov/ct2/show/NCT04367831?cond=covid+anticoagulation&draw=2&rank=13.
58. Spyropoulos A. Full dose heparin vs. prophylactic or intermediate dose heparin in high risk COVID-19 patients: NCT04401293. https://clinicaltrials.gov/ct2/show/results/NCT04401293?cond=covid+anticoagulation&draw=2&rank=18. Accessed 20 Jan 2022. https://clinicaltrials.gov/ct2/show/results/NCT04401293?cond=covid+anticoagulation&draw=2&rank=18.
59. Merli GJ, Galanis P, Ouma GO, Eraso L, Thomson L. Deep vein thrombosis and pulmonary embolism. In: Lee K, editor. The NeuroICU book, 2e. 2nd ed. McGraw Hill; 2017.
60. Centers for Disease Control and Prevention (CDC). Venous thromboembolism in adult hospitalizations—United States, 2007–2009. MMWR Morb Mortal Wkly Rep. 2012;61(22):401–4.
61. Beckman MG, Hooper WC, Critchley SE, Ortel TL. Venous thromboembolism: a public health concern. Am J Prev Med. 2010;38(4 Suppl):S495–501. https://doi.org/10.1016/j.amepre.2009.12.017.
62. Mukhopadhyay S, Johnson TA, Duru N, et al. Fibrinolysis and inflammation in venous thrombus resolution. Front Immunol. 2019;10:1348. https://doi.org/10.3389/fimmu.2019.01348.
63. Spencer FA, Emery C, Joffe SW, et al. Incidence rates, clinical profile, and outcomes of patients with venous thromboembolism. The Worcester VTE study. J Thromb Thrombolysis. 2009;28(4):401–9. https://doi.org/10.1007/s11239-009-0378-3.
64. Huang W, Goldberg RJ, Cohen AT, et al. Declining long-term risk of adverse events after first-time community-presenting venous thromboembolism: the population-based Worcester VTE Study (1999 to 2009). Thromb Res. 2015;135(6):1100–6. https://doi.org/10.1016/j.thromres.2015.04.007.
65. Incidence and outcomes of venous thromboembolism: NCT00005351. https://clinicaltrials.gov/ct2/show/NCT00005351?term=outcomes&cond=Venous+Thromboembolism&draw=4&rank=30. Accessed 9 May 2022.

66. Outpatient treatment of low-risk venous thromboembolism with target specific anticoagulant: NCT02079584. https://clinicaltrials.gov/ct2/show/NCT02079584?term=outcomes&cond=Venous+Thromboembolism&draw=5&rank=38. Accessed 9 May 2022.

67. Ostfold Hospital Trust. Long term outcomes of venous thromboembolism (LOVE): NCT02268630. https://clinicaltrials.gov/ct2/show/NCT02268630. Accessed 9 May 2022.

68. Prevention of symptomatic venous thromboembolism by low molecular weight heparin in hospitalized medical patients aged 70 years and older: a randomized placebo-controlled study. The SYMPTOMS (SYstematic Elderly Medical Patients Thromboprophylaxis: Efficacy on Symptomatic OutcoMeS) study: NCT02379806. https://clinicaltrials.gov/ct2/show/NCT02379806?term=outcomes&cond=Venous+Thromboembolism&draw=2&rank=2. Accessed 9 May 2022.

69. van Hulst M. Safety of DAbigatran and RIvaroxaban Versus NAdroparin in the Prevention of Venous Thromboembolism After Knee Arthroplasty Surgery (DARINA): NCT01431456. https://clinicaltrials.gov/ct2/show/NCT01431456?term=outcomes&cond=Venous+Thromboembolism&draw=2&rank=10. Accessed 9 May 2022.

70. Dauerman HL, Rao SV, Resnic FS, Applegate RJ. Bleeding avoidance strategies. Consensus and controversy. J Am Coll Cardiol. 2011;58(1):1–10. https://doi.org/10.1016/j.jacc.2011.02.039.

71. Dumaine R, Borentain M, Bertel O, et al. Intravenous low-molecular-weight heparins compared with unfractionated heparin in percutaneous coronary intervention: quantitative review of randomized trials. Arch Intern Med. 2007;167(22):2423–30. https://doi.org/10.1001/archinte.167.22.2423.

72. Blankenship JC, Balog C, Sapp SK, et al. Reduction in vascular access site bleeding in sequential abciximab coronary intervention trials. Catheter Cardiovasc Interv. 2002;57(4):476–83. https://doi.org/10.1002/ccd.10322.

73. Seto AH, Abu-Fadel MS, Sparling JM, et al. Real-time ultrasound guidance facilitates femoral arterial access and reduces vascular complications: FAUST (Femoral Arterial Access With Ultrasound Trial). JACC Cardiovasc Interv. 2010;3(7):751–8. https://doi.org/10.1016/j.jcin.2010.04.015.

74. Biancari F, D'Andrea V, di Marco C, Savino G, Tiozzo V, Catania A. Meta-analysis of randomized trials on the efficacy of vascular closure devices after diagnostic angiography and angioplasty. Am Heart J. 2010;159(4):518–31. https://doi.org/10.1016/j.ahj.2009.12.027.

75. Wimmer NJ, Secemsky EA, Mauri L, et al. Effectiveness of arterial closure devices for preventing complications with percutaneous coronary intervention: an instrumental variable analysis. Circ Cardiovasc Interv. 2016;9(4):e003464. https://doi.org/10.1161/CIRCINTERVENTIONS.115.003464.

76. Robertson L, Andras A, Colgan F, Jackson R. Vascular closure devices for femoral arterial puncture site haemostasis. Cochrane Database Syst Rev. 2016;3:CD009541. https://doi.org/10.1002/14651858.CD009541.pub2.

77. Mason PJ, Shah B, Tamis-Holland JE, et al. An update on radial artery access and Best practices for transradial coronary angiography and intervention in acute coronary syndrome: a scientific statement from the American Heart Association. Circ Cardiovasc Interv. 2018;11(9):e000035. https://doi.org/10.1161/HCV.0000000000000035.

78. Jolly SS, Yusuf S, Cairns J, et al. Radial versus femoral access for coronary angiography and intervention in patients with acute coronary syndromes (RIVAL): a randomised, parallel group, multicentre trial. Lancet. 2011;377(9775):1409–20. https://doi.org/10.1016/S0140-6736(11)60404-2.

79. Romagnoli E, Biondi-Zoccai G, Sciahbasi A, et al. Radial versus femoral randomized investigation in ST-segment elevation acute coronary syndrome: the RIFLE-STEACS (Radial Versus Femoral Randomized Investigation in ST-Elevation Acute Coronary Syndrome) study. J Am Coll Cardiol. 2012;60(24):2481–9. https://doi.org/10.1016/j.jacc.2012.06.017.

80. Mehta SR, Jolly SS, Cairns J, et al. Effects of radial versus femoral artery access in patients with acute coronary syndromes with or without ST-segment elevation. J Am Coll Cardiol. 2012;60(24):2490–9. https://doi.org/10.1016/j.jacc.2012.07.050.

81. Bernat I, Horak D, Stasek J, et al. ST-segment elevation myocardial infarction treated by radial or femoral approach in a multicenter randomized clinical trial: the STEMI-RADIAL trial. J Am Coll Cardiol. 2014;63(10):964–72. https://doi.org/10.1016/j.jacc.2013.08.1651.

82. Valgimigli M, Gagnor A, Calabró P, et al. Radial versus femoral access in patients with acute coronary syndromes undergoing invasive management: a randomised multicentre trial. Lancet. 2015;385(9986):2465–76. https://doi.org/10.1016/S0140-6736(15)60292-6.

83. Jolly SS, Amlani S, Hamon M, Yusuf S, Mehta SR. Radial versus femoral access for coronary angiography or intervention and the impact on major bleeding and ischemic events: a systematic review and meta-analysis of randomized trials. Am Heart J. 2009;157(1):132–40. https://doi.org/10.1016/j.ahj.2008.08.023.

84. Hirsh J, Anand SS, Halperin JL, Fuster V. Mechanism of action and pharmacology of unfractionated heparin. Arterioscler Thromb Vasc Biol. 2001;21(7):1094–6. https://doi.org/10.1161/hq0701.093686.

85. Beurskens DMH, Huckriede JP, Schrijver R, Hemker HC, Reutelingsperger CP, Nicolaes GAF. The anticoagulant and nonanticoagulant properties of heparin. Thromb Haemost. 2020;120(10):1371–83. https://doi.org/10.1055/s-0040-1715460.

86. Théroux P, Ouimet H, McCans J, et al. Aspirin, heparin, or both to treat acute unstable angina. N Engl J Med. 1988;319(17):1105–11. https://doi.org/10.1056/NEJM198810273191701.

87. Levine GN, Bates ER, Blankenship JC, et al. 2011 ACCF/AHA/SCAI guideline for percutaneous coronary intervention: a report of the American College of Cardiology Foundation/American Heart Association Task Force on practice guidelines and the Society for Cardiovascular Angiography and Interventions. Circulation. 2011;124(23):e574–651. https://doi.org/10.1161/CIR.0b013e31823ba622.

88. O'Gara PT, Kushner FG, Ascheim DD, et al. 2013 ACCF/AHA guideline for the management of ST-elevation myocardial infarction: a report of the American College of Cardiology Foundation/American Heart Association Task Force on practice guidelines. Circulation. 2013;127(4):e362–425. https://doi.org/10.1161/CIR.0b013e3182742cf6.

89. Amsterdam EA, Wenger NK, Brindis RG, et al. 2014 AHA/ACC guideline for the management of patients with non-ST-elevation acute coronary syndromes: a report of the American College of Cardiology/American Heart Association Task Force on practice guidelines. Circulation. 2014;130(25):e344–426. https://doi.org/10.1161/CIR.0000000000000134.

90. Thomas J, Kostousov V, Teruya J. Bleeding and thrombotic complications in the use of extracorporeal membrane oxygenation. Semin Thromb Hemost. 2018;44(1):20–9. https://doi.org/10.1055/s-0037-1606179.

91. Izzy S, Rubin DB, Ahmed FS, et al. Cerebrovascular accidents during mechanical circulatory support: new predictors of ischemic and hemorrhagic strokes and outcome. Stroke. 2018;49(5):1197–203. https://doi.org/10.1161/STROKEAHA.117.020002.

92. Mack MJ, Leon MB, Smith CR, et al. 5-year outcomes of transcatheter aortic valve replacement or surgical aortic valve replacement for high surgical risk patients with aortic stenosis (PARTNER 1): a randomised controlled trial. Lancet. 2015;385(9986):2477–84. https://doi.org/10.1016/S0140-6736(15)60308-7.

93. Lincoff AM, Bittl JA, Kleiman NS, et al. Comparison of bivalirudin versus heparin during percutaneous coronary intervention (the Randomized Evaluation of PCI Linking Angiomax to Reduced Clinical Events [REPLACE]-1 trial). Am J Cardiol. 2004;93(9):1092–6. https://doi.org/10.1016/j.amjcard.2004.01.033.

94. Gurm HS, Sarembock IJ, Kereiakes DJ, et al. Use of bivalirudin during percutaneous coronary intervention in patients with diabetes mellitus: an analysis from the randomized evaluation in percutaneous coronary intervention linking angiomax to reduced clinical events (REPLACE)-2 trial. J Am Coll Cardiol. 2005;45(12):1932–8. https://doi.org/10.1016/j.jacc.2005.02.074.

95. Mehta SR, Granger CB, Eikelboom JW, et al. Efficacy and safety of fondaparinux versus enoxaparin in patients with acute coronary syndromes undergoing percutaneous coronary intervention: results from the OASIS-5 trial. J Am Coll Cardiol. 2007;50(18):1742–51. https://doi.org/10.1016/j.jacc.2007.07.042.

96. van Rees Vellinga TE, Peters RJG, Yusuf S, et al. Efficacy and safety of fondaparinux in patients with ST-segment elevation myocardial infarction across the age spectrum. Results from the Organization for the Assessment of Strategies for Ischemic Syndromes 6 (OASIS-6) trial. Am Heart J. 2010;160(6):1049–55. https://doi.org/10.1016/j.ahj.2010.08.038.

97. Ageno W, Gallus AS, Wittkowsky A, Crowther M, Hylek EM, Palareti G. Oral anticoagulant therapy: antithrombotic therapy and prevention of thrombosis, 9th ed: American College of Chest Physicians Evidence-Based Clinical Practice Guidelines. Chest. 2012;141(2 Suppl):e44S–88S. https://doi.org/10.1378/chest.11-2292.

98. Weitz JI. Hemostasis, thrombosis, fibrinolysis, and cardiovascular disease. In: Zipes D, Libby P, Bonow R, Mann D, Tomaselli G, Braunwald E, editors. Braunwald's heart disease, vol. 2. 11th ed. Elsevier; 2019. p. 1822–46.

99. Schulman S, Kearon C, Kakkar AK, et al. Dabigatran versus warfarin in the treatment of acute venous thromboembolism. N Engl J Med. 2009;361(24):2342–52. https://doi.org/10.1056/NEJMoa0906598.

100. Schulman S, Kearon C, Kakkar AK, et al. Extended use of dabigatran, warfarin, or placebo in venous thromboembolism. N Engl J Med. 2013;368(8):709–18. https://doi.org/10.1056/NEJMoa1113697.

101. Connolly SJ, Ezekowitz MD, Yusuf S, et al. Dabigatran versus warfarin in patients with atrial fibrillation. N Engl J Med. 2009;361(12):1139–51. https://doi.org/10.1056/NEJMoa0905561.

102. Calkins H, Willems S, Gerstenfeld EP, et al. Uninterrupted dabigatran versus warfarin for ablation in atrial fibrillation. N Engl J Med. 2017;376(17):1627–36. https://doi.org/10.1056/NEJMoa1701005.

103. Garcia D, Barrett YC, Ramacciotti E, Weitz JI. Laboratory assessment of the anticoagulant effects of the next generation of oral anticoagulants. J Thromb Haemost. 2013;11(2):245–52. https://doi.org/10.1111/jth.12096.

104. Siegal DM. Managing target-specific oral anticoagulant associated bleeding including an update on pharmacological reversal agents. J Thromb Thrombolysis. 2015;39(3):395–402. https://doi.org/10.1007/s11239-015-1167-9.

105. Eikelboom JW, Quinlan DJ, van Ryn J, Weitz JI. Idarucizumab: the antidote for reversal of dabigatran. Circulation. 2015;132(25):2412–22. https://doi.org/10.1161/CIRCULATIONAHA.115.019628.

106. Pollack CV, Reilly PA, Eikelboom J, et al. Idarucizumab for dabigatran reversal. N Engl J Med. 2015;373(6):511–20. https://doi.org/10.1056/NEJMoa1502000.

107. Büller HR, Bethune C, Bhanot S, et al. Factor XI antisense oligonucleotide for prevention of venous thrombosis. N Engl J Med. 2015;372(3):232–40. https://doi.org/10.1056/NEJMoa1405760.

108. Eikelboom JW, Hirsh J, Spencer FA, Baglin TP, Weitz JI. Antiplatelet drugs: antithrombotic therapy and prevention of thrombosis, 9th ed: American College of Chest Physicians Evidence-Based Clinical Practice Guidelines. Chest. 2012;141(2 Suppl):e89S–e119S. https://doi.org/10.1378/chest.11-2293.

109. ASCEND Study Collaborative Group, Bowman L, Mafham M, et al. Effects of aspirin for primary prevention in persons with diabetes mellitus. N Engl J Med. 2018;379(16):1529–39. https://doi.org/10.1056/NEJMoa1804988.

110. Gaziano JM, Brotons C, Coppolecchia R, et al. Use of aspirin to reduce risk of initial vascular events in patients at moderate risk of cardiovascular disease (ARRIVE): a randomised, double-blind, placebo-controlled trial. Lancet. 2018;392(10152):1036–46. https://doi.org/10.1016/S0140-6736(18)31924-X.

111. de Berardis G, Lucisano G, D'Ettorre A, et al. Association of aspirin use with major bleeding in patients with and without diabetes. JAMA. 2012;307(21):2286–94. https://doi.org/10.1001/jama.2012.5034.

112. Arnett DK, Blumenthal RS, Albert MA, et al. 2019 ACC/AHA guideline on the primary prevention of cardiovascular disease: a report of the American College of Cardiology/American Heart Association Task Force on clinical practice guidelines. Circulation. 2019;140(11):e596–646. https://doi.org/10.1161/CIR.0000000000000678.

113. Otto CM, Nishimura RA, Bonow RO, et al. 2020 ACC/AHA guideline for the management of patients with valvular heart disease: a report of the American College of Cardiology/American Heart Association Joint Committee on clinical practice guidelines. Circulation. 2021;143(5):e72–e227. https://doi.org/10.1161/CIR.0000000000000923.

114. Gurbel PA, Myat A, Kubica J, Tantry US. State of the art: oral antiplatelet therapy. JRSM Cardiovasc Dis. 2016;5:2048004016652514. https://doi.org/10.1177/2048004016652514.

115. Levine GN, Bates ER, Bittl JA, et al. 2016 ACC/AHA guideline focused update on duration of dual antiplatelet therapy in patients with coronary artery disease: a report of the American College of Cardiology/American Heart Association Task Force on clinical practice guidelines: an update of the 2011 ACCF/AHA/SCAI guideline for percutaneous coronary intervention, 2011 ACCF/AHA guideline for coronary artery bypass graft surgery, 2012 ACC/AHA/ACP/AATS/PCNA/SCAI/STS guidelines. Circulation. 2016;134(10):e123–55. https://doi.org/10.1161/CIR.0000000000000404.

116. Wallentin L, Becker RC, Budaj A, et al. Ticagrelor versus clopidogrel in patients with acute coronary syndromes. N Engl J Med. 2009;361(11):1045–57. https://doi.org/10.1056/NEJMoa0904327.

117. Sabatine MS, Mega JL. Pharmacogenomics of antiplatelet drugs. Hematology Am Soc Hematol Educ Program. 2014;2014(1):343–7. https://doi.org/10.1182/asheducation-2014.1.343.

118. Verro P, Gorelick PB, Nguyen D. Aspirin plus dipyridamole versus aspirin for prevention of vascular events after stroke or TIA: a meta-analysis. Stroke. 2008;39(4):1358–63. https://doi.org/10.1161/STROKEAHA.107.496281.

119. Sacco RL, Diener HC, Yusuf S, et al. Aspirin and extended-release dipyridamole versus clopidogrel for recurrent stroke. N Engl J Med. 2008;359(12):1238–51. https://doi.org/10.1056/NEJMoa0805002.

120. Tantry US, Liu F, Chen G, Gurbel PA. Vorapaxar in the secondary prevention of atherothrombosis. Expert Rev Cardiovasc Ther. 2015;13(12):1293–305. https://doi.org/10.1586/14779072.2015.1109447.

121. Tricoci P, Huang Z, Held C, et al. Thrombin-receptor antagonist vorapaxar in acute coronary syndromes. N Engl J Med. 2012;366(1):20–33. https://doi.org/10.1056/NEJMoa1109719.

122. Morrow DA, Braunwald E, Bonaca MP, et al. Vorapaxar in the secondary prevention of atherothrombotic events. N Engl J Med. 2012;366(15):1404–13. https://doi.org/10.1056/NEJMoa1200933.

123. Chapin JC, Hajjar KA. Fibrinolysis and the control of blood coagulation. Blood Rev. 2015;29(1):17–24. https://doi.org/10.1016/j.blre.2014.09.003.

124. Piazza G, Hohlfelder B, Jaff MR, et al. A prospective, single-arm, multicenter trial of ultrasound-facilitated, catheter-directed, low-dose fibrinolysis for acute massive and submassive pulmonary embolism: the SEATTLE II Study. JACC Cardiovasc Interv. 2015;8(10):1382–92. https://doi.org/10.1016/j.jcin.2015.04.020.

125. Chatterjee S, Chakraborty A, Weinberg I, et al. Thrombolysis for pulmonary embolism and risk of all-cause mortality, major bleeding, and intracranial hemorrhage: a meta-analysis. JAMA. 2014;311(23):2414–21. https://doi.org/10.1001/jama.2014.5990.

126. Engelberger RP, Stuck A, Spirk D, et al. Ultrasound-assisted versus conventional catheter-directed thrombolysis for acute iliofemoral deep vein thrombosis: 1-year follow-up data of a randomized-controlled trial. J Thromb Haemost. 2017;15(7):1351–60. https://doi.org/10.1111/jth.13709.

127. Tapson VF, Sterling K, Jones N, et al. A randomized trial of the optimum duration of acoustic pulse thrombolysis procedure in acute intermediate-risk pulmonary embolism: the OPTALYSE PE trial. JACC Cardiovasc Interv. 2018;11(14):1401–10. https://doi.org/10.1016/j.jcin.2018.04.008.

128. Sista AK, Horowitz JM, Tapson VF, et al. Indigo aspiration system for treatment of pulmonary embolism: results of the EXTRACT-PE trial. JACC Cardiovasc Interv. 2021;14(3):319–29. https://doi.org/10.1016/j.jcin.2020.09.053.

129. Tu T, Toma C, Tapson VF, et al. A prospective, single-arm, multicenter trial of catheter-directed mechanical thrombectomy for intermediate-risk acute pulmonary embolism: the FLARE study. JACC Cardiovasc Interv. 2019;12(9):859–69. https://doi.org/10.1016/j.jcin.2018.12.022.

130. Patel MR, Mahaffey KW, Garg J, et al. Rivaroxaban versus warfarin in nonvalvular atrial fibrillation. N Engl J Med. 2011;365(10):883–91. https://doi.org/10.1056/NEJMoa1009638.

131. Granger CB, Alexander JH, McMurray JJV, et al. Apixaban versus warfarin in patients with atrial fibrillation. N Engl J Med. 2011;365(11):981–92. https://doi.org/10.1056/NEJMoa1107039.

132. Giugliano RP, Ruff CT, Braunwald E, et al. Edoxaban versus warfarin in patients with atrial fibrillation. N Engl J Med. 2013;369(22):2093–104. https://doi.org/10.1056/NEJMoa1310907.

133. Ruff CT, Giugliano RP, Braunwald E, et al. Comparison of the efficacy and safety of new oral anticoagulants with warfarin in patients with atrial fibrillation: a meta-analysis of randomised trials. Lancet. 2014;383(9921):955–62. https://doi.org/10.1016/S0140-6736(13)62343-0.

134. Chen A, Stecker E, Warden BA. Direct oral anticoagulant use: a practical guide to common clinical challenges. J Am Heart Assoc. 2020;9(13):e017559. https://doi.org/10.1161/JAHA.120.017559.

135. Antithrombotic Trialists' Collaboration. Collaborative meta-analysis of randomised trials of antiplatelet therapy for prevention of death, myocardial infarction, and stroke in high risk patients. BMJ. 2002;324(7329):71–86. https://doi.org/10.1136/bmj.324.7329.71.

136. Patrono C, Baigent C, Hirsh J, Roth G. Antiplatelet drugs: American College of Chest Physicians evidence-based clinical practice guidelines (8th Edition). Chest. 2008;133(6 Suppl):199S–233S. https://doi.org/10.1378/chest.08-0672.

137. Mukherjee D, Roffi M. Glycoprotein IIb/IIIa receptor inhibitors in 2008: do they still have a role? J Interv Cardiol. 2008;21(2):118–21. https://doi.org/10.1111/j.1540-8183.2007.00344.x.

138. Michelson AD. P2Y12 antagonism: promises and challenges. Arterioscler Thromb Vasc Biol. 2008;28(3):s33–8. https://doi.org/10.1161/ATVBAHA.107.160689.

139. Wiviott SD, Braunwald E, McCabe CH, et al. Prasugrel versus clopidogrel in patients with acute coronary syndromes. N Engl J Med. 2007;357(20):2001–15. https://doi.org/10.1056/NEJMoa0706482.

140. Sugidachi A, Ogawa T, Kurihara A, et al. The greater in vivo antiplatelet effects of prasugrel as compared to clopidogrel reflect more efficient generation of its active metabolite with similar antiplatelet activity to that of clopidogrel's active metabolite. J Thromb Haemost. 2007;5(7):1545–51. https://doi.org/10.1111/j.1538-7836.2007.02598.x.

141. ESPRIT Study Group, Halkes PHA, van Gijn J, Kappelle LJ, Koudstaal PJ, Algra A. Aspirin plus dipyridamole versus aspirin alone after cerebral ischaemia of arterial origin (ESPRIT): randomised controlled trial. Lancet. 2006;367(9523):1665–73. https://doi.org/10.1016/S0140-6736(06)68734-5.

142. Michelson AD. Antiplatelet therapies for the treatment of cardiovascular disease. Nat Rev Drug Discov. 2010;9(2):154–69. https://doi.org/10.1038/nrd2957.

Blood Pressure and Cardiovascular Outcomes

Steven A. Greenstein and Joseph A. Diamond

Key Points
- The prevalence of hypertension is increasing worldwide.
- Clinical trials were first initiated following the 1965 US President's Commission on Heart Disease recommendations to show evidence of the benefit of treating hypertension. In 1976, the National Heart, Lung, and Blood Institute established the Joint National Committee (JNC) to assess, summarize, and identify areas for future research, thus becoming the guideline on hypertension for the next 27 years.
- In 2003, the JNC-7 guidelines outlined categories of hypertension, redefining normal blood pressure (BP) as <120 mm Hg systolic and <80 mm Hg diastolic. Cutpoints for systolic blood pressure (SBP) of 120-138 mm Hg or diastolic blood pressure (DBP) of 80-89 mm Hg were defined as prehypertension, a finding that triggers the need to address lifestyle.
- Clinical trials regarding the treatment of hypertension in the elderly (e.g., Systolic Hypertension in the Elderly Program [SHEP], Systolic Hypertension in Europe [Syst-Eur], and Hypertension in the Very Elderly Trial [HYVET]) suggested that

The above authors have no relationships with any commercial company that has direct financial interest in subject matter or materials discussed in this chapter. The authors have nothing to disclose.

S. A. Greenstein · J. A. Diamond (✉)
Cardiovascular Institute, Northwell, New Hyde Park, NY, USA
e-mail: jdiamond@northwell.edu

K. C. Maki, D. P. Wilson (eds.), *Cardiovascular Outcomes Research*, Contemporary Cardiology, https://doi.org/10.1007/978-3-031-54960-1_12

treatment to an SBP goal of <150 mm Hg is beneficial compared to higher levels of BP. This helped formulate changes for the JNC-8 guidelines.

- Clinical trials of high-risk populations with co-morbid conditions such as diabetes or chronic kidney disease (e.g., African American Study of Kidney Disease [AASK], Action to Control Cardiovascular Risk in Diabetes [ACCORD], and Systolic Blood Pressure Intervention Trial [SPRINT]) suggested that certain populations require more intensive treatment goals.
- Proper technique for measuring BP is of critical importance. Overestimating BP by as little as 5 mm Hg may lead to inappropriate treatment in almost 30 million Americans, with attendant exposure to adverse drug effects, the psychological effects of misdiagnosis, and unnecessary cost.
- Home BP measurements and 24-h ambulatory BP monitoring are generally more accurate than those obtained in a clinical setting.
- Organizations including the American College of Cardiology (ACC), the American Heart Association (AHA), the American College of Physicians, and the American Academy of Family Physicians are moving toward the incorporation of cardiovascular risk stratification of patients in the treatment of hypertension goals.
- Guidelines should be evidence-based, unbiased, and consistent across organizations, yet comprehensive enough to reflect the complexity of hypertensive disease, easy to understand and implement, and consistent with the way in which clinicians consider the risks and benefits of treatment.

1 Introduction

Hypertension affects billions of individuals, and the prevalence is increasing yearly. It is estimated that by 2025, 1.6 billion people globally will have hypertension. Consequences on the global health environment are staggering. In the United States, approximately 78 million adults have hypertension. Despite aggressive efforts at diagnosis and management, these numbers continue to rise.

Hypertension affects all ages, sexes, and ethnicities, albeit not equally. The incidence in children is becoming alarming and is believed to be linked to a marked rise in childhood obesity. Unlike adult hypertension, childhood values were initially derived based on general population data in youth <18 years of age. Accordingly, the prevalence of childhood hypertension was estimated to be approximately 3.5% based on data from the fourth report on the diagnosis, evaluation, and treatment of high blood pressure (BP) in children and adolescents and other studies [1, 2]. As more attention was paid to childhood hypertension, the guidelines were updated in 2017 [3] to parallel those of adults (Tables 1 and 2). This change was expected to significantly increase the prevalence among the pediatric population [4]. This trend is important for many reasons. Studies demonstrate that higher BP in childhood correlates with the trajectory of hypertension as an adult and worse cardiovascular outcome [5].

Table 1 Updated blood pressure classification for children aged 1–13 years. Definitions are based on normative distribution of healthy children and must be adjusted for age, sex, and height. Therefore, blood pressure stage defined by percentile rank or absolute systolic values. The lower of the two is taken [3]

Children aged 1–13 years	
BP classification	BP level (percentile or SBP/DBP)
Normal	<90th percentile
Elevated BP	≥90th percentile to <95th percentile or 120/80 mm Hg to <95th percentile (whichever is lower)
Stage 1 hypertension	≥95th percentile to <95th percentile +12 mm Hg or 130/80 to 139/89 mm Hg (whichever is lower)
Stage 2 hypertension	≥95th percentile +12 mm Hg or ≥140/90 mm Hg (whichever is lower)

BP blood pressure, *DBP* diastolic blood pressure, *SBP* systolic blood pressure

Table 2 Updated blood pressure classification for children aged ≥13 years. Definitions are based on normative distribution of healthy children and must be adjusted for age, sex, and height. This table is designed as a screening tool for identification of children who need further evaluation and repeat blood pressure measurements. Actual blood pressure cutoffs may be more than 90 mm Hg higher depending on the child's age, length, and weight [3]

Children aged ≥13 years			
BP classification	SBP (mm Hg)		DBP (mm Hg)
Normal	<120	AND	<80
Elevated BP	≥120–129	AND	<80
Stage 1 hypertension	≥130–139	OR	≥80–89
Stage 2 hypertension	≥140	OR	≥90

BP blood pressure, *DBP* diastolic blood pressure, *SBP* systolic blood pressure

The connection of childhood hypertension to other chronic conditions is well recognized. In one study, rapid weight gain and body mass index in the first 6 postnatal months were shown to be related to higher systolic blood pressure (SBP) in mid-childhood [6]. Other studies have shown that among children with obesity, there is a statistically significant increase in both systolic and diastolic blood pressures [7]. Some studies allude to the theory that the early presence of multiple cardiovascular risk factors can lead to a greater increase in cardiovascular risk than each individual risk factor alone [8]. Other associations with childhood hypertension have been made to chronic kidney disease, abnormal birth history, including prematurity, and low birth weight. Regardless, identifying hypertension in childhood is important, as numerous studies have demonstrated increased risk for adult hypertension and metabolic syndrome [3].

For most individuals, the risk of hypertension increases with age. Thus, the prevalence of hypertension is much higher in adults than in children. Data from the National Center for Health Statistics [9] estimated that in a survey period from 2017 to 2018 the age-adjusted prevalence was 45.4% among adults and approximately 75% among those aged 60 years and older. The prevalence of hypertension was 57.1% among non-Hispanic Blacks and 43.7% among non-Hispanic Whites.

Non-Hispanic Blacks had higher BP awareness yet significantly lagged in control of their BP compared to non-Hispanic Whites. Females had lower rates of hypertension than males (51% vs. 39.7%, respectively). However, this difference was not statistically significant for those above age 60, suggesting a possible hormone-mediated etiology. Differences can be seen based on education levels as well. College graduates have significantly lower rates of hypertension than adults with only a high school education. Sex differences remain regardless of race [9].

2 History of Guidelines for Hypertension

Blood pressure was studied as early as 1733 with the advent of sphygmomanometers. The initial evidence that high BP was a risk factor for cardiovascular disease (CVD) came from actuarial data obtained from the insurance industry. Data from a large number of medical examinations performed for individuals applying for life insurance were used. In a publication from 1939, the Actuarial Society of America provided extensive information about the relationship between BP and mortality. Table 3, abstracted from the 1939 report, showed the ratios of actual-to-expected deaths from cardiovascular and renal diseases [10]. For examinations performed on individuals aged ≥40 years, SBP was a more important predictor of death than diastolic blood pressure (DBP), and for examinations performed on individuals aged <30 years, the influence of DBP was more marked than SBP. With the exception of low systolic readings in examinations for individuals aged 10–29 years, the prevailing tendency was an increase in mortality ratio as SBP increased. For relatively low SBP, the mortality was somewhat stable as DBP increased, but at the middle and higher SBP ranges, mortality increased rapidly as DBP readings increased. Of note, a combination of low SBP with high DBP was associated with an increased suicide rate. By the mid-1960s, convincing evidence had accumulated of the cardiovascular effects of elevated BP. The 1965 report of the US President's Commission on Heart Disease recommended increased screening and treatment of hypertension. Over the next 10 years, numerous studies showed evidence of the benefit of treating

Table 3 Abstract from 1939 report: ratios, expressed as percent, of actual-to-expected deaths from cardiovascular and renal disease based on systolic blood pressure (SBP) and diastolic blood pressure (DBP), among insured individuals [10]

Ratio (%) of actual-to-expected deaths					
	For DBP (mm Hg)				
For SBP (mm Hg)	54–78	79–86	87–93	94–98	99–116
108–132	87 ± 2	97 ± 1	111 ± 2	133 ± 6	98 ± 15
133–137	97 ± 3	121 ± 2	132 ± 3	141 ± 6	104 ± 13
138–142	112 ± 4	132 ± 2	152 ± 2	189 ± 5	203 ± 10
143–152	146 ± 8	165 ± 4	193 ± 3	248 ± 5	323 ± 11
153–177	333 ± 35	222 ± 2	285 ± 10	358 ± 12	439 ± 14

hypertension. The National Health and Nutrition Examination Survey (NHANES) community-based surveys were designed to describe the relationships of BP with age and body size in both women and men. This led to the formulation of the National High Blood Pressure Education Program (NHBPEP). This program was designed to be implemented by the National Heart, Lung, and Blood Institute (NHLBI). A few years later, the NHLBI established a task force known as the Joint National Committee (JNC) to assess, summarize, and identify areas for future research, although the data were limited. At its inception, the JNC-1 focused mainly on treating elevated DBP >105 mm Hg. Screening was recommended for SBP >140 mm Hg [11]. The first JNC guideline was published in 1976. While the NHLBI continued to produce task forces and recommendations, the JNC increased awareness and animal research funding. Between 1981 and 2007, animal research increased from $80.6 million to $211.1 million. The JNC continued to publish updated guidelines every 4–6 years. By 2003, the JNC had published seven reports defining acceptable BP levels and treatment strategies for hypertension. In 2011, the Institute of Medicine, an independent, nonprofit organization that works outside of government to provide unbiased and authoritative advice to decision makers and the public, published a report on the importance of guidelines and called for high-quality evidence. The JNC-8 was formed to answer this call; however, the National Institutes of Health (NIH) eventually withdrew from developing guidelines, creating the opportunity for the American Heart Association (AHA) and the American College of Cardiology (ACC) to publish their guideline for hypertension in 2017. Although met with some controversy, the JNC-8 eventually published their updated guidelines.

Considering how the hypertension guidelines have evolved, it is interesting to see how clinical trials have influenced recommendations on the management of hypertension. With the JNC-7, it was clear that the presence of hypertension required treatment, and the Food and Drug Administration developed rigorous methods to evaluate and classify antihypertensive medications. In 2003, the JNC-7 guidelines identified four BP categories (Table 4). Normal BP was defined as SBP <120 mm Hg and DBP <80 mm Hg, prehypertension as SBP 120-138 mm Hg or DBP 80-89 mm Hg, stage 1 hypertension as SBP 140-159 mm Hg or DBP 90-99 mm Hg, and stage 2 hypertension as SBP >160 mm Hg or DBP >100 mm Hg. This reclassification came from data demonstrating that lifetime risk of complications from

Table 4 JNC-7 classification and management of BP for adults aged 18 years or older [34]

JNC-7: adults aged ≥18 years				
BP classification	SBP (mm Hg)		DBP (mm Hg)	Management
Normal	<120	AND	<80	Lifestyle modification
Prehypertension	120-139	OR	80-89	Lifestyle modification
Stage 1 hypertension	140-159	OR	90-99	Lifestyle modification and medication
Stage 2 hypertension	≥160	OR	≥100	Lifestyle modification and medication

BP blood pressure, *DBP* diastolic blood pressure, *JNC* Joint National Committee, *SBP* systolic blood pressure hypertension extends to BP levels previously believed to be normal. The JNC-7's aim was to identify a patient population with prehypertension in which implementation of lifestyle changes would slow progression to hypertension and reduce adverse events. The JNC-7 also attempted to stratify patients based on the presence or absence of risk factors or end-organ damage (compelling factors that influence BP goal and choice of therapy). It was suggested that patients with diabetes or chronic kidney disease target a SBP of <130 mm Hg, preferably using angiotensin-converting enzyme inhibitors (ACEis) or angiotensin receptor blockers (ARBs) to help slow progression of kidney disease. The African American Study of Kidney Disease and Hypertension (AASK) was an instructive trial looking at populations with compelling indications for specific antihypertension medication. This study evaluated 1094 African American individuals who were non-diabetic, but had evidence of hypertensive chronic kidney disease. Baseline glomerular filtration rate (GFR) in this population was between 20 and 65 mL/min/1.73 m^2. The main clinical composite outcome for the trial was time to declining GFR event (50% or 25 mL/min/1.73 m^2 decrease in GFR), progression to end-stage renal disease (ESRD or end-stage kidney disease, defined as initiation of dialysis or receipt of a kidney transplant), or all-cause mortality. There were two BP goals in this trial: the usual goal based on mean arterial pressure (MAP) of 102-107 mm Hg (~140/90 mm Hg) and the strict, or low, goal, with MAP <93 mm Hg (~125/75 mm Hg). Three antihypertensive regimens were employed: dihydropyridine calcium channel blocker (amlodipine), ACEi (ramipril), and beta blocker (metoprolol). The average achieved BP after 5 years of follow-up was 141/85 mm Hg for the usual goal group and 128/78 mm Hg for the strict goal group. With respect to outcomes (decline in renal function, progression to ESRD, or death), there were significantly fewer adverse outcomes in those treated with ramipril than in those treated with either metoprolol or amlodipine (ramipril vs. metoprolol, risk reduction [RR] = 22%, p = 0.04; ramipril vs. amlodipine, RR = 38%, p = 0.004; and metoprolol vs. amlodipine, RR = 20%, p = 0.17). Of note, achieving lower BP goal appeared to be most important for those individuals with baseline proteinuria. Nevertheless, controversy regarding BP targets for the general population and how aggressively to treat high-risk patients, such as the elderly and those with kidney disease or diabetes, remained.

3 Changes in Recommendations Based on the JNC-8 Guidelines

Until the 1980s, it was considered normal for BP to increase with aging. Thus, while younger people were considered to have hypertension if SBP increased above 140 mm Hg, older people were not considered hypertensive until SBP increased to >160 mm Hg. In fact, this "normal" increase in BP with aging was felt necessary to maintain health, giving rise to the clinical term, "essential hypertension." Furthermore, at this time, the risks of high BP were considered greater for elevated

DBP, rather than elevated SBP. Major trial data, particularly in the elderly, were lacking. It is informative, therefore, to briefly review some of the major trials available to the JNC-7 that helped shape the direction and recommendations of later guidelines such as those from the JNC-8 and AHA/ACC.

The Systolic Hypertension in the Elderly Program (SHEP), the results of which were published in 1991, evaluated over 4000 patients between 1985 and 1988 [12]. Participants at least 60 years old with a SBP between 160 and 219 mm Hg were randomized in Step 1 to chlorthalidone or placebo and in Step 2 to atenolol or placebo. Although there was only a small reduction in BP, achieved mean BP was 143/68 mm Hg in the treated group vs. 155/72 mm Hg in the placebo group, and there was a significant reduction in stroke and secondary outcomes of myocardial infarction and heart failure. There was a 36% reduction in strokes, a 32% reduction in cardiovascular events, a 27% reduction in non-fatal myocardial infarction or coronary death, and a 13% reduction in all-cause mortality. Interestingly, there was no increase in serious adverse events (SAEs) in the treatment group, which surprised many as it was expected that treatment of the elderly may result in more complications, such as falling due to treatment-induced orthostatic hypotension. In fact, fracture rates were not significantly different for treatment groups; 2.4% of the treatment group experienced hip fractures vs. 2.0% of the placebo group. Approximately 24% of all participants reported lightheadedness upon standing quickly, and 3% reported loss of consciousness. Orthostatic symptoms did not relate to medication status.

The Swedish Trial in Old Patients with Hypertension (STOP) corroborated these results [13]. These trials began to discredit the theory that lowering BP in the elderly is harmful. However, both trials used low-dose antihypertensive medications and the patients were otherwise relatively healthy, limiting the generalizability to all in the elderly population [14]. At the same time, uncertainties remained about treatment goals and whether or not calcium channel blockers would offer the same results.

In Europe, the Systolic Hypertension in Europe (Syst-Eur) Trial Investigators conducted a trial that included dihydropyridine calcium channel blocker, ACEi, and thiazide diuretic. They found similar results to the SHEP and STOP trials in that this approach reduced stroke and myocardial infarction. The study population included 4695 patients at least 60 years old, with SBP of 160-219 mm Hg and DBP below 95 mm Hg. Average BP of 151/80 mm Hg was achieved in antihypertensive medication-treated subjects and 161/86 mm Hg in the placebo group. There was a 42% reduction in strokes, 26% reduction in cardiac events, and 31% reduction in all cardiovascular events for the treated group. While the data continued to support the reduction in strokes for the elderly, patients in these trials were considered elderly if they were older than 60 years of age. To many, this definition was questionable, which perpetuated the controversy. Using this definition as the threshold for defining the elderly, there was some evidence that adverse events might be higher among the "very elderly" [15]. A meta-analysis of published studies of patients aged 80 years and older suggested that while there was a reduction in stroke risk, there was no treatment benefit for cardiovascular death and a non-significant relative excess of death from all causes.

Soon, the focus changed toward studying patients greater than 80 years of age. This reasoning gave rise to the Hypertension in the Very Elderly Trial (HYVET). The investigators randomly allocated patients greater than 80 years of age to a diuretic-based regimen, an ACEi-based regimen, or no treatment with a target BP of <150/80 mm Hg. It is important to note that providers were able to substitute drugs, and therefore, medications were prescribed according to local practices and to promote the generalizability of the results. Preliminary results published in 2003 suggested a possible reduction in strokes without a significant increase in mortality [16]. The full trial was concluded and published in 2008 [17]. Results from HYVET showed that at two-year follow-up, antihypertensive drug therapy with indapamide, plus perindopril if needed, reduced fatal or non-fatal stroke by 30%, fatal stroke by 39%, all-cause mortality by 21%, cardiovascular death by 23%, and heart failure by 64%. The full data were likely not available to the JNC-7, limiting their conclusions in 2004 to simply "in those older than age 50, systolic blood pressure (SBP) > 140 mm Hg is a more important cardiovascular disease (CVD) risk factor than diastolic BP (DBP)." The results of the HYVET trial were surprising. In contrast to other data available at the time, it was one of the few studies that demonstrated mortality benefit of treating the very elderly. Initial attempts were made to rectify and rationalize this difference. It was speculated that perhaps the medications used in HYVET, or the use of a diuretic-only regimen in other studies, may have led to electrolyte abnormalities or that perhaps the reduction in mortality was related to a reduction in strokes. Despite the results of HYVET, based on limited data that suggested there may not be additional benefit to aggressive reduction in BP [18, 19], the JNC-8 later concluded that a SBP goal of less than 150 mm Hg was beneficial in patients >60 years of age.

The JNC-7 also recommended treatment for diabetic patients with a SBP goal of <130 mm Hg. The data for this decision largely came from randomized controlled trials that included a large number of diabetic patients, such as the UK Prospective Diabetes Study (UKPDS), Hypertension Optimal Treatment (HOT), SHEP, Syst-Eur, Heart Outcomes Prevention Evaluation (HOPE), Losartan Intervention for Endpoint Reduction in Hypertension (LIFE), and the Antihypertensive and Lipid-Lowering Treatment to Prevent Heart Attack (ALLHAT) trials. At the same time, the NHLBI 2003 workshop recommended that the most important trial question was whether treating SBP to a lower level than the recommended goal at that time would reduce CVD mortality and morbidity. Funding was given to two major study groups, the Systolic Blood Pressure Intervention Trial (SPRINT) and the Action to Control Cardiovascular Risk in Diabetes (ACCORD), the latter focusing on patients with diabetes.

In 2010, the ACCORD study group conducted a study to answer the question of whether or not aggressive BP control lowers mortality in hypertensive patients with diabetes [20]. In this trial, over 10,000 patients were randomized to intensive or standard glycemic control. In addition, they were randomized to simvastatin and fenofibrate vs. placebo and intensive (<120 mm Hg) or standard BP control

(<140 mm Hg). The primary endpoint was a composite of non-fatal myocardial infarction, non-fatal stroke, or cardiovascular death observed over the following 5 years. After 1 year, the intensive therapy group had lower BP and no reduction in non-fatal myocardial infarction or death, yet a significant reduction in non-fatal stroke. SAEs were notably higher in the intensive therapy group (3.3% vs. 1.3%, $p < 0.001$). However, while there was a significant difference in hypotension, most of the adverse outcomes were metabolic, such as hypokalemia and changes in GFR. There were no differences in major adverse events such as renal failure, the need for dialysis, or syncope. Because the study failed to demonstrate superiority of lower BP goals and had an increase in adverse events, the results were met with skepticism. The JNC-8, AHA/ACC, American Diabetes Association, and European Association for the Study of Diabetes guidelines retreated from the JNC-7 recommendation of SBP <130 mm Hg to a SBP goal of <140 mm Hg for hypertensive patients with diabetes.

4 Implications for Treatment Goals Based on Newer Clinical Trials

Contemporaneously, the SPRINT study group was funded by the NIH to answer the question of BP goals in high-risk patients. Participants in this trial were at least 50 years of age and had a SBP of 130–180 mm Hg, and an increased risk of cardiovascular events defined by 1 or more of the following: clinical or subclinical CVD, a Framingham Risk Score of ≥15%, chronic kidney disease, or > 75 years of age. Notably, this trial excluded patients with a history of stroke or diabetes. Patients were randomized to an intensive group with a SBP goal of less than 120 mm Hg or to a group with a less intensive goal of 140 mm Hg. The study results were dramatic. On average, BP goals were achieved; the intensive treatment group achieved a mean BP of 121 mm Hg, using an average of one additional drug compared to standard treatment. The intensive treatment group also had a 25% reduction in the composite endpoint of CVD mortality, non-fatal myocardial infarction, stroke, and heart failure. This translated to a number needed to treat (NNT) of 90 to prevent one death and NNT of 61 to prevent one primary cardiovascular outcome. Most notably, there were no significant differences in SAEs, which were defined as events that were fatal or life-threatening, that resulted in clinically significant or persistent disability, that required hospitalization, or, as determined by the investigator, that required medical or surgical intervention. There were, however, higher rates of easily treatable complications in the intensively treated group, such as hypotension, syncope, electrolyte abnormalities, acute kidney injury, and renal failure.

The 2017 ACC/AHA guidelines responded to these new data (Table 5). The guidelines were changed substantially to define elevated SBP as greater than 120 mm Hg and, in addition, recommended non-pharmacologic therapies. For those with CVD, diabetes mellitus, chronic kidney disease, or a 10-year CVD risk of

Table 5 AHA/ACC 2017 classification and management of BP for adults aged 18 years or older. Notable changes include classifying prehypertension as elevated BP and lowering the systolic and diastolic values needed to be classified as stage 1 and stage 2 hypertension [35]

AHA/ACC 2017: adults aged $\geq$18 years				
BP classification	SBP (mm Hg)		DBP (mm Hg)	Management
Normal	<120	AND	<80	Lifestyle modification
Elevated BP	120-129	OR	<80	Lifestyle modification
Stage 1 hypertension	130-139	OR	80-89	Lifestyle modification and medication
Stage 2 hypertension	$\geq$140	OR	$\geq$90	Lifestyle modification and medication

ACC American College of Cardiology, *AHA* American Heart Association, *BP* blood pressure, *DBP* diastolic blood pressure, *SBP* systolic blood pressure

>10%, the BP treatment goal was lowered to less than 130/80 mm Hg as opposed to 150/90. These changes had serious consequences on the population. Using data from NHANES, Bundy et al. [21] estimated the impacts of these changes. By expanding the targeted treatment group using the new 2017 guidelines, the national prevalence of hypertension jumped from 32% to 45% with only a small increase in those for whom treatment was recommended (from 31.1% to 35.9%). This small increase, however, led to the reduction of 340,000 CVD events and 150,000 deaths. Implementation of these guidelines was estimated to increase 62,000 cases of hypotension, 32,000 cases of syncope, 31,000 electrolyte abnormalities, and 79,000 acute kidney injury and renal failure events. Clinicians and patients, therefore, were faced with the dilemma of balancing a reduction in cardiovascular events and death, at the price of adverse events. This treatment-risk paradox in BP management resulted in a reluctance to aggressively lower BP in those most at risk based on an increase in potential adverse events [22].

While SPRINT was informative and changed the way we treated hypertension, it was clear more data were needed as to how we could more appropriately select patients that would benefit from treatment. In a study of data from SPRINT, participants were divided into quartiles based on 10-year CVD risk as determined by the Pooled Cohort Equations commonly used by many clinicians. A predictive model was used to assess the benefit-to-harm ratio of strict BP control as a function of CVD risk [23]. The benefit of intensive BP control was directly related to CVD risk. Within each of the four quartiles of 10-year CVD risk, there was a lower rate of primary adverse outcome events with intensive treatment. However, this difference was more pronounced in the higher risk quartiles. A similar trend was seen with SAEs. While there was no significant difference within each quartile, the absolute difference in all SAEs between treatment groups decreased in the third and fourth quartiles, making the overall number needed to harm 62 in the first quartile and 250 in the fourth quartile. Similar to SPRINT, there were significantly more instances of hypotension, syncope, electrolyte abnormalities, acute kidney injury, and renal failure. With these data in mind, a predictive model on the benefit-to-harm ratio was calculated comparing each quartile. Surprisingly, it was found that in the first and second quartiles the benefit-to-harm ratio was <1.00, suggesting greater harm than benefit. However, in the third and fourth quartiles the benefit-to-harm ratio was >1.00, suggesting that these patients had greater benefit than harm from intensive treatment. Thus, the debate over the benefits of intensive treatment continues.

The American College of Physicians (ACP) and the American Academy of Family Physicians (AAFP) continue to endorse SBP targets of <150 mm Hg. Large-scale observational studies such as the Berlin Initiative Study [24] suggest that intensive treatment results in increased mortality. More recently, results from a Trial of Intensive Blood-Pressure Control in Older Patients with Hypertension were published [25]. These investigators found that intensive BP-lowering therapy was associated with fewer cases of stroke, acute coronary syndrome, heart failure exacerbations, atrial fibrillation, and death from any cause. There were no differences in dizziness, syncope, and adverse renal outcomes; however, the incidence of hypotension was significantly higher in the intensive treatment group.

5 Methods of BP Measurement

Accurate BP measurement is critically important. Overestimating true BP by 5 mm Hg could lead to inappropriate treatment in almost 30 million Americans, with attendant exposure to adverse drug effects, the psychological effects of misdiagnosis, and unnecessary cost. BP has traditionally been measured in the clinical setting using auscultatory measures [26]. Currently, the gold standard for measurement of BP utilizes a calibrated column of mercury. However, given the potential toxicity of mercury, this method has fallen out of favor and replaced with either manual aneroid sphygmomanometers or automatic oscillometric devices, both of which have growing evidence supporting their accuracy. Oscillometer devices use a sensor to detect blood pulsatility during inflation and deflation.

There are many potential errors in the measurement of BP. Most errors can be avoided by following guidelines, which promote a systematic approach to BP measurement. Even when measurement technique is perfect, isolated readings may not reflect the patient's true BP. Therefore, like any other procedure or examination, preparation and repeat measurements are important. The patient should be encouraged to empty their bladder and avoid caffeine, exercise, or smoking for at least 30 min prior to measurement of the BP. After being placed into a clinic room, the patient should sit in a chair for at least 5 min, with both feet on the floor. There should be little, or preferably no, conversation, and the patient's upper arm should be appropriately exposed. The BP measurement device should be applied, and the patient's arm should be supported. It is critically important to use the correct-sized BP cuff. The bladder of the cuff should encircle 80% of the upper arm, and the middle of the cuff should be placed at the level of the right atrium. On a patient's first visit, the BP should be measured in both arms and the arm found to have the higher BP should be used on subsequent visits. For auscultatory readings, the cuff should be deflated at a rate of 2 mm Hg per second to optimize the ability of the provider to hear the Korotkoff sounds. SBP and DBP are defined by the pressure recorded at the first Korotkoff sound and the pressure at the disappearance of all sounds, respectively. For busy providers, this is an arduous process with the potential for many errors. Even when performed with the most precise method, in clinical practice BP measurement tends to be higher than ambulatory or home BP measurements [27, 28].

Automated office BP monitoring is an accepted technique. Current automated outpatient blood pressure (AOBP) devices take multiple readings with a single activation. The device provides an average of these readings. These data can be used with or without staff being present and with the patient in the examination room or waiting room. Studies have shown that results are comparable.

Ambulatory monitoring is often used to obtain BP readings at set intervals. This allows patients to go about their daily activities and provides estimates of mean BP over the entire period of monitoring. It can also identify daytime vs. nighttime pressures, early morning trends in BP and symptomatic hypertension, and estimate BP variability. Although this is generally accepted as the best out-of-hospital approach, home BP monitoring is often more convenient for the patient. Although similar to office techniques, auscultation is difficult, and a validated automated device is recommended [28].

6   Hypertension Categories

Conventional BP measurements in a clinical setting are often misleading. Obtaining accurate data usually requires measurements taken outside the clinic setting, such as by self-measurement at home or by 24-h ambulatory monitoring. The Italian Pressioni Arteriose Monitorate e Loro Associazioni (PAMELA) study compared office/clinic BP measurements, home BP, and 24-h ambulatory BP assessment. Clinic, home, and 24-hour ambulatory BP values were obtained in 2051 subjects between 25 and 74 years of age representative of the general population of Monza (near Milan), Italy. Subjects were followed up for an average of 131 months, during which time cardiovascular and non-cardiovascular fatal events were recorded ($n = 186$). Home BP predicted cardiovascular outcomes better than BP obtained in the clinical setting. Risk of all-cause death increased more with an increase in home or ambulatory BP vs. an increase in clinic BP. The highest correlation between change in BP and risk of death was seen with nighttime ambulatory BP [29].

The availability of ambulatory BP monitoring has facilitated categorization of BP levels. Categories include normotension (normal clinic and ambulatory BP), sustained hypertension (elevated clinic and ambulatory BP), masked hypertension (normal clinic but elevated ambulatory BP), and white-coat hypertension (elevated clinic BP but normal ambulatory BP). It is important to recognize that no matter which technique is used, two things remain clear. No single method has been shown to be either sufficiently sensitive or specific to initiate treatment, and no single method has clearly outperformed the other method. The clinician must use multiple BP values taken at different times, both in office and out of office, to confirm the diagnosis prior to starting treatment. Appropriate categorization is crucial for the treatment of BP as it has prognostic implications. A misdiagnosis of white-coat hypertension may lead to underestimation of the need for BP control and more aggressive treatment. However, not identifying masked hypertension may have consequences as masked hypertension carries a similar all-cause mortality and CVD risk as sustained hypertension. For this reason, the AHA/ACC 2017 guidelines recommended ambulatory BP monitoring or home BP monitoring for those suspected of having either white-coat hypertension or masked hypertension.

7   Future Directions

While many medical societies have offered opinions about and recommendations for optimum BP goals, it is the clinician who is most impacted by the treatment-risk paradox. Their concerns, for the most part, are rational in view of the adverse events found in SPRINT and observational studies. Exposure to moderate- or high-dose antihypertensive medication was associated with an increase in injuries from falls compared with no antihypertensive use [30]. Additionally, in predictive models based on the SPRINT patient population, a 10-year risk of CVD <18.2% led to greater harm of SAEs compared to potential benefit of reduced cardiovascular events, using a higher cutoff than the 10% used in current guidelines [23]. Nevertheless, aggressive treatment of hypertension appears to have significant benefit in lowering cardiovascular events in higher risk patient populations. From low- to high-risk, the same relative risk reduction (RRR) is seen. However, there is a greater absolute risk reduction (ARR) in populations with high underlying cardiovascular risk, because at higher levels of risk, many more untreated individuals will eventually have a cardiovascular event. If the same number of people are treated, many more cardiovascular events and deaths are prevented in higher risk populations than in lower risk populations. In a meta-analysis of BP-lowering trials, over ten times more cardiovascular events and deaths were prevented in the highest risk group, i.e., 5-year cardiovascular risk was >21% for the highest risk group vs. <11% for the lowest risk group [31, 32]. Future clinical cardiovascular outcome trials in hypertension will need to consider the underlying cardiovascular risk of their study populations. The AHA/ACC cutoff of 10-year risk of CVD of 10% is a good start but may inadvertently expose some to the risks of treatment without the benefits. New statistical methods may be applied to assess the impact of BP reductions on cardiovascular outcomes. Mediation analysis is a statistical method in which a quantifiable characteristic, referred to as a mediator, is assessed as a potential cause for a specific intervention leading to a specific outcome. For example, if a dietary intervention for lowering BP causes a reduction in salt intake and this dietary intervention leads eventually to lower BP, then salt intake would be a likely mediator in the effect of the proposed dietary intervention on lowering BP [33]. For the clinician managing hypertension in older patients with high cardiovascular risk, there are strategies to mitigate the risk of adverse events. These may include more frequent office visits to assess for orthostatic hypotension or check for electrolyte abnormalities or telehealth visits with home BP or ambulatory BP monitoring, to better assess BP, and thus move toward a more favorable benefit-to-risk ratio. Future clinical trials will need to better define the population risk level that would be best served by the proposed intervention.

References

1. The fourth report on the diagnosis, evaluation, and treatment of high blood pressure in children and adolescents. Pediatrics. 2004;114(2 Suppl 4th Report):555–76.
2. Hansen ML, Gunn PW, Kaelber DC. Underdiagnosis of hypertension in children and adolescents. JAMA. 2007;298(8):874–9. https://doi.org/10.1001/jama.298.8.874.
3. Flynn JT, Kaelber DC, Baker-Smith CM, et al. Clinical practice guideline for screening and management of high blood pressure in children and adolescents. Pediatrics. 2017;140(3) https://doi.org/10.1542/peds.2017-1904. Erratum in Pediatrics. 2017 Dec;140(6):e20173035. doi:10.1542/peds.2017-3035 and Pediatrics. 2018 Sep;142(3):e20181739. doi:10/1542/peds.2018-1739
4. Bell CS, Samuel JP, Samuels JA. Prevalence of hypertension in children. Hypertension. 2019;73(1):148–52. https://doi.org/10.1161/hypertensionaha.118.11673.
5. Theodore RF, Broadbent J, Nagin D, et al. Childhood to early-midlife systolic blood pressure trajectories: early-life predictors, effect modifiers, and adult cardiovascular outcomes. Hypertension. 2015;66(6):1108–15. https://doi.org/10.1161/hypertensionaha.115.05831.
6. Perng W, Rifas-Shiman SL, Kramer MS, et al. Early weight gain, linear growth, and mid-childhood blood pressure: a prospective study in project viva. Hypertension. 2016;67(2):301–8. https://doi.org/10.1161/hypertensionaha.115.06635.
7. Falkner B, Gidding SS, Ramirez-Garnica G, Wiltrout SA, West D, Rappaport EB. The relationship of body mass index and blood pressure in primary care pediatric patients. J Pediatr. 2006;148(2):195–200. https://doi.org/10.1016/j.jpeds.2005.10.030.
8. Chinali M, de Simone G, Roman MJ, et al. Cardiac markers of pre-clinical disease in adolescents with the metabolic syndrome: the strong heart study. J Am Coll Cardiol. 2008;52(11):932–8. https://doi.org/10.1016/j.jacc.2008.04.013.
9. Ostchega Y, Fryar CD, Nwankwo T, Nguyen DT. Hypertension prevalence among adults aged 18 and over: United States, 2017-2018. NCHS Data Brief. 2020;364:1–8.
10. America ASo, America AoLIMDo. Blood pressure study, 1939. Actuarial Society of America; 1940.
11. Kotchen TA. Historical trends and milestones in hypertension research: a model of the process of translational research. Hypertension. 2011;58(4):522–38. https://doi.org/10.1161/hypertensionaha.111.177766.
12. Prevention of stroke by antihypertensive drug treatment in older persons with isolated systolic hypertension. Final results of the systolic hypertension in the elderly program (SHEP). SHEP Cooperative Research Group. JAMA. 1991;265(24):3255–64.
13. Dahlöf B, Lindholm LH, Hansson L, Scherstén B, Ekbom T, Wester PO. Morbidity and mortality in the Swedish trial in old patients with hypertension (STOP-hypertension). Lancet. 1991;338(8778):1281–5. https://doi.org/10.1016/0140-6736(91)92589-t.
14. Kaplan NM. Systolic hypertension in the elderly program (SHEP) and Swedish trial in old patients with hypertension (STOP). The promises and the potential problems. Am J Hypertens. 1992;5(5 Pt 1):331–4. https://doi.org/10.1093/ajh/5.5.331.

15. Gueyffier F, Bulpitt C, Boissel JP, et al. Antihypertensive drugs in very old people: a subgroup meta-analysis of randomised controlled trials. INDANA Group. Lancet. 1999;353(9155):793–6. https://doi.org/10.1016/s0140-6736(98)08127-6.
16. Bulpitt CJ, Beckett NS, Cooke J, et al. Results of the pilot study for the hypertension in the very elderly trial. J Hypertens. 2003;21(12):2409–17. https://doi.org/10.1097/00004872-200312000-00030.
17. Beckett NS, Peters R, Fletcher AE, et al. Treatment of hypertension in patients 80 years of age or older. N Engl J Med. 2008;358(18):1887–98. https://doi.org/10.1056/NEJMoa0801369.
18. Ogihara T, Saruta T, Rakugi H, et al. Target blood pressure for treatment of isolated systolic hypertension in the elderly: valsartan in elderly isolated systolic hypertension study. Hypertension. 2010;56(2):196–202. https://doi.org/10.1161/hypertensionaha.109.146035.
19. Rakugi H, Ogihara T, Goto Y, Ishii M. Comparison of strict- and mild-blood pressure control in elderly hypertensive patients: a per-protocol analysis of JATOS. Hypertens Res. 2010;33(11):1124–8. https://doi.org/10.1038/hr.2010.144.
20. Cushman WC, Evans GW, Byington RP, et al. Effects of intensive blood-pressure control in type 2 diabetes mellitus. N Engl J Med. 2010;362(17):1575–85. https://doi.org/10.1056/NEJMoa1001286.
21. Bundy JD, Mills KT, Chen J, Li C, Greenland P, He J. Estimating the association of the 2017 and 2014 hypertension guidelines with cardiovascular events and deaths in US adults: an analysis of national data. JAMA Cardiol. 2018;3(7):572–81. https://doi.org/10.1001/jamacardio.2018.1240.
22. Diamond JA, Schussheim AE, Phillips RA. Another nudge to overcome the treatment-risk paradox in blood pressure management. J Am Coll Cardiol. 2021;77(16):1991–3. https://doi.org/10.1016/j.jacc.2021.03.230.
23. Phillips RA, Xu J, Peterson LE, Arnold RM, Diamond JA, Schussheim AE. Impact of cardiovascular risk on the relative benefit and harm of intensive treatment of hypertension. J Am Coll Cardiol. 2018;71(15):1601–10. https://doi.org/10.1016/j.jacc.2018.01.074.
24. Douros A, Tölle M, Ebert N, et al. Control of blood pressure and risk of mortality in a cohort of older adults: the Berlin initiative study. Eur Heart J. 2019;40(25):2021–8. https://doi.org/10.1093/eurheartj/ehz071.
25. Zhang W, Zhang S, Deng Y, et al. Trial of intensive blood-pressure control in older patients with hypertension. N Engl J Med. 2021;385(14):1268–79. https://doi.org/10.1056/NEJMoa2111437.
26. Jones DW, Appel LJ, Sheps SG, Roccella EJ, Lenfant C. Measuring blood pressure accurately: new and persistent challenges. JAMA. 2003;289(8):1027–30. https://doi.org/10.1001/jama.289.8.1027.
27. Handler J. The importance of accurate blood pressure measurement. Perm J. 2009;13(3):51–4. https://doi.org/10.7812/tpp/09-054.
28. Muntner P, Shimbo D, Carey RM, et al. Measurement of blood pressure in humans: a scientific statement from the American Heart Association. Hypertension. 2019;73(5):e35–66. https://doi.org/10.1161/hyp.0000000000000087.
29. Sega R, Facchetti R, Bombelli M, et al. Prognostic value of ambulatory and home blood pressures compared with office blood pressure in the general population: follow-up results from the Pressioni Arteriose Monitorate e Loro Associazioni (PAMELA) study. Circulation. 2005;111(14):1777–83. https://doi.org/10.1161/01.Cir.0000160923.04524.5b.
30. Tinetti ME, Han L, Lee DS, et al. Antihypertensive medications and serious fall injuries in a nationally representative sample of older adults. JAMA Intern Med. 2014;174(4):588–95. https://doi.org/10.1001/jamainternmed.2013.14764.
31. Muntner P, Whelton PK. Using predicted cardiovascular disease risk in conjunction with blood pressure to guide antihypertensive medication treatment. J Am Coll Cardiol. 2017;69(19):2446–56. https://doi.org/10.1016/j.jacc.2017.02.066.
32. Blood pressure-lowering treatment based on cardiovascular risk: a meta-analysis of individual patient data. Lancet. 2014;384(9943):591–8. https://doi.org/10.1016/s0140-6736(14)61212-5.

33. Lee H, Herbert RD, McAuley JH. Mediation analysis. JAMA. 2019;321(7):697–8. https://doi.org/10.1001/jama.2018.21973.
34. Chobanian AV, Bakris GL, Black HR, et al. Seventh report of the Joint National Committee on Prevention, Detection, Evaluation, and Treatment of High Blood Pressure. Hypertension. 2003;42(6):1206–52. https://doi.org/10.1161/01.HYP.0000107251.49515.c2.
35. Whelton PK, Carey RM, Aronow WS, et al. 2017 ACC/AHA/AAPA/ABC/ACPM/AGS/APhA/ASH/ASPC/NMA/PCNA guideline for the prevention, detection, evaluation, and management of high blood pressure in adults: a report of the American College of Cardiology/American Heart Association Task Force on Clinical Practice Guidelines. J Am Coll Cardiol. 2018;71(19):e127–248. https://doi.org/10.1016/j.jacc.2017.11.006.

Pharmacotherapy for Obesity: Recent Evolution and Implications for Cardiovascular Risk Reduction

Kevin C. Maki (iD), Carol F. Kirkpatrick (iD), David B. Allison (iD), and Kishore M. Gadde (iD)

Key Points

- Obesity is highly prevalent in the U.S. and is associated with an increased risk of major adverse cardiovascular events (MACE).
- Modalities for the management of patients with obesity include lifestyle intervention, pharmacotherapy, and bariatric surgery.
- Lifestyle interventions and older antiobesity pharmacotherapies have been associated with body weight reductions of <12% and no clear benefit to reduce MACE risk.
- Some older antiobesity pharmacotherapies had safety issues and are no longer available in the U.S. (fenfluramine, lorcaserin, sibutramine), which has contributed to hesitancy to prescribe available antiobesity pharmacotherapies.
- Bariatric surgery has been associated with significant weight reduction (20-30%), improvements in cardiometabolic risk factors, and a markedly reduced risk of MACE.
- Newer antiobesity pharmacotherapies that are available or in development (semaglutide, tirzepatide) have been associated with greater weight loss efficacy than older agents.

K. C. Maki (✉)
Midwest Biomedical Research, Addison, IL, USA

Midwest Biomedical Research, Bonita Springs, FL, USA

Indiana University School of Public Health-Bloomington, Bloomington, IN, USA
e-mail: kmaki@mbclinicalresearch.com

C. F. Kirkpatrick
Midwest Biomedical Research, Addison, IL, USA

Idaho State University, Pocatello, ID, USA

D. B. Allison
Indiana University School of Public Health-Bloomington, Bloomington, IN, USA

K. M. Gadde
University of California Irvine, Irvine, CA, USA

© The Author(s), under exclusive license to Springer Nature Switzerland AG 2024
K. C. Maki, D. P. Wilson (eds.), *Cardiovascular Outcomes Research*, Contemporary Cardiology, https://doi.org/10.1007/978-3-031-54960-1_13

- Trials are underway to assess the effects of semaglutide and tirzepatide on MACE risk in patients with obesity or overweight plus comorbidities.
- If trials with these newer agents demonstrate reduced MACE risk, this may usher in a new era for management of cardiovascular disease risk in patients with obesity.

1 Introduction

Obesity is common in the U.S., with NHANES data from 2017-2021 showing a prevalence of 41.9% of the population having a body mass index (BMI) of at least 30 kg/m^2 [1]. This represents a dramatic increase from a prevalence of 30.5% in the 1999-2000 NHANES survey [1]. The prevalence of obesity in the U.S. varies by group and is higher in non-Hispanic Black (49.9%) and Hispanic (45.6%) adults, compared to non-Hispanic White (41.4%) and Asian-American (16.1%) adults [1].

Obesity is associated with increased risks for several cardiometabolic diseases, notably coronary heart disease (CHD), stroke, and type 2 diabetes (T2D). In addition, obesity is a risk factor for hypertension, sleep apnea, heart failure, nonalcoholic fatty liver disease, and chronic kidney disease, as well as osteoarthritis and various types of cancer [2].

This narrative review provides an overview of antiobesity interventions and their impacts on cardiovascular (CV) risk and outcomes. The review begins by discussing the challenges related to lifestyle interventions and older antiobesity pharmacotherapies, which have been associated with reductions in body weight of <12% and no clear reduction in risk for major adverse cardiovascular events (MACE) in CV outcomes trials. In contrast, bariatric surgery has been associated with greater and more sustained loss of body weight (20–30%), as well as lower incidence of MACE. This leads to a discussion of newer antiobesity pharmacotherapies for which clinical trials have shown more pronounced weight loss (15–20%) when combined with lifestyle intervention, compared to older pharmacotherapies.

When discussing interventions for patients with overweight or obesity, it is important to understand the difference between efficacy and effectiveness. Efficacy refers to the results of an intervention provided in optimal conditions, such as in randomized controlled trials (RCTs), and effectiveness refers to results of an intervention provided in real-world conditions [3].

2 Lifestyle Intervention for Cardiometabolic Risk Reduction in Obesity

Although patients and healthcare professionals often desire a recommendation for a specific dietary intervention for obesity, the results of studies comparing diets have not demonstrated any one approach to be clearly superior, especially in the long term. Systematic reviews and meta-analyses have examined the effectiveness and efficacy of popular diet programs with a range of macronutrient contents (e.g., low-fat, low-carbohydrate, high-protein, ketogenic, time-restricted eating, intermittent fasting, etc.) on weight loss among adults with overweight or obesity. The results show minor differences regarding short-term (<6 months) weight loss [4–6]. Lower carbohydrate diets were associated with modestly greater weight loss compared to other diets over periods <6 months; however, there was little difference in weight change from baseline between the diets by 12 months [4, 5, 7]. More intensive interventions that include behavioral support and exercise, particularly a structured exercise program, appear to enhance weight loss when included with diet counseling [4, 8–11].

Multicomponent lifestyle intervention programs involving dietary modification, increased physical activity, stress management, and behavior modification strategies, such as coaching on problem solving, motivational interviewing, and behavioral contracts, are recommended for obesity management, but have shown limited results for reducing body weight and improving the cardiometabolic risk factor profile [10, 12]. Meta-analyses of such intervention programs have shown that a majority of participants fail to achieve 5% weight loss at 1 year [12, 13], and, although improvements are generally observed in the cardiometabolic risk factor profile, the magnitudes of these changes are modest [10, 14]. Significant attenuation of effects on body weight and cardiometabolic risk factors is generally observed with longer-term follow-up, particularly after the first year [10, 12]. Although further discussion about differences between categories of diets and lifestyle interventions on weight loss and cardiometabolic risk factors is beyond the scope of this review, readers may find additional details in meta-analyses and clinical practice guidelines [10, 14–16].

The effects of an intensive lifestyle intervention (ILI) on weight loss and improvements in cardiometabolic risk factors are illustrated by the results from the National Institutes of Health-sponsored Look Action for Health in Diabetes (Look AHEAD) trial, which compared an ILI program with general diabetes support and education (control) in patients with overweight or obesity and T2D. After a median follow-up of 9.6 years, the trial was stopped for futility because there was no reduction in the primary outcome of 4-point MACE (death from cardiovascular causes, nonfatal myocardial infarction, nonfatal stroke, and hospitalization for angina) in the ILI group compared with control (hazard ratio [HR]: 0.95, 95% confidence interval [CI] 0.83–1.09, $P = 0.51$). Results were similar for a key secondary outcome of 3-point MACE (HR: 0.93, 95% CI 0.79–1.10, $P = 0.42$) [9].

The ILI employed in Look AHEAD was more successful than most such interventions reported in the literature for inducing and maintaining weight loss. At 1 year, the ILI group had lost a mean of 8.6% of initial body weight compared to 0.7% in the control group [9]. Thus, the goal of achieving at least 7% weight loss with the ILI was achieved. At study end, weight loss was 6% of body weight in the ILI group vs. 3.5% in the control group. Improvements were observed in the ILI group, relative to the control group, in biomarkers of blood glucose metabolism, lipid control, and inflammation, as well as sleep apnea and liver fat. In addition, there were lower frequencies of depression, urinary incontinence, severe kidney disease, and sexual dysfunction in the ILI group, and there were reduced requirements for diabetes medications, greater maintenance of physical mobility, and improved quality of life [17]. Although ILI participants experienced improvements in cardiometabolic risk factors and other health outcomes, the benefit was primarily achieved in the first year of the study, and many of the differences between the ILI and control group did not retain statistical significance through the study end (9.6 years).

Thus, although Look AHEAD failed to demonstrate a reduction in CV events, several benefits were observed that support the use of lifestyle intervention as a cornerstone of obesity management. Also, it should be noted that obesity is typically a progressive condition, with further weight gain occurring over time. Thus, even if lifestyle interventions only arrest weight gain, that is a more favorable outcome than continued increases in body weight and adiposity [2, 15, 16].

3   Bariatric Surgery and Cardiovascular Risk

One possible explanation for the lack of significant reduction in MACE in Look AHEAD is that the degree of weight loss achieved may have been insufficient. Results from studies of the effects of bariatric surgery on CV outcomes support this hypothesis. Although RCTs of bariatric surgery are sparse, results have been published from several large cohort studies and are suggestive of substantial CV risk reduction with surgical interventions.

Bariatric surgery is associated with a mean weight loss of 20–30% of total body weight, with some variation between types of procedures [18–21]. Although some weight regain does occur, a majority of patients maintain significant weight loss following most common types of bariatric surgery (Roux-en-Y gastric bypass and sleeve gastrectomy) over follow-up periods of 5 years or more [18, 21]. For example, in one study of Roux-en-Y gastric bypass surgery, 70% of patients maintained a loss of at least 20% of initial body weight at year 12 [18].

Cardiometabolic risk factors improve after weight loss surgery and bariatric surgery is associated with markedly reduced incidence of new-onset T2D by more than 80% [22]. In addition, a substantial subset (25–45%) of bariatric surgery patients with diabetes presurgery are able to maintain acceptable glycemic control without hypoglycemic medications several years after the procedure [22, 23].

Mentias et al. recently published an analysis of results from a group of 94,885 Medicare beneficiaries who underwent bariatric surgery from 2013 to 2019 [24]. These individuals were matched with a control group for age, sex, BMI, and propensity score based on 87 clinical variables. Mean age and BMI at baseline were 62 years and 44.7 kg/m^2, respectively, and the sample was 70% female. After a median follow-up of 4 years, bariatric surgery was associated with significant reductions ($P < 0.001$) in myocardial infarction (37%), ischemic stroke (39%), heart failure (54%), and all-cause mortality (37%) compared to controls. Adams et al. conducted a retrospective study comparing participants with bariatric surgery

($n = 21,837$) to those without surgery ($n = 21,837$) matched for age, sex, BMI, and surgery date with follow-up extended up to 40 years [25]. The participants were mostly White and female (79%) with a mean age of ~42 years and BMI of ~46.0 kg/m^2. Bariatric surgery (Roux-en-Y gastric bypass, sleeve gastrectomy, adjustable gastric banding, and duodenal switch) was associated with a significantly reduced ($P < 0.001$) rate of death from CV disease (29%) compared to the non-surgery group. These results are consistent with those reported by van Veldhuisen and colleagues, who completed a systematic review and meta-analysis of data from 39 cohort studies [26] and a systematic review and meta-analysis by Wiggins and colleagues of 18 national or regional administrative database cohort studies [27].

4 Pharmacotherapy for Obesity and Cardiovascular Risk

Medications are well accepted in the management of some CV risk factors, such as hypercholesterolemia, hypertension, and diabetes mellitus. However, the use of weight loss medication for the management of obesity and cardiometabolic risk associated with obesity has been minimal because of hesitancy of clinicians to prescribe them, which may be due to concerns about safety and efficacy [28, 29] and/or provider bias and obesity stigmatization [2]. Although it is difficult to quantify, there is a view among some healthcare professionals that obesity is a lifestyle disease related to lack of discipline with eating and physical activity behaviors, which can result in reluctance to prescribe pharmacotherapy [2]. Other reasons for hesitancy to prescribe antiobesity pharmacotherapies include limited experience with available medications, lack of payer coverage, high out-of-pocket costs resulting in patients' inability to afford the therapy, and/or onerous prior authorization procedures [2, 28, 29]. Several antiobesity drugs have been removed from the market in the U.S. and elsewhere due to safety concerns, notably fenfluramine, which was associated with heart valve defects [30, 31]; lorcaserin because of a possible signal for increased risk of cancer [32]; sibutramine due to an increased risk of nonfatal myocardial infarction and nonfatal stroke based on results of the Sibutramine Cardiovascular OUTcomes (SCOUT) trial [33]; and rimonabant because of a higher rate of psychiatric adverse events compared to placebo [34]. Also, until recently, the efficacy of the available antiobesity medications has been modest, with lifestyle intervention plus medication producing average incremental weight loss of <10% of body weight at 1 year relative to lifestyle intervention plus placebo [31].

Five antiobesity pharmacotherapies—orlistat, phentermine/topiramate, naltrexone/bupropion, liraglutide, and semaglutide—are currently Food and Drug Administration (FDA)-approved in the U.S. for long-term (>12 weeks) weight management in patients with a BMI of $\geq$30 kg/m^2 or those with a BMI of at least 27 kg/m^2 with weight-related comorbidities. A summary of the indications and clinical effects of these medications is shown in Table 1.

The use of pharmacotherapy for the management of obesity has recently been evolving rapidly and some newer agents have shown greater efficacy in RCTs than

Table 1 Pharmacotherapies currently approved for short-term and long-term weight loss

Drug	Mechanism of action	Dosage[a]	Placebo-subtracted weight loss	Adverse events	Comments	References
Approved for short-term use (<12 weeks)[b]						
Phentermine	Sympathomimetic amine anorectic	15 mg, 30 mg, or 37.5 mg daily	7.5 mg dose: −3.8% 15 mg dose: −4.4%	Dry mouth, headache, constipation, insomnia	• Contraindications: history of CVD, MOA-i use, agitated states, history of drug abuse, hyperthyroidism, pregnancy or lactation, known hypersensitivity to sympathomimetic amines	[35, 36]
Approved for long-term use (>12 weeks)						
Orlistat (Xenical®)	Gastric and pancreatic lipase inhibitor	120 mg TID	−3.0%	Fecal urgency, fecal incontinence, flatus with discharge, and oily spotting	• Contraindications: pregnancy, chronic malabsorption syndrome, cholestasis, known hypersensitivity to orlistat or its components • Daily multivitamin supplement recommended	[37]
Phentermine/ topiramate ER	Phentermine: sympathomimetic amine anorectic Topiramate: precise mechanism of action unknown	Dose escalation: 3.75 mg/23 mg daily × 14 days, then ↑ to 7.5 mg/46 mg daily × 14 days; if needed, ↑ to 11.25 mg/69 mg × 14 days, then ↑ to 15 mg/92 mg	Obesity: 3.75 mg/23 mg dose: −3.5% 15 mg/92 mg dose: −9.4% Obesity + comorbidities: 7.5 mg/46 mg dose: −6.6% 15 mg/92 mg dose: −8.6 to −9.3%	Paresthesia, dizziness, dysgeusia, insomnia, constipation, and dry mouth	• Contraindications: pregnancy, glaucoma, hyperthyroidism, MOA-i use, known hypersensitivity to sympathomimetic amines • Negative pregnancy test required to start and continue due to increased risk of oral clefts • Monitor for depression, anxiety, and memory/language problems	[38]

Naltrexone/ bupropion ER	Naltrexone: opioid antagonist Bupropion: weak inhibitor of neuronal reuptake of dopamine and norepinephrine	8 mg/90 mg Dose escalation: Wk 1: 1 tablet QAM; 0 QHS Wk 2: 1 tablet QAM and QHS Wk 3: 2 tablets QAM, 1 tablet QHS Wk 4+: 2 tablets QAM and QHS	Obesity: 32/360 mg dose: −4.1% Obesity + T2D: 32/360 mg dose: −2.0%	Nausea, constipation, headache, vomiting, dizziness, insomnia, dry mouth, and diarrhea; neuropsychiatric AEs have been reported with smoking cessation	• Contraindications: uncontrolled HTN, seizure disorders, anorexia nervosa, or bulimia; chronic opioid use; abruptly stopping alcohol, benzodiazepines, barbiturates, or antiepileptic drugs.	[39]
Liraglutide 3.0 mg	GLP-1 receptor agonist	Dose escalation: Wk 1: 0.6 mg s.c. inj. daily; then ↑ 0.6 mg in weekly intervals to 3.0 mg daily	Obesity + comorbidities: −4.5% Obesity + T2D: −3.7%	Nausea, diarrhea, constipation, vomiting, injection site reactions, headache, hypoglycemia, dyspepsia, fatigue, dizziness, abdominal pain, increased lipase, upper abdominal pain, pyrexia, and gastroenteritis	• Contraindications: personal/ family history of medullary thyroid carcinoma or multiple endocrine neoplasia syndrome type 2, hypersensitivity to liraglutide or its components, or pregnancy.	[40]
Semaglutide 2.4 mg	GLP-1 receptor agonist	Dose escalation: 0.25 mg s.c. inj. weekly × 4 wks; then ↑ 0.25 mg in 4-wk intervals to 2.4 mg weekly	Obesity + comorbidities: −12.4% Obesity + T2D: −6.2%	Nausea, diarrhea, vomiting, constipation, abdominal pain, headache, fatigue, dyspepsia, dizziness, abdominal distension, eructation, hypoglycemia in T2D, flatulence, gastroenteritis, and GERD	• Contraindications: personal/ family history of medullary thyroid carcinoma or Multiple Endocrine Neoplasia syndrome type 2 or hypersensitivity to semaglutide or its components.	[41]

AEs adverse events, *CVD* cardiovascular disease, *ER* extended release, *GERD* gastroesophageal reflux disease, *GLP-1* glucagon-like peptide-1, *HTN* hypertension, *MOA-i* monoamine oxidase inhibitors, *QAM* every morning, *QHS* every evening, *s.c. inj.* subcutaneous injection, *T2D* type 2 diabetes, *TID* three times daily, *Wk* week

[a]Refer to the package insert for full prescribing information, including dosage adjustments for patients with renal and/or hepatic impairment and when to consider discontinuing the medication

[b]Three other drugs—diethylpropion, phendimetrazine, and benzphetamine—are also approved in the U.S. for short-term treatment of obesity and have a similar efficacy and adverse event profile as phentermine

was the case for older agents. Newer agents include incretin receptor agonists for glucagon-like peptide-1 (GLP-1) and dual GLP-1 and glucose-dependent insulino-tropic polypeptide (GIP). GLP-1 has insulinotropic and glucagonostatic effects, as well as slowing gastric emptying and affecting neural pathways that promote satiety and reduced food intake [42]. GIP stimulates glucose-dependent insulin secretion and has glucagonotropic effects in normo- and hypoglycemia but glucagonostatic effects in hyperglycemia [42]. Combining GLP-1 and GIP receptor agonists has additive effects for both insulin secretion and weight loss [42, 43].

The drug semaglutide, a GLP-1 receptor agonist, was approved initially for man-agement of glycemia in T2D, then later had its indication expanded for use in weight loss. When combined with lifestyle changes, 2.4 mg of semaglutide given as a sub-cutaneous injection weekly resulted in a mean weight loss of ~15% over 68 weeks, compared with weight loss of ~3% with placebo [44].

Similarly, the drug tirzepatide, a dual GLP-1 and GIP receptor agonist, has recently been approved as an adjunct to lifestyle for control of glycemia in T2D. However, results from a Phase 3 trial for the treatment of obesity have been published showing a dose-dependent reduction in body weight when combined with lifestyle modification [43]. Weekly subcutaneous injections of tirzepatide for 72 weeks reduced body weight by 15.0%, 19.5%, and 20.9% at 5, 10, and 15 mg doses, respectively, compared with a reduction of 3.1% with placebo. Notably, more than half of subjects assigned to the two higher doses of tirzepatide lost ≥20% of body weight, compared to 1.3% of those assigned to placebo.

Several agents in the GLP-1 receptor agonist class have been shown to both pro-mote weight loss and lower risk for MACE in T2D [31, 45]. However, at present, the degree to which the observed benefits can be attributed to weight loss vs. other effects of these medications is unclear. Also, benefits on CV event risk have not been demonstrated to date in patients with obesity who do not have T2D, although clinical trials are underway to assess the impact of both semaglutide (Semaglutide Effects on Heart Disease and Stroke in Patients with Overweight or Obesity [SELECT], NCT03574597) and tirzepatide (A Study of Tirzepatide [LY3298176] on the Reduction on Morbidity and Mortality in Adults with Obesity [SURMOUNT-MMO], NCT05556512) on MACE.

5 Efficacy and Effectiveness of Different Types of Weight Loss Interventions

Figure 1 summarizes the influences of different types of interventions on loss of body weight in patients with overweight or obesity. Lifestyle interventions that gen-erally include advice on consumption of an energy-restricted diet, increased physi-cal activity, and various behavioral strategies, including those employed in clinical trials of pharmacotherapies, have consistently been shown to produce reductions in body weight, although the magnitude is modest, and weight loss typically plateaus

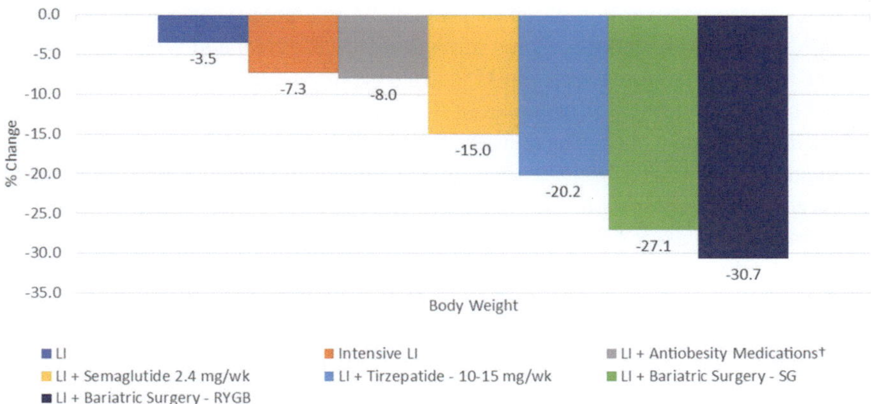

Fig. 1 Representative central tendencies for percent body weight changes for obesity interventions at 6–15 months* [11, 20, 41, 43, 50]. *Percent body weight change with interventions + background lifestyle intervention representative of results from multiple studies. †LI + Antiobesity Medications include orlistat, liraglutide, naltrexone/bupropion, and phentermine/topiramate. *LI* lifestyle interventions, *RYGB* Roux-en-Y gastric bypass, *SG* sleeve gastrectomy

after approximately 6 months. Also, a portion of the weight lost is generally regained in the subsequent 6–24 months [10, 46]. The intensity of the intervention is associated with mean weight change [10, 11, 16, 46]. In less intensive programs, mean weight loss is generally 2–4%, while with more intensive programs that include more in-person counseling sessions, supervised exercise, and behavioral support, mean weight loss has more often been in the range of 6–8% [2, 8–11, 15, 16, 47–49].

Other than semaglutide, when added to lifestyle interventions, antiobesity pharmacotherapies currently available in the U.S. have produced mean additional weight loss of 3–9% compared to placebo in RCTs, thus total weight loss in the active pharmacotherapy groups is typically 5–11% (Fig. 1). Pharmacotherapy extends the period before a weight loss plateau is reached and will often reduce, but not eliminate, weight regain during the second year of follow-up.

One challenge regarding interpretation of results from weight loss trials warrants comment. The control lifestyle intervention in many weight loss pharmacotherapy trials is more intensive than is typically employed in clinical practice. In a meta-analysis of 239 RCTs evaluating interventions for weight loss or prevention of weight regain, Dawson et al. found that, for each kg of weight loss in the control group, the treatment effect (difference in outcome between the active and control conditions) was reduced by 0.31 kg ($p < 0.001$) [51]. Thus, when a pharmacologic intervention is added to a more intensive background treatment, there is somewhat less additional effect than if the intervention was compared to a more modest intensity of background treatment. Therefore, the relatively small incremental effects on weight loss in some RCTs may lead clinicians to underestimate the likely effectiveness of the therapy in practice.

As discussed above, compared to previously available weight loss pharmacotherapies, lifestyle intervention plus semaglutide was associated with substantially greater weight reduction, averaging 15% at a dose of 2.4 mg/week. [44]. Tirzepatide (plus a lifestyle intervention) at doses of 5–10 mg/week was associated with weight reduction of ~20% [43]. These weight reductions, although larger than those obtained with older antiobesity agents, are somewhat smaller than those with bariatric surgery. For example, in the SLEEVEPASS RCT, weight reduction was 31% with Roux-en-Y gastric bypass and 27% with sleeve gastrectomy at the 1-year timepoint [20]. Clinical practice guidelines have been published that outline algorithms for the treatment of obesity, including initiating lifestyle interventions, as well as when to consider pharmacotherapy and bariatric surgery [15, 16].

6 Effects of Currently Approved Antiobesity Medications and Bariatric Surgery on Cardiometabolic Risk Factors

As shown in Table 2 and discussed previously, ILIs improve cardiometabolic risk factors. Regarding the effects of pharmacotherapies, all currently approved drugs for long-term weight management have been shown to reduce hemoglobin A1c

Table 2 Representative central tendencies for changes from baseline in cardiometabolic risk factors associated with obesity interventions[a]

Intervention	LDL-C % Δ[b]	TG % Δ[b]	HDL-C % Δ[b]	SBP Δ (mm Hg)[b]	HbA1c w/o T2D Δ (%)[b]	HbA1c with T2D Δ (%)[b]	References
Intensive lifestyle interventions[c]	−7.3	−3.9	4.4	−3.6	−0.1	−0.7	[8–10]
Orlistat 120 mg (1 y duration)	−4.0	1.3	9.3	−1.0	NR	−0.2	[37]
Phentermine/ topiramate ER 15 mg/92 mg (1 y duration)	−8.4	−5.2	3.5	−2.9	NR	−0.4	[38]
Naltrexone/ bupropion ER 32 mg/360 mg (56 wk duration)	−2.0	−11.6	8.0	−0.1	NR	−0.6	[39]
Liraglutide 3.0 mg s.c. inj. (56 wk duration)	−3.1	−13.0	2.3	−4.3	−0.3	−1.3	[40]

Table 2 (continued)

Intervention	LDL-C % Δ^b	TG % Δ^b	HDL-C % Δ^b	SBP Δ (mm Hg)^b	HbA1c w/o T2D Δ (%)^b	HbA1c with T2D Δ (%)^b	References
Semaglutide 2.4 mg s.c. inj. (68 wk duration)	−2.5	−21.9	5.2	−6.2	−0.4	−1.6	[41]
Tirzepatide 15 mg (72 wk duration)	−8.6	−31.4	8.2	−7.6	−0.5	−1.7	[43, 56]
Bariatric surgery—RYGB and SG^d (1–5 y follow-up)	RYGB: −17.4 SG: −6.3	−33.0	20.4	−12.9	−0.1	−2.9	[19, 23, 52, 54, 55]

Δ change, *ER* extended release, *HbA1c* hemoglobin A1c, *HDL-C* high-density lipoprotein cholesterol, *LDL-C* low-density lipoprotein cholesterol, *NR* not reported, *TG* triglyceride, *RYGB* Roux-en-Y gastric bypass, *SBP* systolic blood pressure, *s.c. inj.* subcutaneous injection, *SG* sleeve gastrectomy, *T2D* type 2 diabetes, *wk* week, *w/o* without, *y* year

[a]Changes from baseline for placebo were generally not clinically meaningful.

[b]Changes from baseline results are reported as means, least-squares means, medians, or approximate midpoints when only ranges were available.

[c]Percent change from baseline for LDL-C, TG, and HDL-C and change from baseline for SBP in lifestyle interventions reflect estimates calculated based on representative studies included in the meta-analysis by Schwingshackl et al. [10]. Change from baseline for HbA1c for participants without T2D reflect 1 y follow-up in the Diabetes Prevention Program [8]. Change from baseline for HbA1c for participants with T2D reflects 1 y follow-up in the Look AHEAD study [9].

[d]Values reported are central tendencies based on results from multiple studies. In general, changes in cardiometabolic risk factor values are slightly larger for RYGB than SG, except for LDL-C where the changes for RYGB have been substantially larger than with SG.

(HbA1c) in 1-year RCTs among adults with overweight or obesity and T2D. Other than orlistat, antiobesity drugs have not been tested specifically in patients with overweight/obesity and comorbid hypertension. Small improvements in systolic blood pressure generally occur with all approved antiobesity drugs, except naltrexone/bupropion, which is associated with small but significant placebo-adjusted increases in systolic and diastolic blood pressure. Most antiobesity drugs have been associated with a clinically significant reduction in serum triglycerides, a small reduction in low-density lipoprotein cholesterol, and a small increase in high-density lipoprotein cholesterol (Table 2). For bariatric surgery, Roux-en-Y gastric bypass results in improvements in all cardiometabolic risk factors at the 2-year follow-up [52], which is maintained at longer durations (5–10 years) and results have been similar for sleeve gastrectomy, although the effect of sleeve gastrectomy on low-density lipoprotein cholesterol is generally smaller than that observed with gastric bypass [19, 53–55] (Table 2).

7   Evidence for the Effects of Weight Loss Interventions on Incident Cardiovascular Outcomes and All-Cause Mortality

Table 3 summarizes results from key studies and meta-analyses that have evaluated the impacts of weight loss interventions on incident CV outcomes and all-cause mortality. Ma and colleagues investigated the effects of lifestyle interventions on weight loss, CV events, and mortality and found no significant reductions in MACE and CV mortality, although all-cause mortality was reduced by 18% (95% CI: 5% to 29%) [57]. In two of the larger lifestyle intervention trials, the Diabetes Prevention Program and Look AHEAD, no significant reductions were observed for MACE, heart failure, CV mortality, or all-cause mortality [9, 58].

Lorcaserin, naltrexone/bupropion, and sibutramine have been examined in studies designed to evaluate the effects of antiobesity pharmacotherapies on MACE as a primary outcome [59–61]. The results of the lorcaserin study showed no evidence of MACE benefit at study end (~2.8% more weight loss than with placebo, HR: 0.99, 95% CI 0.85–1.14) [59]. The naltrexone/bupropion study had similar results at both the 50% interim analysis (HR: 0.88, 95% CI 0.57–1.34) and final end-of-study analysis (HR: 0.95, 95% CI 0.65–1.38) (~2.5% more weight loss with naltrexone/bupropion than placebo) [60]. In the SCOUT CV outcomes trial with sibutramine, the primary outcome event was increased by 16% in the sibutramine group compared with the placebo group (~1.8% more weight loss with sibutramine than placebo, HR: 1.16; 95% CI 1.03–1.31) [61].

Study results for both liraglutide and semaglutide used as treatments for diabetes mellitus have demonstrated lower rates of MACE with these agents compared to placebo. A CV outcomes trial with a median follow-up of 3.8 years among patients with T2D demonstrated that liraglutide 1.8 mg was associated with a lower incidence of 3-point MACE compared to placebo (HR: 0.87, 95% CI 0.78–0.97) [62]. Although a CV outcome trial for liraglutide using the 3.0 mg dose for obesity treatment has not been conducted, a *post hoc* analysis of five RCTs from the weight management clinical development program examined the effect of liraglutide 3.0 mg on CV risk. The results demonstrated a nonsignificantly lower incidence of 3-point MACE for liraglutide 3.0 mg compared to either placebo or orlistat (HR: 0.42, 95% CI 0.17–1.08) [63].

Semaglutide has been investigated in two CV outcomes trials as a treatment for glycemic control in T2D, one with weekly subcutaneous injections of 0.5 or 1.0 mg [64] and another with an orally administered formulation (14 mg/day) [65]. The dosage used as an antiobesity agent is 2.4 mg/day as a weekly subcutaneous injection and a CV outcomes trial (SELECT) is underway with results expected to be available in September 2023. In the two CV outcomes trials published to date, MACE incidence was lower by 21–26%, although this only reached statistical significance with the injectable formulation [64, 65]. In contrast, CV and all-cause mortality were significantly reduced with the oral formulation (CV mortality by 51% [95% CI 8% to 73%], all-cause mortality by 49% [95% CI 16% to 69%]) [65].

Table 3 Cardiovascular disease outcomes associated with obesity or type 2 diabetes interventions that affect body weight compared to control interventions[a]

Treatment	Study population	Total participants/ no. studies	MACE[b] or MACE components ratio (95% CI)	Heart failure ratio (95% CI)	CV mortality ratio (95% CI)	All-cause mortality ratio (95% CI)	References
Lifestyle intervention							
Dietary/lifestyle interventions	Obese with or without IGT or T2D	30,206/54	0.93 (0.83, 1.04)	NR	0.93 (0.67, 1.31)	**0.82 (0.71, 0.95)**	[57]
Look AHEAD	BMI ≥25 + T2D	5145/1	0.93 (0.79, 1.10)	0.80 (0.61, 1.04)	0.88 (0.61, 1.29)	0.85 (0.69, 1.04)	[9]
Pharmacotherapy							
Lorcaserin[c]	Overweight or obese with or without CVD or CV risk	12,000/1	0.99 (0.85, 1.14)	0.95 (0.76, 1.20)	1.04 (0.78, 1.40)	1.08 (0.89, 1.31)	[59]
Naltrexone/ bupropion	Overweight or obese with CV risk	8910/1	0.95 (0.65, 1.38)	NR	0.61 (0.30, 1.27)	0.91 (0.55, 1.50)	[60]
Sibutramine[c]	Overweight or obese with CVD, T2D, or both	10,744/1	**1.16 (1.03, 1.31)**	NR	0.99 (0.82, 1.19)	1.04 (0.91, 1.20)	[61]
GLP-1 receptor agonists[d]	T2D with or without CVD	56,004/7	**0.87 (0.81, 0.93)**	0.93 (0.83, 1.04)	**0.88 (0.80, 0.96)**	**0.90 (0.82, 0.98)**	[45]
Liraglutide— Daily s.c. inj. (1.8 mg)	T2D + high risk for CVD	9340/1	**0.87 (0.78, 0.97)**	0.87 (0.73, 1.05)	**0.78 (0.66, 0.93)**	**0.85 (0.74, 0.97)**	[62]
Semaglutide— weekly s.c. inj. (0.5 or 1.0 mg)	T2D + high risk for CVD	3297/1	**0.74 (0.58, 0.95)**	1.11 (0.77, 1.61)	0.98 (0.65, 1.48)	1.05 (0.74, 1.50)	[64]

(continued)

Table 3 (continued)

Treatment	Study population	Total participants/ no. studies	MACE[b] or MACE components ratio (95% CI)	Heart failure ratio (95% CI)	CV mortality ratio (95% CI)	All-cause mortality ratio (95% CI)	References
Semaglutide— oral administration (14 mg)	T2D with or without CVD or with CV risk	3183/1	0.79 (0.57, 1.11)	0.86 (0.48, 1.55)	**0.49 (0.27, 0.92)**	**0.51 (0.31, 0.84)**	[65]
Tirzepatide (1 to 15 mg/wk)	T2D with or without CVD or with CV risk	7215/7	0.83 (0.58, 1.18)	0.67 (0.26, 1.70)	0.90 (0.50, 1.61)	0.80 (0.51, 1.25)	[66]
Bariatric surgery							
RYGB or SG in adults 18-80 y	Obese with or without T2D	893,044/39	**MI: 0.58 (0.43, 0.76)** **Stroke: 0.37 (0.17, 0.82)**	**0.50 (0.38, 0.66)**	**0.59 (0.47, 0.73)**	**0.55 (0.49, 0.62)**	[26]
Metabolic surgery[e] in adults 18-80 y	Obese with T2D	13,722/1	**0.62 (0.53, 0.72)**	**0.38 (0.30, 0.49)**	NR	**0.59 (0.48, 0.72)**	[67]

Note: Bold font indicates significance

BMI body mass index (kg/m^2), *CI* confidence interval, *CV* cardiovascular, *CVD* cardiovascular disease, *GLP-1* glucagon-like peptide-1, *IGT* impaired glucose intolerance, *Look AHEAD* Look Action for Health in Diabetes, *MACE* major adverse cardiovascular event, *MI* myocardial infarction, *No.* number, *NR* not reported, *RCT* randomized controlled trial, *RYGB* Roux-en-Y gastric bypass, *SG* sleeve gastrectomy, *s.c. inj.* subcutaneous injection, *T2D* type 2 diabetes, *wk* week, *y* year

[a]Effect size reported as hazard ratio, Mantel–Haenszel odds ratio, odds ratio, or risk ratio, and 95% confidence intervals.

[b]MACE defined as cardiovascular death, nonfatal myocardial infarction, or nonfatal stroke, except for the dietary interventions meta-analysis [57], which did not provide a specific definition, and the Aminian study, which defined the secondary outcome of 3-point MACE as all-cause mortality, myocardial infarction, and ischemic stroke [67].

[c]Lorcaserin and sibutramine have been removed from the market in the U.S. due to safety issues [32, 33].

[d]Meta-analysis included one RCT each for albiglutide, dulaglutide, exenatide long-acting release, liraglutide, lixisenatide, semaglutide, and oral semaglutide [45].

[e]Metabolic surgery is defined as "procedures that influence metabolism by inducing weight loss and altering gastrointestinal physiology" [67].

Since the trials only enrolled subjects with T2D and the injectable formulation was used at a lower dosage than is employed for obesity management, the generalizability of these findings to the use of semaglutide for obesity management is uncertain and firm conclusions will need to await results from the ongoing SELECT CV outcomes trial (NCT03574597).

Sattar and colleagues completed a prespecified meta-analysis of the effects of tirzepatide on CV outcomes in the development program for use as an agent to manage T2D [66]. The seven trials included were at least 26 weeks in duration, including a total of 7215 patients with T2D, and dosages of 1–15 mg/week were utilized, with follow-up periods ranging from 30 to 108 weeks. The primary outcome was a 4-point MACE composite (CV death, nonfatal myocardial infarction, nonfatal stroke, hospitalization for unstable angina). Compared to the control conditions, tirzepatide treatment was associated with a numerically lower, but nonstatistically significant, incidence of MACE and other outcomes (10–33%), which allowed a conclusion that the drug was not associated with increased CV risk, but no conclusions could be drawn regarding potential CV benefits [66]. A CV outcomes trial is underway comparing incidence of MACE in patients with T2D randomly assigned to treatment with tirzepatide or the GLP-1 receptor agonist dulaglutide (A Study of Tirzepatide [LY3298176] Compared with Dulaglutide on Major Cardiovascular Events in Participants with Type 2 Diabetes [SURPASS-CVOT], NCT04255433). Based on results from prior studies, tirzepatide is expected to induce greater weight loss than dulaglutide, so this trial, which is expected to be completed in late 2024, will provide additional evidence regarding the extent to which weight loss may contribute to CV risk reduction in T2D. The remainder of this paper will briefly review antiobesity pharmacotherapies in development and discuss important clinical questions that will require additional research.

SELECT Trial Results

As discussed in the original article upon which this chapter is based, the results of the Semaglutide Effects on Heart Disease and Stroke in Patients with Overweight or Obesity (SELECT, NCT03574597) were estimated to be available in the fall of 2023. The results were presented at the American Heart Association Scientific Sessions 2023 and simultaneously published [68] in November 2023.

In SELECT, 17,604 patients were randomized to receive either a once-weekly subcutaneous injection of semaglutide 2.4 mg (n = 8803) or placebo (n = 8801). Patients were eligible for the trial if they were ≥45 years of age, had a BMI ≥27 kg/m^2, and had preexisting CV disease defined as a previous myocardial infarction, stroke, or symptomatic peripheral arterial disease. Patients with preexisting diabetes were excluded from the trial. The mean (±standard deviation [SD]) age of the pooled patient population was 61.6 ± 8.9 years and were primarily male (72.3%) with a mean (±SD) BMI of 33.3 ± 5.0 kg/m^2. The majority of the patients were receiving evidence-based treatments for CV disease. The primary CV end point was a composite of death from CV causes, nonfatal myocardial infarction, or nonfatal stroke (3-point MACE) in a time-to-first-event analysis.

After ~40 months follow-up, there was a 20% reduced risk for the primary CV end point in the semaglutide group compared to the placebo group (hazard ratio: 0.80, 95% confidence interval: 0.72, 0.90, P < 0.001). The mean change in body weight 104 weeks after randomization was −9.4% in the semaglutide group and −0.9% in the placebo group. Serious adverse events were higher with placebo (33.4%) compared to semaglutide (36.4%); however, adverse events that resulted in discontinuation of the study product were more frequent with semaglutide (16.6%) compared to placebo (8.2%). Gastrointestinal disorders were the primary adverse event that led to discontinuation of semaglutide.

The results of SELECT are consistent with those from the Trial to Evaluate Cardiovascular and Other Long-term Outcomes with Semaglutide in Subjects with Type 2 Diabetes (SUSTAIN-6) in which semaglutide reduced the risk for 3-point MACE by 26% compared to placebo in patients with T2D who experienced a modest 4–5% body weight change and at a lower dose of semaglutide [64]. In both SELECT and SUSTAIN-6, it is difficult to estimate the degree to which the benefits are from weight loss vs. the pharmacological effects of semaglutide.

The SURMOUNT-MMO trial (NCT05556512) is underway and has a design similar to that of SELECT and should provide additional information about the effects of pharmacologically induced weight loss on CV risk. The purpose of the study is to investigate the impacts of tirzepatide treatment for weight loss on CV disease morbidity and total mortality in adults with overweight or obesity and known CV disease, who do not have diabetes. The trial has an estimated completion date of October 2027.

8　Drugs in Development for Obesity

8.1　*Tirzepatide*

Tirzepatide, the first dual agonist of GLP-1 and GIP receptors, received fast-track FDA approval for the treatment of T2D in May 2022 on the basis of a robust lowering of HbA1c by an average of 1.6% more than placebo with the 15 mg once-weekly subcutaneous dose in Phase 3 trials. The weight reduction achieved with the various doses of tirzepatide in a Phase 3 RCT was discussed previously (Sect. 4).

Tirzepatide treatment was associated with gastrointestinal adverse events, particularly nausea, which appears to be minimized by use of gradual dose titration, as has been the case for other agents with GLP-1 receptor agonist activity. Discontinuation rates due to adverse events for tirzepatide 5, 10, and 15 mg were 4.3%, 7.1%, and 6.2%, respectively, compared to 2.6% with placebo [43].

Tirzepatide is in late-stage clinical development for the treatment of obesity or overweight with weight-related comorbidities with additional Phase 3 trials to be completed soon. The U.S. FDA has granted fast-track designation to tirzepatide, which is intended to expedite the review of medicines to treat serious conditions and fill an unmet medical need [69]. Similar to GLP-1 receptor agonists, tirzepatide is contraindicated in patients with a personal or family history of medullary thyroid cancer or in patients with multiple endocrine neoplasia syndrome type 2 [56].

8.2 Cagrilintide and Cagrilintide/Semaglutide

Cagrilintide, a long-acting amylin analogue, administered as a once-weekly subcutaneous injection, achieved dose-dependent placebo-subtracted weight loss ranging from 3.0% to 7.8%, but without significant improvements in glycemia, blood pressure, or serum lipids, in a 26-week RCT in patients with overweight or obesity without diabetes [70, 71]. Clinical trials have also been completed to examine the effect of cagrilintide in combination with semaglutide for the management of obesity with or without T2D [72, 73]. A Phase 2 trial (NCT04982575) completed in July 2022 assessed the effects of a fixed dose of cagrilintide (2.4 mg) and semaglutide (2.4 mg), compared to either medication alone, on glycemic control (primary outcome) and change in body weight (secondary outcome) in participants with T2D and BMI $\geq$ 27.0 kg/m^2. Participants who received the cagrilintide + semaglutide achieved a larger body weight reduction (15.6%) compared to semaglutide (5.1%) or cagrilintide (8.1%) alone [73]. Phase 3 trials are now underway to investigate the efficacy and safety of a fixed dose combination of cagrilintide and semaglutide (CagriSema) in persons with obesity with or without T2D (REDEFINE 1, NCT05567796; REDEFINE 2, NCT05394519).

8.3 Cotadutide

In a Phase 2B trial examining the efficacy of various doses, cotadutide, a dual GLP-1 and glucagon receptor agonist administered daily by subcutaneous injection, led to a modest placebo-subtracted weight loss of 2.2–3.3% after 54 weeks in patients with overweight or obesity and T2D [74]. At the time of preparing this manuscript, ClinicalTrials.gov showed an ongoing clinical trial of cotadutide in nonalcoholic steatohepatitis (PROXYMO-ADV, NCT05364931), but no Phase 3 trials for the treatment of obesity or T2D.

8.4 Bimagrumab

In a small Phase 2 trial (75 randomized, 58 completed), an intravenous infusion of bimagrumab, a monoclonal antibody that blocks the activin type II receptor, administered once every 4 weeks was compared against placebo infusion for its effects on body composition and other metabolic outcomes in patients with overweight or obesity and T2D [75]. After 48 weeks, bimagrumab was associated with a placebo-subtracted weight loss of 5.7% along with significant loss of fat mass and gain of lean mass. HbA1c decreased by 0.8% relative to placebo. At the time of preparing this manuscript, ClinicalTrials.gov showed a new RCT (NCT05616013, estimated start date December 2022) to examine the effects of bimagrumab in combination with semaglutide for 48 weeks on waist circumference (primary outcome); however, no trials of bimagrumab monotherapy for the treatment of obesity or T2D were found in the registry.

9 Directions for Future Research

Continued research is needed on safety and effects of antiobesity drugs on CV disease and other outcomes in obesity. Given that obesity is a strong risk factor for adverse CV outcomes, and that bariatric surgery appears to markedly reduce CV risk based on the available evidence, albeit mostly from observational studies, it is reasonable to believe that weight loss pharmacotherapies might also reduce CV risk. However, this needs to be further investigated in prospective, randomized, outcomes trials, particularly in patients with obesity in the absence of T2D.

In recent years, there has been greater recognition that obesity is a chronic disease that requires long-term management, as is the case for other conditions that increase CV risk, such as hypertension, hypercholesterolemia, and T2D [76]. Adequately powered studies are needed that include a sufficient follow-up period to fully assess the effects of antiobesity pharmacotherapies on risk for MACE, as well as other outcomes, such as heart failure and renal disease.

Evidence of safety, efficacy, and effectiveness for weight loss and adverse disease outcomes, as well as cost-effectiveness, will be needed to support reimbursement by health insurers, particularly in light of prior experiences with therapies with safety issues as described in Sect. 4. To assess the overall cost-effectiveness of antiobesity pharmacotherapies, both RCTs and observational studies are needed to document the relationships between long-term use of antiobesity therapies with healthcare costs, including those for medications (for obesity and obesity-related conditions), provider visits, laboratory tests, and procedures to treat comorbidities (e.g., joint replacement, dialysis).

If ongoing RCTs of antiobesity agents show favorable results regarding CV event risk, these would ideally be followed by additional studies in high-risk subgroups, such as those with obesity plus other conditions (e.g., heart failure, resistant hypertension, and renal disease). It will also be of interest to assess the use of combinations of antiobesity agents. Concurrent use of multiple agents is commonly employed for the treatment of other chronic health conditions (e.g., hypertension, T2D) associated with increased CV risk, but this is rare in obesity management. More studies are needed to examine the safety and efficacy of combination antiobesity pharmacotherapy. Additionally, based on currently available evidence, it is reasonable to further investigate potential ancillary benefits of weight loss pharmacotherapy, such as improved quality of life and occupational productivity, as well as lowered risks for depression, incontinence, joint deterioration, and sexual dysfunction [2, 17].

10   Conclusions

Obesity is associated with increased CV risk and adverse changes in several risk factors for CV disease. To date, data from lifestyle intervention studies aimed at producing weight loss have not shown evidence to support a benefit for reducing incident CV events, despite improvements in cardiometabolic risk factors. Studies of bariatric surgery, albeit mostly observational, have shown substantially lower CV risk postsurgery, which supports the hypothesis that greater weight loss than produced by lifestyle interventions may lower CV risk.

Newer drug therapies for obesity, particularly semaglutide and tirzepatide, produce greater weight loss than previously studied pharmacotherapies, and ongoing CV outcomes trials with these agents will provide additional data on safety and efficacy for CV risk reduction in patients with obesity with and without T2D. However, it will still be challenging to determine the degree to which lower CV risk, if observed, is attributable to weight loss vs. other pharmacologic effects of these medications.

Prescribers and payers have been reluctant to employ and reimburse for weight loss medications outside of their use in diabetes management due, in part, to concerns about long-term safety and effectiveness in improving obesity-related disease outcomes. Safety issues with older antiobesity agents have likely contributed to these reservations. Ongoing CV outcomes trials with semaglutide and tirzepatide will provide valuable data regarding potential CV risk reduction in patients with obesity, both with and without T2D, that will inform decision makers about the role of these pharmacotherapies in clinical practice and their reimbursement.

Medications in early-stage development as antiobesity agents include cagrilintide (amylin analogue), cotadutide (GLP-1 and glucagon receptor agonist), and bimagrumab (monoclonal antibody that blocks the activin type II receptor). Thus, the armamentarium available for the management of obesity and its associated risks has evolved rapidly in recent years and may continue to do so.

11 Expert Opinion

Current practice for CV risk reduction in patients with obesity is lifestyle intervention for weight loss, combined with treatment of obesity-related cardiometabolic risk factors individually. Unlike other conditions associated with CV risk, such as dyslipidemia, hypertension, and T2D, use of medications to treat obesity is relatively rare. In part, this reflects concerns about long-term safety and weight loss efficacy, as well as lack of clear evidence of efficacy for CV risk reduction outside of use in the management of T2D. If ongoing outcomes trials demonstrate the efficacy of newer agents, such as semaglutide and tirzepatide, for reducing CV event risk, this will likely lead to expanded use in obesity management. However, even if ongoing trials demonstrate CV risk reduction, questions will remain regarding the role of weight loss per se vs. pharmacologic effects of the medications. Additional investigation will be needed on weight loss induced through other modalities, such as lifestyle intervention plus combinations of different classes of antiobesity medications, to address this question.

Another important issue is the impact of pharmacotherapy for obesity on healthcare costs. It is reasonable to hypothesize that effective weight loss pharmacotherapy might lower healthcare costs by reducing provider visits, hospitalizations, medical procedures (e.g., joint replacement, dialysis, revascularizations), and medications to treat comorbidities (e.g., T2D, dyslipidemia, hypertension, arthritis). Additional data from intervention trials with multiple years of follow-up, as well as observational research, will be needed to allow more definitive inferences regarding cost-effectiveness.

The prevalence of obesity has risen dramatically in the decades since the 1960s from approximately 14% of the population to greater than 40% today [1]. More than 90% of men and women in the U.S. show an upward body weight trajectory from early adulthood to middle age, with average annual weight gain exceeding 0.5 kg [77]. Those with early and/or rapid weight gain are at increased risk for development of obesity, more severe obesity, and obesity-associated comorbidities [77].

The use of weight loss medications in preventing obesity and obesity-associated conditions remains relatively unexplored. It is common to employ pharmacotherapy to treat elevations in blood pressure, cholesterol, and glucose in middle-aged or even younger adults, with the aim of reducing CV risk later in life. Excessive weight gain is implicated in the etiology of these conditions and other metabolic disturbances associated with CV risk [2]. Therefore, it is reasonable to speculate that early pharmacologic intervention as an adjunct to lifestyle to prevent or reduce additional weight gain in those with high-risk weight trajectories might be an effective strategy for CV risk reduction. Recent advances in noninvasive imaging (e.g., coronary computed tomographic angiography) that allow quantification of the degree and rate of progression of atherosclerosis will likely be helpful in such investigations, as this will allow tracking of subclinical atherosclerotic disease [78]. Evidence of reduced appearance and/or progression of subclinical atherosclerosis would provide a strong rationale for larger-scale RCTs to assess the efficacy for the reduction of CV risk.

Funding This paper was not funded.

Financial and Competing Interests Disclosure During the last 24 months, KCM has received research funding and/or consulting fees from Eli Lilly and Co.; Novo Nordisk; 89Bio; New Amsterdam Pharmaceuticals; Acasti Pharmaceuticals; Beren Therapeutics; Matinas Biopharma; North Sea Therapeutics; General Mills; National Dairy Council; Hass Avocado Board; Pharmavite; Campbell's; National Cattleman's Beef Association/Beef Checkoff; Greenyn Biotechnology; Naturmega; Indiana University Foundation; Bragg Live Products; Cargill; Medifast; NeuroEnergy Ventures; PepsiCo; Seed, Inc.

CFK is an employee of Midwest Biomedical Research and has no additional conflicts of interest to report beyond those disclosed for KCM.

During the last 24 months, DBA has received personal payments or promises for same from Alkermes, Inc.; Amin Talati Wasserman for KSF Acquisition Corp (Glanbia); Big Sky Health, Inc.; Clark Hill, PLC; Kaleido Biosciences; Law Offices of Ronald Marron; Medpace/Gelesis; Novo Nordisk Fonden; Sports Research Corp; and Tomasik, Kostin, and Kasserman.

DBA's institution, Indiana University, and the Indiana University Foundation have received funds or donations to support his research or educational activities from: Alliance for Potato Research and Education; American Egg Board; Arnold Ventures; Eli Lilly and Company; Mars, Inc.; National Cattlemen's Beef Association; Pfizer, Inc.; Soleno Therapeutics; USDA; WW (formerly Weight Watchers); and numerous other for-profit and non-profit organizations to support the work of the School of Public Health and the university more broadly.

During the last 24 months, KMG has received grant support from AstraZeneca, BioKier, Indiana University Foundation, and the National Institutes of Health.

The authors have no other relevant affiliations or financial involvement with any organization or entity with a financial interest in or financial conflict with the subject matter or materials discussed in the manuscript apart from those disclosed.

References

1. Centers for Disease Control and Prevention. Adult obesity facts [internet]. Atlanta, GA: Centers for Disease Control and Prevention, U.S. Department of Health and Human Services; 2022. [Cited 2022 Dec 10]. Available from: https://www.cdc.gov/obesity/data/adult.html

2. Bray GA, Heisel WE, Afshin A, et al. The science of obesity management: an Endocrine Society Scientific Statement. Endocr Rev. 2018;39(2):79–132.

3. Gottfredson DC, Cook TD, Gardner FE, et al. Standards of evidence for efficacy, effectiveness, and scale-up research in prevention science: next generation. Prev Sci. 2015;16(7):893–926.

4. Johnston BC, Kanters S, Bandayrel K, et al. Comparison of weight loss among named diet programs in overweight and obese adults: a meta-analysis. JAMA. 2014;312(9):923–33.

5. Ge L, Sadeghirad B, Ball GDC, et al. Comparison of dietary macronutrient patterns of 14 popular named dietary programmes for weight and cardiovascular risk factor reduction in adults: systematic review and network meta-analysis of randomised trials. BMJ. 2020;369:m696.

6. Schwingshackl L, Zähringer J, Nitschke K, et al. Impact of intermittent energy restriction on anthropometric outcomes and intermediate disease markers in patients with overweight and obesity: systematic review and meta-analyses. Crit Rev Food Sci Nutr. 2021;61(8):1293–304.

7. Anton SD, Hida A, Heekin K, et al. Effects of popular diets without specific calorie targets on weight loss outcomes: systematic review of findings from clinical trials. Nutrients. 2017;9(8):822.

8. Knowler WC, Barrett-Connor E, Fowler SE, et al. Reduction in the incidence of type 2 diabetes with lifestyle intervention or metformin. N Engl J Med. 2002;346(6):393–403.

9. Look AHEAD Research Group, Wing RR, Bolin P, et al. Cardiovascular effects of intensive lifestyle intervention in type 2 diabetes. N Engl J Med. 2013;369(2):145–54. Erratum in: N Engl J Med. 2014;370(19):1866.

10. Schwingshackl L, Dias S, Hoffmann G. Impact of long-term lifestyle programmes on weight loss and cardiovascular risk factors in overweight/obese participants: a systematic review and network meta-analysis. Syst Rev. 2014;3:130.
11. LeBlanc ES, Patnode CD, Webber EM, et al. Behavioral and pharmacotherapy weight loss interventions to prevent obesity-related morbidity and mortality in adults: updated evidence report and systematic review for the US Preventive Services Task Force. JAMA. 2018;320(11):1172–91.
12. Madigan CD, Graham HE, Sturgiss E, et al. Effectiveness of weight management interventions for adults delivered in primary care: systematic review and meta-analysis of randomised controlled trials. BMJ. 2022;377:e069719.
13. Khera R, Murad MH, Chandar AK, et al. Association of pharmacological treatments for obesity with weight loss and adverse events: a systematic review and meta-analysis. JAMA. 2016;315(22):2424–34.
14. Sisti LG, Dajko M, Campanella P, Shkurti E, Ricciardi W, de Waure C. The effect of multifactorial lifestyle interventions on cardiovascular risk factors: a systematic review and meta-analysis of trials conducted in the general population and high risk groups. Prev Med. 2018;109:82–97.
15. Garvey WT, Mechanick JI, Brett EM, et al. American Association of Clinical Endocrinologists and American College of Endocrinology Comprehensive Clinical Practice Guidelines for Medical Care of Patients with Obesity. Endocr Pract. 2016;(Suppl 3):1–203.
16. Jensen MD, Ryan DH, Apovian CM, et al. 2013 AHA/ACC/TOS guideline for the management of overweight and obesity in adults: a report of the American College of Cardiology/ American Heart Association Task Force on Practice Guidelines and The Obesity Society. Circulation. 2014;129(25 Suppl 2):S102–S38. Erratum in: Circulation. 2014;129(25 Suppl 2):S139-40.
17. Pi-Sunyer X. The look AHEAD trial: a review and discussion of its outcomes. Curr Nutr Rep. 2014;3(4):387–91.
18. Adams TD, Davidson LE, Litwin SE, et al. Weight and metabolic outcomes 12 years after gastric bypass. N Engl J Med. 2017;377:1143–55.
19. Peterli R, Wölnerhanssen BK, Peters T, et al. Effect of laparoscopic sleeve gastrectomy vs laparoscopic Roux-en-Y gastric bypass on weight loss in patients with morbid obesity: the SM-BOSS randomized clinical trial. JAMA. 2018;319(3):255–65.
20. Salminen P, Grönroos S, Helmiö M, et al. Effect of laparoscopic sleeve gastrectomy vs Roux-en-Y gastric bypass on weight loss, comorbidities, and reflux at 10 years in adult patients with obesity: the SLEEVEPASS randomized clinical trial. JAMA Surg. 2022;157(8):656–66.
21. Sjöström L. Review of the key results from the Swedish Obese Subjects (SOS) trial—a prospective controlled intervention study of bariatric surgery. J Intern Med. 2013;273(3):219–34.
22. Bailly L, Schiavo L, Sebastianelli L, et al. Preventive effect of bariatric surgery on type 2 diabetes onset in morbidly obese inpatients: a national French survey between 2008 and 2016 on 328,509 morbidly obese patients. Surg Obes Relat Dis. 2019;15(3):478–87.
23. Schauer PR, Bhatt DL, Kirwan JP, et al. Bariatric surgery versus intensive medical therapy for diabetes—5-year outcomes. N Engl J Med. 2017;376(7):641–51.
24. Mentias A, Aminian A, Youssef D, et al. Long-term cardiovascular outcomes after bariatric surgery in the Medicare population. J Am Coll Cardiol. 2022;79(15):1429–37.
25. Adams TD, Meeks H, Fraser A, Davidson LE, Holmen J, Newman M, et al. Long-term all-cause and cause-specific mortality for four bariatric surgery procedures. Obesity (Silver Spring). 2023;31(2):574–85.
26. van Veldhuisen SL, Gorter TM, van Woerden G, et al. Bariatric surgery and cardiovascular disease: a systematic review and meta-analysis. Eur Heart J. 2022;43(20):1955–69.
27. Wiggins T, Guidozzi N, Welbourn R, Ahmed AR, Markar SR. Association of bariatric surgery with all-cause mortality and incidence of obesity-related disease at a population level: a systematic review and meta-analysis. PLoS Med. 2020;17(7):e1003206.
28. U.S. Government Accountability Office. Obesity drugs: few adults used prescription drugs for weight loss and insurance coverage varied GAO-19-577, Aug 2019. [Cited 2022 Dec 11]. Available from: https://www.gao.gov/products/GAO-19-577

29. Gadde KM, Atkins KD. The limits and challenges of antiobesity pharmacotherapy. Expert Opin Pharmacother. 2020;21(11):1319–28.
30. Gardin JM, Schumacher D, Constantine G, et al. Valvular abnormalities and cardiovascular status following exposure to dexfenfluramine or phentermine/fenfluramine. JAMA. 2000;283(13):1703–9.
31. Capristo E, Maione A, Lucisano G, et al. Effects of weight loss medications on mortality and cardiovascular events: a systematic review of randomized controlled trials in adults with overweight and obesity. Nutr Metab Cardiovasc Dis. 2021;31(9):2587–95.
32. U.S. Food and Drug Administration. FDA requests the withdrawal of the weight-loss drug Belviq, Belviq XR (lorcaserin) from the market. Potential risk of cancer outweighs the benefits [internet]. Silver Spring, MD: U.S. Food and Drug Administration, U.S. Department of Health and Human Services; 2020. [Cited 2023 Jan 4]. Available from: https://www.fda.gov/drugs/drug-safety-and-availability/fda-requests-withdrawal-weight-loss-drug-belviq-belviq-xr-lorcaserin-market
33. U.S. Food and Drug Administration. FDA Drug Safety Communication: FDA recommends against the continued use of Meridia (sibutramine) [internet]. Silver Spring, MD: U.S. Food and Drug Administration, U.S. Department of Health and Human Services; 2010. [Cited 2023 Jan 4]. Available from: https://www.fda.gov/drugs/drug-safety-and-availability/fda-drug-safety-communication-fda-recommends-against-continued-use-meridia-sibutramine
34. Sam AH, Salem V, Ghatei MA. Rimonabant: from RIO to ban. J Obes. 2011;2011:432607.
35. ADIPEX-P® (phentermine hydrochloride) [package insert]. Parsippany, NJ: Teva Pharmaceuticals USA; 2020. Available from: https://www.adipex.com/globalassets/adipex/adipex_pi.pdf.
36. Aronne LJ, Wadden TA, Peterson C, et al. Evaluation of phentermine and topiramate versus phentermine/topiramate extended-release in obese adults. Obesity (Silver Spring). 2013;21(11):2163–71.
37. XENICAL® (orlistat) [package insert]. Montgomery, AL: H2-Pharma, LLC; 2017. Available from: https://xenical.com/pdf/PI_Xenical-brand_FINAL.PDF.
38. QSYMIA® (phentermine and topiramate) [package insert]. Campbell, CA: VIVUS, LLC; 2022. Available from: https://qsymia.com/patient/include/media/pdf/prescribing-information.pdf?v=0422.
39. CONTRAVE® (naltrexone hydrochloride and bupropion hydrochloride) [package insert]. Brentwood, TN: Nalpropion Pharmaceuticals, LLC; 2021. Available from: https://www.contravehcp.com/wp-content/uploads/Contrave_PI.pdf.
40. SAXENDA® (liraglutide) [package insert]. Plainsboro, NJ: Novo Nordisk, Inc.; 2022. Available from: https://www.novo-pi.com/saxenda.pdf.
41. WEGOVY® (semaglutide) [package insert]. Plainsboro, NJ: Novo Nordisk, Inc.; 2022. Available from: https://www.novo-pi.com/wegovy.pdf.
42. Min T, Bain SC. The role of Tirzepatide, dual GIP and GLP-1 receptor agonist, in the management of Type 2 diabetes: the SURPASS clinical trials. Diabetes Ther. 2021;12(1):143–57.
43. Jastreboff AM, Aronne LJ, Ahmad NN, et al. Tirzepatide once weekly for the treatment of obesity. N Engl J Med. 2022;387(3):205–16.
44. Wilding JPH, Batterham RL, Calanna S, et al. Once-weekly semaglutide in adults with overweight or obesity. N Engl J Med. 2021;384(11):989–1002.
45. Mannucci E, Dicembrini I, Nreu B, et al. Glucagon-like peptide-1 receptor agonists and cardiovascular outcomes in patients with and without prior cardiovascular events: an updated meta-analysis and subgroup analysis of randomized controlled trials. Diabetes Obes Metab. 2020;22(2):203–11.
46. Flore G, Preti A, Carta MG, et al. Weight maintenance after dietary weight loss: systematic review and meta-analysis on the effectiveness of behavioural intensive intervention. Nutrients. 2022;14(6):1259.
47. Wadden TA, Berkowitz RI, Womble LG, et al. Randomized trial of lifestyle modification and pharmacotherapy for obesity. N Engl J Med. 2005;353(20):2111–20.

48. Allison DB, Bier DM, Locher JL. Measurement rigor is not a substitute for design rigor in causal inference: increased physical activity does cause (modest) weight loss. Int J Obes. 2023;47(1):3–4.

49. Pontzer H. Exercise is essential for health but a poor tool for weight loss: a reply to Allison and colleagues. Int J Obes. 2023;47(2):98–9.

50. He K, Guo Q, Zhang H, et al. Once-weekly semaglutide for obesity or overweight: a systematic review and meta-analysis. Diabetes Obes Metab. 2022;24(4):722–6.

51. Dawson JA, Kaiser KA, Affuso O, et al. Rigorous control conditions diminish treatment effects in weight loss-randomized controlled trials. Int J Obes. 2016;40(6):895–8.

52. Adams TD, Pendleton RC, Strong MB, et al. Health outcomes of gastric bypass patients compared to nonsurgical, nonintervened severely obese. Obesity (Silver Spring). 2010;18(1):121–30.

53. Adams TD, Davidson LE, Litwin SE, et al. Health benefits of gastric bypass surgery after 6 years. JAMA. 2012;308(11):1122–31.

54. Salminen P, Helmiö M, Ovaska J, et al. Effect of laparoscopic sleeve gastrectomy vs laparoscopic Roux-en-Y gastric bypass on weight loss at 5 years among patients with morbid obesity: the SLEEVEPASS randomized clinical trial. JAMA. 2018;319(3):241–54.

55. Heffron SP, Parikh A, Volodarskiy A, et al. Changes in lipid profile of obese patients following contemporary bariatric surgery: a meta-analysis. Am J Med. 2016;129(9):952–9.

56. MOUNJARO™ (tirzepatide) [package insert]. Indianapolis, IN: Lilly USA, LLC; 2022. Available from: https://uspl.lilly.com/mounjaro/mounjaro.html?s=pi.

57. Ma C, Avenell A, Bolland M, et al. Effects of weight loss interventions for adults who are obese on mortality, cardiovascular disease, and cancer: systematic review and meta-analysis. BMJ. 2017;359:j4849.

58. Goldberg RB, Orchard TJ, Crandall JP, et al. Effects of long-term metformin and lifestyle interventions on cardiovascular events in the Diabetes Prevention Program and its outcome study. Circulation. 2022;145(22):1632–41.

59. Bohula EA, Wiviott SD, McGuire DK, et al. Cardiovascular safety of lorcaserin in overweight or obese patients. N Engl J Med. 2018;379(12):1107–17.

60. Nissen SE, Wolski KE, Prcela L, et al. Effect of naltrexone-bupropion on major adverse cardiovascular events in overweight and obese patients with cardiovascular risk factors: a randomized clinical trial. JAMA. 2016;315(10):990–1004.

61. James WP, Caterson ID, Coutinho W, et al. Effect of sibutramine on cardiovascular outcomes in overweight and obese subjects. N Engl J Med. 2010;363(10):905–17.

62. Marso SP, Daniels GH, Brown-Frandsen K, et al. Liraglutide and cardiovascular outcomes in type 2 diabetes. N Engl J Med. 2016;375(4):311–22.

63. Davies MJ, Aronne LJ, Caterson ID, et al. Liraglutide and cardiovascular outcomes in adults with overweight or obesity: a post hoc analysis from SCALE randomized controlled trials. Diabetes Obes Metab. 2018;20(3):734–9.

64. Marso SP, Bain SC, Consoli A, et al. Semaglutide and cardiovascular outcomes in patients with type 2 diabetes. N Engl J Med. 2016;375(19):1834–44.

65. Husain M, Birkenfeld AL, Donsmark M, et al. Oral semaglutide and cardiovascular outcomes in patients with type 2 diabetes. N Engl J Med. 2019;381(9):841–51.

66. Sattar N, McGuire DK, Pavo I, et al. Tirzepatide cardiovascular event risk assessment: a prespecified meta-analysis. Nat Med. 2022;28(3):591–8.

67. Aminian A, Zajichek A, Arterburn DE, et al. Association of metabolic surgery with major adverse cardiovascular outcomes in patients with type 2 diabetes and obesity. JAMA. 2019;322(13):1271–82.

68. Lincoff AM, Brown-Frandsen K, Colhoun HM, et al. Semaglutide and cardiovascular outcomes in obesity without diabetes. N Engl J Med. 2023;389(24):2221–32.

69. Lilly. News release—Lilly receives U.S. FDA Fast Track designation for tirzepatide for the treatment of adults with obesity, or overweight with weight-related comorbidities [internet]. Indianapolis, IN: Lilly USA, LLC; 2022. [Cited 2023 Jan 6]. Available from:

https://investor.lilly.com/news-releases/news-release-details/lilly-receives-us-fda-fast-track-designation-tirzepatide
70. Lau DCW, Erichsen L, Francisco AM, et al. Once-weekly cagrilintide for weight management in people with overweight and obesity: a multicentre, randomised, double-blind, placebo-controlled and active-controlled, dose-finding phase 2 trial. Lancet. 2021;398(10317):2160–72.
71. Gadde KM, Allison DB. Long-acting amylin analogue for weight reduction. Lancet. 2021;398(10317):2132–4.
72. Enebo LB, Berthelsen KK, Kankam M, et al. Safety, tolerability, pharmacokinetics, and pharmacodynamics of concomitant administration of multiple doses of cagrilintide with semaglutide 2·4 mg for weight management: a randomised, controlled, phase 1b trial. Lancet. 2021;397(10286):1736–48.
73. Novo Nordisk. Company announcement. Novo Nordisk successfully completes phase 2 trial with CagriSema in people with type 2 diabetes [internet]. Bagsværd, Denmark: Novo Nordisk A/S; 2022. [Cited 2023 April 25]. Available from: https://www.novonordisk.com/news-and-media/news-and-ir-materials/news-details.html?id=131155
74. Nahra R, Wang T, Gadde KM, et al. Effects of cotadutide on metabolic and hepatic parameters in adults with overweight or obesity and type 2 diabetes: a 54-week randomized phase 2b study. Diabetes Care. 2021;44(6):1433–42.
75. Heymsfield SB, Coleman LA, Miller R, et al. Effect of bimagrumab vs placebo on body fat mass among adults with type 2 diabetes and obesity: a phase 2 randomized clinical trial. JAMA Netw Open. 2021;4(1):e2033457.
76. Perdomo CM, Cohen RV, Sumithran P, et al. Contemporary medical, device, and surgical therapies for obesity in adults. Lancet. 2023;401(10382):1116–30.
77. Malhotra R, Ostbye T, Riley CM, et al. Young adult weight trajectories through midlife by body mass category. Obesity (Silver Spring). 2013;21(9):1923–34. Erratum in: Obesity (Silver Spring). 2014;22(7):1770
78. Gu H, Lu B, Gao Y, et al. Prognostic value of atherosclerosis progression for prediction of cardiovascular events in patients with nonobstructive coronary artery disease. Acad Radiol. 2021;28(7):980–7.

Cardiovascular Disease Risk and Risk Reduction Strategies in Diabetes Mellitus

Don P. Wilson, Luke Hamilton, and Kevin C. Maki

Key Points
- The prevalence of diabetes has increased dramatically in recent years, primarily type 2 diabetes (T2D), and has paralleled the increases in prevalence of overweight and obesity.
- Diabetes is an independent risk factor for atherosclerotic cardiovascular disease (ASCVD), accounting for approximately 70% of all mortality in individuals with diabetes.
- The relative risk of cardiovascular (CV) mortality for individuals with diabetes is 2–3-fold higher for men and 3–4-fold higher for women, compared to those without diabetes.
- Improved glycemic control in T2D reduces the risk of microvascular disease; treatment of other CV risk factors appears to be more effective in preventing macrovascular disease than treatment of hyperglycemia.
- Numerous studies have shown the efficacy of controlling individual risk factors in preventing or slowing ASCVD in individuals with diabetes, particularly when they are addressed simultaneously.
- For prevention and optimum management of both ASCVD and heart failure, risk factors should be systematically assessed at least annually in all individuals with diabetes, including children.

D. P. Wilson
Pediatric Endocrinology and Diabetes, Cook Children's Medical Center, Fort Worth, TX, USA

L. Hamilton
Research Data Science & Analytics, Cook Children's Health Care System, Fort Worth, TX, USA

K. C. Maki (✉)
Midwest Biomedical Research, Addison, IL, USA
e-mail: kmaki@mbclinicalresearch.com

© The Author(s), under exclusive license to Springer Nature Switzerland AG 2024
K. C. Maki, D. P. Wilson (eds.), *Cardiovascular Outcomes Research*, Contemporary Cardiology, https://doi.org/10.1007/978-3-031-54960-1_14

- Most of the evidence supporting interventions to reduce CV risk in diabetes comes from trials of individuals with T2D, while randomized controlled trials designed to assess risk reduction strategies in type 1 diabetes are lacking.
- Concurrent evidence-based approaches to the management of glycemia, blood pressure, and lipids, and the incorporation of specific therapies with CV and kidney outcomes benefit, are fundamental components of global risk reduction in diabetes.
- In addition to traditional, guideline-based preventive medical therapies, individuals with T2D with/or at high risk for ASCVD, heart failure, or chronic kidney disease should be treated with a sodium glucose cotransporter 2 inhibitor and/or a glucagon-like peptide-1 receptor agonist as part of the comprehensive approach to CV and kidney risk reduction.
- Healthcare professionals who provide care to adults and children with diabetes should be aware of the strong clinical evidence regarding therapies with a demonstrated ability to lower CV risk.

1 Diabetes Mellitus

Diabetes mellitus is a disease characterized by dysregulation of plasma glucose, resulting in chronic hyperglycemia. Type 1 diabetes (T1D) results from destruction of pancreatic beta-cells, most often secondary to an autoimmune process. An inability to secrete insulin necessitates exogenous insulin to maintain normal or near-normal levels of plasma glucose. Type 2 diabetes (T2D) typically results from a combination of insulin resistance in a variety of tissues (skeletal muscle, adipose, liver) combined with relative insulin deficiency. Insulin resistance is often present for many years prior to diagnosis of T2D, creating a need for compensatory hyperinsulinemia to maintain plasma glucose at normal or near-normal levels. Over time, pancreatic beta-cells progressively lose the ability to produce insulin (beta-cell exhaustion), resulting in relative hypoinsulinemia and hyperglycemia. In T2D, pancreatic beta-cell function is generally 80% or more below that observed in individuals with normal glucose tolerance. While insulin resistance leading to progressive pancreatic beta-cell exhaustion is the most common pathophysiologic process, a subset of individuals appears to have a primary beta-cell defect that results in T2D [1]. Other forms of diabetes, such as maturity-onset diabetes in youth and gestational diabetes, are not included in this review. Given the lack of clear evidence, we have also limited our discussion of prediabetes.

2 Prevalence and Incidence of Diabetes Mellitus

Globally, in 2023, it was estimated that more than 530 million people had diabetes, of which a large majority (~95%) was T2D [2]. The prevalence of diabetes has increased dramatically in recent years, with global age-adjusted prevalence nearly doubling from an estimated 3.2% of the population in 1990 to 6.1% in 2021 [2]. The increase in prevalence of diabetes has been mainly from T2D and has paralleled the increases in prevalence of overweight and obesity, which are the strongest risk factors for T2D development [1, 3]. In the United States, where the prevalence of overweight and obesity in adults was 74% in 2018 [4], the estimated prevalence of diabetes was 37.2 million in 2019, which represents more than 11% of the total population. This includes 1.9 million with T1D, as well as ~2.8 million people with undiagnosed diabetes (primarily T2D) [5]. At current rates, by 2050, 1.3 billion individuals worldwide are projected to have diabetes [2].

While T1D remains the predominant form of diabetes in youth, the estimated prevalence of diabetes in this population has increased for both T1D and T2D. Among youth ≤19 years of age, 4958 of 3.35 million had T1D in 2001 compared with 6672 of 3.46 million in 2009, and 7759 of 3.61 million in 2017. The estimated prevalence of T1D per 1000 youth ≤19 years of age increased significantly from 1.48 in 2001 to 2.15 in 2017, a 45.1% relative increase over 16 years. The greatest absolute increases were observed among non-Hispanic White and non-Hispanic Black youth [6].

The estimated prevalence of T2D per 1000 youth 10–19 years of age also increased significantly from 0.34 in 2001 to 0.67 in 2017, a 95.3% relative increase over 16 years [6]. Racial and ethnic minority populations carried the largest burden of the disease, with the greatest absolute increases among non-Hispanic Black and Hispanic youth. In several non-White racial and ethnic groups, the incidence of T2D in adolescents is twice that of T1D [7, 8]. There has been a steady rise in the incidence of T2D in youth, with 9 new cases per 100,000 individuals/year in 2002–2003 and 13.8 in 2014–2016 [7], corresponding to an age- and sex-adjusted annual percent change in incidence of 4.8% from 2002 to 2015.

3 Cardiovascular Disease Risk and Diabetes Mellitus

Cardiovascular (CV) diseases, including atherosclerotic cardiovascular disease (ASCVD), hypertension, and heart failure, are the leading causes of morbidity and mortality in individuals with T1D and T2D. The presence of diabetes and coexisting risk factors (e.g., dyslipidemia, hypertension) confer increased risk for a variety of adverse CV outcomes, including myocardial infarction (MI), stroke, incident peripheral arterial disease, heart failure hospitalization, and CV death [9]. In addition to macrovascular events, chronic hyperglycemia is strongly associated with microvascular diseases, including retinopathy, neuropathy, and nephropathy, which can result in sequelae such as blindness, chronic kidney disease, neuropathic pain, and erectile dysfunction [10].

The development of ASCVD is accelerated by diabetes in youth as well as in adults. It is important to note that the epidemiology, pathophysiology, and management of T2D in youth differ from T1D, as well as T2D in adults. Because clinical research in youth with diabetes is limited by a lack of long-term outcome studies, recommendations are often based upon a review of available experimental data, epidemiologic observations, and expert opinion.

In contrast to T1D, the clinical presentation of T2D in youth is slower in onset. Consequently, comorbid conditions may already be present at the time of diagnosis [11, 12]. In the SEARCH for Diabetes in Youth (SEARCH) study, youth from minority groups with diabetes had a higher prevalence of having two or more CV risk factors compared with non-Hispanic White youth. At least two CV risk factors were present in 92% of youth with T2D and 14% of those with T1D and were independently associated with age, race/ethnicity, and diabetes type [13]. Compared to those with T1D, elevated apolipoprotein B and small, dense low-density lipoprotein (LDL) are common lipoprotein abnormalities in youth with T2D; the prevalence of these risk factors is substantially increased with poor glycemic control in both groups [14]. Despite shorter duration of diabetes and lower glycated hemoglobin (HbA1c) values, comorbidities in youth with T2D appear to be higher, and the progression of vascular abnormalities more pronounced, than in youth with T1D [12].

Age-adjusted mortality is increased 30–200% in those with vs. those without diabetes. Duration of diabetes is an important determinant of mortality. Those with T1D diagnosed before 20 years of age have a life expectancy that is 15–27 years shorter than that of persons without diabetes. No life expectancy studies are available among youth with T2D [15].

4 When Does the Clock Start Ticking for Cardiovascular Risk in T2D?

Although hyperglycemia is believed to play a key role in the development of microvascular complications in diabetes, the relationship of glycemia per se to macrovascular risk in diabetes is not as strong. Particularly in T2D, risk factors other than hyperglycemia are key determinants of ASCVD event risk, such as hypertension, dyslipidemia, overweight/obesity, chronic inflammation, and renal impairment [16]. A cluster of cardiometabolic disturbances associated with insulin resistance and increased adiposity are often present for years or decades prior to the onset of sufficient hyperglycemia for a diagnosis of T2D. This cluster has been referred to as the metabolic syndrome and includes prediabetes (impaired fasting glucose and impaired glucose tolerance), increased waist circumference, increased triglyceride concentration, low high-density lipoprotein cholesterol (HDL-C) concentration, and elevated blood pressure (BP). Additional cardiometabolic disturbances include insulin resistance, hyperuricemia, chronic low-grade inflammation, excess hepatic fat, and an imbalance of factors involved in coagulation and fibrinolysis [17, 18]. Thus, although T2D is a major ASCVD risk factor, it should be recognized that cardiometabolic disturbances that contribute to increased ASCVD risk have often been present for decades before the onset of hyperglycemia [19].

5   Impact of Diabetes on ASCVD Risk

The presence of diabetes is associated with approximately a doubling of ASCVD event risk in primary prevention patients. As an example, using the ASCVD risk calculator from the American College of Cardiology (ACC) [20], 10-year ASCVD risk was estimated for an African American man, 55 years of age, with resting BP of 130/85 mm Hg, who is currently not taking antihypertensive medication, aspirin, or statin. Total cholesterol, HDL-C, and LDL cholesterol (LDL-C) for this patient were entered as 180, 50, and 105 mg/dL, respectively. The 10-year risk estimate for such a patient is 6.7% without diabetes and 12.3% with diabetes. Using the same parameters for a woman, the corresponding values are 3.4% and 7.9%, respectively. The presence of diabetes is also associated with ~20% higher residual ASCVD risk in secondary prevention patients after adjustment for other major ASCVD risk factors [21].

6   Cardiovascular Risk Factor Screening

In addition to glycemic control, ample evidence demonstrates a reduction of ASCVD-related morbidity and mortality with early identification and aggressive management of concomitant risk factors in this high-risk population [22–24]. CV risk assessment in individuals with diabetes should include a careful review of the medical and family history, symptoms, findings from examination, laboratory and other diagnostic tests, and the presence of ASCVD or severe target organ damage (diminished estimated glomerular filtration rate with or without microalbuminuria, proteinuria, and evidence of microvascular disease in at least three different sites).

The American Diabetes Association and others have published clinical guidelines for ASCVD risk assessment and recommendations for optimal management of both adults and youth [9]. Most organizations recommend global risk assessment at least annually in all adults and children with diabetes. These risk factors include duration of diabetes, obesity/overweight, hypertension, dyslipidemia, smoking, a family history of premature coronary disease, chronic kidney disease, and the presence of albuminuria. There is also growing awareness of the role of social determinants of health and an ongoing need to ensure accessible and affordable healthcare.

The ACC/American Heart Association (AHA), American Diabetes Association, and United States Preventive Services Task Force all endorse the use of the Pooled Cohort Equations to estimate 10-year ASCVD risk for primary prevention [25–27]. This calculation includes age, sex, race, BP, total cholesterol, HDL-C, smoking status, and history of diabetes, the latter of which significantly increases predicted 10-year ASCVD risk for all race-sex groups. Since age plays a critical role in these algorithms, use of a risk calculator is not appropriate in youth. The ACC/AHA guidelines include prolonged duration of disease (>10 years), albuminuria >30 mg/ mg of creatinine, reduced estimated glomerular filtration rate (<60 mL/min/1.73 m^2), retinopathy, neuropathy, and reduced ankle-brachial index (<0.90) as diabetes-specific risk enhancers. While the Pooled Cohort Equations have been validated for individuals 40–79 years of age, no such validation is available for younger individuals and those ≥80 years of age [28].

The European Society of Cardiology/European Atherosclerosis Society utilizes a risk stratification model similar to that of the ACC/AHA, with the exception of including left ventricular hypertrophy and excluding neuropathy and reduced ankle-brachial index. ASCVD risk is classified as either "moderate", "high", or "very high", based upon the person's age, duration of diabetes, and the presence of ASCVD risk factors, target organ damage, or established ASCVD. The SCORE2-Diabetes algorithm is recommended to estimate 10-year ASCVD risk in patients aged ≥40 years with T2D without ASCVD or severe target organ damage [29]. SCORE2-Diabetes integrates information on conventional ASCVD risk factors (i.e., age, smoking status, systolic BP [SBP], total cholesterol, and HDL-C) with diabetes-specific information (e.g., age at diabetes diagnosis, HbA1c, and estimated glomerular filtration rate) [30].

7 Clinical Management of Cardiovascular Risk in Diabetes

Guidance for management of ASCVD risk in adults and youth with diabetes has been published by a number of professional organizations and is beyond the scope of this chapter [31].

8 Lifestyle Intervention and Weight Loss (See Chap. "Lifestyle Interventions and Atherosclerotic Cardiovascular Disease Outcomes")

Weight loss through decreased caloric intake and increased physical activity is recommended for individuals with T2D who are overweight or obese, including children [3, 32]. Benefits of weight loss include improved glycemic control, quality of life, and other obesity-related comorbidities. However, these benefits are based upon short-term studies with little knowledge about the ability of weight loss to reduce morbidity and mortality in T2D.

A randomized trial of overweight or obese adults with T2D compared the effects of an intensive lifestyle intervention to achieve weight loss vs. diabetes support and education (control group) [33]. The primary outcome in this study was the first post-randomization occurrence of a composite CV outcome (CV death, nonfatal MI, nonfatal stroke, or hospitalization for angina). While weight loss was greater in the intervention group than the control group throughout the study (8.6% vs. 0.7% at 1 year; 6.0% vs. 3.5% at study end), and the intervention group achieved greater reductions in HbA1c and improvements in fitness and all CV risk factors except for LDL-C, no reduction in ASCVD-related events was noted. Therefore, the trial was stopped early based on a futility analysis. Nonetheless, several subgroups showed improved CV outcomes, including those who achieved >10% weight loss [34] and those with moderately or poorly managed diabetes (HbA1c >6.8%) at baseline [35].

9 Pharmacotherapy for Weight Loss

Pharmacotherapy for weight loss in diabetes was covered in Chap. "Pharmacotherapy for Obesity: Recent Evolution and Implications for Cardiovascular Risk Reduction", thus will not be discussed in detail in this chapter.

10 Surgical Weight Loss

Metabolic surgery encompasses a wide range of surgical procedures designed to address obesity and its related comorbidities. A growing number of randomized controlled trials, observational studies, and meta-analyses have demonstrated the benefits of metabolic surgery for the treatment of obesity and indicate it should be considered a treatment option in adults [36] and children [37–39] with T2D who are appropriate surgical candidates. Compared with various lifestyle/medical interventions, metabolic surgery achieves better glycemic control as well as a reduction of CV risk factors, including body weight, BP, and triglycerides, in those with T2D and obesity [40–42]. Improvements in ASCVD, CV mortality, and all-cause mortality have been observed following surgically induced weight loss (ranging from ~40% to 80% risk reduction) with potentially greater benefits for mortality among patients with vs. without diabetes [42–44]. In those with T1D undergoing metabolic surgery, a 49-unit decrease in insulin requirement, 0.93% reduction in HbA1c, and 11.04 kg/m^2 decrease in body mass index were observed [45], along with reduced CV risk [46].

Metabolic surgery has also been shown to be safe and effective in obese youth, resulting in durable weight loss and improved comorbid conditions. Adolescents with severe obesity (body mass index ≥40, or ≥ 35 kg/m^2 with comorbidity) undergoing metabolic surgery were reported to have significantly greater weight loss and improvements in BP and dyslipidemia for up to 8 years after surgery compared with adolescents undergoing medical management [47], a finding supported by the Teen-Longitudinal Assessment of Bariatric Surgery database (Teen-LABS). Of note, current evidence suggests that the benefits of surgical weight loss on T2D and hypertension are greater in youth than adults [48–51]. Such data, although short-term, seem to support the idea of better outcomes with earlier implementation of safe and effective therapies.

11 Lipid and Lipoprotein Management

Dyslipidemia is common in diabetes, particularly in T2D. Insulin resistance, life-style factors, and genetic predisposition are all important determinants of dyslipid-emia in diabetes [52]. The pattern of dyslipidemia in T2D is most often moderately elevated plasma triglycerides, triglyceride-rich lipoproteins, and triglyceride-rich lipoprotein cholesterol levels, normal-to-mildly elevated LDL-C, and low HDL-C. Small, dense LDL particles are often increased, which are likely more athero-genic, and associated with a higher rate of nephropathy. Similar patterns are reported in adults and children with T1D, in whom prolonged exposure to dyslipidemia might induce atherosclerosis as early as adolescence. In addition, high levels of LDL-C can be seen in patients with T1D with poor glycemic control. LDL-C is predictive of ASCVD outcomes, and the prevalence of elevated LDL-C is similar between individuals with and without diabetes [53].

While LDL-C is the primary target of lipid-lowering therapies, non-HDL-C should be considered in patients with diabetes. Elevated levels of non-HDL-C cor-relate with the severity of coronary atherosclerosis [54] and are a significant and independent risk factor for MI [55]. Additionally, non-HDL-C appears to be more sensitive and specific than Friedewald-calculated LDL-C for coronary artery dis-ease risk [56] and has been found to be a better correlated surrogate marker for apolipoprotein B than LDL-C [57].

Lifestyle and behavior-focused approaches are critically important and represent the cornerstone of treatment to lower ASCVD risk in patients with diabetes [58, 59]. Lifestyle changes have been shown to lower triglycerides, elevate HDL-C, and lower LDL-C levels. However, lipid-lowering medication is warranted in primary prevention, when estimated ASCVD risk is sufficiently high, and in secondary prevention.

Statins remain the first line of pharmacotherapy in those with dyslipidemia, with and without diabetes. Abundant evidence supports CV risk reduction with timely and aggressive use of statins, which are generally well tolerated by adults and chil-dren [60, 61]. High-intensity statins are indicated for patients with diabetes at high- or very-high ASCVD risk and reduce both LDL-C (40% to 63%) and incidence of coronary and cerebral complications [29]. Accordingly, in 2018, the AHA, ACC, and several additional societies recommended moderate intensity statin therapy in patients 40 to 75 years without calculation of 10-year ASCVD risk, with the goal of reducing LDL-C by at least 50% [62], or non-HDL-C < 100 mg/dL [63]. Similar benefits have been observed in both adults and youth with T1D and T2D [64–66].

Most patients who report statin intolerance, mainly myalgias, are able to take some form of statin regimen, which may involve a change in dosage, agent, or dosing frequency [67, 68]. A meta-analysis of randomized controlled trials comparing different types and intensities of statins in adults with T1D or T2D found the greatest reductions in non-HDL-C levels with rosuvastatin, atorvastatin, and simvastatin and strong evidence of reduced risk for major vascular events [69].

Ezetimibe, a cholesterol absorption inhibitor, taken alone or in combination with statins, improves the lipid profile and reduces CV risk [70, 71]. Bempedoic acid, an ATP citate lyase inhibitor, is also shown to reduce ASCVD event risk in patients with statin intolerance and is available as a monotherapy and as a combination therapy with ezetimibe [72].

Proprotein convertase subtilisin/kexin type 9 (PCSK9) inhibitors regulate the presence of the LDL receptor on the cell surface and have been shown to significantly reduce LDL-C. In the Further Cardiovascular Outcomes Research with PCSK9 Inhibition in Subjects with Elevated Risk (FOURIER) trial [73], evolocumab, a monoclonal antibody to PCSK9, reduced the relative risk of composite CV death, MI, stroke, hospitalization for unstable angina, and coronary revascularization by 17% in patients with diabetes. Monoclonal antibody PCSK9 inhibitors are recommended in high-risk patients with LDL-C levels persistently above target, both in combination with statins or ezetimibe, or in patients with statin intolerance [74]. Inclisiran, a small interfering RNA molecule, inhibits PCSK9 production in the liver, thereby prolonging activity of LDL receptors. It is FDA-approved to lower LDL-C in adults with ASCVD or heterozygous familial hypercholesterolemia as adjunct to diet and maximally tolerated statin therapy. CV outcomes trials of inclisiran have not yet been completed, but are anticipated by 2026–2027 [63].

The role of triglyceride lowering in diabetes remains controversial, with conflicting evidence regarding its ASCVD benefits [75]. Neither fenofibrate nor niacin, in combination with a statin, has been shown to improve ASCVD and thus they are generally not recommended for ASCVD risk reduction [9]. Furthermore, niacin may increase the risk of stroke and has side effects which are difficult to tolerate. Pemafibrate, a selective peroxisome proliferator-activated receptor alpha modulator, showed a favorable benefit-risk balance in a phase 2 trial, but the large, phase 3 Pemafibrate to Reduce Cardiovascular Outcomes by Reducing Triglycerides in Patients with Diabetes (PROMINENT) trial was recently stopped for futility [76].

Omega-3 fatty acids have also been used as add-on therapy in statin-treated patients to help reduce triglycerides and CV risk [77, 78]. The Reduction of Cardiovascular Events With Icosapent Ethyl-Intervention Trial (REDUCE-IT) reported a 25% relative risk reduction in major adverse CV events (MACE) with use of icosapent ethyl compared with pharmaceutical grade mineral oil [79]. To date, the strongest evidence for ASCVD risk reduction with omega-3 fatty acid pharmacotherapy has been from studies of icosapent ethyl (a form of eicosapentaenoic acid ethyl esters), whereas results from studies with eicosapentaenoic acid plus docosahexaenoic acid have not shown clear evidence of reduced ASCVD risk [80].

Lipoprotein (a) is an independent, causative risk factor for ASCVD [81]. In patients with diabetes, the risk of CV events is positively associated with lipoprotein (a) levels [82–84]. Although targeted lipoprotein (a) lowering therapies have not been evaluated in patients with diabetes, analysis of the large PCSK9 inhibitor clinical trials suggests lipoprotein (a) lowering may be beneficial for CV outcomes [85]. Guidelines recommend consideration of additional lipid-lowering therapy, including PCSK9 inhibitors, in patients with diabetes, ASCVD, and elevated LDL-C levels despite maximally tolerated statin therapy [9].

12 Blood Pressure Management

High BP levels significantly contribute to CV risk and adverse outcomes in individuals with diabetes. Evidence supports a reduction in nonfatal stroke rates and microvascular events with intensive BP lowering [86]. Nonetheless, notable differences in guidelines exist and optimal BP levels continue to be debated. For example, the American Diabetes Association promotes the use of risk stratification to determine individual BP goals to avoid overtreatment of vulnerable patients and to decrease the potential of polypharmacy and adverse drug events [9, 87, 88]. Early identification and appropriate management of BP following a shared decision model is encouraged [9].

The Systolic Blood Pressure Intervention Trial (SPRINT) compared standard vs. intensive BP treatment in individuals without diabetes, with SBP $\geq$130 mm Hg, and with increased ASCVD risk. On-treatment SBP targets were <140 mm Hg (standard) vs. <120 mm Hg (intensive treatment group). Compared to standard treatment, those who received intensive treatment were found to have a 25% lower risk of the primary composite outcome (stroke, acute coronary syndrome [acute MI and hospitalization for unstable angina], acute decompensated heart failure, coronary revascularization, atrial fibrillation, or death from CV causes) and a 27% reduction in CV death. However, intensive therapy was associated with increased risks of hypotension, syncope, electrolyte abnormality, and acute kidney injury [89, 90].

The Hypertension Optimal Treatment (HOT) trial targeted diastolic BP (DBP) in 18,790 patients, ~8% with diabetes. No significant differences were found between DBP <90 mm Hg, <85 mm Hg, or <80 mm Hg for fatal or nonfatal MI, fatal and nonfatal strokes, and all other CV events. The lowest incidence of CV events occurred with an achieved DBP of 82 mm Hg. For study participants with diabetes, a 51% reduction in CV events was noted in the treatment group with a target DBP of <80 mm Hg compared with a target DBP of <90 mm Hg [91].

In the Action to Control Cardiovascular Risk in Diabetes (ACCORD) Blood Pressure trial, individuals with T2D were assigned to intensive therapy (targeting a SBP <120 mm Hg) or standard therapy (targeting a SBP <140 mm Hg). While no significant reduction was found in the primary composite outcome of nonfatal MI, nonfatal stroke, or death from CV causes, in those receiving intensive treatment, a 41% reduction of stroke was reported in a prespecified secondary outcome analysis. This clinical trial, however, was viewed as underpowered because the composite primary end point was less sensitive to BP regulation [89]. Compared with standard treatment, intensive treatment was associated with a higher frequency of adverse events, including hypotension, syncope, bradycardia, hyperkalemia, and elevated serum creatinine [92].

The Strategy of Blood Pressure Intervention in the Elderly Hypertensive Patients (STEP) trial compared a SBP target of 110 to <130 mm Hg (intensive treatment) vs. 130 to <150 mm Hg (standard treatment). Of the study participants with hypertension (aged 60–80 years), 18.9% in the intensive treatment arm and 19.4% in the standard treatment arm had T2D. In the intensive treatment group, there was a 26% reduction in the primary composite outcome of stroke, acute coronary syndrome, acute decompensated heart failure, coronary revascularization, atrial fibrillation, or death from CV causes. Hypotension occurred more frequently in the intensive treatment group (3.4%) compared with the standard treatment group (2.6%). No significant differences were observed in other adverse events, including dizziness, syncope, or fractures [93].

13 Glycemic Control

The rates of both micro- and macrovascular events are associated with increasing average blood glucose levels [94–97]. Epidemiologic analyses suggest that each 1% increase in HbA1c is associated with an 18% increase in the risk for ASCVD [96]. Ideally, lifestyle changes and available medical therapies would facilitate achievement of glycemic control. A growing number of these therapeutic agents are becoming available for use in youth, particularly those with T2D. Medical therapies are often delayed, expensive, or inaccessible to a large segment of those with diabetes, especially children [98, 99].

Numerous clinical trials have investigated the ability of improved glycemic control to reduce diabetes-related micro- and macrovascular disease. Randomized controlled trials have conclusively demonstrated that intensive glycemic control can reduce the risk of microvascular complications, including diabetic retinopathy, nephropathy, and neuropathy, in both T1D and T2D [100–103].

Long-term follow-up of adults with T1D who received intensive glycemic control early in the course of their disease has shown evidence suggestive of CV benefit. A trend toward lower risk of ASCVD-related events was noted in those who received intensive control during the Diabetes Control and Complications Trial (DCCT), which persisted during the observational follow-up study (Epidemiology of Diabetes Interventions and Complications). Compared to the standard treatment group, those who received intensive therapy had a 57% reduction of nonfatal MI, stroke, and CV death in the 9 years following participation in the DCCT, which persisted and was associated with a modest reduction of all-cause mortality [104–106].

In contrast, results from studies investigating whether intensive glycemic control in adults with T2D may reduce the rate of long-term ASCVD have been mixed. For example, the UK Prospective Diabetes Study (UKPDS) was a landmark randomized, multicenter, 20-year trial of glycemic therapies in patients with newly diagnosed T2D. It demonstrated conclusively that the complications of T2D could be reduced by improving blood glucose and/or BP control. The results showed a non-statistically significant 16% reduction in combined fatal and nonfatal MI and sudden death with no suggested benefit on other CV outcomes, such as stroke. Nonetheless, when the intervention trial was completed, all surviving UKPDS subjects were entered into a 10-year, posttrial monitoring program during which those who received intensive glycemic control were found to have a significant long-term reduction in MI and all-cause mortality. Furthermore, an epidemiologic analysis of the study cohort found a continuous association such that for every percentage point of lower median on-study HbA1c (e.g., a change from 8% to 7%), there was a statistically significant 18% reduction in ASCVD events, with no glycemic threshold [99]. Other short-term (3.5–5.6 years) studies (ACCORD, Action in Diabetes and Vascular Disease: Preterax and Diamicron Modified Release Controlled Evaluation [ADVANCE], and Veterans Affairs Diabetes Trial [VADT]) of intensive glycemic control showed no significant reduction in ASCVD outcomes. It should be noted, however, that in each of these trials, participants were older, had longer duration of diabetes, and multiple CV risk factors or ASCVD. The ACCORD trial was halted due to an increased mortality rate in the intensive vs. standard treatment arms, while long-term follow-up of the ADVANCE trial showed no evidence of ASCVD benefit. During a 10-year follow-up, participants in the VADT cohort demonstrated a 17% reduction in the risk of CV events with no benefit in CV-related or overall mortality. It has been suggested that the heterogeneity of mortality effects across studies may reflect differences in glycemic goals, therapeutic approaches, and population characteristics. Characteristics of glucose-lowering medications are shown in Table 1 [107].

Table 1 Characteristics of glucose-lowering medications

	Efficacy[1]	Hypogly-caemia	Weight change[2]	CV effects		Renal effects		Oral/SQ	Cost	Clinical considerations
				Effect on MACE	HF	Progression of DKD	Dosing/use considerations*			
Metformin	High	No	Neutral (potential for modest loss)	Potential benefit	Neutral	Neutral	• Contraindicated with eGFR <30 ml/min per 1.73 m²	Oral	Low	• GI side effects common; to mitigate GI side effects, consider slow dose titration, extended release formulations and administration with food • Potential for vitamin B₁₂ deficiency; monitor at regular intervals
SGLT2 Inhibitors	Intermediate to high	No	Loss (intermediate)	Benefit: canagliflozin, empagliflozin	Benefit: canagliflozin, dapagliflozin, empagliflozin, ertugliflozin	Benefit: canagliflozin, dapagliflozin, empagliflozin	• See labels for renal dose considerations of individual agents • Glucose-lowering effect is lower for SGLT2 inhibitors at lower eGFR	Oral	High	• DKA risk, rare in T2DM: discontinue, evaluate and treat promptly if suspected; be aware of predisposing risk factors and clinical presentation (including euglycaemic DKA); discontinue before scheduled surgery (e.g. 3–4 days), during critical illness, or during prolonged fasting to mitigate potential risk • Increased risk of genital mycotic infections • Necrotising fasciitis of the perineum (Fournier's gangrene), rare reports: institute prompt treatment if suspected • Attention to volume status, blood pressure; adjust other volume-contracting agents as applicable
GLP-1 RAs	High to very high	No	Loss (intermediate to very high)	Benefit: dulaglutide, liraglutide, semaglutide (SQ) — Neutral: exenatide once weekly, lixisenatide	Neutral	Benefit for renal endpoints in CVOTs, driven by albuminuria outcomes: dulaglutide, liraglutide, semaglutide (SQ)	• See labels for renal dose considerations of individual agents • No dose adjustment for dulaglutide, liraglutide, semaglutide • Monitor renal function when initiating or escalating doses in patients with renal impairment reporting severe adverse GI reactions	SQ; oral (semaglutide)	High	• Risk of thyroid C-cell tumours in rodents; human relevance not determined (liraglutide, dulaglutide, exenatide extended release, semaglutide) • Counsel patients on potential for GI side effects and their typically temporary nature; provide guidance on dietary modifications to mitigate GI side effects [reduction in meal size, mindful eating practices (e.g. stop eating once full), decreasing intake of high-fat or spicy food]; consider slower dose titration for patients experiencing GI challenges • Pancreatitis has been reported in clinical trials but causality has not been established. Discontinue if pancreatitis is suspected • Evaluate for gallbladder disease if cholelithiasis or cholecystitis are suspected
GIP and GLP-1 RA	Very high	No	Loss (very high)	Under investigation	Under investigation	Under investigation	• See label for renal dose considerations • No dose adjustment • Monitor renal function when initiating or escalating doses in patients with renal impairment reporting severe adverse GI reactions	SQ	High	• Risk of thyroid C-cell tumours in rodents; human relevance not determined • Counsel patients on potential for GI side effects and their typically temporary nature; provide guidance on dietary modifications to mitigate GI side effects [reduction in meal size, mindful eating practices (e.g. stop eating once full), decreasing intake of high-fat or spicy food]; consider slower dose titration for patients experiencing GI challenges • Pancreatitis has been reported in clinical trials but causality has not been established. Discontinue if pancreatitis is suspected • Evaluate for gallbladder disease if cholelithiasis or cholecystitis are suspected
DPP-4 Inhibitors	Intermediate	No	Neutral	Neutral	Neutral (potential risk, saxagliptin)	Neutral	• Renal dose adjustment required (sitagliptin, saxagliptin, alogliptin); can be used in renal impairment • No dose adjustment required for linagliptin	Oral	High	• Pancreatitis has been reported in clinical trials but causality has not been established. Discontinue if pancreatitis is suspected • Joint pain • Bullous pemphigoid (postmarketing): discontinue if suspected
Thiazolidinediones	High	No	Gain	Potential benefit: pioglitazone	Increased risk	Neutral	• No dose adjustment required • Generally not recommended in renal impairment due to potential for fluid retention	Oral	Low	• Congestive heart failure (pioglitazone, rosiglitazone) • Fluid retention (oedema; heart failure) • Benefit in NASH • Risk of bone fractures • Weight gain: consider lower doses to mitigate weight gain and oedema
Sulfonylureas (2nd Generation)	High	Yes	Gain	Neutral	Neutral	Neutral	• Glyburide: generally not recommended in chronic kidney disease • Glipizide and glimepiride: initiate conservatively to avoid hypoglycaemia	Oral	Low	• FDA Special Warning on increased risk of CV mortality based on studies of an older sulfonylurea (tolbutamide); glimepiride shown to be CV safe (see text) • Use with caution in persons at risk for hypoglycaemia
Insulin — Human / Analogues	High to very high	Yes	Gain	Neutral	Neutral	Neutral	• Lower insulin doses required with a decrease in eGFR; titrate per clinical response	SQ; inhaled / SQ	Low (SQ) / High	• Injection site reactions • Higher risk of hypoglycaemia with human insulin (NPH or premixed formulations) vs analogues

CV, Cardiovascular; CVOT, Cardiovascular Outcomes Trial; DKA, Diabetic Ketoacidosis; DKD, Diabetic Kidney Disease; DPP-4, Dipeptidyl peptidase-4; eGFR, Estimated Glomerular Filtration Rate; GI, Gastrointestinal; GIP, Gastric Inhibitory Polypeptide; GLP-1 RA, Glucagon-Like Peptide-1 Receptor Agonist; HF, Heart Failure; NASH, Non-Alcoholic Steatohepatitis; MACE, Major Adverse Cardiovascular Events; SGLT2, Sodium-glucose Cotransporter-2; SQ, Subcutaneous; T2DM, Type 2 Diabetes Mellitus

* For agent-specific dosing recommendations, please refer to manufacturers' prescribing information

1. Tsapas A, Avgerinos I, Karagiannis T et al. Comparative Effectiveness of Glucose-Lowering Drugs for Type 2 Diabetes: A Systematic Review and Network Meta-analysis. Ann Intern Med. 2020 Aug 18;173(4):278–86; 2. Tsapas A, Karagiannis T, Kakotrichi P et al. Comparative efficacy of glucose-lowering medications on body weight and blood pressure in patients with type 2 diabetes: A systematic review and network meta-analysis. Diabetes Obes Metab. 2021;23(9):2116–24.

14 Effects of Medications on ASCVD Event Risk in Diabetes Mellitus

14.1 Metformin

Metformin is widely used in the treatment of individuals with T2D, either as monotherapy or in combination with other antidiabetic drugs. In a meta-analysis of 13 randomized controlled trials evaluating the CV effects of metformin vs. placebo or active control, none of the differences in assessed CV outcomes were statistically significant [108].

14.2 Pioglitazone

Despite the increased risk of hospitalization for heart failure due to fluid retention, pioglitazone use has been consistently associated with reduced risk of MI and ischemic stroke, both in primary and secondary prevention, without any proven direct harm on the myocardium. Moreover, it reduces atherosclerosis progression, in-stent restenosis after coronary stent implantation, progression rate from persistent to permanent atrial fibrillation, and re-ablation rate in diabetic patients with paroxysmal atrial fibrillation after catheter ablation [109].

The Diabetes Reduction Assessment with Ramipril and Rosiglitazone Medication (DREAM) trial evaluated whether pioglitazone could prevent the development of T2D in individuals with impaired glucose tolerance [110]. The study found that pioglitazone reduced the risk of developing diabetes by 62% compared to placebo over an average of 3 years of follow-up. It also improved insulin sensitivity and beta-cell function. However, the study also reported an increased risk of edema and heart failure with pioglitazone use.

The Insulin Resistance Intervention after Stroke (IRIS) trial assessed whether pioglitazone could reduce the risk of recurrent stroke or CV events in patients with insulin resistance and a recent history of ischemic stroke or transient ischemic attack [111]. The results indicated that pioglitazone use was associated with a 24% reduction in the risk of recurrent stroke or CV events compared to placebo over a median follow-up of 4.8 years (hazard ratio [HR], 0.76; 95% confidence interval [CI], 0.62–0.93, $P = 0.007$). This suggests that pioglitazone might have a beneficial effect on reducing CV risk in this specific high-risk population.

The Actos Now for Prevention of Diabetes (ACT-NOW) trial examined the effects of early intervention with pioglitazone in individuals with impaired glucose tolerance and early-stage T2D [112]. The trial found that pioglitazone use improved beta-cell function and significantly reduced the risk of progression to overt diabetes by 72% compared to placebo over a median follow-up of 2.4 years (HR, 0.28; 95% CI, 0.16–0.49; $P < 0.001$).

In 2016, the US Food and Drug Administration announced the results of an updated review that concluded that use of pioglitazone in patients with T2D may be linked to an increased risk of bladder cancer [113]. Despite its potential benefits, health care professionals should carefully consider the benefits and risks before using pioglitazone in patients with a history of bladder cancer.

14.3 Alpha-Glucosidase Inhibitors

Alpha-glucosidase inhibitors competitively inhibit enzymes that convert complex nonabsorbable carbohydrates into simple absorbable carbohydrates, thus delaying carbohydrate absorption and reducing the rise in postprandial blood glucose concentrations by about 3 mmol/L. In the Study to Prevent (STOP)-NIDDM, acarbose was associated with a 49% relative risk reduction in the development of CV events (HR, 0.51; 95% CI, 0.28–0.95; $P = 0.03$) and a 2.5% absolute risk reduction in participants with impaired glucose tolerance compared to placebo [114].

14.4 Dipeptidyl Peptidase-4 Inhibitors

This class of drugs inhibits the dipeptidyl peptidase-4 enzyme, prolonging the action of the incretin hormones glucagon-like peptide-1 (GLP-1) and glucose-dependent insulinotropic polypeptide, leading to inhibition of glucagon release, increased insulin secretion, decreased gastric emptying, and lower glucose. Several drugs within this class have been studied in CV outcomes trials (saxagliptin [115], alogliptin [116], sitagliptin [117], and linagliptin [118, 119]) with median follow-up of 1.5–3 years in populations of T2D with high CV risk and known ASCVD. Although dipeptidyl peptidase-4 inhibitors reduced HbA1c, there was no reduction in MACE. Use of saxagliptin has been associated with increased risk of heart failure [120, 121].

14.5 Glucagon-like Peptide-1 Receptor Agonist Agents

Several large clinical trials have shown that GLP-1 receptor agonists (GLP-1 RAs) can reduce the risk of ASCVD in people with T2D. For example, the Liraglutide Effect and Action in Diabetes: Evaluation of Cardiovascular Outcome Results (LEADER) trial found that liraglutide (Victoza) reduced the risk of MACE by 13% in people with T2D and established ASCVD. The Trial to Evaluate Cardiovascular and Other Long-term Outcomes with Semaglutide in Subjects with Type 2 Diabetes (SUSTAIN 6) found that semaglutide (Ozempic) reduced the risk of MACE by 12% in people with T2D and at high risk for CVD [122].

14.6 Combination Glucose-Dependent Insulinotropic Polypeptide and Glucagon-like Peptide-1 Receptor Agonists

Combination glucose-dependent insulinotropic polypeptide and GLP-1 RAs demonstrated superior glycemic efficacy and weight reduction vs. comparators [123, 124], improved liver fat content, and reduced visceral and subcutaneous abdominal adipose tissue volume [125]. Understanding the potential long-term CV benefits awaits completion of the Study of Tirzepatide Compared with Dulaglutide on Major Cardiovascular Events in Participants with Type 2 Diabetes (SURPASS-CVOT) [126].

14.7 Sodium-Glucose Cotransporter 2 Inhibitors

Sodium-glucose cotransporter 2 (SGLT2) in the proximal tubule of the nephron is responsible for approximately 90% of urinary glucose reabsorption. SGLT2 inhibitors are oral therapies which lower blood glucose levels through induction of glycosuria. Large randomized controlled trials have shown that many of these agents reduce MACE and the risk of heart failure hospitalizations in adults with T2D who have established ASCVD and/or diabetes-related kidney disease (Table 2) [127]. While the benefits of agents within this class appear to be similar, the results of CV outcomes trials may reflect the unique patient populations enrolled in each study.

Table 2 SGLT2 inhibitor cardiovascular and renal outcome trials

	EMPA-REG OUTCOME (12)	CANVAS/ CANVAS-R (16)	DECLARE-TIMI 58 (17)	CREDENCE (19)	DAPA-HF[a] (47)
Patients enrolled, n	7020	10,142	17,160	4401	4744
Drug	Empagliflozin	Canagliflozin	Dapagliflozin	Canagliflozin	Dapagliflozin
Dose	10 or 25 mg PO daily	100 or 300 mg PO daily	10 mg PO daily	100 mg PO daily	10 mg PO daily
Median duration of follow-up (years)	3.1	2.4	4.2	2.6	1.5
Mean baseline HbA1c (%)	8.1	8.2	8.3	8.3	a
Mean duration of diabetes (years)	N/A[b]	13.5	11.0	15.8	a
Baseline statin use (%)	77	75	75	69	n/a
Baseline prevalence of CV disease/HF (%)	99	72	41	50	Not reported
Baseline prevalence of HF (%)	10	14	10	15	100[a]
MACE outcome, HR (95% CI)[c]	0.86 (0.74–0.99)	0.86 (0.75–0.97)	0.93 (0.84–1.03)	0.80 (0.67–0.95)	Not reported
Hospitalization for HF or CV death, HR (95% CI)[d]	0.66 (0.55–0.79)	0.78 (0.67–0.91)	0.83 (0.73–0.95)	0.69 (0.57–0.83)	0.75 (0.65–0.85)
CV death, HR (95% CI)	0.62 (0.49–0.77)	0.87 (0.72–1.06)	0.98 (0.82–1.17)	0.78 (0.61–1.00)	0.82 (0.69–0.98)
Fatal or nonfatal MI, HR (95% CI)	0.87 (0.70–1.09)	0.89 (0.73–1.09)	0.89 (0.77–1.01)	Not reported	Not reported
Fatal or nonfatal stroke, HR (95% CI)	1.18 (0.89–1.56)	0.87 (0.69–1.09)	1.01 (0.84–1.21)	Not reported	Not reported

(continued)

Table 2 (continued)

	EMPA-REG OUTCOME (12)	CANVAS/ CANVAS-R (16)	DECLARE-TIMI 58 (17)	CREDENCE (19)	DAPA-HF[a] (47)
All-cause mortality, HR (95% CI)	0.68 (0.57–0.82)	0.87 (0.74–1.01)	0.93 (0.82–1.04)	0.83 (0.68–1.02)	0.83 (0.71–0.97)
HF hospitalization, HR (95% CI)	0.65 (0.50–0.85)	0.67 (0.52–0.87)	0.73 (0.61–0.88)	0.61 (0.47–0.80)	0.70 (0.59–0.83)
Renal composite endpoint,[e] HR (95% CI)	0.54 (0.40–0.75)	0.60 (0.47–0.77)	0.53 (0.43–0.66)	0.70 (0.59–0.82)	0.71 (0.44–1.16)

Reprinted from Journal of the American College of Cardiology, 76, Das SR, Everett BM, Birtcher, KK, et al., 2020 Expert Consensus Decision Pathway on Novel Therapies for Cardiovascular Risk Reduction in Patients with Type 2 Diabetes: A Report of the American College of Cardiology Solution Set Oversight Committee, 1117–1145, 2020, with permission from Elsevier [127]

CANVAS/CANVAS-R Canagliflozin CV Assessment Study/A Study of the Effects of Canagliflozin (JNJ-28431754) on Renal Endpoints in Adult Participants With T2D, *CI* confidence interval, *CREDENCE* Evaluation of the Effects of Canagliflozin on Renal and CV Outcomes in Participants With Diabetic Nephropathy, *CV* cardiovascular, *DAPA-HF* Study to Evaluate the Effect of Dapagliflozin on the Incidence of Worsening HF or CV Death in Patients With Chronic HF, *DECLARE-TIMI 58* Multicenter Trial to Evaluate the Effect of Dapagliflozin on the incidence of CV Events-Thrombolysis In Myocardial Infarction 58, *eGFR* estimated glomerular filtration rate, *EMPA-REG OUTCOME* (Empagliflozin) CV Outcome Event Trial in T2D Patients, *HbA1c* hemoglobin A1c, *HF* heart failure, *HFrEF* heart failure with reduced ejection fraction, *HR* hazard ratio, *MACE* major adverse cardiovascular event, *MI* myocardial infarction, *PO* "per os," by mouth, *SGLT2* sodium-glucose cotransporter-2

[a]58.2% of patients enrolled in DAPA-HF did not have diabetes mellitus. All patients enrolled in DAPA-HF had HFrEF

[b]Mean duration of diabetes was not provided for EMPA-REG OUTCOME, but 57% of patients enrolled had diabetes for more than 10 years

[c]This outcome was the primary outcome for CANVAS and EMPA-REG OUTCOME and was a dual primary outcome for DECLARE-TIMI 58. It was a secondary outcome for CREDENCE. It consists of 3-point MACE, a composite of nonfatal MI, nonfatal stroke, and CV death. The p value for superiority for the primary endpoint for empagliflozin (all doses) vs. placebo was 0.04, and the *p* value for superiority for the primary endpoint for canagliflozin (all doses) vs. placebo was 0.02. The p values for the other comparisons are available in the primary EMPA-REG OUTCOME report but were not published in the CANVAS/CANVAS-R report. DECLARE-TIMI 58 had dual primary endpoints of MACE and hospitalization for HF or CV death. MACE was not assessed in DAPA-HF, which was an HF outcome trial

[d]Hospitalization for HF or CV death was a dual primary endpoint of the DECLARE-TIMI 58 trial. In EMPA-REG OUTCOME, this endpoint excluded fatal stroke events. The primary endpoint of DAPAHF was worsening HF (urgent HF visit or hospitalization for HF) or CV death. Dapagliflozin, 10 mg dally was associated with a 26% reduction in the primary endpoint (HR: 0.74; 95% CI: 0.65 to 0.85)

[e]A renal endpoint reported in a recent meta-analysis was a composite of sustained doubling of serum creatinine or a 40% decline in eGFR, end-stage kidney disease, or death of renal cause (49). The DAPAHF renal composite endpoint was defined as a sustained decline in eGFR of 50% or greater, end-stage kidney disease, renal transplantation, renal death, and death from any cause

Multiple clinical trials have shown CV benefits of SGLT2 inhibitors independent of glycemic control and diminished risks of heart failure hospitalization and progression of diabetic kidney disease. Use of these agents has received strong recommendations [26, 127–129]; although some limit their recommendation to patients with underlying chronic kidney disease [130–132]. Safety concerns include an increased risk of genital mycotic infections [133, 134], rare cases of necrotizing fasciitis of the perineum, diabetic ketoacidosis [135], increase in bone fracture, and risk of volume depletion and hypotension. No significant risk of acute kidney injury has been observed in trials of SGLT2 inhibitors; studies of chronic use are in progress [31].

14.8   Antiplatelet Therapy

Aspirin therapy has been shown to be effective in reducing CV-related morbidity and mortality in secondary prevention, while the net benefits in primary prevention are less well defined [136–138]. In individuals with diabetes, aspirin failed to consistently show a significant reduction in overall ASCVD end points, although some sex differences were suggested [139–142]. Evidence regarding the benefits of aspirin is summarized in Table 3. There appears to be a modest effect on ischemic

Table 3 Selected studies of aspirin in adults with diabetes

Study	Type of study	Patient population (*N*)	Findings
Antithrombotic Trialist Collaboration [137]	Meta-analysis of 6 large trials of aspirin for primary prevention in the general population	95,000 subjects; 4000 with diabetes	Aspirin reduced the risk of serious vascular events by 12% (relative risk 0.88 [95% CI 0.82–0.94]). The largest reduction was for nonfatal MI, with little effect on CHD death (relative risk 0.95 [95% CI 0.78–1.15]) or total stroke
ASCEND (A Study of Cardiovascular Events in Diabetes) [142]	Placebo-controlled, randomized trial	15,480 subjects with diabetes but no evident CVD	During a mean follow-up of 7.4 years, there was a significant 12% reduction in the primary efficacy end point (8.5% vs. 9.6%; *P* = 0.01). In contrast, major bleeding was significantly increased from 3.2 to 4.1% in the aspirin group (rate ratio 1.29; *P* = 0.003), with most of the excess being gastrointestinal bleeding and other extracranial bleeding

(continued)

Table 3 (continued)

Study	Type of study	Patient population (*N*)	Findings
ARRIVE (Aspirin to Reduce Risk of Initial Vascular Events) [143]	Randomized trial of aspirin for primary prevention	12,546 subjects; Men aged ≥55 years or women ≥60 years with average CVD risk, without diabetes	No benefit of aspirin on the primary efficacy end point and an increased risk of bleeding
ASPREE (Aspirin In Reducing Events in the Elderly) [144]	Randomized trial of aspirin for primary prevention	19,114 subjects; ≥70 years of age or older (or ≥65 years of age among blacks and Hispanics in the U.S.) and did not have CVD	No benefit of aspirin on the primary efficacy end point and an increased risk of bleeding

CHD coronary heart disease, *CI* confidence interval, *CVD* cardiovascular disease, *MI* myocardial infarction

vascular events, with the absolute decrease in events depending on the underlying ASCVD risk [9]. Aspirin therapy was associated with an increased risk of gastrointestinal bleeding.

Given the available evidence, the use of aspirin for primary prevention needs to be carefully considered and may generally not be recommended. It is not recommended for men and women <50 years of age at low risk of ASCVD and is contraindicated in those <21 years of age. In secondary prevention, aspirin is still recommended based on greater benefit than risk [9, 137]. Dual antiplatelet or antiplatelet plus anticoagulant treatment strategies may be helpful in selected patients.

15 Summary

Individuals with diabetes are highly susceptible to the development and progression of ASCVD. Chronic hyperglycemia triggers a cascade of pathophysiological changes, including oxidative stress, endothelial dysfunction, and inflammation, which promote atherosclerosis, endothelial injury, and vascular remodeling. Evidence of diabetes-related vascular changes may be present prior to diagnosis. Consequently, patients with diabetes face a substantially elevated risk of ASCVD manifestations, such as MI, stroke, peripheral artery disease, and heart failure. Furthermore, the presence of diabetes in patients with ASCVD confers worse outcomes and complicates treatment strategies due to its influence on the underlying disease pathogenesis and response to interventions. Understanding and effectively managing the intricate interplay between diabetes and ASCVD remains of paramount importance in both clinical practice and public health initiatives to improve outcomes and reduce the burden of these chronic and intertwined conditions. Healthcare professionals who provide care to adults and children with diabetes should be aware of the strong clinical evidence regarding therapies with a demonstrated ability to lower CV risk. Critical steps for improving outcomes include: (1) early identification of those at risk or affected by diabetes; (2) initial and ongoing screening of CV risk factors, starting at diagnosis; (3) aggressive and timely management of CV risk factors to reach recommended goals; and (4) empathetic follow-up to encourage lifelong adherence.

References

1. ElSayed NA, Aleppo G, Aroda VR, et al. 2. classification and diagnosis of diabetes: standards of Care in Diabetes-2023. Diabetes Care. 2023;46:S19–40.
2. G. B. D. Diabetes Collaborators. Global, regional, and national burden of diabetes from 1990 to 2021, with projections of prevalence to 2050: a systematic analysis for the Global Burden of Disease Study 2021. Lancet. 2023;402:203–34.
3. ElSayed NA, Aleppo G, Aroda VR, et al. 8. Obesity and weight management for the prevention and treatment of type 2 diabetes: standards of care in diabetes-2023. Diabetes Care. 2023;46:S128–39.
4. Fryar CD, Carroll MD, Afful J. Prevalence of overweight, obesity, and severe obesity among adults aged 20 and over: United States, 1960-1962 through 2017-2018. https://www.cdc.gov/nchs/data/hestat/obesity-adult-17-18/obesity-adult.htm. Accessed: Feb 15 2024.
5. American Diabetes Association. Statistics about diabetes [internet]. https://diabetes.org/about-diabetes/statistics/about-diabetes. Accessed: 04 July 2023.
6. Lawrence JM, Divers J, Isom S, et al. Trends in prevalence of type 1 and type 2 diabetes in children and adolescents in the US, 2001-2017. JAMA. 2021;326:717–27.
7. Divers J, Mayer-Davis EJ, Lawrence JM, et al. Trends in incidence of type 1 and type 2 diabetes among youths—selected counties and Indian reservations, United States, 2002–2015. MMWR Morb Mortal Wkly Rep. 2020;69:161–5.
8. Mayer-Davis EJ, Lawrence JM, Dabelea D, et al. Incidence trends of type 1 and type 2 Diabetes among youths, 2002-2012. N Engl J Med. 2017;376:1419–29.
9. ElSayed NA, Aleppo G, Aroda VR, et al. 10. Cardiovascular disease and risk management: standards of care in diabetes-2023. Diabetes Care. 2023;46:S158–90.
10. Faselis C, Katsimardou A, Imprialos K, Deligkaris P, Kallistratos M, Dimitriadis K. Microvascular complications of type 2 Diabetes mellitus. Curr Vasc Pharmacol. 2020;18:117–24.
11. Copeland KC, Zeitler P, Geffner M, et al. Characteristics of adolescents and youth with recent-onset type 2 diabetes: the TODAY cohort at baseline. J Clin Endocrinol Metab. 2011;96:159–67.
12. Eppens MC, Craig ME, Cusumano J, et al. Prevalence of diabetes complications in adolescents with type 2 compared with type 1 diabetes. Diabetes Care. 2006;29:1300–6.
13. Rodriguez BL, Fujimoto WY, Mayer-Davis EJ, et al. Prevalence of cardiovascular disease risk factors in U.S. children and adolescents with diabetes: the SEARCH for diabetes in youth study. Diabetes Care. 2006;29:1891–6.
14. Albers JJ, Marcovina SM, Imperatore G, et al. Prevalence and determinants of elevated apolipoprotein B and dense low-density lipoprotein in youths with type 1 and type 2 diabetes. J Clin Endocrinol Metab. 2008;93:735–42.
15. Dabelea D, Hamman RF, Knowler WC. Diabetes in youth. In: Cowie CC, Casagrande SS, Menke A, et al., editors. Diabetes in America. 3rd ed. Bethesda (MD); 2018.

16. Viigimaa M, Sachinidis A, Toumpourleka M, Koutsampasopoulos K, Alliksoo S, Titma T. Macrovascular complications of type 2 diabetes mellitus. Curr Vasc Pharmacol. 2020;18:110–6.
17. Yanai H, Adachi H, Hakoshima M, Katsuyama H. Molecular biological and clinical understanding of the pathophysiology and treatments of hyperuricemia and its association with metabolic syndrome, cardiovascular diseases and chronic kidney disease. Int J Mol Sci. 2021;22
18. Li X, Weber NC, Cohn DM, et al. Effects of hyperglycemia and diabetes mellitus on coagulation and hemostasis. J Clin Med. 2021;10
19. Haffner SM, Stern MP, Hazuda HP, Mitchell BD, Patterson JK. Cardiovascular risk factors in confirmed prediabetic individuals. Does the clock for coronary heart disease start ticking before the onset of clinical diabetes? JAMA. 1990;263:2893–8.
20. American College of Cardiology. ASCVD risk estimator plus. https://tools.acc.org/ascvd-risk-estimator-plus/#!/calculate/estimate/. Accessed 2 Nov 2023.
21. Zhao Y, Xiang P, Coll B, Lopez JAG, Wong ND. Diabetes associated residual atherosclerotic cardiovascular risk in statin-treated patients with prior atherosclerotic cardiovascular disease. J Diabetes Complicat. 2021;35:107767.
22. Ali MK, Bullard KM, Gregg EW. Achievement of goals in U.S. Diabetes Care, 1999-2010. N Engl J Med. 2013;369:287–8.
23. Buse JB, Ginsberg HN, Bakris GL, et al. Primary prevention of cardiovascular diseases in people with diabetes mellitus: a scientific statement from the American Heart Association and the American Diabetes Association. Diabetes Care. 2007;30:162–72.
24. Gaede P, Lund-Andersen H, Parving HH, Pedersen O. Effect of a multifactorial intervention on mortality in type 2 diabetes. N Engl J Med. 2008;358:580–91.
25. U. S. Preventive Services Task Force, Bibbins-Domingo K, Grossman DC, et al. Statin Use for the Primary Prevention of Cardiovascular Disease in Adults: US Preventive Services Task Force Recommendation Statement. JAMA. 2016;316:1997–2007.
26. American Diabetes Association Professional Practice Committee. 10. Cardiovascular disease and risk management: standards of medical care in diabetes-2022. Diabetes Care. 2022;45:S144–74.
27. Arnett DK, Blumenthal RS, Albert MA, et al. 2019 ACC/AHA guideline on the primary prevention of cardiovascular disease: a report of the American College of Cardiology/American Heart Association Task Force on Clinical Practice Guidelines. J Am Coll Cardiol. 2019;74:e177–232.
28. Sattar N, Rawshani A, Franzen S, et al. Age at diagnosis of type 2 diabetes mellitus and associations with cardiovascular and mortality risks. Circulation. 2019;139:2228–37.
29. Marx N, Federici M, Schutt K, et al. 2023 ESC Guidelines for the management of cardiovascular disease in patients with diabetes. Eur Heart J. 2023;44:4043–140.
30. SCORE2-Diabetes Working Group, ESC Cardiovascular Risk Collaboration. SCORE2-Diabetes: 10-year cardiovascular risk estimation in type 2 diabetes in Europe. Eur Heart J. 2023;44:2544–56.
31. Kelsey MD, Nelson AJ, Green JB, et al. Guidelines for cardiovascular risk reduction in patients with type 2 Diabetes: JACC guideline comparison. J Am Coll Cardiol. 2022;79:1849–57.
32. Samson SL, Vellanki P, Blonde L, et al. American Association of Clinical Endocrinology Consensus Statement: comprehensive type 2 diabetes management algorithm—2023 update. Endocr Pract. 2023;29:305–40.
33. Look Ahead Research Group, Wing RR, Bolin P, et al. Cardiovascular effects of intensive lifestyle intervention in type 2 diabetes. N Engl J Med. 2013;369:145–54.
34. Look Ahead Research Group, Gregg EW, Jakicic JM, et al. Association of the magnitude of weight loss and changes in physical fitness with long-term cardiovascular disease outcomes in overweight or obese people with type 2 diabetes: a post-hoc analysis of the Look AHEAD randomised clinical trial. Lancet Diabetes Endocrinol. 2016;4:913–21.
35. Baum A, Scarpa J, Bruzelius E, Tamler R, Basu S, Faghmous J. Targeting weight loss interventions to reduce cardiovascular complications of type 2 diabetes: a machine learning-

based post-hoc analysis of heterogeneous treatment effects in the Look AHEAD trial. Lancet Diabetes Endocrinol. 2017;5:808–15.

36. Rubino F, Nathan DM, Eckel RH, et al. Metabolic surgery in the treatment algorithm for type 2 diabetes: a joint statement by International Diabetes Organizations. Obes Surg. 2017;27:2–21.

37. Hampl SE, Hassink SG, Skinner AC, et al. Clinical practice guideline for the evaluation and treatment of children and adolescents with obesity. Pediatrics. 2023;151:e2022060640.

38. Eisenberg D, Shikora SA, Aarts E, et al. 2022 American Society for Metabolic and Bariatric Surgery (ASMBS) and International Federation for the Surgery of Obesity and Metabolic Disorders (IFSO): indications for metabolic and bariatric surgery. Surg Obes Relat Dis. 2022;18:1345–56.

39. Pratt JSA, Browne A, Browne NT, et al. ASMBS pediatric metabolic and bariatric surgery guidelines, 2018. Surg Obes Relat Dis. 2018;14:882–901.

40. Khorgami Z, Shoar S, Saber AA, Howard CA, Danaei G, Sclabas GM. Outcomes of bariatric surgery versus medical management for type 2 diabetes mellitus: a meta-analysis of randomized controlled trials. Obes Surg. 2019;29:964–74.

41. O'Brien PE, Hindle A, Brennan L, et al. Long-term outcomes after bariatric surgery: a systematic review and meta-analysis of weight loss at 10 or more years for all bariatric procedures and a single-centre review of 20-year outcomes after adjustable gastric banding. Obes Surg. 2019;29:3–14.

42. Arterburn DE, Telem DA, Kushner RF, Courcoulas AP. Benefits and risks of bariatric surgery in adults: a review. JAMA. 2020;324:879–87.

43. Fisher DP, Johnson E, Haneuse S, et al. Association between bariatric surgery and macrovascular disease outcomes in patients with type 2 diabetes and severe obesity. JAMA. 2018;320:1570–82.

44. Dicker D, Greenland P, Leibowitz M, et al. All-cause mortality of patients with and without diabetes following bariatric surgery: comparison to non-surgical matched patients. Obes Surg. 2021;31:755–62.

45. Ashrafian H, Harling L, Toma T, et al. Type 1 Diabetes mellitus and bariatric surgery: a systematic review and meta-analysis. Obes Surg. 2016;26:1697–704.

46. Dirksen C, Jacobsen SH, Bojsen-Moller KN, et al. Reduction in cardiovascular risk factors and insulin dose, but no beta-cell regeneration 1 year after Roux-en-Y gastric bypass in an obese patient with type 1 diabetes: a case report. Obes Res Clin Pract. 2013;7:e269–74.

47. Olbers T, Beamish AJ, Gronowitz E, et al. Laparoscopic Roux-en-Y gastric bypass in adolescents with severe obesity (AMOS): a prospective, 5-year, Swedish nationwide study. Lancet Diabetes Endocrinol. 2017;5:174–83.

48. Inge TH, Jenkins TM, Xanthakos SA, et al. Long-term outcomes of bariatric surgery in adolescents with severe obesity (FABS-5+): a prospective follow-up analysis. Lancet Diabetes Endocrinol. 2017;5:165–73.

49. Michalsky MP, Inge TH, Jenkins TM, et al. Cardiovascular risk factors after adolescent bariatric surgery. Pediatrics. 2018;141:e20172485.

50. Inge TH, Laffel LM, Jenkins TM, et al. Comparison of surgical and medical therapy for type 2 diabetes in severely obese adolescents. JAMA Pediatr. 2018;172:452–60.

51. Inge TH, Courcoulas AP, Jenkins TM, et al. Five-year outcomes of gastric bypass in adolescents as compared with adults. N Engl J Med. 2019;380:2136–45.

52. Warraich HJ, Rana JS. Dyslipidemia in diabetes mellitus and cardiovascular disease. Cardiovasc Endocrinol. 2017;6:27–32.

53. Almdal T, Scharling H, Jensen JS, Vestergaard H. The independent effect of type 2 diabetes mellitus on ischemic heart disease, stroke, and death: a population-based study of 13,000 men and women with 20 years of follow-up. Arch Intern Med. 2004;164:1422–6.

54. Pischon T, Girman CJ, Sacks FM, Rifai N, Stampfer MJ, Rimm EB. Non-high-density lipoprotein cholesterol and apolipoprotein B in the prediction of coronary heart disease in men. Circulation. 2005;112:3375–83.

55. Bittner V, Hardison R, Kelsey SF, et al. Non-high-density lipoprotein cholesterol levels predict five-year outcome in the Bypass Angioplasty Revascularization Investigation (BARI). Circulation. 2002;106:2537–42.

56. Kathariya G, Aggarwal J, Garg P, Singh S, Manzoor S. Is evaluation of non-HDL-C better than calculated LDL-C in CAD patients? MMIMSR experiences. Indian Heart J. 2020;72:189–91.

57. Levinson SS. High density- and beta-lipoprotein screening for risk of coronary artery disease in the context of new findings on reverse cholesterol transport. Ann Clin Lab Sci. 2002;32:123–36.

58. American Diabetes Association. Physical activity/exercise and diabetes. Diabetes Care. 2004;27(Suppl 1):S58–62.

59. Franz MJ, Bantle JP, Beebe CA, et al. Nutrition principles and recommendations in diabetes. Diabetes Care. 2004;27(Suppl 1):S36–46.

60. Moon J, Cohen Sedgh R, Jackevicius CA. Examining the nocebo effect of statins through statin adverse events reported in the food and drug administration adverse event reporting system. Circ Cardiovasc Qual Outcomes. 2021;14:e007480.

61. Luirink IK, Wiegman A, Kusters DM, et al. 20-year follow-up of statins in children with familial hypercholesterolemia. N Engl J Med. 2019;381:1547–56.

62. Grundy SM, Stone NJ, Bailey AL, et al. 2018 AHA/ACC/AACVPR/AAPA/ABC/ACPM/ADA/AGS/APhA/ASPC/NLA/PCNA guideline on the management of blood cholesterol: a report of the American College of Cardiology/American Heart Association Task Force on Clinical Practice Guidelines. Circulation. 2019;139:e1082–143.

63. Writing Committee, Lloyd-Jones DM, Morris PB, et al. ACC expert consensus decision pathway on the role of nonstatin therapies for LDL-cholesterol lowering in the management of atherosclerotic cardiovascular disease risk: a report of the American College of Cardiology Solution Set Oversight Committee. J Am Coll Cardiol. 2022;2022(80):1366–418.

64. Hero C, Rawshani A, Svensson AM, et al. Association between use of lipid-lowering therapy and cardiovascular diseases and death in individuals with type 1 diabetes. Diabetes Care. 2016;39:996–1003.

65. Collins R, Armitage J, Parish S, Sleigh P, Peto R, Heart Protection Study Collaborative G. MRC/BHF Heart Protection Study of cholesterol-lowering with simvastatin in 5963 people with diabetes: a randomised placebo-controlled trial. Lancet. 2003;361:2005–16.

66. Marcovecchio ML, Chiesa ST, Bond S, et al. ACE inhibitors and statins in adolescents with type 1 Diabetes. N Engl J Med. 2017;377:1733–45.

67. Reston JT, Buelt A, Donahue MP, Neubauer B, Vagichev E, McShea K. Interventions to improve statin tolerance and adherence in patients at risk for cardiovascular disease : a systematic review for the 2020 U.S. Department of Veterans Affairs and U.S. Department of Defense Guidelines for Management of Dyslipidemia. Ann Intern Med. 2020;173:806–12.

68. Cheeley MK, Saseen JJ, Agarwala A, et al. NLA scientific statement on statin intolerance: a new definition and key considerations for ASCVD risk reduction in the statin intolerant patient. J Clin Lipidol. 2022;16:361–75.

69. Hodkinson A, Tsimpida D, Kontopantelis E, Rutter MK, Mamas MA, Panagioti M. Comparative effectiveness of statins on non-high density lipoprotein cholesterol in people with diabetes and at risk of cardiovascular disease: systematic review and network meta-analysis. BMJ. 2022;376:e067731.

70. Giugliano RP, Cannon CP, Blazing MA, et al. Benefit of adding ezetimibe to statin therapy on cardiovascular outcomes and safety in patients with versus without diabetes mellitus: results from IMPROVE-IT (improved reduction of outcomes: vytorin efficacy international trial). Circulation. 2018;137:1571–82.

71. Ouchi Y, Sasaki J, Arai H, et al. Ezetimibe lipid-lowering trial on prevention of atherosclerotic cardiovascular disease in 75 or older (EWTOPIA 75): a randomized, controlled trial. Circulation. 2019;140:992–1003.

72. Nissen SE, Lincoff AM, Brennan D, et al. Bempedoic acid and cardiovascular outcomes in statin-intolerant patients. N Engl J Med. 2023;388:1353–64.

73. Sabatine MS, Giugliano RP, Keech AC, et al. Evolocumab and clinical outcomes in patients with cardiovascular disease. N Engl J Med. 2017;376:1713–22.

74. Ray KK, Colhoun HM, Szarek M, et al. Effects of alirocumab on cardiovascular and metabolic outcomes after acute coronary syndrome in patients with or without diabetes: a prespecified analysis of the ODYSSEY OUTCOMES randomised controlled trial. Lancet Diabetes Endocrinol. 2019;7:618–28.

75. Rodriguez V, Newman JD, Schwartzbard AZ. Towards more specific treatment for diabetic dyslipidemia. Curr Opin Lipidol. 2018;29:307–12.

76. Bavry AA. Pemafibrate to reduce cardiovascular outcomes by reducing triglycerides in patients with diabetes—PROMINENT. https://www.acc.org/Latest-in-Cardiology/Clinical-Trials/2022/11/04/14/15/prominent. Accessed 1 Nov 2023.

77. Ballantyne CM, Bays HE, Kastelein JJ, et al. Efficacy and safety of eicosapentaenoic acid ethyl ester (AMR101) therapy in statin-treated patients with persistent high triglycerides (from the ANCHOR study). Am J Cardiol. 2012;110:984–92.

78. Orringer CE, Jacobson TA, Maki KC. National Lipid Association Scientific Statement on the use of icosapent ethyl in statin-treated patients with elevated triglycerides and high or very-high ASCVD risk. J Clin Lipidol. 2019;13:860–72.

79. Bhatt DL, Steg PG, Miller M, et al. Cardiovascular risk reduction with icosapent ethyl for hypertriglyceridemia. N Engl J Med. 2019;380:11–22.

80. Sweeney TE, Gaine SP, Michos ED. Eicosapentaenoic acid vs. docosahexaenoic acid for the prevention of cardiovascular disease. Curr Opin Endocrinol Diabetes Obes. 2023;30:87–93.

81. Arsenault BJ, Kamstrup PR. Lipoprotein(a) and cardiovascular and valvular diseases: a genetic epidemiological perspective. Atherosclerosis. 2022;349:7–16.

82. Waldeyer C, Makarova N, Zeller T, et al. Lipoprotein(a) and the risk of cardiovascular disease in the European population: results from the BiomarCaRE consortium. Eur Heart J. 2017;38:2490–8.

83. Zhang HW, Zhao X, Guo YL, et al. Elevated lipoprotein (a) levels are associated with the presence and severity of coronary artery disease in patients with type 2 diabetes mellitus. Nutr Metab Cardiovasc Dis. 2018;28:980–6.

84. Saeed A, Sun W, Agarwala A, et al. Lipoprotein(a) levels and risk of cardiovascular disease events in individuals with diabetes mellitus or prediabetes: the atherosclerosis risk in communities study. Atherosclerosis. 2019;282:52–6.

85. Lamina C, Ward NC. Lipoprotein (a) and diabetes mellitus. Atherosclerosis. 2022;349:63–71.

86. Adler AI, Stratton IM, Neil HA, et al. Association of systolic blood pressure with macrovascular and microvascular complications of type 2 diabetes (UKPDS 36): prospective observational study. BMJ. 2000;321:412–9.

87. Karmali KN, Lloyd-Jones DM. Global risk assessment to guide blood pressure management in cardiovascular disease prevention. Hypertension. 2017;69:e2–9.

88. de Boer IH, Bangalore S, Benetos A, et al. Diabetes and hypertension: a position statement by the American Diabetes Association. Diabetes Care. 2017;40:1273–84.

89. Sprint Research Group, Wright JT Jr, Williamson JD, et al. A randomized trial of intensive versus standard blood-pressure control. N Engl J Med. 2015;373:2103–16.

90. Sink KM, Evans GW, Shorr RI, et al. Syncope, hypotension, and falls in the treatment of hypertension: results from the randomized clinical systolic blood pressure intervention trial. J Am Geriatr Soc. 2018;66:679–86.

91. Hansson L, Zanchetti A, Carruthers SG, et al. Effects of intensive blood-pressure lowering and low-dose aspirin in patients with hypertension: principal results of the Hypertension Optimal Treatment (HOT) randomised trial. HOT Study Group. Lancet. 1998;351:1755–62.

92. Accord Study Group, Cushman WC, Evans GW, et al. Effects of intensive blood-pressure control in type 2 diabetes mellitus. N Engl J Med. 2010;362:1575–85.

93. Zhang W, Zhang S, Deng Y, et al. Trial of intensive blood-pressure control in older patients with hypertension. N Engl J Med. 2021;385:1268–79.

94. Khaw KT, Wareham N, Bingham S, Luben R, Welch A, Day N. Association of hemoglobin A1c with cardiovascular disease and mortality in adults: the European prospective investigation into cancer in Norfolk. Ann Intern Med. 2004;141:413–20.
95. Kirkman MS, McCarren M, Shah J, Duckworth W, Abraira C, Group VS. The association between metabolic control and prevalent macrovascular disease in type 2 diabetes: the VA Cooperative Study in diabetes. J Diabetes Complicat. 2006;20:75–80.
96. Selvin E, Marinopoulos S, Berkenblit G, et al. Meta-analysis: glycosylated hemoglobin and cardiovascular disease in diabetes mellitus. Ann Intern Med. 2004;141:421–31.
97. Stratton IM, Adler AI, Neil HA, et al. Association of glycaemia with macrovascular and microvascular complications of type 2 diabetes (UKPDS 35): prospective observational study. BMJ. 2000;321:405–12.
98. Zoungas S, Woodward M, Li Q, et al. Impact of age, age at diagnosis and duration of diabetes on the risk of macrovascular and microvascular complications and death in type 2 diabetes. Diabetologia. 2014;57:2465–74.
99. Skyler JS, Bergenstal R, Bonow RO, et al. Intensive glycemic control and the prevention of cardiovascular events: implications of the ACCORD, ADVANCE, and VA diabetes trials: a position statement of the American Diabetes Association and a scientific statement of the American College of Cardiology Foundation and the American Heart Association. Diabetes Care. 2009;32:187–92.
100. Reichard P, Nilsson BY, Rosenqvist U. The effect of long-term intensified insulin treatment on the development of microvascular complications of diabetes mellitus. N Engl J Med. 1993;329:304–9.
101. Diabetes Control Complications Trial Research Group, Nathan DM, Genuth S, et al. The effect of intensive treatment of diabetes on the development and progression of long-term complications in insulin-dependent diabetes mellitus. N Engl J Med. 1993;329:977–86.
102. Ohkubo Y, Kishikawa H, Araki E, et al. Intensive insulin therapy prevents the progression of diabetic microvascular complications in Japanese patients with non-insulin-dependent diabetes mellitus: a randomized prospective 6-year study. Diabetes Res Clin Pract. 1995;28:103–17.
103. Intensive blood-glucose control with sulphonylureas or insulin compared with conventional treatment and risk of complications in patients with type 2 diabetes (UKPDS 33). UK Prospective Diabetes Study (UKPDS) Group. Lancet. 1998;352:837–53.
104. Nathan DM, Cleary PA, Backlund JY, et al. Intensive diabetes treatment and cardiovascular disease in patients with type 1 diabetes. N Engl J Med. 2005;353:2643–53.
105. Diabetes Control Complications Trial/Epidemiology of Diabetes Interventions and Complications (DCCT/EDIC) Research Group, Nathan DM, Zinman B, et al. Modern-day clinical course of type 1 diabetes mellitus after 30 years' duration: the diabetes control and complications trial/epidemiology of diabetes interventions and complications and Pittsburgh epidemiology of diabetes complications experience (1983–2005). Arch Intern Med. 2009;169:1307–16.
106. Emerging Risk Factors Collaboration, Di Angelantonio E, Kaptoge S, et al. Association of Cardiometabolic Multimorbidity with Mortality. JAMA. 2015;314:52–60.
107. Davies MJ, Aroda VR, Collins BS, et al. Management of hyperglycaemia in type 2 diabetes, 2022. A consensus report by the American Diabetes Association (ADA) and the European Association for the Study of Diabetes (EASD). Diabetologia. 2022;65:1925–66.
108. Griffin SJ, Leaver JK, Irving GJ. Impact of metformin on cardiovascular disease: a meta-analysis of randomised trials among people with type 2 diabetes. Diabetologia. 2017;60:1620–9.
109. Nesti L, Trico D, Mengozzi A, Natali A. Rethinking pioglitazone as a cardioprotective agent: a new perspective on an overlooked drug. Cardiovasc Diabetol. 2021;20:109.
110. Dream Trial Investigators, Gerstein HC, Yusuf S, et al. Effect of rosiglitazone on the frequency of diabetes in patients with impaired glucose tolerance or impaired fasting glucose: a randomised controlled trial. Lancet. 2006;368:1096–105.
111. Kernan WN, Viscoli CM, Furie KL, et al. Pioglitazone after ischemic stroke or transient ischemic attack. N Engl J Med. 2016;374:1321–31.

112. DeFronzo RA, Tripathy D, Schwenke DC, et al. Pioglitazone for diabetes prevention in impaired glucose tolerance. N Engl J Med. 2011;364:1104–15.
113. U.S. Food & Drug Administration. FDA Drug Safety Communication: updated FDA review concludes that use of type 2 diabetes medicine pioglitazone may be linked to an increased risk of bladder cancer. https://www.fda.gov/drugs/drug-safety-and-availability/fda-drug-safety-communication-updated-fda-review-concludes-use-type-2-diabetes-medicine-pioglitazone. Accessed 2 Nov 2023.
114. Chiasson JL, Josse RG, Gomis R, et al. Acarbose treatment and the risk of cardiovascular disease and hypertension in patients with impaired glucose tolerance: the STOP-NIDDM trial. JAMA. 2003;290:486–94.
115. Scirica BM, Bhatt DL, Braunwald E, et al. Saxagliptin and cardiovascular outcomes in patients with type 2 diabetes mellitus. N Engl J Med. 2013;369:1317–26.
116. White WB, Cannon CP, Heller SR, et al. Alogliptin after acute coronary syndrome in patients with type 2 diabetes. N Engl J Med. 2013;369:1327–35.
117. Green JB, Bethel MA, Armstrong PW, et al. Effect of sitagliptin on cardiovascular outcomes in type 2 diabetes. N Engl J Med. 2015;373:232–42.
118. Rosenstock J, Kahn SE, Johansen OE, et al. Effect of Linagliptin vs glimepiride on major adverse cardiovascular outcomes in patients with type 2 diabetes: the CAROLINA randomized clinical trial. JAMA. 2019;322:1155–66.
119. Rosenstock J, Perkovic V, Johansen OE, et al. Effect of Linagliptin vs placebo on major cardiovascular events in adults with type 2 diabetes and high cardiovascular and renal risk: the CARMELINA randomized clinical trial. JAMA. 2019;321:69–79.
120. Li L, Li S, Deng K, et al. Dipeptidyl peptidase-4 inhibitors and risk of heart failure in type 2 diabetes: systematic review and meta-analysis of randomised and observational studies. BMJ. 2016;352:i610.
121. Secrest MH, Udell JA, Filion KB. The cardiovascular safety trials of DPP-4 inhibitors, GLP-1 agonists, and SGLT2 inhibitors. Trends Cardiovasc Med. 2017;27:194–202.
122. Kristensen SL, Rorth R, Jhund PS, et al. Cardiovascular, mortality, and kidney outcomes with GLP-1 receptor agonists in patients with type 2 diabetes: a systematic review and meta-analysis of cardiovascular outcome trials. Lancet Diabetes Endocrinol. 2019;7:776–85.
123. Rosenstock J, Wysham C, Frias JP, et al. Efficacy and safety of a novel dual GIP and GLP-1 receptor agonist tirzepatide in patients with type 2 diabetes (SURPASS-1): a double-blind, randomised, phase 3 trial. Lancet. 2021;398:143–55.
124. Dahl D, Onishi Y, Norwood P, et al. Effect of subcutaneous tirzepatide vs placebo added to titrated insulin glargine on glycemic control in patients with type 2 diabetes: the SURPASS-5 randomized clinical trial. JAMA. 2022;327:534–45.
125. Gastaldelli A, Cusi K, Fernandez Lando L, Bray R, Brouwers B, Rodriguez A. Effect of tirzepatide versus insulin degludec on liver fat content and abdominal adipose tissue in people with type 2 diabetes (SURPASS-3 MRI): a substudy of the randomised, open-label, parallel-group, phase 3 SURPASS-3 trial. Lancet Diabetes Endocrinol. 2022;10:393–406.
126. Sattar N, McGuire DK, Pavo I, et al. Tirzepatide cardiovascular event risk assessment: a pre-specified meta-analysis. Nat Med. 2022;28:591–8.
127. Das SR, Everett BM, Birtcher KK, et al. 2020 expert consensus decision pathway on novel therapies for cardiovascular risk reduction in patients with type 2 diabetes: a report of the American College of Cardiology Solution Set Oversight Committee. J Am Coll Cardiol. 2020;76:1117–45.
128. Garber AJ, Handelsman Y, Grunberger G, et al. Consensus statement by the American Association of Clinical Endocrinologists and American College of Endocrinology on the Comprehensive Type 2 Diabetes Management Algorithm—2020 executive summary. Endocr Pract. 2020;26:107–39.
129. Cosentino F, Grant PJ, Aboyans V, et al. 2019 ESC Guidelines on diabetes, pre-diabetes, and cardiovascular diseases developed in collaboration with the EASD. Eur Heart J. 2020;41:255–323.

130. Zelniker TA, Wiviott SD, Raz I, et al. SGLT2 inhibitors for primary and secondary prevention of cardiovascular and renal outcomes in type 2 diabetes: a systematic review and meta-analysis of cardiovascular outcome trials. Lancet. 2019;393:31–9.

131. Zelniker TA, Wiviott SD, Raz I, et al. Comparison of the effects of glucagon-like peptide receptor agonists and sodium-glucose cotransporter 2 inhibitors for prevention of major adverse cardiovascular and renal outcomes in type 2 Diabetes mellitus. Circulation. 2019;139:2022–31.

132. Furtado RHM, Bonaca MP, Raz I, et al. Dapagliflozin and cardiovascular outcomes in patients with type 2 Diabetes mellitus and previous myocardial infarction. Circulation. 2019;139:2516–27.

133. Li D, Wang T, Shen S, Fang Z, Dong Y, Tang H. Urinary tract and genital infections in patients with type 2 diabetes treated with sodium-glucose co-transporter 2 inhibitors: a meta-analysis of randomized controlled trials. Diabetes Obes Metab. 2017;19:348–55.

134. Jabbour S, Seufert J, Scheen A, Bailey CJ, Karup C, Langkilde AM. Dapagliflozin in patients with type 2 diabetes mellitus: a pooled analysis of safety data from phase IIb/III clinical trials. Diabetes Obes Metab. 2018;20:620–8.

135. Erondu N, Desai M, Ways K, Meininger G. Diabetic ketoacidosis and related events in the canagliflozin type 2 diabetes clinical program. Diabetes Care. 2015;38:1680–6.

136. Collaborative overview of randomised trials of antiplatelet therapy--I: prevention of death, myocardial infarction, and stroke by prolonged antiplatelet therapy in various categories of patients. Antiplatelet Trialists' Collaboration. BMJ. 1994;308:81–106.

137. Antithrombotic Trialists Collaboration, Baigent C, Blackwell L, et al. Aspirin in the primary and secondary prevention of vascular disease: collaborative meta-analysis of individual participant data from randomised trials. Lancet. 2009;373:1849–60.

138. Perk J, De Backer G, Gohlke H, et al. European Guidelines on cardiovascular disease prevention in clinical practice (version 2012). The Fifth Joint Task Force of the European Society of Cardiology and Other Societies on cardiovascular disease prevention in clinical practice (constituted by representatives of nine societies and by invited experts). Eur Heart J. 2012;33:1635–701.

139. Belch J, MacCuish A, Campbell I, et al. The prevention of progression of arterial disease and diabetes (POPADAD) trial: factorial randomised placebo controlled trial of aspirin and antioxidants in patients with diabetes and asymptomatic peripheral arterial disease. BMJ. 2008;337:a1840.

140. Zhang C, Sun A, Zhang P, et al. Aspirin for primary prevention of cardiovascular events in patients with diabetes: a meta-analysis. Diabetes Res Clin Pract. 2010;87:211–8.

141. De Berardis G, Sacco M, Strippoli GF, et al. Aspirin for primary prevention of cardiovascular events in people with diabetes: meta-analysis of randomised controlled trials. BMJ. 2009;339:b4531.

142. Ascend Study Collaborative Group, Bowman L, Mafham M, et al. Effects of aspirin for primary prevention in persons with diabetes mellitus. N Engl J Med. 2018;379:1529–39.

143. Gaziano JM, Brotons C, Coppolecchia R, et al. Use of aspirin to reduce risk of initial vascular events in patients at moderate risk of cardiovascular disease (ARRIVE): a randomised, double-blind, placebo-controlled trial. Lancet. 2018;392:1036–46.

144. McNeil JJ, Wolfe R, Woods RL, et al. Effect of aspirin on cardiovascular events and bleeding in the healthy elderly. N Engl J Med. 2018;379:1509–18.

Cardiac Rhythms and Cardiovascular Outcomes

Bahij Kreidieh, Ali Keramati, and Peter R. Kowey

Key Points

- The field of cardiac electrophysiology is young and rapidly evolving with a wealth of outcomes data continually added to the literature.
- Bradyarrhythmias are common and occur from various etiologies including congenital, iatrogenic, and others.
- Cardiac pacing largely mitigates the deleterious effects of bradyarrhythmia, and it continues to progress with the evolution of modern technology.
- Supraventricular arrhythmias are mostly benign, but may cause significant symptomatic discomfort.
- Modern treatments of most supraventricular arrhythmias via ablative and drug therapy are highly effective with low complication rates.
- Atrial fibrillation and atrial flutter are very prevalent and cause increased morbidity and mortality through various pathophysiologic means.
- The optimal treatment strategy of atrial fibrillation, in terms of rhythm vs rate control, remains poorly defined.
- Catheter ablation of atrial fibrillation has proven effective in many patients and adds a crucial tool in the management of this disease entity.
- Over the last two decades, there has been substantial improvement in the field of stroke prevention in atrial fibrillation, both with pharmacologic and procedural techniques.

B. Kreidieh · A. Keramati
The Lankenau Institute for Medical Research, Wynnewood, PA, USA
e-mail: KeramatiA@mlhs.org

P. R. Kowey (✉)
The Lankenau Institute for Medical Research, Wynnewood, PA, USA

Department of Medicine, Thomas Jefferson University, Philadelphia, PA, USA
e-mail: koweyp@mlhs.org

K. C. Maki, D. P. Wilson (eds.), *Cardiovascular Outcomes Research*, Contemporary Cardiology, https://doi.org/10.1007/978-3-031-54960-1_15

- Ventricular arrhythmias may be a source of significant morbidity as well as a cause of sudden death.
- Implantable cardioverter-defibrillators (ICDs) have proven instrumental in preventing sudden death from ventricular tachycardia, whereas medical and ablative therapy play a role in the reduction of ICD shocks.

1   Introduction

Since its inception with the recording of the His bundle in 1969, the field of cardiac electrophysiology has evolved dramatically. Over the ensuing 50 years, a wealth of basic and clinical studies revolutionized our understanding of the electrophysiologic properties of the heart. Originally confined to the operating room, ablation procedures have slowly expanded into the cardiac catheterization laboratory. With this transition, cardiac electrophysiology has developed into its own sub-specialty within the field of cardiology. Today, electrophysiology involves pacemaker implantation and complex percutaneous catheter-based ablations of supraventricular and ventricular arrhythmias. Additionally, with the invention of the implantable cardioverter-defibrillator (ICD) and cardiac resynchronization therapy, electrophysiologists have helped mitigate the outcomes of ischemic and non-ischemic cardiomyopathies. Contemporaneously, the use of pharmacologic agents by electrophysiologists has evolved with the development of various anti-arrhythmic drugs and novel anticoagulants.

In this chapter, we provide a contemporary review of the different cardiac arrhythmias, and delve into their impact on cardiovascular outcomes. In doing so, we focus our attention on epidemiologic trends over time, as well as the impact of common interventions meant to mitigate the adversities of arrhythmic disease. The outcomes of greatest interest in modern-day studies, and thus the focus of most of our analysis, relate to cardiovascular and overall mortality as well as hospitalization and cost.

2   Bradyarrhythmias

Bradycardia is defined as a heart rate below the normal range appropriate for one's age. Bradyarrhythmias result from abnormal impulse formation and/or conduction. This occurs at the sinoatrial (SA) node in sinus node dysfunction or at the level of the atrioventricular (AV) node or the distal His-Purkinje system in the AV block. While epidemiologic data are available in several global locations and at various timepoints, outcomes data are more difficult to track over time. In view of its proven benefit, it is both unnecessary and unethical to withhold pacing in a control group when conducting traditional randomized controlled trials in this population. We provide a review of bradyarrhythmias and highlight the advancements that have impacted disease outcomes in recent years.

2.1 Sinus Node Dysfunction

The true incidence of sinus node dysfunction in the general population is poorly defined. In 1997, sinus node dysfunction was the indication for 48% of permanent pacemaker (PPM) implantations in the US. In 1998, for Medicare patients older than 65 years, the rate of hospitalization for sinus node dysfunction was 207 per 100,000 person-years. In the US, 78,000 cases of sick sinus syndrome occurred in 2012, a number that is projected to increase to 172,000 in 2060. The risk increases with age and is lower in African Americans as compared to Whites. Other associated factors include increased body mass index (BMI), height, hypertension, right bundle branch block, and a prior cardiovascular event.

The presence of sick sinus syndrome is associated with increased risk of AF, heart failure (HF), stroke, PPM implantation, and death [1]. PPM implantation has proven beneficial in this population, and mortality becomes comparable to controls with its use. Notably, mortality does not differ significantly with the use of ventricular-only vs dual-chamber pacing [2].

2.2 Atrioventricular (AV) Block

The prevalence of the first-degree AV block within the healthy population varies in observational studies, anywhere from 0.1 to 7.8%, with higher likelihood occurring with advancing age, male gender, and black race as compared to white. The clinical presentation of the first-degree AV block is not generally associated with symptoms. In rare cases, marked PR prolongation results in atrial contraction following a preceding ventricular contraction. This may present as "pacemaker syndrome." Overall, the first-degree AV block is associated with an increased risk of AF, need for PPM implantation, and death [3]. PPM implantation has not been shown to improve survival in patients with the first-degree AV block [4]. Although the Heart Rhythm Society (HRS)/American College of Cardiology (ACC) guidelines do not recommend a pacemaker for the first-degree AV block, pacemaker implantation can potentially be considered if the symptoms are suggestive of "pacemaker syndrome" in the setting of markedly prolonged PR interval. This phenomenon is exceedingly rare and infrequently seen in clinical practice.

The second-degree AV block is defined as intermittent transmission of impulse from the atria to the ventricles. The second-degree AV block can be further classified as Mobitz I or Mobitz II. The site of block in Mobitz I is generally in the AV node and, for this reason, it typically does not progress to the high-grade AV block. Mobitz I is relatively common in young and healthy individuals, especially at night

(1–2%). Similar to the first-degree AV block, the clinical presentation of Mobitz I is benign and it rarely produces symptoms. The management of Mobitz I depends on the presence and severity of symptoms. In a small subset of patients who are symptomatic from Mobitz I and in whom no reversible causes were identified, implantation of a pacemaker may be indicated.

Mobitz II manifests as an abrupt loss of conduction from the atria to the ventricle. The third-degree AV block manifests as complete dissociation between the atrial and ventricular electrical activity. Mobitz II and third-degree AV block are very rare in otherwise healthy people (<0.01%) and, when present, they are typically harbingers of underlying cardiovascular disease. Generally, pacemaker implantation is indicated in patients with the high-grade AV block in the presence or absence of symptoms. In those with the third-degree AV block, the intervention has proven to reduce mortality [5] and represents the cornerstone of therapy.

As an alternative to electronic device implantation, biological pacing technology, using somatic gene transfer, cell transplantation or cell fusion, has been in preclinical development over the last two decades [6]. It may prove advantageous in the treatment of congenital heart block, atrial fibrillation (AF) with slow ventricular response, and electronic device-related infection. However, it is yet unclear when this technology will be ready for clinical application.

2.3 Conduction Disturbances Post-Trans-Catheter Aortic Valve Replacement (TAVR)

Conduction disease after trans-catheter aortic valve replacement (TAVR) merits special consideration. In the last few years, there has been an expansion in the indications for this procedure and, as such, a substantial rise in the volume of TAVR cases performed worldwide. The procedure is frequently associated with the iatrogenic development of the left bundle branch block (LBBB), as well as high-grade AV block/complete heart block (CHB). New onset LBBB has been reported in 4–65% of patients after TAVR. The association between LBBB development and increased 1-year mortality after TAVR is inconsistent in the literature [7], while the presence of LBBB with wide QRS duration has been associated with sudden cardiac death (SCD) [8], all-cause mortality [9] and rehospitalization for HF [9] during follow-up.

A meta-analysis of 41 studies (11,210 patients) showed male sex, first-degree AV block, preprocedural left anterior fascicular block, preprocedural right bundle branch block, intra-operative heart block, and the use of self-expandable prosthesis to be predictors of the need for pacemaker implantation after TAVR. Like LBBB, there are conflicting data about the association of pacemaker implantation and 1-year mortality after TAVR [10, 11]. At this point, there is no unified recommendation for the management of post-TAVR conduction disturbances and indications may vary according to operator and center-specific policies [7].

3 Supraventricular Tachycardia

Supraventricular tachycardia (SVT) is a broad term used to describe any arrhythmia that requires an atrial structure for arrhythmia maintenance. It encompasses a multitude of tachy-arrhythmias with varying mechanisms. With the exception of AF and atrial flutter (AFL), many of these arrhythmias share a common diagnostic and treatment algorithm, and will be discussed jointly in this section. AF and AFL will be covered separately.

The majority of SVTs are considered benign arrhythmias and an infrequent cause of mortality. In this setting, the treatment outcomes generally relate to symptomatology, and large-scale patient randomization is scarce as it is considered superfluous. We provide an overview of the available disease trends and pertinent outcomes data mostly derived from observational studies.

3.1 *Epidemiology*

The prevalence of SVT within the general population is estimated at 0.225% [4]. It is more common among females and in individuals who are 65 years and older. Patients with SVT in the absence of structural heart disease are typically younger and have higher arrhythmic rates compared to those with cardiovascular disease [12]. SVT accounts for approximately 50,000 emergency department (ED) visits a year, 24% of which require hospital admission. Intermediate-term monitoring suggests that clinically undetected SVT is likely much more common than data from the ED visits suggested [4].

SVTs can be divided into three main subcategories: AV nodal reentrant tachycardia (AVNRT), AV re-entrant (or reciprocating) tachycardia (AVRT), and atrial tachycardia (AT) [13] (Fig. 1). Other subcategories are rare and beyond the scope of this chapter.

AVNRT is more common in middle-aged and older patients, whereas AVRT is equally prevalent or more common in younger patients. A bypass tract may or may not manifest itself as delta waves in the ECG. The prevalence of delta waves (manifest bypass tract) is approximately 0.1–0.3% in the general population, although it does not necessarily result in clinically relevant arrhythmia [14]. Atrial tachycardia constitutes the third most common SVT. Multi-focal atrial tachycardia (MAT) is rare overall and most common among older patients (average onset 70–72 years) with underlying pulmonary disease. MAT is associated with higher mortality, but this is attributed to co-existent medical conditions as opposed to the tachycardia itself [15].

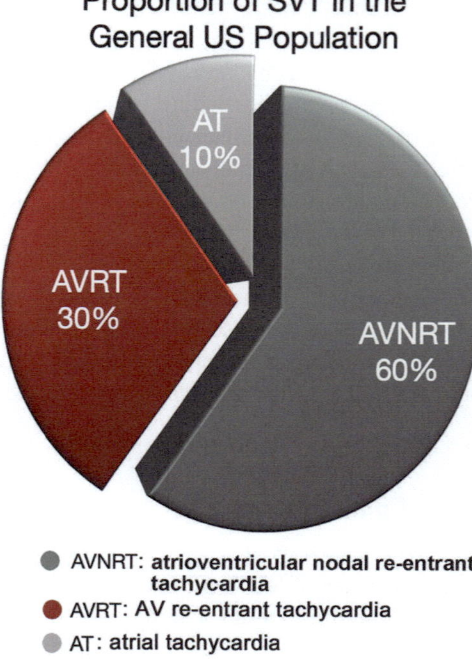

Fig. 1 Proportion of supraventricular tachycardia (SVT) within the US population. Other subtypes of SVT are very rare. Abbreviations: *AT* atrial tachycardia, *AVRT* AV re-entrant tachycardia, *AVNRT* atrioventricular nodal re-entrant tachycardia

3.2 SVTs and Outcomes

Paroxysmal SVT is often associated with symptoms of palpitations and patient discomfort. In very rare cases, incessant SVT may lead to tachycardia-induced cardiomyopathy or even SCD [16, 17]. It is also associated with increased stroke risk, although the absolute risk of stroke is low. Despite their benign nature in the general population, the occurrence of SVTs during pregnancy needs to be managed carefully. Paroxysmal SVT during pregnancy is associated with worse maternal and fetal outcomes including maternal morbidity, preterm birth, cesarean delivery, low birth weight, and fetal stress [18].

Wolff-Parkinson-White (WPW) syndrome carries an increased risk of SCD. Atrial fibrillation occurs in 10–30% of patients with WPW syndrome [19]. The risk of SCD is attributed to rapid conduction of AF through an accessory pathway, resulting in ventricular fibrillation [4]. While the majority of patients with WPW syndrome have no added risk of SCD compared to controls, electrophysiologic properties have been found that correlate with increased risk and are useful for patient stratification. These include the inducibility of AVRT, short accessory pathway refractory period, inducibility of AF, and its shortest RR interval during atrial fibrillation [20].

3.3 SVT Treatments

In the acute setting, the initial treatment of SVT is vagal maneuvers or adenosine to terminate the tachycardia. Intravenous beta blocker (BB) and calcium channel blocker (CCB) therapy may also be attempted. If a wide complex rhythm is present, recognizing pre-excited AF is crucial to avoid ventricular fibrillation. Generally, AV nodal agents are contraindicated in pre-excited atrial fibrillation, and flecainide or procainamide is utilized to slow down conduction through the bypass tract. In the setting of hemodynamic instability or drug-refractory SVT, synchronized cardioversion is indicated.

For the ongoing management of paroxysmal SVT, treatment strategy is individually tailored based on symptomatology, frequency of episodes, and patient preference regarding medical vs ablative strategy. BB and CCB therapies are reasonable and effective first-line therapies in patients who do not desire electrophysiology study (EPS) and ablation [14]. Alternatively, anti-arrhythmic drug (AAD) therapy may be effective, but frequently has significant side effects and contraindications, and is thus reserved as second-line therapy for those who fail BB/CCB treatment. Flecainide or propafenone may be utilized in the absence of structural heart disease. Within a year of treatment, the incidence of effective arrhythmia suppression (<2 episodes) and drug safety is 93% for flecainide and 86% for propafenone [21]. These drugs have been found to be pro-arrhythmic in the setting of ischemic or structural heart disease and are contraindicated in this population. Sotalol and dofetilide are useful options for patients with structural and/or ischemic heart disease, but also carry a pro-arrhythmic risk and are similarly considered as second-line therapy. If the above therapy is ineffective, amiodarone may be used in select patient populations but comes with an increased risk of multi-organ toxicity.

3.4 Catheter Ablation

For patients willing to undergo the procedure, catheter ablation is the keystone of SVT treatment. It offers a "curative" option for most subtypes of SVT and has a long-standing, well-established safety and efficacy profile. In the setting of SVT, where resultant mortality is rare, and the symptomatic benefit of a curative procedure is obvious, there has been no clear need for large-scale prospective randomization trials. As such, outcomes data are estimated from observational studies, although in contemporary clinical practice, the numbers may vary slightly from prior observational reports (Fig. 2) [14, 22–24]. Catheter ablation of AVNRT has a 96–97% acute procedural efficacy rate with a 5% recurrence rate [22, 23]. AVRT ablation carries a 93% acute success rate and an 8% recurrence rate [22, 23]. Ablation of focal AT has an 80–100% acute success rate and a 4–27% recurrence rate [14, 24]. Overall, catheter ablation of SVT is safe and has a less than 3% major

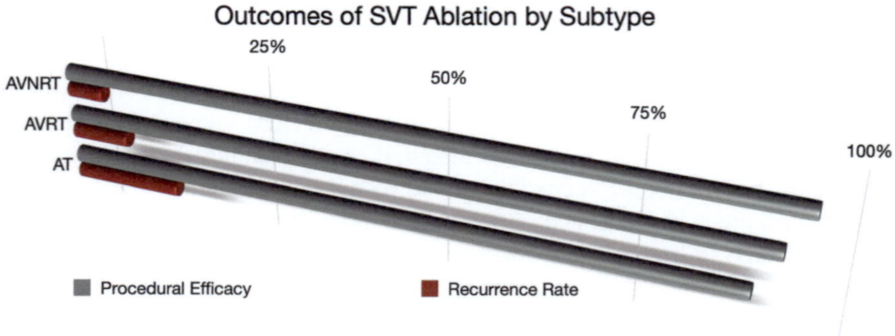

Fig. 2 Catheter ablation of atrioventricular nodal re-entrant tachycardia (AVNRT) has a 96–97% acute procedural efficacy with a 5% recurrence rate [22, 23]. Atrioventricular re-entrant tachycardia (AVRT) ablation carries a 93% acute success rate and 8% recurrence rate [22, 23]. Ablation of focal atrial tachycardia (AT) has an 80–100% acute success rate and 4–27% recurrence rate [14, 24]. Abbreviation: *SVT* supraventricular tachycardia

complication rate, which includes vascular complications, pericardial effusion, need for PPM, and death [14].

4 Atrial Fibrillation and Atrial Flutter

Atrial fibrillation is the most common sustained arrhythmia in humans, with a substantial impact on the global healthcare system. It is associated with increased risk of HF, stroke, dementia, and overall mortality. Considerable efforts are ongoing to delineate the mechanism of AF and its downstream effects, as well as to halt its progression and reduce its burden. We provide a broad review of the current state of AF and AFL, as well as the relevant contemporary trials in the field of AF/AFL treatment.

4.1 *Epidemiology*

In 2010, the prevalence of AF was estimated to be 2.7–6.1 million in the US and 8.8 million in adults aged >55 years in the European Union [4]. These numbers are projected to rise to 12.1 million in the US by 2030 and 17.9 million in European adults by 2060. The lifetime risk of incident AF in individuals of European ancestry is approximated to be as high as 1 in 3. This risk appears to vary significantly between races. In the Atherosclerosis Risk in Communities (ARIC) study, the lifetime risk of developing AF is approximately 1 in 3 in Whites and 1 in 5 African Americans [25]. Even after adjustment for AF risk factors, the incidence of AF is lower in African American, Hispanic, and Asian populations as compared to Whites.

In recent years, with the prominence of implantable rhythm monitoring devices including pacemakers and defibrillators, as well as the advent of wearable rhythm detection devices, the true incidence of subclinical AF has come into question. While not yet well quantified, the implications of a subclinical AF diagnosis and the need for more widespread screening are poorly defined. No existing studies have proven a benefit of AF screening in the reduction of stroke or mortality. Multiple studies are ongoing in efforts to evaluate the risks and benefits of anticoagulant therapy in the high stroke-risk population in the absence of known AF history. These efforts are expected to help guide future decision algorithms regarding the need and process of AF screening [4].

4.2 Atrial Fibrillation Risk Factors

Many risk factors have been linked to a higher incidence of AF. These include age, hypertension, elevated BMI, smoking, diabetes, cardiovascular disease including congenital heart disease, hyperthyroidism, chronic kidney disease, excessive alcohol consumption, central sleep apnea, etc. [4]. Similarly, AF may be triggered by reversible conditions such as cardiac surgery (30%), sepsis (23%), acute myocardial infarction (MI) (18%), and others. AF that occurs in the setting of a precipitant condition remains clinically relevant, as it recurs frequently afterwards [4].

Multiple tools have been developed over time to predict AF. The most recent and well-validated model is CHARGE-AF, developed by the Cohorts for Heart Aging and Research in Genomic Epidemiology (CHARGE)-AF Consortium [26]. It provides a 5-year predictive tool derived from clinical characteristics including age, diastolic and systolic blood pressures, race, height, weight, treatment of hypertension, diabetes, history of MI, smoking, and HF. The prediction model was validated within multi-ethnic populations, both in the US and Europe.

4.3 Atrial Fibrillation and Outcomes

In 2016, AF was the cause of death in 24,855 people in the US, and was listed on 154,816 death certificates [27]. The number of global AF/AFL-attributable deaths within the same year was estimated at 200,000. The adjusted risk of death is stronger in females than males and is thought to reduce the survival advantage that is normally seen in females. Overall, the risk of death is higher in African Americans and Hispanics with AF; however, after adjustment for comorbid conditions, these populations had a lower risk of death than their White counterparts. Mortality varies substantially between counties within the US. Similarly, on a global scale, significant regional variations were observed in prospective registries, whereby South

American and African countries had double the annual AF mortality rate compared to North America, Western Europe, and Australia ($p < 0.001$). A Swedish study also noted higher mortality within lower socioeconomic groups.

Limited observational studies suggest high early mortality from the time of diagnosis of AF. While stroke death has classically been of greatest concern, the Randomized Evaluation of Long-Term Anticoagulation Therapy (RE-LY) trial showed that as a proportion of all AF deaths, stroke constituted 7%, whereas SCD accounted for 22.25%, progressive HF accounted for 15.1%, and 35.8% were related to non-cardiovascular causes [28]. AF is considered to be an independent risk factor for all-cause mortality in patients with other cardiovascular comorbidities including peripheral vascular disease [29], hypertrophic cardiomyopathy [30], MI [31], post-coronary artery bypass graft [32], post-TAVR [33], heart failure with reduced ejection fraction (HFrEF) [34], and heart failure with preserved ejection fraction (HFpEF) [34, 35]. Furthermore, AF is associated with higher all-cause mortality in patients with diabetes [36], end-stage kidney disease [37], cerebrovascular accidents (CVA) [38], and sepsis [39].

4.4   Atrial Fibrillation and Embolic Events

AF is associated with an increased risk of both CVA and extracranial systemic emboli. The aggregate of four large randomized anticoagulation trials reported a rate of systemic emboli of 0.24 per 100 person-years, as compared to 1.92 ischemic strokes per 100 person-years [4]. Both events were associated with increased mortality when compared to AF patients who had neither. Prior to widespread adoption of anticoagulant therapy, AF was associated with 4–5 times increased risk of stroke. The risk of stroke is variable across studies, largely due to the heterogeneity of comorbidities within them. In studies conducted in Medicare recipients, African American and Hispanic race were associated with an increased risk of stroke within AF patients as compared to Whites. Notably, among stroke patients overall, the presence of AF is associated with increased CVA severity and higher mortality, as well as increased ischemic recurrence rates. Higher AF burden is also associated with an increased incidence of stroke and worse outcomes [40].

The CHADS2-VASC score has been widely adopted by the American and European guidelines and remains the main stroke prediction tool in routine clinical practice [41]. It has high specificity for low and intermediate stroke risk, but low specificity for high risk. Specific biomarkers have also been associated with an increased incidence of stroke including high sensitivity troponin and N-terminal fragment B-type natriuretic peptide [42]. When age, biomarkers, and prior clinical history of transient ischemic attack/stroke are combined into the ABC (Age, Biomarkers, Clinical History) stroke score, they perform better than the traditional CHADS2-VASC score in predicting stroke in patients with AF.

4.5 Atrial Fibrillation and Heart Failure

AF-mediated cardiomyopathy (AMC) is a term often utilized when AF is established as the sole cause or precipitating factor in ventricular dysfunction. It is defined as the development of otherwise unexplained HF or the exacerbation of pre-existing HF in the presence of uncontrolled AF [43].

The acute hemodynamic effects of AF are particularly relevant in the intensive care setting, where AF remains the most commonly encountered arrhythmia [44]. The acute loss of atrial systole, as well as rapid ventricular rates, have been shown to lead to hemodynamic compromise and drop in the cardiac output [44]. In fact, 37% of critically ill patients develop immediate hemodynamic instability with new onset AF [45]. Cardioversion and restoration of sinus rhythm can lead to a 15–25% acute increase in cardiac output [46, 47]. Over the long term, AF causes both atrial and ventricular remodeling. In the atrium, electrical and structural remodeling leads to the perpetuation of atrial fibrillation. Ultimately, ventricular remodeling from AF results in systolic and diastolic dysfunction, as well as tricuspid and mitral regurgitation. Numerous studies have examined the interplay of HF and AF and have documented the deleterious effect this combination has on cardiovascular outcomes, as well as the benefit attained from the restoration of sinus rhythm (Table 1) [28, 48–52].

Table 1 Major findings of the studies examining the effect of coexistent HF and AF on cardiovascular outcomes

Study	Study type	Major outcomes
ORBIT-AF [94]	Registry	3.6% of AF patients developed HF over 2 years (64% HFpEF; 13.5% HfrEF). PeAF was more strongly associated with the occurrence of HF as compared to PAF
Framingham [48]	Registry	AF was strongly associated with the development of both HfpEF (HR of 2.3) and HfrEF (HR of 1.3). The combination of AF and HF was associated with increased all-cause mortality (HR of 1.6 for men; 95% CI, 1.2–2.1 and HR of 2.7 for women; 95% CI, 2.0–3.6)
RE-LY [95]	RCT	HF and SCD accounted for 15.1% and 22% of deaths in AF, respectively
PABA-CHF [51]	RCT	76% of patients who underwent ablation had significantly improved LVEF vs 25% in those who underwent AV nodal ablation and biventricular pacing
CAMERA-MRI [52]	RCT	57% of patients in the catheter ablation arm had normalization of LVEF vs 9% in the rate control medical therapy arm ($p = 0.0002$)

Abbreviations: *AF* atrial fibrillation, *AV* atrioventricular, *CAMERA-MRI* Catheter Ablation Versus Medical Rate Control in Atrial Fibrillation and Heart Failure—An MRI-Guided Multicenter Randomized Controlled Trial, *CI* confidence interval, *HF* heart failure, *HfpEF* heart failure with preserved ejection fraction, *HfrEF* heart failure with reduced ejection fraction, *HR* hazard ratio, *LVEF* left ventricular ejection fraction, *ORBIT-AF* Outcomes Registry for Better Informed Treatment of Atrial Fibrillation, *PABA-CHF* Pulmonary Vein Antrum Isolation Versus AV Node Ablation with Bi-Ventricular Pacing for Treatment of Atrial Fibrillation in Patients With Congestive Heart Failure, *PAF* paroxysmal atrial fibrillation, *PeAF* persistent atrial fibrillation, *RCT* randomized controlled trial, *RE-LY* Randomized Evaluation of Long-Term Anticoagulation Therapy, *SCD* sudden cardiac death

4.6 Impact of Atrial Fibrillation Treatment Strategy on Outcomes

The primary objective of AF treatment is symptom relief and the prevention of the downstream effects associated with progressive AF burden. The optimal treatment strategy for AF has been debated for multiple decades and remains largely inconclusive. Two primary treatment strategies have been utilized. Rhythm control seeks to establish and maintain sinus rhythm via anti-arrhythmic drug (AAD) and ablative therapy (see below). Rate control, on the other hand, focuses on the suppression of high ventricular rates during episodes of AF. Multiple large randomized trials compared these strategies head-to-head (Table 2) [53–58], but have failed to show a mortality benefit in either treatment arm. Overall, there was some symptomatic benefit from rhythm control, but this came at the expense of increased hospitalization for anti-arrhythmic drug titration. These trials were carried out prior to the widespread adoption of catheter ablation, bringing into question the applicability of their results. More recently, the Early Treatment of Atrial Fibrillation for Stroke Prevention Trial 4 (EAST-AFNET 4) randomized patients to early (within a year of diagnosis) rhythm control vs usual care [59]. It showed a significant reduction in the primary composite outcome of death from cardiovascular causes, stroke, or cardiovascular hospitalization. The findings suggest there may be an optimal time for the institution of rhythm control prior to the development of atrial myopathy and more persistent AF. To date, no reliable comparison of catheter ablation with rate control therapy has been conducted, but it will be instrumental in answering the rhythm vs rate control question more conclusively.

4.7 Atrial Fibrillation and Catheter Ablation

Ablation of AF has evolved over the last 20 years. From a procedural standpoint, the achievement of successful AF ablation requires isolation of the pulmonary vein antra (Fig. 3) using radiofrequency, cryoballoon, or laser. Multiple randomized trials have proven the superiority of catheter ablation over AAD therapy in the maintenance of sinus rhythm for paroxysmal atrial fibrillation (PAF). The Radiofrequency Ablation vs Antiarrhythmic Drugs as First-line Therapy of Atrial Fibrillation 2 (RAAFT-2) trial compared radiofrequency catheter ablation to anti-arrhythmic drug therapy in patients with PAF who were AAD-naïve [60]. It showed a lower arrhythmia recurrence rate at 2 years with radiofrequency catheter ablation. Similarly, the STOP-AF First: Cryoballoon Catheter Ablation in Antiarrhythmic Drug Naïve Paroxysmal Atrial Fibrillation study showed a decreased recurrence of atrial arrhythmias post-cryoballoon ablation in a similar PAF patient population as compared to AAD therapy [61]. Although catheter ablation is more efficacious compared to AADs, freedom from recurrence remains lower than 80–90% in PAF and significantly lower in the presence of persistent AF (PeAF)/permanent AF (PerAF) or structural heart disease [62–65].

Table 2 Major trials comparing various outcomes of rate vs rhythm control strategy in the treatment of AF

Trial	Primary endpoint	Major outcomes
AFFIRM [53]	Overall mortality	There was a trend toward a decrease in all-cause mortality in the rate control arm (HR 0.87, $p = 0.08$), without differences in cardiac death, stroke, or arrhythmic death
RACE [96]	A composite of death from cardiovascular causes, HF, thromboembolic complications, bleeding, pacemaker implants, and severe adverse effects of drugs	No significant difference between rate and rhythm control arms in patients with PeAF (90% CI, -11.0 to 0.4%)
AF-CHF [55]	Time to death from cardiovascular causes	Rhythm control strategy did not reduce the rate of death from cardiovascular causes in patients with AF and HfrEF (LVEF $\leq$ 35%) as compared to rate control strategy (HR 1.06; 95% CI, 0.86–1.30; $p = 0.59$)
PIAF [56]	Improvement in symptoms related to AF	Similar symptomatic improvement in rhythm vs rate control arms ($p = 0.317$). Increased hospital admission with rhythm control ($p = 0.001$)
STAF [57]	Combination of death, cardiopulmonary resuscitation, cerebrovascular event, and systemic embolism	No differences between the two treatment strategies in all end points except hospitalizations ($p = 0.99$)
HOT CAFE [97]	Composite of all-cause mortality, number of thromboembolic events, or major bleeding	No significant difference in primary endpoint between rhythm and rate control for chronic AF (OR, 1.98; 95% CI, 0.28–22.3; $p > 0.71$). Lower hospitalization in rate control arm (12% vs 74%, respectively; $p < 0.001$)
EAST-AFNET 4 [59]	Composite of death, stroke, or serious adverse events related to rhythm-control therapy	Trial stopped early for improved efficacy in early rhythm control arm as compared to usual care (HR, 0.79; 95% CI, 0.66–0.94; $p = 0.005$)

Abbreviations: *AF* atrial fibrillation, *AF-CHF* Atrial Fibrillation and Congestive Heart Failure, *AFFIRM* Atrial Fibrillation Follow-Up Investigation of Rhythm Management, *CI* confidence interval, *EAST-AFNET 4* Early Treatment of Atrial Fibrillation for Stroke Prevention Trial, *HOT CAFE* How to Treat Chronic Atrial Fibrillation, *HFrEF* heart failure with reduced ejection fraction, *HR* hazard ratio, *LVEF* left ventricular ejection fraction, *OR* odds ratio, *PeAF* persistent atrial fibrillation, *PIAF* Pharmacological Intervention in Atrial Fibrillation, *RACE* Rate Control Versus Electrical Cardioversion for Persistent Atrial Fibrillation Study, *STAF* Strategies of Treatment of Atrial Fibrillation

It is thought that as AF progresses from paroxysmal to more persistent forms, the contribution of extra-PV triggers substantiates and ablation outcomes are considerably worse. The etiology of arrhythmia recurrence may include new triggers, fibrotic

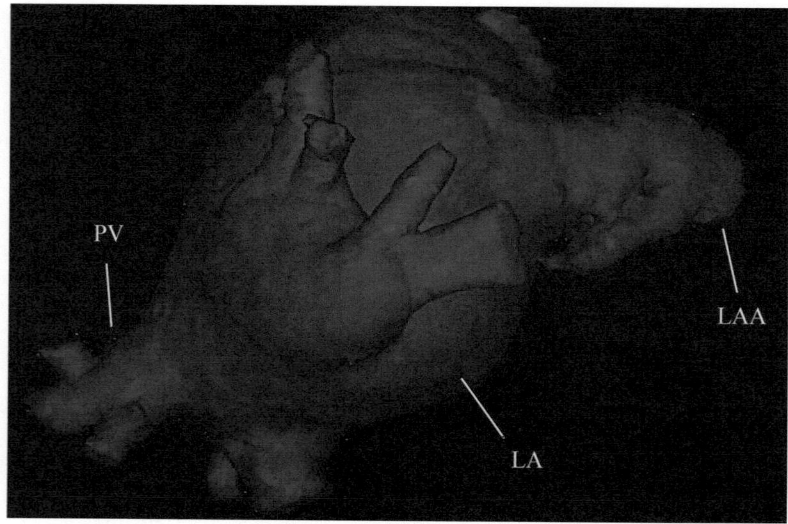

Fig. 3 3D reconstruction of left atrial (LA) anatomy derived from computed tomography. The left atrial appendage (LAA) and pulmonary veins (PV), targets for procedural stroke prevention and AF ablation, respectively, are depicted

scar or recovery across isolation lines. The extent of ablation required remains unclear and is the subject of active investigation [62]. Possible additional ablative targets include the superior vena cava, linear ablation (roofline, posterior line, etc.), the vein of Marshall, the left atrial appendage (LAA), and areas with complex fractionated atrial electrograms (CFAE). Targeting these sites is technically challenging and has relatively low efficacy and significant hazard, without clearly defined predictors for success. In fact, the Substrate and Trigger Ablation for Reduction of Atrial Fibrillation Trial Part II (STAR AF II) randomized persistent AF patients to receive pulmonary vein isolation (PVI) alone, PVI plus focal ablation of areas that demonstrate complex fractional activity (CFAE), or PVI plus linear ablation of the left atrial roof and mitral valve isthmus. The study found no difference in outcomes with atrial substrate modification. We have since seen the emergence of multiple procedural augmentations in attempts to improve PeAF ablation outcomes. The Convergence of Epicardial and Endocardial Ablation for the Treatment of Symptomatic AF (CONVERGE) [66] trial achieved improved efficacy when endocardial and epicardial ablation were combined in a hybrid approach. The Vein of Marshall Ethanol for Untreated Persistent AF (VENUS) [67] trial utilized ethanol ablation of the vein of Marshall in addition to standard catheter ablation to reduce PeAF recurrence and the need for repeat ablation procedures. While promising, these techniques entail considerable operator training, cost, and procedural duration, as well as carry a higher complication rate. Substantial efforts are ongoing in search of improved and unified ablation protocols in the treatment of PeAF.

Data on the effect of AF catheter ablation on mortality are inconclusive. In the Catheter Ablation Versus Antiarrhythmic Drug Therapy for Atrial Fibrillation

(CABANA) trial [15], catheter ablation for AF did not significantly reduce the primary composite end point of death, disabling stroke, serious bleeding, or cardiac arrest, compared with medical therapy in the general AF population. However, the estimated treatment effect of catheter ablation in this study was affected by the lower-than-expected event rates and treatment crossovers.

Catheter ablation, however, may potentially improve outcomes in patients with AF and HFrEF. The Catheter Ablation for Atrial Fibrillation with Heart Failure (CASTLE-AF) trial randomized symptomatic paroxysmal and PeAF patients with HFrEF to receive catheter ablation or medical therapy with rate and rhythm control agents [63]. It showed a reduction in death from any cause (hazard ratio [HR] 0.53, $p = 0.01$) and HF hospitalization (HR 0.56, $p = 0.004$) with catheter ablation. In PeAF patients with LVEF < 50% and symptomatic HF, catheter ablation reduced symptoms, improved functional capacity and LVEF when compared with a rate control strategy (CAMTAF) [68]. Similarly, in PeAF, the Ablation vs Amiodarone for Treatment of Atrial Fibrillation in Patients with Congestive Heart Failure and an Implanted ICD/CRTD (AATAC) trial demonstrated the superiority of catheter ablation to AAD therapy with amiodarone in HFrEF (LVEF < 40%) patients [69] in reducing AF recurrence, hospitalization, and mortality.

4.8 Stroke Prevention in Atrial Fibrillation

The most common site for thrombogenesis and embolic source in the setting of non-valvular AF [70] is the LAA (Fig. 3). The underlying mechanisms for this are not yet completely understood. Predominantly, and as derived from years of robust data (Table 3), the approach to stroke prevention in AF relies on systemic anticoagulation (AC). In those intolerant of AC, procedural alternatives have been developed and remain under active investigation.

Table 3 Investigations of pharmacologic stroke prevention in non-valvular AF

Study	Agent investigated	Control/ comparator	Major outcomes
Meta-analysis of 7 trials [98]	Asa	Placebo	19% stroke-risk reduction with Asa as compared to placebo (95% CI, 1–35%)
ACTIVE-A [99]	Asa (75–100 mg daily) and clopidogrel (75 mg daily)	Asa (75–100 mg daily)	Addition of clopidogrel reduced the risk of major vascular events and increased the risk of major hemorrhage (RR, 0.89; 95% CI, 0.81–0.98; $p = 0.01$)
ACTIVE-W [100]	Warfarin (INR 2–3)	Asa (75–100 mg daily) and clopidogrel (75 mg daily)	Warfarin was superior to Asa + clopidogrel for prevention of vascular events (RR, 1.44; 95% CI, 1.18–1.76; $p = 0.0003$)

(continued)

Table 3 (continued)

Study	Agent investigated	Control/comparator	Major outcomes
RE-LY [95]	Dabigatran (110 and 150 mg twice daily)	Warfarin (INR 2–3)	Dabigatran 110 mg had similar rates of stroke and systemic embolism (RR, 0.91; 95% CI, 0.74–1.11; $p < 0.001$); lower rates of major hemorrhage ($p = 0.003$). Dabigatran 150 mg had lower rates of stroke and systemic embolism (RR, 0.66; 95% CI, 0.53–0.82; $p < 0.001$ for superiority); similar rates of major hemorrhage ($p = 0.31$)
ROCKET-AF [101]	Rivaroxaban 20 mg daily	Warfarin (INR 2–3)	Rivaroxaban was noninferior to warfarin for the prevention of stroke or systemic embolism (HR, 0.79; 95% CI, 0.66–0.96; $p < 0.001$ for noninferiority); less intracranial ($p = 0.02$) and fatal ($p = 0.003$) bleeding with rivaroxaban
ARISTOTLE [102]	Apixaban 5 mg twice daily	Warfarin (INR 2–3)	Apixaban was superior to warfarin in preventing stroke or systemic embolism (HR, 0.79; 95% CI, 0.66–0.95; $p < 0.001$ for noninferiority; $p = 0.01$ for superiority) caused less bleeding (HR, 0.69; 95% CI, 0.60–0.80; $p < 0.001$), and resulted in lower mortality (HR, 0.89; 95% CI, 0.80–0.99; $p = 0.047$)
ENGAGE-AF TIMI 48 [103]	Edoxaban (60 mg and 30 mg daily)	Warfarin (INR 2–3)	Edoxaban was non-inferior to warfarin at both doses (HR, 0.79; 97.5% CI for high-dose, 0.63–0.99; $p < 0.001$ and HR, 1.07; 97.5% CI, 0.87–1.31; $p = 0.005$ for low dose) with lower risk of major bleeding (HR, 0.80; 95% CI, 0.71–0.91; $p < 0.001$ for high dose and HR, 0.47; 95% CI, 0.41–0.55; $p < 0.001$ for low dose) and death from cardiovascular causes (HR, 0.86; 95% CI, 0.77–0.97; $p = 0.01$ for high dose and HR, 0.85; 95% CI, 0.76–0.96; $p = 0.008$ for low dose)

Abbreviations: *ACTIVE* Atrial Fibrillation Clopidogrel Trial with Irbesartan for Prevention of Vascular Events, *AF* atrial fibrillation, *ARISTOTLE* Apixaban for Reduction in Stroke and Other Thromboembolic Events in Atrial Fibrillation, *Asa* acetylsalicylic acid, *CI* confidence interval, *ENGAGE AF-TIMI 48* Effective Anticoagulation With Factor Xa Next Generation in Atrial Fibrillation-Thrombolysis in Myocardial Infarction 48, *HR* hazard ratio, *INR* international normalized ratio, *RE-LY* Randomized Evaluation of Long-Term Anticoagulation Therapy, *ROCKET-AF* Rivaroxaban Once Daily Oral Direct Factor Xa Inhibition Compared with Vitamin K Antagonism for Prevention of Stroke and Embolism Trial in Atrial Fibrillation, *RR* relative risk

While vitamin K antagonists were the only oral anticoagulant available for 60 years prior to the development of the direct oral anticoagulant agents (DOACs), their use was somewhat impractical due to the narrow therapeutic window, multiple drug-drug interactions, dietary restrictions, and need for routine international normalized ratio (INR) monitoring. More recently, we have seen the advent of the

DOACs. These agents have a more predictable dose-response and do not require routine surveillance [71]. Phase III clinical trials for dabigatran (RE-LY study), rivaroxaban (Rivaroxaban Once Daily Oral Direct Factor Xa Inhibition Compared with Vitamin K Antagonism for Prevention of Stroke and Embolism Trial in Atrial Fibrillation [ROCKET-AF]), and apixaban (Apixaban for Reduction in Stroke and Other Thromboembolic Events in Atrial Fibrillation [ARISTOTLE] study) were conducted to assess the efficacy of these drugs in stroke prevention. The three studies comprised 50,578 patients and compared the DOAC agents (dabigatran $n = 12,091$; rivaroxaban $n = 7131$; apixaban $n = 9120$) to warfarin ($n = 22,236$). In terms of the primary efficacy endpoint, the DOACs were not more effective than warfarin in preventing non-hemorrhagic strokes and systemic embolism (relative risk [RR] = 0.93; 95% CI 0.83–1.04). They did however achieve a reduction in risk of intracranial bleed in comparison with warfarin (RR = 0.46; 95% CI 0.33–0.65). There was heterogeneity within the trials, however, and rivaroxaban had lower reduction in the risk of intracranial bleed than dabigatran and apixaban. There was also a trend towards lower rates of major bleeding with DOACs in RE-LY and ARISTOTLE. On the other hand, there was a trend towards higher gastrointestinal bleeding with DOACs in RE-LY and ROCKET-AF. Overall, DOACs reduced the risk of death when compared to warfarin. However, this effect was heterogenous; whereby, it was significant in centers whose patients' average warfarin time in therapeutic range (TTR) was <64% and non-significant in centers with average patient TTR >64% [71], highlighting the impact of AC compliance on its efficacy in stroke prevention.

Globally, underutilization of anticoagulant therapy is a well-documented problem [4]. In a retrospective analysis by the Get With The Guidelines-Stroke (GWTG-Stroke) program (2012–2015), 83% of 94,474 patients with CVA and known AF were not receiving therapeutic anticoagulation [72]; 13.5% were subtherapeutic, while the remainder of patients were on antiplatelet therapy or were receiving no antithrombotic therapy. In meta-analyses, factors that increased likelihood of undertreatment included alcohol and drug abuse, non-compliance, advanced age, dementia, falls, major bleeding, renal disease, and contraindications to anticoagulant therapy. In the PINNACLE registry of outpatients with AF, females were found to be significantly less likely to receive oral anticoagulant therapy [73].

There is a small subset of AF patients with contraindications to oral anticoagulation, such as major bleeding risk. Multiple procedural interventions have been utilized to mitigate stroke risk in this specific population. Over 90% of embolic strokes in AF originate in the LAA [70]. As such, all procedural interventions are based on the exclusion or obliteration of this structure to reduce stroke risk. Multiple surgical techniques have been utilized over the years for this purpose, including excision and exclusion of the appendage via staples and sutures. Unfortunately, a large number of retrospective studies have shown inconsistent and incomplete closure with these techniques, without reliable evidence of stroke reduction [74]. More recently, the AtriClip (AtriCure, Mason, Ohio), an epicardial closure device, has been employed in open and minimally invasive surgery, and has proven to be safe and durable [75]. Its efficacy in stroke prevention in randomized trials is still under investigation.

Multiple percutaneous devices have also been developed, including Watchman (Boston Scientific, Natick, Massachusetts), Amplatzer Cardiac Plug/Amulet (Abbott, Golden Valley, Minnesota), and others. The most robust randomized clinical trial data for the efficacy of LAA exclusion derive from two consecutive trials, the Watchman Left Atrial Appendage System for Embolic Protection in Atrial Fibrillation (PROTECT-AF) and the Prospective Randomized Evaluation of Watchman Left Atrial Appendage Closure Device in Patients with Atrial Fibrillation Versus Long-Term Warfarin Therapy (PREVAIL-AF), along with their respective continued access registries [76]. They showed non-inferiority of LAA exclusion in the prevention of stroke as compared to warfarin. Furthermore, they showed a cumulative advantage of LAA occlusion over warfarin in major bleeding and death combined [62]. Unfortunately, all data available from randomized trials are in non-valvular AF patients without absolute contraindication to anticoagulation, due to the need for post-procedural anticoagulation, at least in the short-term, to ensure appropriate device endothelialization. For those with absolute contraindication to anticoagulation, the LARIAT suture ligation (SentreHEART Inc., Redwood City, California) has been used off-label. It is Food and Drug Administration approved for soft tissue approximation and utilizes a combined epicardial/endocardial approach to deliver a suture for LAA ligation without the need for post-procedural anticoagulation. Its efficacy in stroke prevention has yet to be investigated in randomized trials.

5   Ventricular Arrhythmias

Premature ventricular contractions (PVCs) and ventricular tachycardia (VT) are heart rhythms originating within the ventricles. If sustained, then ventricular arrhythmias can be immediately life threatening. Consequently, an objective assessment of treatment outcomes has been fraught with challenges. Patient participation in trials is low, and in many cases, enrollment into a traditional control arm may be considered unethical. In the realm of VT ablation in particular, there is low patient participation, high patient crossover, heterogeneity in procedure techniques, controversy in defining clinical endpoints, and constant technological development over time that makes trial outcomes rapidly obsolete [77]. We provide an overview of the epidemiologic trends in ventricular arrhythmias, as well as the available literature on treatment outcomes.

5.1   *Epidemiology*

Approximately 40% of adults have premature ventricular contractions (PVCs) [78]. The prevalence of monomorphic VT (MVT) in the general population is difficult to quantify due to its association with SCD. MVTs can be divided into idiopathic VT (in a structurally normal heart) and scar mediated VT (in a structurally abnormal heart) (Table 4). In patients with structural heart disease and ICD implantation, 81%

Table 4 Common sites of ventricular tachycardia

VT in the structurally normal heart	VT in structural heart disease
Right and left outflow tract VT (most common)	Post-myocardial infarction—localized to the site of scar with predilection for sub-endocardium
Papillary muscle VT (5–12%)	Dilated cardiomyopathy—mostly basal anteroseptal and inferolateral LV—may be mid-myocardial or epicardial
Fascicular VT (10–20%)	Arrhythmogenic right ventricular dysplasia—predominantly involves the RV, although left dominant and biventricular variants occur
	Hypertrophic cardiomyopathy—site of myocardial scar or LV aneurysm
	Cardiac sarcoidosis—sites of myocardial scar and inflammation
	Chagas cardiomyopathy—80% in inferolateral LV. Endocardial involvement is most common, but up to 37% have epicardial circuits

Abbreviations: *LV* left ventricle, *RV* right ventricle, *VT* ventricular tachycardia

developed clinically relevant MVT within 11 months of follow-up [79]. Polymorphic VT (PVT) is a notoriously more malignant arrhythmia. In fact, PVT occurs in 30–43% [4] of patients who develop SCD during ambulatory monitoring. It was observed in 4.4% of acute MIs [80] and portends higher mortality in this setting. The development of torsade de pointes is commonly associated with medications that prolong QTc [81]. The risk is higher in females, advanced age, patients with QT prolongation, bradycardia, systolic dysfunction, electrolyte disturbances, drug interactions, as well as kidney and liver disease [4].

5.2   PVCs and Cardiovascular Outcomes

The majority of PVCs in adults with structurally normal hearts are thought to be benign, and the risk of SCD is exceedingly low in the absence of PVC-triggered polymorphic VT/VF [82]. However, an increased burden of PVCs is associated with a higher risk of developing PVC-induced cardiomyopathy. A PVC burden of 24% has been shown to have high sensitivity and specificity for the development of PVC-cardiomyopathy. PVC QRS >150 ms also correlates with a higher incidence of PVC-cardiopathy, while an excessively long QRS duration predicts lower likelihood of LV function recovery after PVC ablation [78]. The development of PVT in the setting of acute MI increases the risk of mortality by 17.8% [80].

5.3   PVC/VT Treatment

A PVC burden of <10% without symptoms does not normally warrant treatment. For patients with a higher burden and symptoms and/or cardiomyopathy, as well as those with elevated burden impeding optimal cardiac resynchronization therapy, treatment is recommended. The best course of action for patients who remain asymptomatic despite a high PVC burden is unknown, and typically requires shared decision-making, as well as close clinical and echocardiographic follow-up.

5.4   Drug Therapy

The first-line therapies for PVC and VT treatment are beta blockers, both in the normal heart and most etiologies of structural heart disease. Non-dihydropyridine calcium channel blockers are also frequently used. AAD therapy is effective in suppressing ventricular arrhythmias (VA), but its use is limited by adverse and pro-arrhythmia side effects. The combined use of BB therapy with AAD has been shown to reduce recurrent ICD shocks in ischemic cardiomyopathy. The combination of amiodarone and BB therapy is utilized most frequently, with addition of mexiletine in refractory cases. Dofetilide and sotalol may also be useful but are considered second-line therapy. When drug therapy fails, or is poorly tolerated, catheter ablation is an effective alternative option for VA suppression.

5.5   ICD Therapy

The mainstay of primary and secondary preventive therapy for patients with structural heart disease is ICD implantation [83, 84]. This is based on a large number of trials that consistently showed a survival benefit including the Sudden Cardiac Death in Heart Failure (SCD-HeFT) [85], Comparison of Medical Therapy, Pacing and Defibrillation in Heart Failure (COMPANION) [86], Multicenter Automatic Defibrillator Implantation (MADIT II) [87] and Defibrillators in Non-ischemic Cardiomyopathy Treatment Evaluation (DEFINITE) [88] trials, among others. More recently, the Defibrillator Implantation in Patients with Non-ischemic Systolic Heart Failure (DANISH) [89] trial failed to show a mortality benefit in a non-ischemic population, but did show a reduction in SCD. Nonetheless, overall, the aggregate of available data suggests a mortality benefit to ICD therapy in non-ischemic cardiomyopathy [90].

5.6   Cather Ablation in Ventricular Arrhythmias

Catheter ablation has been proven to be highly successful in treating VT in individuals with a structurally normal heart. While not as effective as VT ablation in a normal heart, the catheter ablation of VT is frequently performed in patients with structural heart disease as well (Fig. 4). Despite the abundance of retrospective and prospective data, there is a paucity of randomized clinical trials comparing ablation

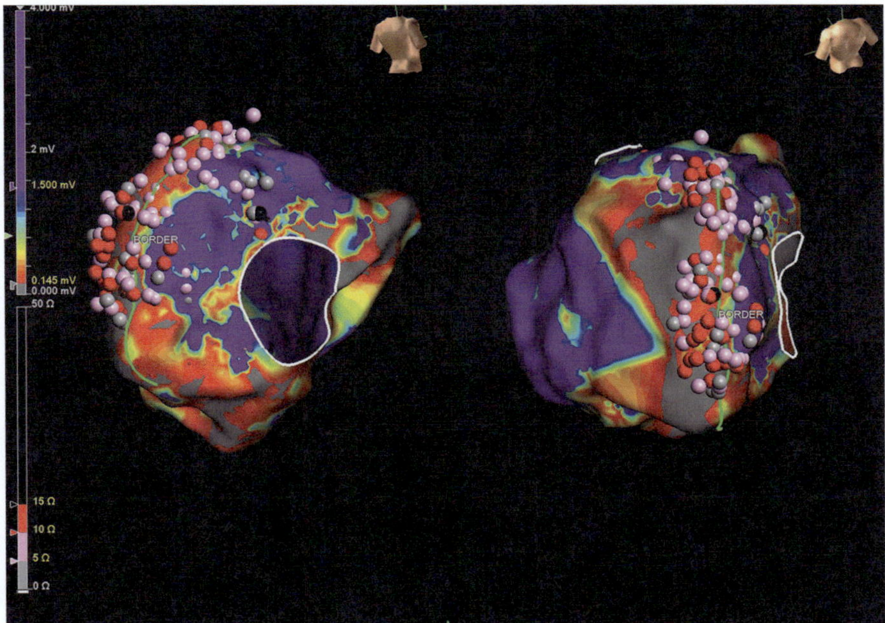

Fig. 4 Voltage map demonstrating the radiofrequency ablation lesions delivered during a case of scar-mediated ventricular tachycardia ablation

to AAD therapy in the treatment of VT in structural heart disease patients. The Substrate Mapping and Ablation in Sinus Rhythm to Halt Ventricular Tachycardia (SMASH-VT) trial included a cohort of patients with prior MI and ICD and compared catheter ablation to standard medical therapy, although the medical therapy cohort did not receive AAD therapy [91]. The study showed a reduction in appropriate ICD shocks as a result of the ablation. The Ventricular Tachycardia Ablation in Coronary Heart Disease (VTACH) trial similarly enrolled patients with prior MI, reduced LVEF (<50%) and ICD to receive catheter ablation vs medical therapy, but did allow the medical therapy arm to receive AADs [92]. It showed longer freedom from recurrent VT and reduction in ICD shocks in the ablation arm. There was no reduction in mortality noted in any of the trials, and recurrent VT/ICD shocks did occur, highlighting the inadequacy of ablative therapy alone in preventing mortality in this patient population. The Ventricular Tachycardia Ablation Versus Escalated Anti-Arrhythmic Drug Therapy in Ischemic Heart Disease (VANISH) trial enrolled patients with prior MI and ICD who had recurrent VT despite AAD therapy and compared the utility of escalation of AADs to catheter ablation. The ablation group had a reduction in the composite endpoint of ICD shocks, VT storm, and mortality, primarily driven by ICD shocks and VT storm, again with no difference in mortality between groups. The Ablation of Clinical Ventricular Tachycardia versus Addition of Substrate Ablation on the Long-Term Success Rate of VT Ablation (VISTA) trial compared clinical/mappable VT ablation to more extensive substrate ablation [93].

The substrate ablation group had lower VT recurrence rates and less required AAD therapy; however, there was no difference in mortality between groups. As such, in the setting of structural heart disease, ablative therapy is widely adopted for refractory VT and for the reduction of ICD shocks but does not provide a mortality benefit.

6 Conclusion

We have only begun to understand the fundamentals of cardiac electrophysiology within the last few decades. However, as summarized in this chapter, we have uncovered a tremendous global disease burden associated with heart rhythm problems. As a consequence, the field of cardiac electrophysiology has grown at a remarkable pace. This chapter highlights its most substantial impacts on cardiovascular outcomes. Ongoing research and innovation continue to mitigate the adversities of arrhythmic disease and thrive to alleviate the morbidity and excess mortality associated with it.

Funding The authors have no funding sources to disclose.

Disclosures Dr. Kowey is a consultant for Medtronic, Sanofi, InCarda, Milestone, Novartis, Acesion, Johnson & Johnson, BMS, Boehringer, Anthos, Huya and Pfizer; he chairs the NCDR EP steering committee at the ACC; he has served on the steering committee of the CABANA trial; and he was a sub-investigator for the AFFIRM trial. All other authors have reported that they have no relationships relevant to the contents of this chapter to disclose.

References

1. Alonso A, Jensen PN, Lopez FL, et al. Association of sick sinus syndrome with incident cardiovascular disease and mortality: the Atherosclerosis Risk in Communities study and Cardiovascular Health Study. PLoS One. 2014;9(10):e109662. (In Eng). https://doi.org/10.1371/journal.pone.0109662.
2. Lamas GA, Lee KL, Sweeney MO, et al. Ventricular pacing or dual-chamber pacing for sinus-node dysfunction. N Engl J Med. 2002;346(24):1854–62. (In Eng). https://doi.org/10.1056/NEJMoa013040.
3. Cheng S, Keyes MJ, Larson MG, et al. Long-term outcomes in individuals with prolonged PR interval or first-degree atrioventricular block. JAMA. 2009;301(24):2571–7. (In Eng). https://doi.org/10.1001/jama.2009.888.
4. Benjamin EJ, Muntner P, Alonso A, et al. Heart disease and stroke statistics-2019 update: a report from the American Heart Association. Circulation. 2019;139(10):e56–e528. (In Eng). https://doi.org/10.1161/cir.0000000000000659.
5. Epstein AE, DiMarco JP, Ellenbogen KA, et al. 2012 ACCF/AHA/HRS focused update incorporated into the ACCF/AHA/HRS 2008 guidelines for device-based therapy of cardiac rhythm abnormalities: a report of the American College of Cardiology Foundation/American Heart Association Task Force on practice guidelines and the Heart Rhythm Society. J Am Coll Cardiol. 2013;61(3):e6–75. (In Eng). https://doi.org/10.1016/j.jacc.2012.11.007.

6. Cingolani E, Goldhaber JI, Marbán E. Next-generation pacemakers: from small devices to biological pacemakers. Nat Rev Cardiol. 2018;15(3):139–50. (In Eng). https://doi.org/10.1038/nrcardio.2017.165.

7. Auffret V, Puri R, Urena M, et al. Conduction disturbances after transcatheter aortic valve replacement: current status and future perspectives. Circulation. 2017;136(11):1049–69. (In Eng). https://doi.org/10.1161/circulationaha.117.028352.

8. Urena M, Webb JG, Eltchaninoff H, et al. Late cardiac death in patients undergoing transcatheter aortic valve replacement: incidence and predictors of advanced heart failure and sudden cardiac death. J Am Coll Cardiol. 2015;65(5):437–48. (In Eng). https://doi.org/10.1016/j.jacc.2014.11.027.

9. Meguro K, Lellouche N, Yamamoto M, et al. Prognostic value of QRS duration after transcatheter aortic valve implantation for aortic stenosis using the CoreValve. Am J Cardiol. 2013;111(12):1778–83. (In Eng). https://doi.org/10.1016/j.amjcard.2013.02.032.

10. Regueiro A, Abdul-Jawad Altisent O, Del Trigo M, et al. Impact of new-onset left bundle branch block and periprocedural permanent pacemaker implantation on clinical outcomes in patients undergoing transcatheter aortic valve replacement: a systematic review and meta-analysis. Circ Cardiovasc Interv. 2016;9(5):e003635. (In Eng). https://doi.org/10.1161/circinterventions.115.003635.

11. Fadahunsi OO, Olowoyeye A, Ukaigwe A, et al. Incidence, predictors, and outcomes of permanent pacemaker implantation following transcatheter aortic valve replacement: analysis from the U.S. Society of Thoracic Surgeons/American College of Cardiology TVT Registry. JACC Cardiovasc Interv. 2016;9(21):2189–99. (In Eng). https://doi.org/10.1016/j.jcin.2016.07.026.

12. Orejarena LA, Vidaillet H Jr, DeStefano F, et al. Paroxysmal supraventricular tachycardia in the general population. J Am Coll Cardiol. 1998;31(1):150–7. (In Eng). https://doi.org/10.1016/s0735-1097(97)00422-1.

13. Sohinki D, Obel OA. Current trends in supraventricular tachycardia management. Ochsner J. 2014;14(4):586–95. (In Eng). https://pubmed.ncbi.nlm.nih.gov/25598724; https://www.ncbi.nlm.nih.gov/pmc/articles/PMC4295736/.

14. Page RL, Joglar JA, Caldwell MA, et al. 2015 ACC/AHA/HRS guideline for the management of adult patients with supraventricular tachycardia: a report of the American College of Cardiology/American Heart Association Task Force on clinical practice guidelines and the Heart Rhythm Society. Circulation. 2016;133(14):e506–74. (In Eng). https://doi.org/10.1161/CIR.0000000000000311.

15. McCord J, Borzak S. Multifocal atrial tachycardia. Chest. 1998;113(1):203–9. (In Eng). https://doi.org/10.1378/chest.113.1.203.

16. Wu EB, Chia HM, Gill JS. Reversible cardiomyopathy after radiofrequency ablation of lateral free-wall pathway-mediated incessant supraventricular tachycardia. Pacing Clin Electrophysiol. 2000;23(8):1308–10. (In Eng). https://doi.org/10.1111/j.1540-8159.2000.tb00951.x.

17. Wang YS, Scheinman MM, Chien WW, Cohen TJ, Lesh MD, Griffin JC. Patients with supraventricular tachycardia presenting with aborted sudden death: incidence, mechanism and long-term follow-up. J Am Coll Cardiol. 1991;18(7):1711–9. (In Eng). https://doi.org/10.1016/0735-1097(91)90508-7.

18. Chang SH, Kuo CF, Chou IJ, et al. Outcomes associated with paroxysmal supraventricular tachycardia during pregnancy. Circulation. 2017;135(6):616–8. (In Eng). https://doi.org/10.1161/circulationaha.116.025064.

19. Campbell RWF, Smith RA, Gallagher JJ, Pritchett ELC, Wallace AG. Atrial fibrillation in the preexcitation syndrome. Am J Cardiol. 1977;40(4):514–20. https://doi.org/10.1016/0002-9149(77)90065-0.

20. Leitch JW, Klein GJ, Yee R, Murdock C. Prognostic value of electrophysiology testing in asymptomatic patients with Wolff-Parkinson-White pattern. Circulation. 1990;82(5):1718–23. (In Eng). https://doi.org/10.1161/01.cir.82.5.1718.

21. Chimienti M, Cullen MT Jr, Casadei G. Safety of flecainide versus propafenone for the long-term management of symptomatic paroxysmal supraventricular tachyarrhythmias. Report from the Flecainide and Propafenone Italian Study (FAPIS) Group. Eur Heart J. 1995;16(12):1943–51. (In Eng). https://doi.org/10.1093/oxfordjournals.eurheartj.a060852.
22. Spector P, Reynolds MR, Calkins H, et al. Meta-analysis of ablation of atrial flutter and supraventricular tachycardia. Am J Cardiol. 2009;104(5):671–7. (In Eng). https://doi.org/10.1016/j.amjcard.2009.04.040.
23. Calkins H, Yong P, Miller JM, et al. Catheter ablation of accessory pathways, atrioventricular nodal reentrant tachycardia, and the atrioventricular junction: final results of a prospective, multicenter clinical trial. The Atakr Multicenter Investigators Group. Circulation. 1999;99(2):262–70. (In Eng). https://doi.org/10.1161/01.cir.99.2.262.
24. Collins KK, Van Hare GF, Kertesz NJ, et al. Pediatric nonpost-operative junctional ectopic tachycardia medical management and interventional therapies. J Am Coll Cardiol. 2009;53(8):690–7. (In Eng). https://doi.org/10.1016/j.jacc.2008.11.019.
25. Mou L, Norby FL, Chen LY, et al. Lifetime risk of atrial fibrillation by race and socioeconomic status: ARIC study (atherosclerosis risk in communities). Circ Arrhythm Electrophysiol. 2018;11(7):e006350. (In Eng). https://doi.org/10.1161/circep.118.006350.
26. Christophersen IE, Yin X, Larson MG, et al. A comparison of the CHARGE-AF and the CHA2DS2-VASc risk scores for prediction of atrial fibrillation in the Framingham Heart Study. Am Heart J. 2016;178:45–54. (In Eng). https://doi.org/10.1016/j.ahj.2016.05.004.
27. Abugroun A, Taha A, Abdel-Rahman M, Volgman AS. Economic impact of atrial fibrillation on hospitalization outcomes of acute heart failure in the United States. Am J Cardiol. 2021;138:124–7. (In Eng). https://doi.org/10.1016/j.amjcard.2020.10.023.
28. Marijon E, Le Heuzey JY, Connolly S, et al. Causes of death and influencing factors in patients with atrial fibrillation: a competing-risk analysis from the randomized evaluation of long-term anticoagulant therapy study. Circulation. 2013;128(20):2192–201. (In Eng). https://doi.org/10.1161/circulationaha.112.000491.
29. Vrsalović M, Presečki AV. Atrial fibrillation and risk of cardiovascular events and mortality in patients with symptomatic peripheral artery disease: a meta-analysis of prospective studies. Clin Cardiol. 2017;40(12):1231–5. (In Eng). https://doi.org/10.1002/clc.22813.
30. Masri A, Kanj M, Thamilarasan M, et al. Outcomes in hypertrophic cardiomyopathy patients with and without atrial fibrillation: a survival meta-analysis. Cardiovasc Diagn Ther. 2017;7(1):36–44. (In Eng). https://doi.org/10.21037/cdt.2016.11.23.
31. Jabre P, Jouven X, Adnet F, et al. Atrial fibrillation and death after myocardial infarction: a community study. Circulation. 2011;123(19):2094–100. (In Eng). https://doi.org/10.1161/circulationaha.110.990192.
32. Phan K, Ha HS, Phan S, Medi C, Thomas SP, Yan TD. New-onset atrial fibrillation following coronary bypass surgery predicts long-term mortality: a systematic review and meta-analysis. Eur J Cardiothorac Surg. 2015;48(6):817–24. (In Eng). https://doi.org/10.1093/ejcts/ezu551.
33. Mojoli M, Gersh BJ, Barioli A, et al. Impact of atrial fibrillation on outcomes of patients treated by transcatheter aortic valve implantation: a systematic review and meta-analysis. Am Heart J. 2017;192:64–75. https://doi.org/10.1016/j.ahj.2017.07.005.
34. Cheng M, Lu X, Huang J, Zhang J, Zhang S, Gu D. The prognostic significance of atrial fibrillation in heart failure with a preserved and reduced left ventricular function: insights from a meta-analysis. Eur J Heart Fail. 2014;16(12):1317–22. (In Eng). https://doi.org/10.1002/ejhf.187.
35. Zakeri R, Chamberlain AM, Roger VL, Redfield MM. Temporal relationship and prognostic significance of atrial fibrillation in heart failure patients with preserved ejection fraction: a community-based study. Circulation. 2013;128(10):1085–93. (In Eng). https://doi.org/10.1161/circulationaha.113.001475.
36. Echouffo-Tcheugui JB, Shrader P, Thomas L, et al. Care patterns and outcomes in atrial fibrillation patients with and without diabetes: ORBIT-AF registry. J Am Coll Cardiol. 2017;70(11):1325–35. (In Eng). https://doi.org/10.1016/j.jacc.2017.07.755.
37. Zimmerman D, Sood MM, Rigatto C, Holden RM, Hiremath S, Clase CM. Systematic review and meta-analysis of incidence, prevalence and outcomes of atrial fibrillation in patients on

dialysis. Nephrol Dial Transplant. 2012;27(10):3816–22. (In Eng). https://doi.org/10.1093/ndt/gfs416.

38. Lin HJ, Wolf PA, Kelly-Hayes M, et al. Stroke severity in atrial fibrillation. The Framingham Study. Stroke. 1996;27(10):1760–4. (In Eng). https://doi.org/10.1161/01.str.27.10.1760.

39. Walkey AJ, Hammill BG, Curtis LH, Benjamin EJ. Long-term outcomes following development of new-onset atrial fibrillation during sepsis. Chest. 2014;146(5):1187–95. (In Eng). https://doi.org/10.1378/chest.14-0003.

40. de Vos CB, Pisters R, Nieuwlaat R, et al. Progression from paroxysmal to persistent atrial fibrillation clinical correlates and prognosis. J Am Coll Cardiol. 2010;55(8):725–31. (In Eng). https://doi.org/10.1016/j.jacc.2009.11.040.

41. Lip GY, Nieuwlaat R, Pisters R, Lane DA, Crijns HJ. Refining clinical risk stratification for predicting stroke and thromboembolism in atrial fibrillation using a novel risk factor-based approach: the euro heart survey on atrial fibrillation. Chest. 2010;137(2):263–72. (In Eng). https://doi.org/10.1378/chest.09-1584.

42. Hijazi Z, Lindbäck J, Alexander JH, et al. The ABC (age, biomarkers, clinical history) stroke risk score: a biomarker-based risk score for predicting stroke in atrial fibrillation. Eur Heart J. 2016;37(20):1582–90. (In Eng). https://doi.org/10.1093/eurheartj/ehw054.

43. Qin D, Mansour MC, Ruskin JN, Heist EK. Atrial fibrillation-mediated cardiomyopathy. Circ Arrhythm Electrophysiol. 2019;12(12):e007809. (In Eng). https://doi.org/10.1161/circep.119.007809.

44. Bosch NA, Cimini J, Walkey AJ. Atrial fibrillation in the ICU. Chest. 2018;154(6):1424–34. (In Eng). https://doi.org/10.1016/j.chest.2018.03.040.

45. Kanji S, Williamson DR, Yaghchi BM, Albert M, McIntyre L. Epidemiology and management of atrial fibrillation in medical and noncardiac surgical adult intensive care unit patients. J Crit Care. 2012;27(3):326.e1–8. (In Eng). https://doi.org/10.1016/j.jcrc.2011.10.011.

46. Shapiro W, Klein G. Alterations in cardiac function immediately following electrical conversion of atrial fibrillation to normal sinus rhythm. Circulation. 1968;38(6):1074–84. (In Eng). https://doi.org/10.1161/01.cir.38.6.1074.

47. Orlando JR, van Herick R, Aronow WS, Olson HG. Hemodynamics and echocardiograms before and after cardioversion of atrial fibrillation to normal sinus rhythm. Chest. 1979;76(5):521–6. (In Eng). https://doi.org/10.1378/chest.76.5.521.

48. Santhanakrishnan R, Wang N, Larson MG, et al. Atrial fibrillation begets heart failure and vice versa: temporal associations and differences in preserved versus reduced ejection fraction. Circulation. 2016;133(5):484–92. (In Eng). https://doi.org/10.1161/circulationaha.115.018614.

49. Wang TJ, Larson MG, Levy D, et al. Temporal relations of atrial fibrillation and congestive heart failure and their joint influence on mortality: the Framingham Heart Study. Circulation. 2003;107(23):2920–5. (In Eng). https://doi.org/10.1161/01.Cir.0000072767.89944.6e.

50. Pandey A, Kim S, Moore C, et al. Predictors and prognostic implications of incident heart failure in patients with prevalent atrial fibrillation. JACC Heart Fail. 2017;5(1):44–52. (In Eng). https://doi.org/10.1016/j.jchf.2016.09.016.

51. Khan MN, Jaïs P, Cummings J, et al. Pulmonary-vein isolation for atrial fibrillation in patients with heart failure. N Engl J Med. 2008;359(17):1778–85. (In Eng). https://doi.org/10.1056/NEJMoa0708234.

52. Prabhu S, Taylor AJ, Costello BT, et al. Catheter ablation versus medical rate control in atrial fibrillation and systolic dysfunction: the CAMERA-MRI study. J Am Coll Cardiol. 2017;70(16):1949–61. (In Eng). https://doi.org/10.1016/j.jacc.2017.08.041.

53. Wyse DG, Waldo AL, DiMarco JP, et al. A comparison of rate control and rhythm control in patients with atrial fibrillation. N Engl J Med. 2002;347(23):1825–33. (In Eng). https://doi.org/10.1056/NEJMoa021328.

54. Van Gelder IC, Hagens VE, Bosker HA, et al. A comparison of rate control and rhythm control in patients with recurrent persistent atrial fibrillation. N Engl J Med. 2002;347(23):1834–40. (In Eng). https://doi.org/10.1056/NEJMoa021375.

55. Roy D, Talajic M, Nattel S, et al. Rhythm control versus rate control for atrial fibrillation and heart failure. N Engl J Med. 2008;358(25):2667–77. https://doi.org/10.1056/NEJMoa0708789.

56. Hohnloser SH, Kuck KH, Lilienthal J. Rhythm or rate control in atrial fibrillation—Pharmacological Intervention in Atrial Fibrillation (PIAF): a randomised trial. Lancet. 2000;356(9244):1789–94. (In Eng). https://doi.org/10.1016/s0140-6736(00)03230-x.

57. Carlsson J, Miketic S, Windeler J, et al. Randomized trial of rate-control versus rhythm-control in persistent atrial fibrillation: the Strategies of Treatment of Atrial Fibrillation (STAF) study. J Am Coll Cardiol. 2003;41(10):1690–6. (In Eng). https://doi.org/10.1016/s0735-1097(03)00332-2.

58. Opolski G, Torbicki A, Kosior D, et al. Rhythm control versus rate control in patients with persistent atrial fibrillation. Results of the HOT CAFE Polish Study. Kardiol Pol. 2003;59(7):1–16; discussion 15–16. (In Eng).

59. Kirchhof P, Camm AJ, Goette A, et al. Early rhythm-control therapy in patients with atrial fibrillation. N Engl J Med. 2020;383(14):1305–16. https://doi.org/10.1056/NEJMoa2019422.

60. Kaba RA, Cannie D, Ahmed O. RAAFT-2: Radiofrequency ablation vs antiarrhythmic drugs as first-line treatment of paroxysmal atrial fibrillation. Glob Cardiol Sci Pract. 2014;2014(2):53–5. https://doi.org/10.5339/gcsp.2014.26. PMID: 25405179; PMCID: PMC4220435.

61. Wazni OM, Dandamudi G, Sood N, et al. Cryoballoon ablation as initial therapy for atrial fibrillation. N Engl J Med. 2020;384(4):316–24. https://doi.org/10.1056/NEJMoa2029554.

62. Chung MK, Refaat M, Shen WK, et al. Atrial fibrillation: JACC council perspectives. J Am Coll Cardiol. 2020;75(14):1689–713. (In Eng). https://doi.org/10.1016/j.jacc.2020.02.025.

63. Morillo CA, Verma A, Connolly SJ, et al. Radiofrequency ablation vs antiarrhythmic drugs as first-line treatment of paroxysmal atrial fibrillation (RAAFT-2): a randomized trial. JAMA. 2014;311(7):692–700. (In Eng). https://doi.org/10.1001/jama.2014.467.

64. Natale A, Reddy VY, Monir G, et al. Paroxysmal AF catheter ablation with a contact force sensing catheter: results of the prospective, multicenter SMART-AF trial. J Am Coll Cardiol. 2014;64(7):647–56. (In Eng). https://doi.org/10.1016/j.jacc.2014.04.072.

65. Conti S, Weerasooriya R, Novak P, et al. Contact force sensing for ablation of persistent atrial fibrillation: a randomized, multicenter trial. Heart Rhythm. 2018;15(2):201–8. (In Eng). https://doi.org/10.1016/j.hrthm.2017.10.010.

66. DeLurgio DB, Crossen KJ, Gill J, et al. Hybrid convergent procedure for the treatment of persistent and long-standing persistent atrial fibrillation: results of CONVERGE clinical trial. Circ Arrhythm Electrophysiol. 2020;13(12):e009288. (In Eng). https://doi.org/10.1161/circep.120.009288.

67. Valderrábano M, Peterson LE, Swarup V, et al. Effect of catheter ablation with vein of Marshall ethanol infusion vs catheter ablation alone on persistent atrial fibrillation: the VENUS randomized clinical trial. JAMA. 2020;324(16):1620–8. (In Eng). https://doi.org/10.1001/jama.2020.16195.

68. Hunter RJ, Berriman TJ, Diab I, et al. A randomized controlled trial of catheter ablation versus medical treatment of atrial fibrillation in heart failure (the CAMTAF trial). Circ Arrhythm Electrophysiol. 2014;7(1):31–8. (In Eng). https://doi.org/10.1161/circep.113.000806.

69. Biase LD, Mohanty P, Mohanty S, et al. Ablation versus amiodarone for treatment of persistent atrial fibrillation in patients with congestive heart failure and an implanted device. Circulation. 2016;133(17):1637–44. https://doi.org/10.1161/CIRCULATIONAHA.115.019406.

70. Blackshear JL, Odell JA. Appendage obliteration to reduce stroke in cardiac surgical patients with atrial fibrillation. Ann Thorac Surg. 1996;61(2):755–9. (In Eng). https://doi.org/10.1016/0003-4975(95)00887-x.

71. Gómez-Outes A, Terleira-Fernández AI, Calvo-Rojas G, Suárez-Gea ML, Vargas-Castrillón E. Dabigatran, rivaroxaban, or apixaban versus warfarin in patients with nonvalvular atrial fibrillation: a systematic review and meta-analysis of subgroups. Thrombosis. 2013;2013:640723. (In Eng). https://doi.org/10.1155/2013/640723.

72. Xian Y, O'Brien EC, Liang L, et al. Association of preceding antithrombotic treatment with acute ischemic stroke severity and in-hospital outcomes among patients with atrial fibrillation. JAMA. 2017;317(10):1057–67. (In Eng). https://doi.org/10.1001/jama.2017.1371.

73. Thompson LE, Maddox TM, Lei L, et al. Sex differences in the use of oral anticoagulants for atrial fibrillation: a report from the National Cardiovascular Data Registry (NCDR(®))

PINNACLE Registry. J Am Heart Assoc. 2017;6(7):e005801. (In Eng). https://doi. org/10.1161/jaha.117.005801.

74. Kanderian AS, Gillinov AM, Pettersson GB, Blackstone E, Klein AL. Success of surgical left atrial appendage closure: assessment by transesophageal echocardiography. J Am Coll Cardiol. 2008;52(11):924–9. (In Eng). https://doi.org/10.1016/j.jacc.2008.03.067.

75. Caliskan E, Sahin A, Yilmaz M, et al. Epicardial left atrial appendage AtriClip occlusion reduces the incidence of stroke in patients with atrial fibrillation undergoing cardiac surgery. Europace. 2018;20(7):e105–14. (In Eng). https://doi.org/10.1093/europace/eux211.

76. Holmes DR Jr, Doshi SK, Kar S, et al. Left atrial appendage closure as an alternative to warfarin for stroke prevention in atrial fibrillation: a patient-level meta-analysis. J Am Coll Cardiol. 2015;65(24):2614–23. (In Eng). https://doi.org/10.1016/j.jacc.2015.04.025.

77. Pokorney SD, Friedman DJ, Calkins H, et al. Catheter ablation of ventricular tachycardia: lessons learned from past clinical trials and implications for future clinical trials. Heart Rhythm. 2016;13(8):1748–54. (In Eng). https://doi.org/10.1016/j.hrthm.2016.04.001.

78. Dukkipati SR, Choudry S, Koruth JS, Miller MA, Whang W, Reddy VY. Catheter ablation of ventricular tachycardia in structurally normal hearts: indications, strategies, and outcomes-part I. J Am Coll Cardiol. 2017;70(23):2909–23. (In Eng). https://doi.org/10.1016/j. jacc.2017.10.031.

79. Wathen MS, DeGroot PJ, Sweeney MO, et al. Prospective randomized multicenter trial of empirical antitachycardia pacing versus shocks for spontaneous rapid ventricular tachycardia in patients with implantable cardioverter-defibrillators: Pacing Fast Ventricular Tachycardia Reduces Shock Therapies (PainFREE Rx II) trial results. Circulation. 2004;110(17):2591–6. (In Eng). https://doi.org/10.1161/01.Cir.0000145610.64014.E4.

80. Hai JJ, Un KC, Wong CK, et al. Prognostic implications of early monomorphic and non-monomorphic tachyarrhythmias in patients discharged with acute coronary syndrome. Heart Rhythm. 2018;15(6):822–9. (In Eng). https://doi.org/10.1016/j.hrthm.2018.02.016.

81. Drew BJ, Ackerman MJ, Funk M, et al. Prevention of torsade de pointes in hospital settings: a scientific statement from the American Heart Association and the American College of Cardiology Foundation. Circulation. 2010;121(8):1047–60. (In Eng). https://doi.org/10.1161/ circulationaha.109.192704.

82. Lemery R, Brugada P, Bella PD, Dugernier T, van den Dool A, Wellens HJ. Nonischemic ventricular tachycardia. Clinical course and long-term follow-up in patients without clinically overt heart disease. Circulation. 1989;79(5):990–9. (In Eng). https://doi.org/10.1161/01. cir.79.5.990.

83. Epstein AE, DiMarco JP, Ellenbogen KA, et al. ACC/AHA/HRS 2008 guidelines for device-based therapy of cardiac rhythm abnormalities: American College of Cardiology/ American Heart Association Task Force on practice guidelines (writing committee to revise the ACC/AHA/NASPE 2002 guideline update for implantation of cardiac pacemakers and antiarrhythmia devices) developed in collaboration with the American Association for Thoracic Surgery and Society of Thoracic Surgeons. Heart Rhythm. 2008;5(6):e1–e62. https://doi.org/10.1016/j.hrthm.2008.04.014.

84. Al-Khatib SM, Stevenson WG, Ackerman MJ, et al. 2017 AHA/ACC/HRS guideline for management of patients with ventricular arrhythmias and the prevention of sudden cardiac death. Circulation. 2018;138(13):e272–391. https://doi.org/10.1161/CIR.0000000000000549.

85. Bardy GH, Lee KL, Mark DB, et al. Amiodarone or an implantable cardioverter–defibrillator for congestive heart failure. N Engl J Med. 2005;352(3):225–37. https://doi.org/10.1056/ NEJMoa043399.

86. Bristow MR, Saxon LA, Boehmer J, et al. Cardiac-resynchronization therapy with or without an implantable defibrillator in advanced chronic heart failure. N Engl J Med. 2004;350(21):2140–50. https://doi.org/10.1056/NEJMoa032423.

87. Moss AJ, Zareba W, Hall WJ, et al. Prophylactic implantation of a defibrillator in patients with myocardial infarction and reduced ejection fraction. N Engl J Med. 2002;346(12):877–83. https://doi.org/10.1056/NEJMoa013474.

88. Kadish A, Dyer A, Daubert JP, et al. Prophylactic defibrillator implantation in patients with nonischemic dilated cardiomyopathy. N Engl J Med. 2004;350(21):2151–8. (In Eng). https:// doi.org/10.1056/NEJMoa033088.

89. Køber L, Thune JJ, Nielsen JC, et al. Defibrillator implantation in patients with nonischemic systolic heart failure. N Engl J Med. 2016;375(13):1221–30. https://doi.org/10.1056/NEJMoa1608029.
90. Golwala H, Bajaj NS, Arora G, Arora P. Implantable cardioverter-defibrillator for nonischemic cardiomyopathy: an updated meta-analysis. Circulation. 2017;135(2):201–3. (In Eng). https://doi.org/10.1161/circulationaha.116.026056.
91. Reddy VY, Reynolds MR, Neuzil P, et al. Prophylactic catheter ablation for the prevention of defibrillator therapy. N Engl J Med. 2007;357(26):2657–65. https://doi.org/10.1056/NEJMoa065457.
92. Kuck K-H, Schaumann A, Eckardt L, et al. Catheter ablation of stable ventricular tachycardia before defibrillator implantation in patients with coronary heart disease (VTACH): a multicentre randomised controlled trial. Lancet. 2010;375(9708):31–40. https://doi.org/10.1016/S0140-6736(09)61755-4.
93. Di Biase L, Burkhardt JD, Lakkireddy D, et al. Ablation of stable VTs versus substrate ablation in ischemic cardiomyopathy: the VISTA randomized multicenter trial. J Am Coll Cardiol. 2015;66(25):2872–82. (In Eng). https://doi.org/10.1016/j.jacc.2015.10.026.
94. Steinberg BA, Peterson ED, Kim S, et al. Use and outcomes associated with bridging during anticoagulation interruptions in patients with atrial fibrillation: findings from the Outcomes Registry for Better Informed Treatment of Atrial Fibrillation (ORBIT-AF). Circulation. 2015;131(5):488–94. (In Eng). https://doi.org/10.1161/circulationaha.114.011777.
95. Connolly SJ, Ezekowitz MD, Yusuf S, et al. Dabigatran versus warfarin in patients with atrial fibrillation. N Engl J Med. 2009;361(12):1139–51. https://doi.org/10.1056/NEJMoa0905561.
96. Hagens VE, Ranchor AV, Van Sonderen E, et al. Effect of rate or rhythm control on quality of life in persistent atrial fibrillation. Results from the Rate Control Versus Electrical Cardioversion (RACE) Study. J Am Coll Cardiol. 2004;43(2):241–7. (In Eng). https://doi.org/10.1016/j.jacc.2003.08.037.
97. Opolski G, Torbicki A, Kosior DA, et al. Rate control vs rhythm control in patients with nonvalvular persistent atrial fibrillation: the results of the Polish How to Treat Chronic Atrial Fibrillation (HOT CAFE) Study. Chest. 2004;126(2):476–86. (In Eng). https://doi.org/10.1378/chest.126.2.476.
98. Meta-analysis: antithrombotic therapy to prevent stroke in patients who have nonvalvular atrial fibrillation. Ann Intern Med. 2007;146(12):857–67. https://doi.org/10.7326/0003-4819-146-12-200706190-00007. PMID: 17577005.
99. Effect of clopidogrel added to aspirin in patients with atrial fibrillation. N Engl J Med. 2009;360(20):2066–78. https://doi.org/10.1056/NEJMoa0901301.
100. Clopidogrel plus aspirin versus oral anticoagulation for atrial fibrillation in the Atrial fibrillation Clopidogrel Trial with Irbesartan for prevention of Vascular Events (ACTIVE W): a randomised controlled trial. Lancet. 2006;367(9526):1903–12. https://doi.org/10.1016/S0140-6736(06)68845-4.
101. Patel MR, Mahaffey KW, Garg J, et al. Rivaroxaban versus warfarin in nonvalvular atrial fibrillation. N Engl J Med. 2011;365(10):883–91. https://doi.org/10.1056/NEJMoa1009638.
102. Granger CB, Alexander JH, McMurray JJV, et al. Apixaban versus warfarin in patients with atrial fibrillation. N Engl J Med. 2011;365(11):981–92. https://doi.org/10.1056/NEJMoa1107039.
103. Giugliano RP, Ruff CT, Braunwald E, et al. Edoxaban versus warfarin in patients with atrial fibrillation. N Engl J Med. 2013;369(22):2093–104. https://doi.org/10.1056/NEJMoa1310907.

Chronic Kidney Disease and Cardiovascular Outcomes

Gates B. Colbert, Lovy Gaur, Mohamed Elrggal, Hector Madariaga, and Edgar Lerma

Key Points

- Cardiovascular disease is the primary cause of mortality in patients with chronic kidney disease (CKD).
- The kidneys receive 25% of cardiac output and are completely dependent on proper cardiac function.
- Several cardiorenal syndromes exist, revealing the pathophysiologic interplay of the kidneys and heart.
- Multiple biomarkers are being studied to determine risks and outcomes in patients experiencing worsening kidney function with CKD.
- Renin-angiotensin-aldosterone system inhibitor (RAASi) medications are the foundation of lowering proteinuria, controlling hypertension, and limiting cardiovascular complications in those with CKD.

G. B. Colbert (✉)
Division of Nephrology, Texas A&M College of Medicine, Dallas, TX, USA
e-mail: gates.colbert@bswhealth.org

L. Gaur
Department of Nephrology and Kidney Transplant, Max Superspeciality Hospital, Vaishali, Delhi-NCR, Ghaziabad, Uttar Pradesh, India

M. Elrggal
Nephrology Department, AlQabbary Hospital, Alexandria, Egypt

Nephrology Department, Kidney and Urology Center, Alexandria, Egypt

H. Madariaga
Lahey Hospital and Medical Center, Burlington, MA, USA

E. Lerma
Section of Nephrology, Department of Medicine, University of Illinois at Chicago College of Medicine, Associates in Nephrology, SC, Chicago, IL, USA

© The Author(s), under exclusive license to Springer Nature Switzerland AG 2024
K. C. Maki, D. P. Wilson (eds.), *Cardiovascular Outcomes Research*, Contemporary Cardiology, https://doi.org/10.1007/978-3-031-54960-1_16

- Sodium-glucose cotransporter inhibitor medications have become a new cornerstone of cardioprotection in CKD.
- 3-hydroxy-3-methylglutaryl coenzyme A reductase inhibitor (statin) class medications have been shown to provide benefits to patients with CKD, but are controversial for outcomes in patients with end-stage kidney disease
- Controlling blood pressure to a goal of <130/80 mm Hg is recommended in those with CKD.
- Smoking cessation, exercise, and a low salt diet have been associated with better outcomes in patients with CKD.
- Second-generation mineralocorticoid antagonists and endothelin antagonists are being studied and approved recently as new classes to add to aggressive RAASi therapies.

1 Introduction

As a widely recognized public health issue, chronic kidney disease (CKD) poses a significant burden that affects various aspects of societal and healthcare systems on a global scale. With almost 700 million people worldwide with CKD [1], there is also a corollary increase in the number of patients reaching advanced stages of CKD who may require kidney replacement therapy. About three million patients worldwide are receiving kidney replacement therapy, including dialysis and transplants, and these numbers are expected to grow by 50–100% in the coming decade [2]. There are a myriad of reasons for this increase; some of them are growth of the elderly population, increased prevalence of type 2 diabetes and hypertension, and lack of screening earlier stages of CKD.

Although, as of late, there has been improved recognition of the increasing burden of CKD, as manifested by increasing allocation of healthcare resources for the early diagnosis and treatment of CKD, those affected continue to have a significantly decreased life expectancy as compared to that of the general population. In a report published in 2017 [3], globally, CKD accounted for 2,968,600 (1.1%) of disability-adjusted life years (DALYs) and 2,546,700 (1.3%) of life years lost in 2012.

Moreover, a meta-analysis of cohort studies [4, 5] involving >1.4 million individuals showed an association between low estimated glomerular filtration rate (eGFR) and higher degree of albuminuria with cardiovascular disease (CVD). These analyses demonstrate that the risk of developing CVD in patients with CKD surpasses the risk of reaching end-stage kidney disease (ESKD), and, therefore, CKD must be considered one of the strongest risk factors for the development of CVD [6].

In this chapter, we discuss the intricate interrelationships between CKD and CVD from a pathophysiological standpoint, and also take a more in-depth look at the current landscape as influenced by various landmark cardiovascular (CV) outcome trials involving novel therapeutic agents.

2 Mechanisms and Pathophysiology

The association and organ cross talk between the heart and kidneys was first observed by Robert Bright in 1836, based on his observations of cardiac structural changes in patients with CKD [7]. Ancient Chinese medicine textbooks describe patients with dyspnea, abdominal distention, palpitations, and "water Qi disorder" similar to what we know as a cardiorenal syndrome in contemporary or Western medicine. In addition, the heart is described as the "dominant fire" and the kidneys as the "subordinate fire." If there is dysregulation or incoordination of these two organs, it results in a condition called "xin shen bu jiao," which leads to heart failure or "heart water" (Xinshui) and kidney failure typically described as "guan" or oliguria, which is very similar to today's cardiorenal syndrome [8].

Cardiorenal syndromes (CRS) are disorders of the heart and kidneys in which one organ induces disease in the other organ. It is a bidirectional disorder and was first described in a 2004 National, Heart, Lung, and Blood Institute Working Group conference [9], in which the main focus was a better understanding of the connection between the heart and the kidneys based on observations in patients with cardiac dysfunction abnormalities that were not preceded by a known diagnosis of CKD. Until that time, it was suspected that acute and chronic kidney responses were due primarily to a cardiac function impairment. At first, it was described as "cardiorenal dysregulation," which later became known as "cardio-renal syndrome" in which the attempt to relieve symptoms of congestive heart failure was limited by a decrease in kidney function.

In 2008, the Acute Dialysis Quality Initiative [10] recognized that there was a wider clinical spectrum of this syndrome and the consensus was to expand and phenotype the CRS into two groups: CRS and renocardiac syndromes (Table 1), which

Table 1 Cardiorenal syndromes with descriptions

Cardiorenal syndrome	Time frame	Characterization	Phenotypes
Type 1	Acute	Acute heart decompensation resulting in acute kidney injury	1. Coronary syndrome resulting in cardiogenic shock and resultant acute kidney injury 2. Cardiac outflow problem resulting in acute kidney injury
Type 2	Chronic	Chronic heart failure resulting in chronic kidney disease	Chronic heart failure with resultant fluid overload and electrolyte abnormalities
Type 3	Acute	Acute kidney injury leading to acute heart decompensation	1. Elevated creatinine resulting in acute cardiogenic shock 2. Inflammatory cascade 3. Hyperkalemia, metabolic acidosis, hypocalcemia leading to myocyte compromise

(continued)

Table 1 (continued)

Cardiorenal syndrome	Time frame	Characterization	Phenotypes
Type 4	Chronic	Chronic kidney disease resulting in chronic heart failure	Chronic loss of eGFR leading to right sided heart failure with fluid overload
Type 5	Secondary causes	Systemic process resulting in heart failure and kidney failure	1. Amyloidosis 2. Sepsis syndrome 3. Chronic liver disease

eGFR estimated glomerular filtration rate

later became five categories or subgroups, based on the acuity of heart or kidney disease and sequential organ involvement. These categories facilitated an approach to the different clinical presentations of cardiorenal dysregulation, simplified the diagnosis, and gave more options for therapeutic interventions. However, diagnosis continues to be challenging for clinicians as phenotypes tend to overlap in clinical practice and it is difficult to distinguish whether the heart or the kidney is the primary source of pathology adversely affecting the other organ. Furthermore, in general, the categorization does not help to guide therapy, particularly if the patient has other comorbidities such as hypertension, diabetes mellitus, liver cirrhosis, or sepsis.

A simplified case scenario to explain CRS is based on the fact that the heart pumps blood to other organs, including the kidney. The kidneys receive a large proportion of the entire cardiac output, 25%, which is due to a circumstantial low resistance circuit within the kidney that facilitates adequate glomerular filtration. This low resistance predisposes the kidney vasculature to a low oxygen tension in the outer medulla, making it susceptible to injuries, such as damage resulting from hypotension. When the heart fails, there is reduced ejection fraction and reduced cardiac output, which impair the ability to move blood forward leading to kidney hypoperfusion. This phenomenon results in the activation of the renin-angiotensin-aldosterone axis due to the poor blood flow to the renal afferent arteriole, which leads to vasoconstriction and activation of the sympathetic nervous system. This in turn results in arginine vasopressin secretion, which subsequently results in increased preload due to fluid retention causing worsening of pump failure [11]. However, this low-flow state or "underfilling" theory does not entirely explain the sequential phenomena taking place in CRS.

More recent evidence, including results from clinical trials, has shown that it is actually venous congestion or increased central venous pressure, right heart failure, and fluid overload that result in kidney dysfunction. In patients with acute heart failure, it has been established that there is a relative preservation of GFR even in the presence of reduced blood flow to the kidney. This is supported by an increase in the filtration fraction from elevated intraglomerular pressures in the setting of increased renin levels. On the other hand, severely elevated kidney venous pressures with decreased kidney blood flow and an increase in the filtration fraction lead to a decline in GFR which is caused by the intense neurohumoral axis activation along with the renin-angiotensin-aldosterone system (RAAS). In this situation, there is increased sodium and water reabsorption in the proximal tubule to maintain effective plasma volumes which results in oliguria and venous congestion. These hemodynamic changes are reflected by elevations in serum creatinine in the setting of decreased glomerular filtration. It has also been observed that an increase in right atrial pressure is associated with kidney impairment. In addition, an increase in intra-abdominal pressure during an episode of acute heart failure causes kidney compression, reduced perfusion, and poor filtration.

Other mechanisms in CRS that are considered non-hemodynamic pathways include elevated circulating levels of tumor necrosis factor-α (TNF-α), interleukin (IL)-1, and IL-6 observed in experimental models of acute kidney injury (AKI). These markers may have a direct effect on the left ventricular ejection fraction. Most recently, the fibroblast growth factor (FGF)-23 was shown to be associated with CRS type IV or uremic cardiomyopathy, which can lead to left ventricular hypertrophy. Hypertrophy in these cases leads to microvascular ischemia due to capillary density reduction. The long-term effects have not been well studied; nonetheless, some experimental AKI-CKD transition models in mice have demonstrated that despite normalization of GFR, inflammation continues after the initial episode, with elevated biomarkers such as the fibrosis marker α-smooth muscle actin (α-SMA) and the kidney injury molecule (KIM)-1, leading to loss of function, delayed fibrosis after ischemic-reperfusion, proximal tubule injuries, as well as unilateral obstruction impairment [12].

3 Cardiorenal Biomarkers

Soluble biomarkers can help in the diagnosis and prognosis of CRS and to guide therapy (Table 2). There are different approaches to the timing and frequency of measurement of specific biomarkers. For instance, some studies have utilized single

Table 2 Biomarkers for CRS

Biomarker	Description
Brain natriuretic peptide (BNP)	– Widely used for diagnosis of decompensated HF – Has been associated with AKI – Higher cutoff values have been suggested for patients with kidney dysfunction
Kidney injury molecule-1 (KIM1)	– Has been shown to be an AKI marker after cardiopulmonary surgery – When combined with other AKI markers (CysC, NGAL), detection of AKI improves
Neutrophil gelatinase-associated lipocalin (NGAL)	– Widely accepted as a marker of AKI – Serum NGAL levels associated with worsening kidney function in patients admitted for ADHF

(continued)

Table 2 (continued)

Biomarker	Description
Angiopoietin	– Elevated plasma levels of Ang-2 (usually in ACS) has been associated as a strong and independent predictor of mortality in patients with AKI in ICU
ST2 (soluble ST2, sST2)	– Increased sST2 levels correlate with LVEF, hemodynamics and severity in acute MI – ST2 elevations are predictive of AKI in patients with STEMI
Soluble thrombomodulin	– When combined with Ang-2, it can serve as an independent predictor of development of AKI in patients with acute MI
Cystatin C (CysC)	– Levels increase earlier than serum creatinine in patients with AKI – Elevated CysC levels are associated with AKI in patients after cardiopulmonary bypass – Increased CysC levels are associated with mortality in patients with ADHF
Interleukin-18 (IL-18)	Increased levels associated with adverse cardiovascular outcomes in chronic dialysis patients
Calprotectin	In patients with CRS 1, it has shown high sensitivity and specificity in patients at risk of AKI – Interpretation might be difficult as it is also elevated in some malignancies and in urinary tract infections
High-sensitivity cardiac troponin (hs-cTn)	– Elevated in patients with CKD, even in the absence of AHF or ACS, however higher peak levels have a greater risk of cardiorenal rehospitalization – In CKD patients, without prevalent HF, elevated levels are associated with five-fold risk of incident HF [13, 14]

Fan et al. [15]

ACS acute coronary syndrome, *ADHF* acute decompensated heart failure, *AHF* acute heart failure, *AKI* acute kidney injury, *Ang-2* angiopoietin, *BNP* brain natriuretic peptide, *CKD* chronic kidney disease, *CRS* cardiorenal syndrome, *CysC* cystatin C, *HF* heart failure, *ICU* intensive care unit, *IL* interleukin, *KIM-1* kidney injury molecule-1, *LVEF* left ventricular ejection fraction, *MI* myocardial infarction, *NGAL* neutrophil gelatinase-associated lipocalin, *sST2* soluble ST2, *STEMI* ST-elevation myocardial infarction

measurements at the time of acute heart failure with decompensation. In these cases, interpretation is limited as levels might be affected by the degree of renal function; worsening kidney function may not be a good indicator of cardiorenal morbidity [13] (Fig. 1).

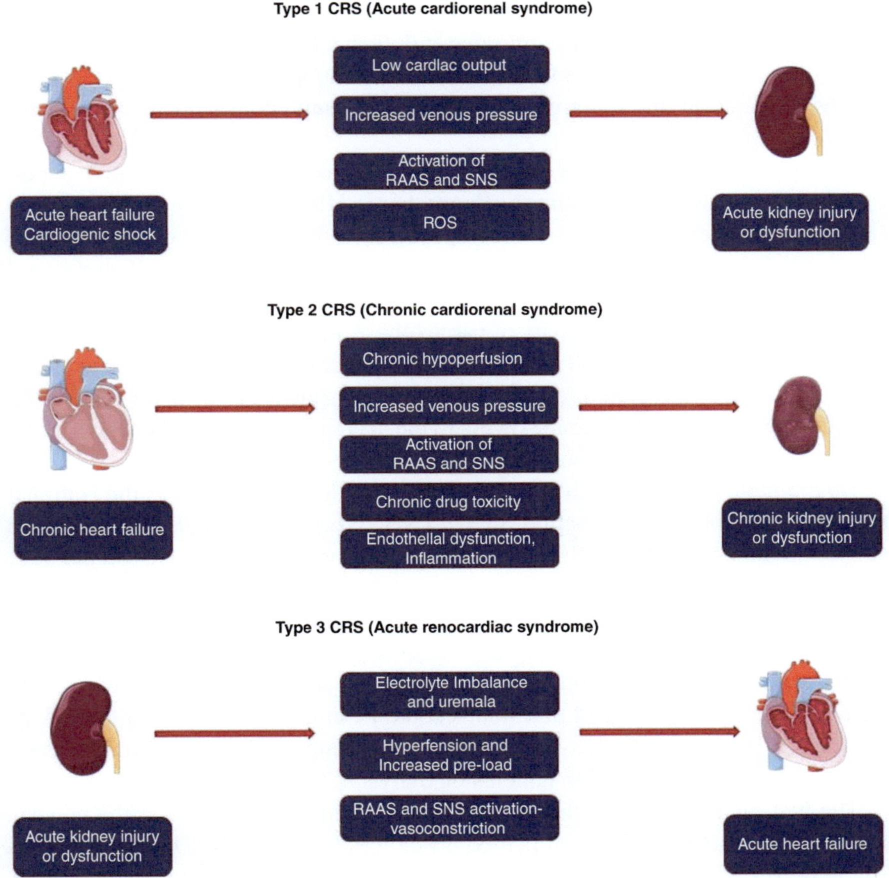

Fig. 1 Cardiorenal Syndromes Types 1-3 with primary and secondary organ impact. Figure from [16]

4 Low-Density Lipoprotein Cholesterol (LDL-C)-Lowering Drugs and CV Outcomes in CKD

Statins inhibit 3-hydroxy-3-methylglutaryl coenzyme A reductase (HMG Co-A reductase), an enzyme which catalyzes the rate-limiting step in the *de novo* synthesis of cholesterol. This leads to a reduction in cholesterol levels within the hepatocytes which, in turn, promotes the transcription of genes for the synthesis of the low-density lipoprotein receptor (LDLR). The upregulation of the LDLR on the cell surface facilitates clearance of LDL from the bloodstream, resulting in reduced circulating LDL-C [17]. In addition to LDL-lowering benefits, statins are known to exert pleiotropic effects, such as improve endothelial function, stabilize atherosclerotic plaques, and alter anti-inflammatory and immunomodulatory functions, primarily mediated by the inhibition of synthesis of isoprenoid intermediates of the mevalonate pathway [18].

Dyslipidemia is common in patients with CKD, as are certain qualitative abnormalities in cholesterol-containing lipoproteins [19]. High-density lipoprotein (HDL) levels decline due to decreased production of apolipoprotein A, impaired activity of lecithin-cholesterol acyltransferase, and increased activity of cholesteryl ester transfer protein. Furthermore, the anti-oxidative property of HDL is compromised due to the decreased activity of paraoxonase and glutathione peroxidase [20]. LDL-C is generally not elevated, but the level of a distinct subclass known as small, dense LDL may be elevated, and may be an independent predictor of CVD [21]. Hypertriglyceridemia also occurs, owing to the decreased activity of hepatic triglyceride lipase and peripheral lipoprotein lipase [22].

Dyslipidemia worsens with the progression of CKD. According to the National Health and Nutrition Examination Survey (NHANES) 2001–2010, the prevalence of dyslipidemia was 45.5%, 53.5%, 55.1%, 63.4%, and 67.8% in CKD Stages 1, 2, 3a, 3b, and 4, respectively [23]. The first major trials that studied the efficacy of statins to reduce CV events excluded patients with kidney failure (eGFR <30 mL/min/1.73 m^2). Therefore, the potential benefits of statins in CKD patients were initially derived from retrospective studies, post-hoc analyses of major trials, and meta-analyses which signaled that statins could be effective in lowering the risk of incident CV events in patients with CKD not requiring dialysis [24–26]. However, no benefit was demonstrated in patients on dialysis [27, 28].

The first randomized trial that demonstrated the futility of statins in the prevention of CV events in patients on hemodialysis was the Deutsche Diabetes Dialyse Studie (4D) [29], though the post-hoc data suggested a benefit in the patients with LDL-C levels in the highest quartile [30]. These results were nearly replicated when rosuvastatin was studied in dialysis patients [31]. The Study of Heart and Renal Protection (SHARP) [32] was the largest randomized controlled trial (RCT) undertaken to study statins (plus ezetimibe) in a CKD population. One-third of patients were receiving maintenance dialysis at randomization. At a median follow-up of 4.9 years, there was a significant reduction (17%) in major atherosclerotic events (non-fatal myocardial infarction [MI], coronary death, non-hemorrhagic stroke, or arterial revascularization) in the statin plus ezetimibe arm, mainly driven by reductions in non-fatal MI and revascularization procedures. There was no difference in CV mortality. A more recent meta-analysis examined the effects of statin and ezetimibe combination therapy in 14,016 patients with CKD [33]. Statin and ezetimibe combination had beneficial effects on serum total cholesterol, LDL-C, and triglycerides compared to statin monotherapy. All-cause mortality and major adverse cardiovascular events (MACE) were also significantly reduced (RR 0.86, $p = 0.01$). However, patients were not stratified according to non-dialysis and dialysis. Thus, this was an encouraging retrospective study of CV event reduction, but prospective studies supporting a CV benefit in patients on dialysis remain elusive. At this time, statins are recommended in patients with CKD except those on dialysis in which there is limited evidence of benefit. If a patient transitions from CKD to dialysis, statins may provide benefit and the current recommendation is to continue their use in this circumstance, but not to initiate new statin therapy. While individuals who require dialysis have an increased risk of CVD, the risk is a result of non-atherosclerotic changes to the heart, i.e., left ventricular hypertrophy, volume overload, and, with time, micro-ischemia.

Experimental evidence suggests that proprotein convertase subtilisin/kexin type 9 (PCSK9) plays an important role in LDL metabolism. It regulates the degradation of the LDLR on the surface of hepatocytes, thereby reducing clearance of LDL from circulation. The inhibition of PCSK9 is a novel mechanism to lower lipids. At the time of this writing, there are two agents available for clinical use—evolocumab and alirocumab. The Further Cardiovascular Outcomes Research with PCSK9 Inhibition in Subjects with Elevated Risk (FOURIER) [34] and the Evaluation of Cardiovascular Outcomes After an Acute Coronary Syndrome During Treatment With Alirocumab (ODYSSEY Outcomes) [35] trials demonstrated the efficacy of evolocumab and alirocumab, respectively, in reducing MACE in patients who failed to achieve the LDL-C target of <70 mg/dL despite a maximal tolerated dose of statins. While the original studies excluded patients with eGFR <30 mL/min/1.73 m^2, the post-hoc analysis of FOURIER showed that the absolute reduction in CV death, MI, or stroke with evolocumab was numerically greater with more advanced CKD (stage $\geq$3 CKD, median [interquartile range] eGFR 51.1 (43.6–56.2) mL/min/1.73 m^2) [36]. Thus, PCSK9 inhibitors represent an attractive strategy to reduce CV morbidity in patients with CKD, but larger prospective studies are needed to evaluate their safety and efficacy. Combining the above studies, we still lack sufficient outcomes data in patients with CKD receiving lipid-lowering therapies. Guidelines recommend lowering LDL-C levels in line with CVD risk, but evidence of mortality benefit is lacking.

5 Diabetes: Antihyperglycemic Agents and CV Outcomes in CKD

Good glycemic control is key to prevent microvascular and macrovascular complications. However, the impact of glycemic control on CV outcomes remains a subject of controversy. While the Epidemiology of Diabetes Interventions and Complications (EDIC) [37] study demonstrated reduction in CV events with intensive glucose control, the Action in Diabetes and Vascular Disease-Preterax and Diamicron Modified Release Controlled Evaluation (ADVANCE) [38] and the Veterans Affairs Glycemic Control and Complications in Diabetes Mellitus Type 2 (VADT) [39] studies showed no CV benefit. Rather, the Action to Control Cardiovascular Disease in Diabetes (ACCORD) [40] trial demonstrated increased mortality in the intensive-glucose-control group. Results of a post-hoc analysis of ACCORD in patients with kidney dysfunction mirrored those of the original study and reaffirmed that intensive glucose lowering was associated with an increase in all-cause mortality [41].

Patients with CKD are at a greater risk of hypoglycemia because of dysregulated insulin metabolism. A cohort study done in Canada demonstrated a U-shaped association of glycated hemoglobin (HbA1c) levels with all-cause mortality in patients with underlying CKD, though a graded increase in CV events was noted with increasing HbA1c levels [42]. Based on these observations, the Kidney Disease: Improving Global Outcomes (KDIGO) recommends that the targets of HbA1c in CKD patients may range from <6.5% to <8.0%, governed by factors such as: potential hypoglycemic risks of medications, hypoglycemic awareness, and availability of resources to detect and intervene in case hypoglycemia occurs. Metformin is an antihyperglycemic agent which has stood the test of time since its first introduction. Reduction in HbA1c with metformin monotherapy is comparable to that with sulfonylureas and insulin, albeit with a lower risk of hypoglycemia [41]. Furthermore, a study conducted in China [43] demonstrated reduced CV mortality in patients receiving metformin vs. glipizide. However, there is no randomized trial that has evaluated the role of metformin for cardioprotection in a CKD population. Given the safety of metformin in the general population, it is recommended as the first agent in patients with GFR >45 mL/min/1.73 m^2 and the treatment can be continued as long as the eGFR remains above 30 mL/min/1.73 m^2.

Sodium-glucose cotransporter-2 inhibitors (SGLT2i) are novel additions to the armory of antihyperglycemic agents. Various theories have been put forth to explain the mechanisms of cardioprotection offered by SGLT2i, which include natriuresis, glycemic moderation, reduction of blood pressure, weight loss, inhibition of the sympathetic nervous system, prevention of cardiac remodeling, prevention of ischemia-reperfusion injury, restoration of vascular progenitor cells, and decrease in oxidative stress. There is ample evidence to confirm their cardioprotective and reno-protective potential. Two early trials—the Empagliflozin Cardiovascular Outcome Event Trial in Type 2 Diabetes Mellitus Patients–Removing Excess Glucose (EMPA-REG OUTCOME) trial [44] and the Canagliflozin Cardiovascular Assessment Study (CANVAS) [45] showed that empagliflozin and canagliflozin reduced the 3-point MACE by 14% in patients with pre-existing CVD. The trend for benefit was also noted in 26% and 20% of those enrolled in the EMPA-REG OUTCOME and CANVAS trials, respectively, who had underlying CKD (eGFR <20 mL/min/1.73 m^2). Likewise, dapagliflozin met the primary safety endpoint of non-inferiority for MACE (not significant when tested for superiority) in the Dapagliflozin Effect on Cardiovascular Events–Thrombolysis in Myocardial Infarction 58 (DECLARE-TIMI 58) trial [46]. Though the inclusion criteria mandated eGFR >60 mL/min/1.73 m^2, about 7.4% of the patients had lower eGFR. Nevertheless, the CV benefit was demonstrated in all subgroups stratified by eGFR. The CV benefit was again shown in the "primarily-renal" Canagliflozin and Renal Events in Diabetes with Established Nephropathy Clinical Evaluation (CREDENCE) trial using canagliflozin in patients with CKD [47].

While a trend for reduction in hospitalization for heart failure was noted in all the trials discussed above, this was further explored as a primary outcome in two notable trials—the Dapagliflozin and Prevention of Adverse Outcomes in Heart Failure (DAPA-HF) trial [48] and the Empagliflozin Outcome Trial in Patients With Chronic Heart Failure With Reduced Ejection Fraction (EMPEROR-Reduced) [49]. There was a significant reduction in the primary outcome (worsening heart failure or CV death) in the group receiving SGLT2i which extended to even those with eGFR <60 mL/min/1.73 m^2 at baseline. Even in patients with heart failure and preserved ejection fraction (HFpEF), SGLT2i class medications have demonstrated improvements. As an important quality indicator for heart failure therapies, the ability of the SGLT2i class to reduce hospitalization rates is, thus, a significant milestone. Studying further possibilities of empagliflozin in HFpEF, EMPERIAL-PRESERVED showed that it did not meet the primary endpoint at 12 weeks of 6-min walk test distance change [50], but it was well tolerated and these results should prove helpful to design future trials. In the PRESERVED-HF trial of 324 patients on dapagliflozin vs placebo, dapagliflozin met the primary endpoint of improvement in the Kansas City Cardiomyopathy Questionnaire Clinical Summary Score (KCCQ-CS) at 12 weeks with an increase in score of 5.8 [51]. KDIGO recommends that the first-line glycemic management for patients with CKD should include metformin and a SGLT2i.

In patients who are unable to achieve individualized glycemic targets, a glucagon-like peptide-1 (GLP-1) receptor agonist is recommended in view of the CV and kidney benefits associated with this class of drugs. GLP-1 is an incretin produced by L-cells of ileum and colon in response to eating. It performs a multitude of functions like augmentation of glucose-stimulated insulin secretion by pancreatic islet cells, inhibition of glucagon and gastric acid secretion, and promotion of satiety. Four of the available injectable GLP-1 receptor agonist agents, liraglutide [52], semaglutide [53], albiglutide outside of the United States [54], and dulaglutide [55], have been shown to confer cardioprotective effects. In contrast, lixisenatide [56] and oral semaglutide [57] were found to be non-inferior to placebo in reduction of MACE. It is important to note that the CV benefit from SGLT2i appears to be mainly from the reduced incidence of hospitalization for HF and cardiac mortality, in contrast to benefits of GLP-1 agonists, which appear to mainly be reduction in MI and stroke.

Additional medications may be required to achieve glycemic targets. However, there is no evidence of cardioprotection with other classes of antihyperglycemic drugs (Table 3).

Table 3 SGLT2i studies

Study	Population	Intervention	Mean eGFR at inclusion	Median follow-up	Primary outcomes	Results
EMPA-REG [44] 2015	7020 patients with T2DM and established CVD and eGFR >30 mL/min/1.73 m^2	Empagliflozin 10 mg or 25 mg vs. placebo	26% had GFR <60 mL/min/1.73 m^2	3.1 years	Composite of death from CV causes, non-fatal MI, or non-fatal stroke	14% reduction in primary outcome (HR 0.86, 95% CI 0.74–0.99; $p = 0.04$)
CANVAS [45] 2017	10,142 T2DM patients with high CV risk and eGFR >30 mL/min/1.73 m^2	Canagliflozin 100 mg or 300 mg vs. placebo	76.5 mL/min/1.73 m^2 (20% had GFR <60 mL/min/1.73 m^2)	126 weeks	Composite of death from CV causes, non-fatal MI, or non-fatal stroke	14% reduction in primary outcome (HR 0.86, 95% CI 0.75–0.97; $p = 0.02$)
DECLARE-TIMI-58 [46] 2019	17,160 patients with T2DM and CVD (41%) or at high risk of developing atherosclerotic CVD (59%)	Dapagliflozin 10 mg vs. placebo	85.2 mL/min/1.73 m^2 (7.4% had GFR <60 mL/min/1.73 m^2)	4.2 years	Two primary efficacy outcomes were MACE (defined as CV death, MI, or ischemic stroke) and a composite of CV death or hospitalization for heart failure	Dapagliflozin met the prespecified criterion for noninferiority with respect to MACE (upper boundary of the 95% CI <1.3, $p < 0.001$ for non-inferiority) Lower rate of composite of CV death or hospitalization for heart failure (HR 0.83, 95% CI 0.73–0.95, $p = 0.005$)—Mainly driven by a reduction in hospitalization for heart failure
DAPA-HF [47] 2019	4744 patients with NYHA Class II-IV heart failure and EF < =40%. 45% had T2DM	Dapagliflozin	65.7 mL/min/1.73 m^2	18.2 months	Composite of worsening heart failure or CV death	26% reduction in primary outcome (HR 0.74, 95% CI 0.65–0.85, $p < 0.001$)

Table 3 (continued)

Study	Population	Intervention	Mean eGFR at inclusion	Median follow-up	Primary outcomes	Results
CREDENCE [47] 2019	4401 patients with GFR 30–90 mL/min/1.73 m^2	Canagliflozin	56 mL/min/1.73 m^2	2.62 years	CV events were assessed as secondary outcomes in hierarchical testing	31% reduction in composite of CV death or hospitalization for heart failure (HR 0.69, 95% CI 0.57–0.983, $p < 0.001$) 20% reduction in risk of composite of CV death, MI or stroke (HR 0.80, 95% CI 0.67–0.95, $p = 0.01$)
VERTIS CV [58] 2020	8246 patients with established atherosclerotic CVD with GFR >30 mL/min/1.73 m^2	Ertugliflozin	76 mL/min/1.73 m^2	3.5 years	Composite of death from CV causes, nonfatal MI, or nonfatal stroke	Non-inferior to placebo
DAPA-CKD [59] 2020	4303 patients with GFR 25–75 mL/min/1.73 m^2 and UACR 200–5000	Dapagliflozin	43 mL/min/1.73 m^2	2.4 years	CV outcome (hospitalization for heart failure or death from CV causes) as secondary outcome	29% reduction in CV deaths and hospitalization due to heart failure (0.71, 95% CI 0.55–0.92; $p = 0.009$)
EMPEROR-Reduced [49] 2020	3730 patients with Class II–IV with EF < =40%	Empagliflozin 10 mg/day vs. placebo	62 mL/min/1.73 m^2 (48% had GFR <60 mL/min/1.73 m^2)	16 months	Composite of adjudicated CV death or hospitalization for heart failure	25% reduction in risk of primary outcome (HR 0.75, 95% CI 0.65–0.86, $p < 0.001$)

CANVAS Canagliflozin Cardiovascular Assessment Study, *CI* confidence interval, *CREDENCE* Canagliflozin and Renal Events in Diabetes with Established Nephropathy Clinical Evaluation, *CV* Cardiovascular, *DAPA-CKD* Dapagliflozin and Prevention of Adverse Outcomes in Chronic Kidney Disease, *DAPA-HF* Dapagliflozin and Prevention of Adverse Outcomes in Heart Failure, *DECLARE-TIMI 58* The Dapagliflozin Effect on Cardiovascular Events–Thrombolysis in Myocardial Infarction 58, *EMPEROR-reduced* Empagliflozin Outcome Trial in Patients With Chronic Heart Failure With Reduced Ejection Fraction, *EF* Ejection fraction, *eGFR* estimated glomerular filtration rate, *EMPA-REG* Empagliflozin Cardiovascular Outcome Event Trial in Type 2 Diabetes Mellitus Patients–Removing Excess Glucose (EMPA-REG) OUTCOME trial, *HR* hazard ratio, *MACE* major adverse cardiovascular event, *MI* myocardial infarction, *NYHA* New York Heart Association, *T2DM* Type 2 diabetes mellitus, *UACR* urine albumin-to-creatinine ratio, *VERTIS-CV* Evaluation of Ertugliflozin Efficacy and Safety Cardiovascular Outcomes Trial

6 Antiplatelet Agents

Patients with CKD are at increased risk for thrombotic and hemorrhagic complications, often due to effects of uremic toxins on platelet function. Although long-term antiplatelet therapies have been shown to reduce the risk of MI, stroke and vascular death among the general population [60–62], patients with moderate to severe CKD were excluded from most clinical trials. Thus, fewer data are available to inform clinical practice in patients with CKD. For primary prevention, i.e., in adult patients with CKD and no history of CVD, a meta-analysis of five trials of aspirin therapy were pooled ($n = 7852$ total, $n = 3935$ aspirin, $n = 3917$ placebo). Overall, 434 CVD events were cited but there was no statistically significant reduction in CVD events (hazard ratio [HR] 0.76, 95% confidence interval [CI] 0.54–1.08; $p = 0.13$, $I^2 = 63\%$), all-cause mortality (HR 0.94, 95% CI 0.74–1.19; $p = 0.60$, $I^2 = 21\%$), coronary heart disease events (HR 0.66, 95% CI 0.27–1.63; $p = 0.37$, $I^2 = 64\%$), or stroke (HR 0.87, 95% CI 0.6–1.27; $p = 0.48$, $I^2 = 24\%$) from aspirin therapy versus placebo [63]. The Aspirin to Target Arterial Events in Chronic Kidney Disease (ATTACK) trial (NCT03796156, Clinicaltrials.gov) is an open label, multi-center primary prevention trial of aspirin in CKD currently underway that may help clarify the role of aspirin in this setting.

There is somewhat better evidence to support the use of antiplatelet therapy in secondary prevention of CVD in CKD. A Cochrane systematic review and meta-analysis including 50 RCTs, enrolling 27,139 participants, examined the efficacy and safety of antiplatelets (mainly aspirin) in secondary prevention of CVD in CKD patients [64]. Compared to placebo or no treatment, antiplatelet agents reduced the risk of MI (17 studies; relative risk [RR] 0.87, 95% CI 0.76–0.99), but not all-cause mortality (30 studies; RR 0.93, 95% CI 0.81–1.06), CV mortality (19 studies; RR 0.89, 95% CI 0.70–1.12), or stroke (11 studies; RR 1.00, 95% CI 0.58–1.72). Again, antiplatelet agents increased the risk of major (27 studies; RR 1.33, 95% CI 1.10–1.65) and minor bleeding (18 studies; RR 1.49, 95% CI 1.12–1.97). These results did not differ according to the CKD stage. Specific recommendations for the use of dual antiplatelet therapy among CKD patients are lacking.

In summary, patients with CKD have uremic platelet dysfunction and antiplatelets agents have continuously been shown to increase risk of bleeding, which may contribute to iron deficiency anemia. However, it is unlikely that the benefits of aspirin as demonstrated in other high-risk, non-CKD populations would be completely nullified in patients with CKD, and the guidelines consistently recommend its use for secondary prevention of CVD in patients with CKD.

7 Direct Oral Anticoagulants

Patients with CKD are at increased risk of developing atrial fibrillation and venous thromboembolism [65, 66]. Therapeutic anticoagulation options include both vitamin K antagonists (VKAs), such as warfarin, and direct oral anticoagulants

(DOACs), such as dabigatran. DOACs are favorable due to lower bleeding risk, lack of monitoring requirement, less drug and dietary interactions, and lower risk of vascular calcifications with their use. However, all of the DOACs have some degree of kidney excretion and, therefore, require dose adjustment in kidney impairment. Many studies have provided assuring data about the safety of DOACs in CKD patients, however, whether they have CV benefits is still an unanswered question. A retrospective study compared 27,552 new DOAC users matched to 27,552 new VKA users for a composite CV outcome (MI, revascularization, or ischemic stroke) or mortality [67]. There was a significantly lower risk of CV events or mortality among DOAC users compared with warfarin users (HR 0.82, 95% CI 0.75–0.90) with lower risk for hemorrhage. Another observational study examined whether DOACs are a safe alternative to warfarin across different CKD stages [68]. Among 351,407 patients on anticoagulation therapy, 45% were on DOACs. CKD stages 3–5 and ESKD patients represented 12% of the cohort. DOACs, compared with warfarin, were associated with a 22% decrease in the risk of CV outcomes (HR 0.78, 95% CI 0.77–0.80; $p < 0.001$) and a 10% decrease in the risk of bleeding outcomes (HR 0.90, 95% CI 0.88–0.92; $p < 0.001$) after adjustment. This study suggests that DOACs might be a safe alternative to warfarin in patients with CKD.

8 Lifestyle Interventions to Reduce CVD Risk in CKD Patients

Lifestyle interventions to reduce CVD risk in CKD patients include diet, exercise, weight loss, and smoking cessation.

8.1 Smoking Cessation

Smoking is a known risk factor for both development and progression of CKD, and for CV-related morbidity and mortality in kidney patients [69]. While no randomized clinical trials have examined the effect of smoking on CV outcomes in CKD patients, many prospective cohorts have examined the CV risk associated with smoking in patients with CKD. An analysis of baseline smoking status among participants in SHARP compared the CV risk of current/prior smokers against never smokers in patients with diabetes and CKD [70]. Smoking significantly increased the risks for vascular and nonvascular morbidity and mortality compared to non-smoking. Results from another large cohort showed that non-smoking was associated with lower risk of atherosclerotic events (MI, stroke, or peripheral arterial disease) and all-cause mortality [71]. On the other hand, few data are present to evaluate the effect of smoking cessation in patients with CKD on CV morbidity and mortality. One prospective cohort study investigated the associations between smoking and new-onset CV outcomes and death in approximately 4000 patients with ESKD initiating dialysis [72]. As expected, active smokers were 59% more likely to develop new-onset heart failure and 68% more likely to develop peripheral artery disease compared to non-smokers. Interestingly, former smokers had adjusted event risks similar to nonsmokers, suggesting that smoking cessation can substantially lower CVD risk in this population. Therefore, patients with CKD who smoke should be counseled to quit smoking to lower their CV risks [73].

8.2 Exercise and Weight Loss

Unintentional weight loss has been associated with increased mortality in patients with CKD/ESKD [74, 75]. This is probably due to uremia, malnutrition, and sarcopenia being the main drivers of unintentional weight loss and, therefore, increasing mortality [76]. This leads to the use of the common term "obesity paradox" in these patients by reverse epidemiology, i.e., patients who are obese often have better outcomes than patients who are not obese [77]. A meta-analysis suggested that higher body mass index, waist circumference, and waist-to-height ratio are independent risk factors for decline in GFR and death in those with and without CKD [78].

On the other hand, bariatric surgery has been associated with decreased mortality in patients with obesity and CKD/ESKD [79, 80]. Moreover, the use of liraglutide to treat obesity reduced the risk for major CV events and all-cause mortality in patients with type 2 diabetes mellitus and CKD [81]. Until prospective trials are available, intentional weight loss is recommended in patients with obesity and CKD.

Physical inactivity and loss of muscle mass are the important correlates of frailty and mortality in CKD patients [82]. Therefore, physical exercise is vital for patients with CKD. It improves eGFR, reduces systolic and diastolic blood pressures, and decreases adiposity [83]. Exercise has also been associated with improved quality of life, increased exercise and walking capacity, decreased arterial stiffness, lower CV morbidity and mortality, and decreased all-cause mortality [84–87]. A recent RCT implementing caloric restriction and aerobic exercises for patients with moderate to severe CKD in a 2×2 factorial design found that these interventions had significant benefits on body weight, fat mass, and markers of oxidative stress and inflammatory response [88]. Given the multitude of benefits demonstrated for intentional weight loss and physical activity in patients with and without CKD, methods to implement these interventions should always be encouraged with CKD patients.

8.3 Dietary Intervention

Dietary modifications are recommended in the management of CKD due to the fact that significant comorbid conditions, such as high blood pressure, diabetes, CVD, and obesity respond to diet [89]. Dietary sodium, potassium, phosphorus, protein, acid load, and fiber contents usually need modifications in patients with advanced CKD. However, how much these changes affect CV outcomes is still an area of scarce data and low evidence.

8.3.1 Sodium

Excess sodium intake has been identified as a major health problem. All hypertension guidelines in both CKD and non-CKD populations recommend low salt intake. Nevertheless, cross-sectional studies have repeatedly shown worse outcomes with low-sodium diets. In an observational analysis of two large cohorts ($n = 28,880$) included in the Ongoing Telmisartan Alone and in Combination with Ramipril Global Endpoint Trial (ONTARGET) and the Telmisartan Randomized Assessment Study in ACE Intolerant Subjects with Cardiovascular Disease (TRANSCEND) trial, sodium excretion of less than 3 g per day was associated with an increased risk of CV mortality and hospitalization for congestive heart failure [90]. As expected, increased sodium intake was associated with an increased risk of all CV events. The European Project on Genes in Hypertension (EPOGH) study found the same results; lower sodium excretion was associated with higher CVD mortality [91]. Possible mechanisms behind this include that low sodium diets increase renin, aldosterone, and sympathetic nervous system activity.

On the other hand, high salt intake remains a risk factor for hypertension. A Cochrane systematic review and meta-analysis of randomized trials found that a modest reduction in salt intake causes significant decreases in blood pressure in both hypertensive and normotensive individuals [92]. Another, more recent, the Cochrane systematic review of RCTs evaluated the benefits and harms of altering dietary salt for adults with CKD [93]. This study found, with high certainty evidence, that salt reduction reduced blood pressure and albuminuria in the short term among people with CKD. Long-term benefits could not be established due to scarcity of data. Given the prognostic role of blood pressure reduction, these results will likely translate into clinically significant reductions in CKD progression and CV events. Therefore, moderation, but not severe restriction, of salt and total sodium intake appears prudent in CKD patients.

8.3.2 Potassium

While there is plenty of evidence highlighting the health benefits of a potassium-rich diet in the general population (i.e., lower blood pressure, stroke, and CV mortality) [94, 95], it is not known whether these benefits outweigh the risk of hyperkalemia in patients with CKD. Food rich in potassium such as fruits and vegetables is usually an excellent source for alkali and fiber, which are important for CKD patients as metabolic acidosis can potentiate hyperkalemia [96] and CKD progression [97]. Moreover, a diet rich in potassium citrate can prevent incident nephrolithiasis [98].

Many studies have shown the effect of a potassium-rich diet on CV outcomes in CKD patients. In the Chronic Renal Insufficiency Cohort (CRIC) study, the risks for atherosclerotic events and all-cause mortality were reduced among patients with mild to moderate CKD with a healthy lifestyle [71]. In another observational cohort study, a diet rich in fruits and vegetables was associated with lower risk for all-cause mortality and ESKD [99]. An RCT demonstrated that, compared to sodium bicarbonate treatment, a diet rich in fruits and vegetables in non-diabetic CKD patients with metabolic acidosis improved CVD risk factors, including body mass index, systolic blood pressure, LDL-C, lipoprotein(a), and serum vitamin K levels [100]. The ongoing Potassium Supplementation in CKD (K+ in CKD) study investigating the renoprotective effects of dietary potassium, with secondary outcomes of blood pressure, CV events, all-cause mortality, and incidence of hyperkalemia, may help answer some questions about dietary potassium in patients with CKD (NCT03253172, Clinicaltrials.gov).

9 Blood Pressure Management in CKD with CV Outcomes

Blood pressure management is one of the cornerstones of curbing morbidity and mortality of CVD. Patients with CKD have even greater risk than the general population of compounding risks associated with mortality as a consequence of uncontrolled hypertension and CVD [101]. These risks are increased further by proteinuria, which is present in many patients with CKD [101]. Prior to 2015, a well-known hypertension guidance trial, the ACCORD trial, showed that aggressive systolic blood pressure control targeting <120 mm Hg, compared with <140 mm Hg, did not reduce the primary composite outcome of non-fatal MI, non-fatal stroke, or death [40]. Thus, the accepted guidelines recommended a blood pressure target of <140/90 mm Hg for most patients, rather than stricter systolic blood pressure control [102]. This changed in 2015 with the publication of the Systolic Blood Pressure Intervention Trial (SPRINT), which included 9631 non-diabetic patients with hypertension. This showed that patients with a systolic blood pressure target of <120 mm Hg had fewer CV events and mortality than patients with looser control of hypertension (HR 0.75, 95% CI 0.64–0.89) [103]. While there was a worse rate of eGFR decline and AKI in patients with systolic blood pressure <120 mm Hg, the overall CV event improvement and no greater risk of ESKD helped to justify the push towards stricter blood pressure control in patients considered high risk. These trials have been heralded as gold standard trials for hypertension management given that they have been the only randomized trials looking at primary CV endpoints with blood pressure lowering. The landmark SPRINT trial helped lead to the guidelines by the American College of Cardiology (ACC)/American Heart Association (AHA) in 2017 recommending a blood pressure goal of <130/80 mm Hg in patients with CKD [104]. KDIGO guidelines, as of this publication, still recommend <140/90 mm Hg in those with low albumin excretion, <30 mg/24 h, and <130/80 mm Hg in those with albumin >30 mg/24 h [105], but this is expected to be revised with the next updated guideline publication.

Based on previous large studies, angiotensin converting enzyme inhibitors (ACEi) and angiotensin receptor blockers (ARB) are the accepted first choice medications for controlling blood pressure in patients with CKD, especially those with proteinuria [106]. The Reduction of Endpoints in Non-insulin Dependent Diabetes Mellitus with Angiotensin II Antagonist Losartan (RENAAL) study and the Heart Outcomes and Prevention Evaluation (HOPE) study investigated CV outcomes in patients using an ACEi or ARB vs. placebo [107, 108]. RENAAL showed no difference in CV outcomes, but did have less hospitalization for heart failure with ACEi or ARB. HOPE using ramipril reported improvements in patients in regard to CV outcomes. A subsequent Bayesian meta-analysis of these trials along with other studies totaling 119 trials with 64,768 patients noted that ACEi or ARB reduced the risk of CKD and CV events, thus helping hoist ACEi or ARB to the top of the CKD hypertension management [106]. A further hypothesis suggested that if one ACEi or ARB is good, then the combination of both might increase the CV benefit while controlling blood pressure to a maximal effect. The Ongoing Telmisartan Alone and in Combination with Ramipril Global Endpoint Trial (ONTARGET) and the Veterans Affairs Nephropathy in Diabetes (VA NEPHRON-D) trial studied the concept of combination of ACEi and ARB [109, 110]. Both studies demonstrated no benefit of combination therapy with ACEi/ARB as AKI and hyperkalemia risk were increased. Thus, combination therapy with ACEi and ARB is not recommended, which is reflected in the 2017 ACC/AHA guidelines.

Other classes of medications have been studied in head-to-head randomized trials. The Antihypertensive and Lipid-Lowering Treatment to Prevent Heart Attack Trial (ALLHAT) did not show a difference in CV outcomes between amlodipine, chlorthalidone, and lisinopril in patients with CKD [111]. In the Candesartan Antihypertensive Survival Evaluation in Japan (CASE-J) trial of 2720 Japanese patients, improved CV outcomes (HR 0.45) were reported in those with Stage 4 CKD treated with candesartan vs. amlodipine [112]. Yet, other studies have shown mixed results in head-to-head comparisons. A 2013 meta-analysis of trials comparing medication classes to either placebo or head-to-head in those with eGFR <60 mL/min/1.73 m^2 showed CV outcomes were improved with ACEis vs. placebo and either ACEi or calcium channel blocker (CCB) vs. placebo, but when comparing ACEis to diuretics, beta-blockers, or CCBs, no differences in CV outcomes between groups were found [113].

As of this publication, there have been no dedicated hypertension trials investigating exclusively CKD patients and CV outcomes. The best trials, SPRINT and ACCORD, showed discordant results; current guidelines rely on subgroup analyses in the CKD patients that were included in the total cohorts. Lower blood pressure is not without risks, and it is associated with higher risk of AKI, hyperkalemia, volume depletion, and dizziness [114]. Larger comparative trials are needed to investigate the CKD population exclusively, classified by the degree of proteinuria, to help clinical decision-making. Each patient should be monitored with multi-pronged goals of lowering blood pressure to guideline-driven values and maximizing RAASi dosing to tolerated levels to achieve the best CV outcomes, while minimizing adverse events and side effects.

10 Future

The development of novel therapeutic interventions and ongoing clinical trials designed to reduce CV events offer hope to patients with CKD. Some of the most promising and well-studied options on the horizon are described below.

Finerenone is a nonsteroidal, selective mineralocorticoid receptor antagonist (MRA) approved by the Food and Drug Administration in 2021 [115]. It has been shown to have potent anti-inflammatory and antifibrotic effects compared to the previous MRA agents, spironolactone and eplerenone. Additionally, finerenone has been shown to reduce the urinary albumin-to-creatinine ratio in patients with CKD already on a RAASi with less risk of hyperkalemia. The Finerenone in Reducing Kidney Failure and Disease Progression in Diabetic Kidney Disease (FIDELIO-DKD) trial was a randomized trial of 5734 patients that showed an improved primary composite outcome, defined as kidney failure, sustained decrease of at least 40% in the eGFR from baseline, or death from renal causes, in the finerenone group vs. placebo (HR = 0.82) [116]. Additionally, the finerenone group had a lower risk of secondary events including death from CV causes, nonfatal MI, nonfatal stroke, or hospitalization for heart failure (HR 0.86). The Cardiovascular Events with Finerenone in Kidney Disease and Type 2 Diabetes (FIGARO-DKD) trial studied 7437 patients with eGFR of 25–90 mL/min/1.73 m^2 with diabetes in which finerenone vs. placebo was added to maximal tolerated ACEi or ARB. The primary outcome of the composite of death from CV causes, nonfatal MI, nonfatal stroke, or hospitalization for heart failure occurred in 12.4% of the finerenone group and 14.2% of the placebo group with a HR of 0.87 [117]. Both trials are promising because they show that adding finerenone to the standard of care in patients with CKD and diabetes may reduce CV events and progression of CKD. A pooled analysis trial, FIDELITY, showed that among the 13,026 patients who received finerenone, the composite CV outcome was less than placebo (HR 0.86, $p = 0.0018$) and the composite kidney outcome with finerenone was better as well (HR 0.77, $p = 0.0002$) [118].

Endothelins (ET) are a group of peptides that behave as potent vasoconstrictors and have been shown to be pro-fibrotic growth factors. Specifically, ET-1 is integral for vascular tone, is associated with kidney and CV pathophysiology, and is tied to activation of aldosterone, catecholamines, and angiotensin [119]. Endothelin antagonists (ETA), such as bosentan, have been shown to be helpful in treating pulmonary hypertension [120]. ET activation can escalate progression of CKD via pro-fibrotic pathways, and is also associated with diabetic nephropathy, focal segmental glomerular sclerosis, and polycystic kidney disease [121]. ETA have been shown in preliminary studies to delay glomerular injury and podocyte effacement and reduce proteinuria and scarring. An experimental ETA class drug, atrasentan, reduced albuminuria in patients with diabetic nephropathy; withdrawal of the agent caused albuminuria to rise to baseline [122]. The Avosentan for Overt Diabetic Nephropathy (ASCEND) trial tested another ETA, avosentan, vs. placebo added to RAASi in 1392 patients, but the study was halted early at 4 months because fluid retention was pervasive and led to increased CV events [123]. As atrasentan, avosentan, and bosentan are not highly selective, they frequently cause fluid overload and are contraindicated with severe edema, heart failure, or advanced CKD. ETA agents show a lot of promise physiologically, but are not ready for clinical use until they can become more selective for target receptors and have been proven safe. Studies of two newer agents, sparsentan and sitaxsentan, are ongoing and may yield better results [119]. Sparsentan is currently approved by the FDA for use in IgA nephropathy only, but may have off-label, real-world use in the future for other glomerular diseases.

Another area that is under investigation is microvascular damage of end organs in patients with CKD. Systemic microvascular rarefaction is described in patients with CKD. It is attributed to a multitude of compounding risk factors including: uremic angiopathy, dysfunctional microcirculation, tissue shunting, hypoxia, and micro-ischemia [124]. Endothelial losses have been studied in patients with early CKD, and this may represent the tip of the iceberg for further microvascular loss [124]. Hypoxia inducible factor (HIF)-1a is important for promoting angiogenesis, but it has been shown to be downregulated in the skeletal muscle and heart of patients with CKD. In the kidney, HIF-1a accumulation promotes fibrosis, without the increased angiogenesis needed to counteract the losses caused by rarefaction [125]. This tissue injury then further leads to fibrosis, and progressively more rarefaction has been demonstrated in several animal models [126]. Apoptosis is associated with capillary rarefaction in animal models of hypertension [127]. As most patients with CKD die from CVD, microvascular disease of other organs, principally the heart and brain, has been a target of study and hypotheses to promote decreased morbidity and mortality. Currently, there are no approved vascular agents to reverse or halt progressive rarefaction, fibrosis, and eventual end organ damage.

11 Conclusion

Recent years have yielded a number of advances with regard to limiting CVD and death in patients with CRS. Our understanding of the pathophysiology and link between the heart and the kidney continues to improve. As new tools are used, individually or in combination, such as maximizing RAASi dosing and adding SGLT2i and additional new generation MRA agents, long-term outcomes may continue to improve. To date, there are no randomized trial data combining all the available medications along with a complete understanding of the optimum management of patients with CKD. Hopefully, this will change as new trials are planned in which all agents available at optimized dosing will be administered to drive guideline recommendations.

References

1. GBD Chronic Kidney Disease Collaboration. Global, regional, and national burden of chronic kidney disease, 1990-2017: a systematic analysis for the Global Burden of Disease Study 2017. Lancet. 2020;395(10225):709–33. https://doi.org/10.1016/S0140-6736(20)30045-3. Epub 2020 Feb 13.
2. International Society of Nephrology. ISN Global Health Atlas. 2019. https://www.theisn.org/initiatives/global-kidney-health-atlas. Accessed 26 Aug 2021; United States Renal Data System, Annual Data Report. 2018. https://www.usrdsorg/2018/view/v2_01aspx. Accessed 25 Feb 2021.
3. Webster AC, Nagler EV, Morton RL, Masson P. Chronic kidney disease. Lancet. 2017;389:1238–52. https://doi.org/10.1016/S0140-6736(16)32064-5.
4. Matsushita K, van der Velde M, Astor BC, Woodward M, Levey AS, de Jong PE, Coresh J, Gansevoort RT. Association of estimated glomerular filtration rate and albuminuria with all-cause and cardiovascular mortality in general population cohorts: a collaborative meta-analysis. Lancet. 2010;375:2073–81. https://doi.org/10.1016/S0140-6736(10)60674-5.
5. van der Velde M, Matsushita K, Coresh J, Astor BC, Woodward M, Levey A, de Jong P, Gansevoort RT, van der Velde M, Matsushita K, et al. Chronic Kidney Disease Prognosis Consortium. Lower estimated glomerular filtration rate and higher albuminuria are associated with all-cause and cardiovascular mortality. A collaborative meta-analysis of high-risk population cohorts. Kidney Int. 2011;79:1341–52. https://doi.org/10.1038/ki.2010.536.
6. Jankowski J, Floege J, Fliser D, Böhm M, Marx N. Cardiovascular disease in chronic kidney disease: pathophysiological insights and therapeutic options. Circulation. 2021;143(11):1157–72. https://doi.org/10.1161/CIRCULATIONAHA.120.050686. Epub 2021 Mar 15.
7. R. Cases and observations illustrative of renal disease accompanied with the secretion of albuminous urine. Guy's Hosp Trans. 1836;1:338–79. https://ci.nii.ac.jp/naid/10030343458/.
8. Dai X, Zhou B, Fan S, Xiao HB. Cardiorenal syndrome: a Bright idea with earlier roots. Br J Cardiol. 2021;28:51–2. https://doi.org/10.5837/bjc.2021.022.
9. Cardio-renal connections in heart failure and cardiovascular disease. https://www.nhlbi.nih.gov/events/2004/cardio-renal-connections-heart-failure-and-cardiovascular-disease. Accessed 13 Sept 2021.
10. Ronco C, McCullough P, Anker SD, Anand I, Aspromonte N, Bagshaw SM, Bellomo R, Berl T, Bobek I, Cruz DN, Daliento L, Davenport A, Haapio M, Hillege H, House AA, Katz N, Maisel A, Mankad S, Zanco P, Mebazaa A, Palazzuoli A, Ronco F, Shaw A, Sheinfeld G, Soni S, Vescovo G, Zamperetti N, Ponikowski P, Acute Dialysis Quality Initiative (ADQI) Consensus Group. Cardio-renal syndromes: report from the consensus conference of the acute dialysis quality initiative. Eur Heart J. 2010;31(6):703–11. https://doi.org/10.1093/eurheartj/ehp507. Epub 2009 Dec 25.
11. Schrier RW, Abraham WT. Hormones and hemodynamics in heart failure. N Engl J Med. 1999;341(8):577–85. https://doi.org/10.1056/NEJM199908193410806.
12. Matsushita K, Saritas T, Eiwaz MB, McClellan N, Coe I, Zhu W, Ferdaus MZ, Sakai LY, McCormick JA, Hutchens MP. The acute kidney injury to chronic kidney disease transition in a mouse model of acute cardiorenal syndrome emphasizes the role of inflammation. Kidney Int. 2020;97(1):95–105. https://doi.org/10.1016/j.kint.2019.06.022. Epub 2019 Aug 1.
13. Seliger S. The cardiorenal syndrome: mechanistic insights and prognostication with soluble biomarkers. Curr Cardiol Rep. 2020;22(10):114. https://doi.org/10.1007/s11886-020-01360-8.
14. Triposkiadis F, Starling RC, Boudoulas H, Giamouzis G, Butler J. The cardiorenal syndrome in heart failure: cardiac? renal? syndrome? Heart Fail Rev. 2012;17(3):355–66. https://doi.org/10.1007/s10741-011-9291-x.

15. Fan PC, Chang CH, Chen YC. Biomarkers for acute cardiorenal syndrome. Nephrology (Carlton). 2018;23(Suppl 4):68–71. https://doi.org/10.1111/nep.13473.

16. Mitsas AC, Elzawawi M, Mavrogeni S, Boekels M, Khan A, Eldawy M, Stamatakis I, Kouris D, Daboul B, Gunkel O, et al. Heart failure and cardiorenal syndrome: a narrative review on pathophysiology, diagnostic and therapeutic regimens—from a cardiologist's view. J Clin Med. 2022;11(23):7041. https://doi.org/10.3390/jcm11237041.

17. Ward NC, Watts GF, Eckel RH. Statin toxicity: mechanistic insights and clinical implications. Circ Res. 2019;124(2):328–50.

18. Buhaescu I, Izzedine H. Mevalonate pathway: a review of clinical and therapeutical implications. Clin Biochem. 2007;40(9–10):575–84.

19. Keane WF, Tomassini JE, Neff DR. Lipid abnormalities in patients with chronic kidney disease: implications for the pathophysiology of atherosclerosis. J Atheroscler Thromb. 2013;20(2):123–33.

20. Moradi H, Pahl MV, Elahimehr R, Vaziri ND. Impaired antioxidant activity of high-density lipoprotein in chronic kidney disease. Transl Res. 2009;153(2):77–85.

21. Shen H, Xu Y, Lu J, Ma C, Zhou Y, Li Q, Chen X, Zhu A, Shen G. Small dense low-density lipoprotein cholesterol was associated with future cardiovascular events in chronic kidney disease patients. BMC Nephrol. 2016;17(1):1–7.

22. Mikolasevic I, Žutelija M, Mavrinac V, Orlic L. Dyslipidemia in patients with chronic kidney disease: etiology and management. Int J Nephrol Renov Dis. 2017;10:35.

23. Kuznik A, Mardekian J, Tarasenko L. Evaluation of cardiovascular disease burden and therapeutic goal attainment in US adults with chronic kidney disease: an analysis of national health and nutritional examination survey data, 2001–2010. BMC Nephrol. 2013;14(1):1–1.

24. Scandinavian Simvastatin Survival Study Group. Randomised trial of cholesterol lowering in 4444 patients with coronary heart disease: the Scandinavian Simvastatin Survival Study (4S). Lancet. 1994;344(8934):1383–9.

25. Tonelli M, Isles C, Curhan GC, Tonkin A, Pfeffer MA, Shepherd J, Sacks FM, Furberg C, Cobbe SM, Simes J, Craven T. Effect of pravastatin on cardiovascular events in people with chronic kidney disease. Circulation. 2004;110(12):1557–63.

26. Palmer SC, Navaneethan SD, Craig JC, Johnson DW, Perkovic V, Hegbrant J, Strippoli GF. HMG CoA reductase inhibitors (statins) for people with chronic kidney disease not requiring dialysis. Cochrane Database Syst Rev. 2014;5.

27. Messow CM, Isles C. Meta-analysis of statins in chronic kidney disease: who benefits? QJM. 2017;110(8):493–500.

28. Palmer SC, Craig JC, Navaneethan SD, Tonelli M, Pellegrini F, Strippoli GF. Benefits and harms of statin therapy for persons with chronic kidney disease: a systematic review and meta-analysis. Ann Intern Med. 2012;157(4):263–75.

29. Wanner C, Krane V, März W, Olschewski M, Mann JF, Ruf G, Ritz E. Atorvastatin in patients with type 2 diabetes mellitus undergoing hemodialysis. N Engl J Med. 2005;353(3):238–48.

30. März W, Genser B, Drechsler C, Krane V, Grammer TB, Ritz E, Stojakovic T, Scharnagl H, Winkler K, Holme I, Holdaas H. Atorvastatin and low-density lipoprotein cholesterol in type 2 diabetes mellitus patients on hemodialysis. Clin J Am Soc Nephrol. 2011;6(6):1316–25.

31. Fellström BC, Jardine AG, Schmieder RE, Holdaas H, Bannister K, Beutler J, Chae DW, Chevaile A, Cobbe SM, Grönhagen-Riska C, De Lima JJ. Rosuvastatin and cardiovascular events in patients undergoing hemodialysis. N Engl J Med. 2009;360(14):1395–407.

32. Baigent C, Landray MJ, Reith C, Emberson J, Wheeler DC, Tomson C, Wanner C, Krane V, Cass A, Craig J, Neal B. The effects of lowering LDL cholesterol with simvastatin plus ezetimibe in patients with chronic kidney disease (Study of Heart and Renal Protection): a randomised placebo-controlled trial. Lancet. 2011;377(9784):2181–92.

33. Lin YC, Lai TS, Wu HY, Chou YH, Chiang WC, Lin SL, Chen YM, Chu TS, Tu YK. Effects and safety of statin and ezetimibe combination therapy in patients with chronic kidney disease: a systematic review and meta-analysis. Clin Pharmacol Ther. 2020;108(4):833–43. https://doi.org/10.1002/cpt.1859.

34. Sabatine MS, Giugliano RP, Keech AC, Honarpour N, Wiviott SD, Murphy SA, Kuder JF, Wang H, Liu T, Wasserman SM, Sever PS. Evolocumab and clinical outcomes in patients with cardiovascular disease. N Engl J Med. 2017;376(18):1713–22.
35. Schwartz GG, Steg PG, Szarek M, Bhatt DL, Bittner VA, Diaz R, Edelberg JM, Goodman SG, Hanotin C, Harrington RA, Jukema JW. Alirocumab and cardiovascular outcomes after acute coronary syndrome. N Engl J Med. 2018;379(22):2097–107.
36. Charytan DM, Sabatine MS, Pedersen TR, Im K, Park JG, Pineda AL, Wasserman SM, Deedwania P, Olsson AG, Sever PS, Keech AC. Efficacy and safety of evolocumab in chronic kidney disease in the FOURIER trial. J Am Coll Cardiol. 2019;73(23):2961–70.
37. Nathan DM, For the Diabetes Control and Complications Trial/Epidemiology of Diabetes Interventions and Complications (DCCT/EDIC) Study Research Group. Intensive diabetes treatment and cardiovascular disease in patients with type 1 diabetes. N Engl J Med. 2005;353:2643–53.
38. ADVANCE Collaborative Group. Intensive blood glucose control and vascular outcomes in patients with type 2 diabetes. N Engl J Med. 2008;358(24):2560–72.
39. Duckworth W, Abraira C, Moritz T, Reda D, Emanuele N, Reaven PD, Zieve FJ, Marks J, Davis SN, Hayward R, Warren SR. Glucose control and vascular complications in veterans with type 2 diabetes. N Engl J Med. 2009;360(2):129–39.
40. ACCORD Study Group, Cushman WC, Evans GW, Byington RP, Goff DC Jr, Grimm RH Jr, et al. Effects of intensive blood-pressure control in type 2 diabetes mellitus. N Engl J Med. 2010;362(17):1575–85.
41. Papademetriou V, Lovato L, Doumas M, Nylen E, Mottl A, Cohen RM, Applegate WB, Puntakee Z, Yale JF, Cushman WC, ACCORD Study Group. Chronic kidney disease and intensive glycemic control increase cardiovascular risk in patients with type 2 diabetes. Kidney Int. 2015;87(3):649–59. https://doi.org/10.1038/ki.2014.296.
42. Shurraw S, Hemmelgarn B, Lin M, Majumdar SR, Klarenbach S, Manns B, Bello A, James M, Turin TC, Tonelli M, Alberta Kidney Disease Network. Association between glycemic control and adverse outcomes in people with diabetes mellitus and chronic kidney disease: a population-based cohort study. Arch Intern Med. 2011;171(21):1920–7.
43. Hong J, Zhang Y, Lai S, Lv A, Su Q, Dong Y, Zhou Z, Tang W, Zhao J, Cui L, Zou D. Effects of metformin versus glipizide on cardiovascular outcomes in patients with type 2 diabetes and coronary artery disease. Diabetes Care. 2013;36(5):1304–11.
44. Zinman B, Wanner C, Lachin JM, Fitchett D, Bluhmki E, Hantel S, Mattheus M, Devins T, Johansen OE, Woerle HJ, Broedl UC. Empagliflozin, cardiovascular outcomes, and mortality in type 2 diabetes. N Engl J Med. 2015;373(22):2117–28.
45. Neal B, Perkovic V, Mahaffey KW, De Zeeuw D, Fulcher G, Erondu N, Shaw W, Law G, Desai M, Matthews DR. Canagliflozin and cardiovascular and renal events in type 2 diabetes. N Engl J Med. 2017;377(7):644–57.
46. Wiviott SD, Raz I, Bonaca MP, Mosenzon O, Kato ET, Cahn A, Silverman MG, Zelniker TA, Kuder JF, Murphy SA, Bhatt DL. Dapagliflozin and cardiovascular outcomes in type 2 diabetes. N Engl J Med. 2019;380(4):347–57.
47. Perkovic V, Jardine MJ, Neal B, Bompoint S, Heerspink HJ, Charytan DM, Edwards R, Agarwal R, Bakris G, Bull S, Cannon CP. Canagliflozin and renal outcomes in type 2 diabetes and nephropathy. N Engl J Med. 2019;380(24):2295–306.
48. McMurray JJ, Solomon SD, Inzucchi SE, Køber L, Kosiborod MN, Martinez FA, Ponikowski P, Sabatine MS, Anand IS, Bělohlávek J, Böhm M. Dapagliflozin in patients with heart failure and reduced ejection fraction. N Engl J Med. 2019;381(21):1995–2008.
49. Packer M, Anker SD, Butler J, Filippatos G, Pocock SJ, Carson P, Januzzi J, Verma S, Tsutsui H, Brueckmann M, Jamal W. Cardiovascular and renal outcomes with empagliflozin in heart failure. N Engl J Med. 2020;383(15):1413–24.
50. Abraham WT, Lindenfeld J, Ponikowski P, Agostoni P, Butler J, Desai AS, Filippatos G, Gniot J, Fu M, Gullestad L, Howlett JG, Nicholls SJ, Redon J, Schenkenberger I, Silva-Cardoso J, Störk S, Krzysztof Wranicz J, Savarese G, Brueckmann M, Jamal W, Nordaby

M, Peil B, Ritter I, Ustyugova A, Zeller C, Salsali A, Anker SD. Effect of empagliflozin on exercise ability and symptoms in heart failure patients with reduced and preserved ejection fraction, with and without type 2 diabetes. Eur Heart J. 2021;42(6):700–10. https://doi.org/10.1093/eurheartj/ehaa943.

51. Nassif ME, Windsor SL, Borlaug BA, Kitzman DW, Shah SJ, Tang F, Khariton Y, Malik AO, Khumri T, Umpierrez G, Lamba S, Sharma K, Khan SS, Chandra L, Gordon RA, Ryan JJ, Chaudhry SP, Joseph SM, Chow CH, Kanwar MK, Pursley M, Siraj ES, Lewis GD, Clemson BS, Fong M, Kosiborod MN. The SGLT2 inhibitor dapagliflozin in heart failure with preserved ejection fraction: a multicenter randomized trial. Nat Med. 2021;27(11):1954–60. https://doi.org/10.1038/s41591-021-01536-x. Epub 2021 Oct 28.

52. Marso SP, Daniels GH, Brown-Frandsen K, Kristensen P, Mann JF, Nauck MA, Nissen SE, Pocock S, Poulter NR, Ravn LS, Steinberg WM. Liraglutide and cardiovascular outcomes in type 2 diabetes. N Engl J Med. 2016;375(4):311–22.

53. Marso SP, Bain SC, Consoli A, Eliaschewitz FG, Jódar E, Leiter LA, Lingvay I, Rosenstock J, Seufert J, Warren ML, Woo V. Semaglutide and cardiovascular outcomes in patients with type 2 diabetes. N Engl J Med. 2016;375:1834–44.

54. Hernandez AF, Green JB, Janmohamed S, D'Agostino RB Sr, Granger CB, Jones NP, Leiter LA, Rosenberg AE, Sigmon KN, Somerville MC, Thorpe KM. Albiglutide and cardiovascular outcomes in patients with type 2 diabetes and cardiovascular disease (Harmony Outcomes): a double-blind, randomised placebo-controlled trial. Lancet. 2018;392(10157):1519–29.

55. Gerstein HC, Colhoun HM, Dagenais GR, Diaz R, Lakshmanan M, Pais P, Probstfield J, Riesmeyer JS, Riddle MC, Rydén L, Xavier D. Dulaglutide and cardiovascular outcomes in type 2 diabetes (REWIND): a double-blind, randomised placebo-controlled trial. Lancet. 2019;394(10193):121–30.

56. Pfeffer MA, Claggett B, Diaz R, Dickstein K, Gerstein HC, Køber LV, Lawson FC, Ping L, Wei X, Lewis EF, Maggioni AP. Lixisenatide in patients with type 2 diabetes and acute coronary syndrome. N Engl J Med. 2015;373(23):2247–57.

57. Husain M, Birkenfeld AL, Donsmark M, Dungan K, Eliaschewitz FG, Franco DR, Jeppesen OK, Lingvay I, Mosenzon O, Pedersen SD, Tack CJ. Oral semaglutide and cardiovascular outcomes in patients with type 2 diabetes. N Engl J Med. 2019;381(9):841–51.

58. Cannon CP, Pratley R, Dagogo-Jack S, Mancuso J, Huyck S, Masiukiewicz U, Charbonnel B, Frederich R, Gallo S, Cosentino F, Shih WJ. Cardiovascular outcomes with ertugliflozin in type 2 diabetes. N Engl J Med. 2020;383(15):1425–35.

59. Heerspink HJ, Stefánsson BV, Correa-Rotter R, Chertow GM, Greene T, Hou FF, Mann JF, McMurray JJ, Lindberg M, Rossing P, Sjöström CD. Dapagliflozin in patients with chronic kidney disease. N Engl J Med. 2020;383(15):1436–46.

60. Rothwell PM, et al. Effects of aspirin on risk and severity of early recurrent stroke after transient ischaemic attack and ischaemic stroke: time-course analysis of randomised trials. Lancet. 2016;388(10042):365–75. https://doi.org/10.1016/S0140-6736(16)30468-8.

61. Berger JS. Oral antiplatelet therapy for secondary prevention of acute coronary syndrome. Am J Cardiovasc Drugs. 2018;18(6):457. https://doi.org/10.1007/S40256-018-0291-2.

62. Hackam DG, Spence JD. Antiplatelet therapy in ischemic stroke and transient ischemic attack. Stroke. 2019;50(3):773–8. https://doi.org/10.1161/STROKEAHA.118.023954.

63. Pallikadavath S, Ashton L, Brunskill NJ, Burton JO, Gray LJ, Major RW. Aspirin for the primary prevention of cardiovascular disease in individuals with chronic kidney disease: a systematic review and meta-analysis. Eur J Prev Cardiol. 2022;28(17):1953–60. https://doi.org/10.1093/eurjpc/zwab132.

64. Palmer SC, et al. Antiplatelet agents for chronic kidney disease. Cochrane Database Syst Rev. 2013;(4). https://doi.org/10.1002/14651858.CD008834.PUB3.

65. Christiansen CF, et al. Kidney disease and risk of venous thromboembolism: a nationwide population-based case-control study. J Thromb Haemost. 2014;12(9):1449–54. https://doi.org/10.1111/JTH.12652.

66. Lau YC, et al. Atrial fibrillation and thromboembolism in patients with chronic kidney disease. J Am Coll Cardiol. 2016;68(13):1452–64. https://doi.org/10.1016/J.JACC.2016.06.057.

67. Ashley J, et al. Risk of cardiovascular events and mortality among elderly patients with reduced GFR receiving direct oral anticoagulants. Am J Kidney Dis. 2020;76(3):311–20. https://doi.org/10.1053/J.AJKD.2020.02.446.

68. Sy J, et al. Cardiovascular and bleeding outcomes with anticoagulants across kidney disease stages: analysis of a national US cohort. Am J Nephrol. 2021;52(3):199–208. https://doi.org/10.1159/000514753.

69. Orth SR, Hallan SI. Smoking: a risk factor for progression of chronic kidney disease and for cardiovascular morbidity and mortality in renal patients—absence of evidence or evidence of absence? Clin J Am Soc Nephrol. 2008;3(1):226–36. https://doi.org/10.2215/CJN.03740907.

70. Staplin N, et al. Smoking and adverse outcomes in patients with CKD: the Study of Heart and Renal Protection (SHARP). Am J Kidney Dis. 2016;68(3):371–80. https://doi.org/10.1053/J.AJKD.2016.02.052.

71. Ricardo AC, et al. Healthy lifestyle and risk of kidney disease progression, atherosclerotic events, and death in CKD: findings from the Chronic Renal Insufficiency Cohort (CRIC) study. Am J Kidney Dis. 2015;65(3):412–24. https://doi.org/10.1053/J.AJKD.2014.09.016.

72. Foley RN, Herzog CA, Collins AJ. Smoking and cardiovascular outcomes in dialysis patients: the United States Renal Data System Wave 2 study. Kidney Int. 2003;63(4):1462–7. https://doi.org/10.1046/J.1523-1755.2003.00860.X.

73. Stack AG, Murthy BVR. Cigarette use and cardiovascular risk in chronic kidney disease: an unappreciated modifiable lifestyle risk factor. Semin Dial. 2010;23(3):298–305. https://doi.org/10.1111/J.1525-139X.2010.00728.X.

74. Molnar MZ, et al. Associations of body mass index and weight loss with mortality in transplant-waitlisted maintenance hemodialysis patients. Am J Transplant. 2011;11(4):725–36. https://doi.org/10.1111/J.1600-6143.2011.03468.X.

75. Harhay MN, et al. Association between weight loss before deceased donor kidney transplantation and posttransplantation outcomes. Am J Kidney Dis. 2019;74(3):361–72. https://doi.org/10.1053/J.AJKD.2019.03.418.

76. Wilkinson TJ, et al. Association of sarcopenia with mortality and end-stage renal disease in those with chronic kidney disease: a UK Biobank study. J Cachexia Sarcopenia Muscle. 2021;12(3):586–98. https://doi.org/10.1002/JCSM.12705.

77. Kalantar-Zadeh K, et al. The obesity paradox in kidney disease: how to reconcile it with obesity management. Kidney Int Rep. 2017;2(2):271. https://doi.org/10.1016/J.EKIR.2017.01.009.

78. Chang AR, et al. Adiposity and risk of decline in glomerular filtration rate: meta-analysis of individual participant data in a global consortium. BMJ. 2019;364:5301. https://doi.org/10.1136/BMJ.K5301.

79. Docherty NG, le Roux CW. Bariatric surgery for the treatment of chronic kidney disease in obesity and type 2 diabetes mellitus. Nat Rev Nephrol. 2020;16:709–20. https://doi.org/10.1038/s41581-020-0323-4.

80. Sheetz KH, et al. Bariatric surgery and long-term survival in patients with obesity and end-stage kidney disease. JAMA Surg. 2020;155(7):581–8. https://doi.org/10.1001/JAMASURG.2020.0829.

81. Mann JFE, et al. Effects of liraglutide versus placebo on cardiovascular events in patients with type 2 diabetes mellitus and chronic kidney disease. Circulation. 2018;138(25):2908–18. https://doi.org/10.1161/CIRCULATIONAHA.118.036418.

82. Watson EL, et al. The association of muscle size, strength and exercise capacity with all-cause mortality in non-dialysis-dependent CKD patients. Clin Physiol Funct Imaging. 2020;40(6):399–406. https://doi.org/10.1111/CPF.12655.

83. Zhang L, et al. Exercise therapy improves eGFR, and reduces blood pressure and BMI in non-dialysis CKD patients: evidence from a meta-analysis. BMC Nephrol. 2019;20(1):398. https://doi.org/10.1186/S12882-019-1586-5.

84. Heiwe S, Jacobson SH. Exercise training in adults with CKD: a systematic review and meta-analysis. Am J Kidney Dis. 2014;64(3):383–93. https://doi.org/10.1053/J.AJKD.2014.03.020.

85. Tsai Y-C, et al. Association of physical activity with cardiovascular and renal outcomes and quality of life in chronic kidney disease. PLoS One. 2017;12(8):e0183642. https://doi.org/10.1371/JOURNAL.PONE.0183642.

86. Greenwood SA, et al. Mortality and morbidity following exercise-based renal rehabilitation in patients with chronic kidney disease: the effect of programme completion and change in exercise capacity. Nephrol Dial Transplant. 2019;34(4):618–25. https://doi.org/10.1093/NDT/GFY351.

87. Kuo C-P, et al. Dose–response effects of physical activity on all-cause mortality and major cardiorenal outcomes in chronic kidney disease. Eur J Prev Cardiol. 2021;29:452–61. https://doi.org/10.1093/EURJPC/ZWAA162.

88. Ikizler TA, et al. Metabolic effects of diet and exercise in patients with moderate to severe CKD: a randomized clinical trial. J Am Soc Nephrol. 2018;29(1):250–9. https://doi.org/10.1681/ASN.2017010020.

89. Anderson CAM, Nguyen HA, Rifkin DE. Nutrition interventions in chronic kidney disease. Med Clin North Am. 2016;100(6):1265–83. https://doi.org/10.1016/J.MCNA.2016.06.008.

90. O'Donnell MJ, et al. Urinary sodium and potassium excretion and risk of cardiovascular events. JAMA. 2011;306(20):2229–38. https://doi.org/10.1001/JAMA.2011.1729.

91. Stolarz-Skrzypek K, et al. Fatal and nonfatal outcomes, incidence of hypertension, and blood pressure changes in relation to urinary sodium excretion. JAMA. 2011;305(17):1777–85. https://doi.org/10.1001/JAMA.2011.574.

92. Feng J He, Jiafu Li, Graham A Macgregor. (2013) Effect of longer term modest salt reduction on blood pressure: Cochrane systematic review and meta-analysis of randomised trials. BMJ, 346(7903):f1325. doi: https://doi.org/10.1136/BMJ.F1325.

93. McMahon EJ, et al. Altered dietary salt intake for people with chronic kidney disease. Cochrane Database Syst Rev. 2021;2021(6). https://doi.org/10.1002/14651858.CD010070.PUB3.

94. Kieneker LM, et al. Urinary potassium excretion and risk of developing hypertension: the prevention of renal and vascular end-stage disease study. Hypertension. 2014;64(4):769–76. https://doi.org/10.1161/HYPERTENSIONAHA.114.03750.

95. Seth A, et al. Potassium intake and risk of stroke in women with hypertension and non-hypertension in the Women's Health Initiative. Stroke. 2014;45(10):2874–80. https://doi.org/10.1161/STROKEAHA.114.006046.

96. Aronson PS, Giebisch G. Effects of pH on potassium: new explanations for old observations. J Am Soc Nephrol. 2011;22(11):1981–9. https://doi.org/10.1681/ASN.2011040414.

97. Tangri N, et al. Metabolic acidosis is associated with increased risk of adverse kidney outcomes and mortality in patients with non-dialysis dependent chronic kidney disease: an observational cohort study. BMC Nephrol. 2021;22(1):185. https://doi.org/10.1186/S12882-021-02385-Z.

98. Ferraro PM, et al. Dietary protein and potassium, diet-dependent net acid load, and risk of incident kidney stones. Clin J Am Soc Nephrol. 2016;11(10):1834–44. https://doi.org/10.2215/CJN.01520216.

99. Gutiérrez OM, et al. Dietary patterns and risk of death and progression to ESRD in individuals with CKD: a cohort study. Am J Kidney Dis. 2014;64(2):204–13. https://doi.org/10.1053/J.AJKD.2014.02.013.

100. Goraya N, et al. Fruit and vegetable treatment of chronic kidney disease-related metabolic acidosis reduces cardiovascular risk better than sodium bicarbonate. Am J Nephrol. 2019;49(6):438–48. https://doi.org/10.1159/000500042.

101. Ali S, Dave N, Virani SS, Navaneethan SD. Primary and secondary prevention of cardiovascular disease in patients with chronic kidney disease. Curr Atheroscler Rep. 2019;21(9):32.

102. James PA, Oparil S, Carter BL, Cushman WC, Dennison-Himmelfarb C, Handler J, et al. 2014 Evidence-based guideline for the management of high blood pressure in adults: report from the panel members appointed to the Eighth Joint National Committee (JNC 8). JAMA. 2014;311(5):507–20.

103. SPRINT Research Group, Wright JT Jr, Williamson JD, Whelton PK, Snyder JK, Sink KM, et al. A randomized trial of intensive versus standard blood-pressure control. N Engl J Med. 2015;373(22):2103–16.

104. Whelton PK, Carey RM, Aronow WS, Casey DE Jr, Collins KJ, Dennison Himmelfarb C, et al. 2017 ACC/AHA/AAPA/ABC/ ACPM/AGS/APhA/ASH/ASPC/NMA/PCNA guideline for the prevention, detection, evaluation, and management of high blood pressure in adults: executive summary: a report of the American College of Cardiology/American Heart Association Task Force on clinical practice guidelines. Hypertension. 2018;71(6):1269–324.
105. Kidney Disease: Improving Global Outcomes (KDIGO) Blood Pressure Work Group. KDIGO clinical practice guideline for the management of blood pressure in chronic kidney disease. Kidney Int Suppl. 2012;337–414.
106. Xie X, Liu Y, Perkovic V, Li X, Ninomiya T, Hou W, et al. Renin-angiotensin system inhibitors and kidney and cardiovascular outcomes in patients with CKD: a Bayesian network meta-analysis of randomized clinical trials. Am J Kidney Dis. 2016;67(5):728–41.
107. Brenner BM, Cooper ME, de Zeeuw D, Keane WF, Mitch WE, Parving HH, et al. Effects of losartan on renal and cardiovascular outcomes in patients with type 2 diabetes and nephropathy. N Engl J Med. 2001;345(12):861–9.
108. Mann JF, Gerstein HC, Pogue J, Bosch J, Yusuf S. Renal insufficiency as a predictor of cardiovascular outcomes and the impact of ramipril: the HOPE randomized trial. Ann Intern Med. 2001;134(8):629–36.
109. Tobe SW, Clase CM, Gao P, McQueen M, Grosshennig A, Wang X, et al. Cardiovascular and renal outcomes with telmisartan, ramipril, or both in people at high renal risk: results from the ONTARGET and TRANSCEND studies. Circulation. 2011;123(10):1098–107.
110. Fried LF, Emanuele N, Zhang JH, Brophy M, Conner TA, Duckworth W, et al. Combined angiotensin inhibition for the treatment of diabetic nephropathy. N Engl J Med. 2013;369(20):1892–903.
111. Rahman M, Ford CE, Cutler JA, Davis BR, Piller LB, Whelton PK, et al. Long-term renal and cardiovascular outcomes in antihypertensive and lipid-lowering treatment to prevent heart attack trial (ALLHAT) participants by baseline estimated GFR. Clin J Am Soc Nephrol. 2012;7(6):989–1002.
112. Saruta T, Hayashi K, Ogihara T, Nakao K, Fukui T, Fukiyama K, et al. Effects of candesartan and amlodipine on cardiovascular events in hypertensive patients with chronic kidney disease: subanalysis of the CASE-J study. Hypertens Res. 2009;32(6):505–12.
113. Blood Pressure Lowering Treatment Trialists' Collaboration, Ninomiya T, Perkovic V, Turnbull F, et al. Blood pressure lowering and major cardiovascular events in people with and without chronic kidney disease: meta-analysis of randomised controlled trials. BMJ. 2013;347:f5680.
114. Gregg LP, Hedayati SS. Management of traditional cardiovascular risk factors in CKD: what are the data? Am J Kidney Dis. 2018;72(5):728–44.
115. FDA approves drug to reduce risk of serious kidney and heart complications in adults with chronic kidney disease associated with type 2 diabetes. Published 9 Jul 2021. https://www.fda.gov/drugs/drug-safety-and-availability/fda-approves-drug-reduce-risk-serious-kidney-and-heart-complications-adults-chronic-kidney-disease. Accessed 20 Jul 2021.
116. Bakris GL, Agarwal R, Anker SD, Pitt B, Ruilope LM, Rossing P, Kolkhof P, Nowack C, Schloemer P, Joseph A, Filippatos G, FIDELIO-DKD Investigators. Effect of finerenone on chronic kidney disease outcomes in type 2 diabetes. N Engl J Med. 2020;383(23):2219–29. https://doi.org/10.1056/NEJMoa2025845.
117. Pitt B, Filippatos G, Agarwal R, Anker SD, Bakris GL, Rossing P, Joseph A, Kolkhof P, Nowack C, Schloemer P, Ruilope LM, FIGARO-DKD Investigators. Cardiovascular events with finerenone in kidney disease and type 2 diabetes. N Engl J Med. 2021;385:2252–63. https://doi.org/10.1056/NEJMoa2110956.
118. Agarwal R, Filippatos G, Pitt B, Anker SD, Rossing P, Joseph A, Kolkhof P, Nowack C, Gebel M, Ruilope LM, Bakris GL, FIDELIO-DKD and FIGARO-DKD Investigators. Cardiovascular and kidney outcomes with finerenone in patients with type 2 diabetes and

chronic kidney disease: the FIDELITY pooled analysis. Eur Heart J. 2022;43(6):474–84. https://doi.org/10.1093/eurheartj/ehab777.

119. Raina R, Chauvin A, Chakraborty R, Nair N, Shah H, Krishnappa V, Kusumi K. The role of endothelin and endothelin antagonists in chronic kidney disease. Kidney Dis. 2020;6(1):22–34. https://doi.org/10.1159/000504623.

120. Kuang HY, Wu YH, Yi QJ, Tian J, Wu C, Shou WN, Lu TW. The efficiency of endothelin receptor antagonist bosentan for pulmonary arterial hypertension associated with congenital heart disease: a systematic review and meta-analysis. Medicine (Baltimore). 2018;97(10):e0075. https://doi.org/10.1097/MD.0000000000010075.

121. Wesson DE. Endothelin role in kidney acidification. Semin Nephrol. 2006;26(5):393–8.

122. Gagliardini E, Zoja C, Benigni A. Et and diabetic nephropathy: preclinical and clinical studies. Semin Nephrol. 2015;35(2):188–96.

123. Mann JF, Green D, Jamerson K, Ruilope LM, Kuranoff SJ, Littke T, et al. ASCEND Study Group. Avosentan for overt diabetic nephropathy. J Am Soc Nephrol. 2010;21(3):527–35.

124. Querfeld U, Mak RH, Pries AR. Microvascular disease in chronic kidney disease: the base of the iceberg in cardiovascular comorbidity. Clin Sci. 2020;134:1333–56.

125. Tanaka S, Tanaka T, Nangaku M. Hypoxia and dysregulated angiogenesis in kidney disease. Kidney Dis (Basel). 2015;1:80–9. https://doi.org/10.1159/000381515.

126. Ehling J, et al. Quantitative micro-computed tomography imaging of vascular dysfunction in progressive kidney diseases. J Am Soc Nephrol. 2016;27:520–32. https://doi.org/10.1681/ASN.2015020204.

127. Kobayashi N, DeLano FA, Schmid-Schonbein GW. Oxidative stress promotes endothelial cell apoptosis and loss of microvessels in the spontaneously hypertensive rats. Arterioscler Thromb Vasc Biol. 2005;25:2114–21. https://doi.org/10.1161/01.ATV.0000178993.13222.f2.

Index